Clinical Aspects of Dental Materials

Theory, Practice, and Cases

FIFTH EDITION

Clinical Aspects of Dental Materials

Theory, Practice, and Cases

FIFTH EDITION

Marcia (Gladwin) Stewart, R.D.H., Ed.D.
Professor Emerita
Department of Dental Hygiene
School of Dentistry
West Virginia University
Morgantown, West Virginia

Michael Bagby, D.D.S., Ph.D.
Professor
Department of Pediatric Dentistry
School of Dentistry
West Virginia University
Morgantown, West Virginia

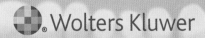

Philadelphia • Baltimore • New York • London
Buenos Aires • Hong Kong • Sydney • Tokyo

Acquisitions Editor: Jonathan Joyce
Development Editor: Amy Millholen
Editorial Coordinator: John Larkin
Marketing Manager: Leah Thomson
Production Project Manager: Bridgett Dougherty
Design Coordinator: Elaine Kasmer
Manufacturing Coordinator: Margie Orzech
Prepress Vendor: SPi Global

Fifth edition

Copyright © 2018 Wolters Kluwer

9 8 7 6 5 4 3 2 1

Printed in China

Library of Congress Cataloging-in-Publication Data
Names: Stewart, Marcia (Marcia A.), author. | Bagby, Michael (Michael D.), author.
Title: Clinical aspects of dental materials : theory, practice and cases / Marcia (Gladwin) Stewart, Michael Bagby.
Description: Fifth edition. | Philadelphia : Wolters Kluwer Health, [2018] | Includes bibliographical references and index.
Identifiers: LCCN 2017022076 | ISBN 9781496360083
Subjects: | MESH: Dental Materials | Dental Casting Technique | Dental Impression Technique | Case Reports
Classification: LCC RK652.5 | NLM WU 190 | DDC 617.6/95—dc23 LC record available at https://lccn.loc.gov/2017022076

LWW.com

The authors wish to dedicate the fifth edition to two groups of individuals:

*To all of the dental hygiene students for making the effort to grasp
the basic principles and manipulation techniques of dental materials
along with your other coursework. With dedication and determination
you will meet your career goals!*

and

*To the dental materials instructors for continuously updating and presenting lectures,
for preparing the lab, for demonstrating techniques, and for grading
and helping students in lab sessions.*

We have experienced these same challenges.

Contributors

Linda Bagby, B.A., B.S.
Consultant
Morgantown, West Virginia

Michael Bagby, D.D.S., Ph.D.
Professor
Department of Pediatric Dentistry
School of Dentistry
West Virginia University
Morgantown, West Virginia

Caren M. Barnes, R.D.H., M.S.
Professor (retired)
College of Dentistry
University of Nebraska Medical Center
Lincoln, Nebraska

Cathryn Frere, B.S.D.H., M.S.Ed.
Professor (retired)
Department of Dental Hygiene
School of Dentistry
West Virginia University
Morgantown, West Virginia

Aurora M. Graves DeMarco, BA, RDH, CDA
Dedicated to Mary Anne Butler, DMD
Private Practice
Orlando, Florida
Ancillaries

Christine Nathe, R.D.H., M.S.
Professor and Director
Division of Dental Hygiene
Vice Chair
Department of Dental Medicine
University of New Mexico
Albuquerque, New Mexico

Ashlee Sowards, M.S.D.H., T.T.S.
Assistant Professor
Department of Dental Hygiene
School of Dentistry
West Virginia University
Morgantown, West Virginia

Carol Spear, B.S.D.H., M.S.
Professor Emerita
Department of Dental Hygiene
School of Dentistry
West Virginia University
Morgantown, West Virginia

Marcia (Gladwin) Stewart, R.D.H., Ed.D.
Professor Emerita
Department of Dental Hygiene
Department of Periodontics
School of Dentistry
West Virginia University
Morgantown, West Virginia

Michele R. Sweeney, R.D.H., M.S.D.H.
Professor
Sarah Whitaker Glass School of Dental Hygiene
West Liberty State College
West Liberty, West Virginia

Andrea Warzynski, R.D.H., M.Ed.
Technical Advisor
Patterson Dental
Pittsburgh, Pennsylvania

PAST CONTRIBUTORS

Marylou Gutmann, R.D.H., M.A.
The Texas A&M University
College Station, Texas

Joan Gibson Howell, R.D.H., Ed.D.
Cambridge, Ohio

Jacqueline Harper, R.D.H., M.S.
West Virginia University
Morgantown, West Virginia

William R. Howard, D.D.S., M.P.H.
Western Kentucky University
Bowling Green, Kentucky

James Overberger, D.D.S., M.S.
West Virginia University
Morgantown, West Virginia

Norton P. Smith
West Virginia University
Morgantown, West Virginia

Preface

The objective of the fifth edition of *Clinical Aspects of Dental Materials: Theory, Practice, and Cases* is, first, to provide a dental materials background that emphasizes the clinical aspects of dental materials and, second, to introduce concepts of materials science. It is our hope that the student will become more familiar with the practice of dentistry through the use of this textbook.

In too many instances, the practice of dentistry and dental hygiene in an office setting becomes separated and disjointed. As a member of the dental team, the hygienist must be an advocate of dentistry. Although knowledge of caries, periodontology, and oral pathology are basic to the hygienist's daily responsibilities, a basic understanding of general dentistry and dental materials allows the hygienist to become a more effective member of the general dentistry team.

As new dental materials and techniques are continuously being developed, it can be difficult to keep abreast of all the new products, improvements, and their applications. And, as a member of the dental hygiene profession, the hygienist is obligated by our Code of Ethics to be a lifelong learner. This continual effort to "stay current" includes the science of dental materials. We need to understand the behavior of materials, how to handle materials, and how to assess the patient's oral condition. This knowledge then allows us to treat and educate the patient so that optimum oral health is achieved.

The authors hope that this publication provides a basic foundation for that lifelong learning.

ORGANIZATION

The text continues to be divided into three distinct parts: Theoretical Perspectives, Laboratory and Clinical Applications, and Case Studies. All chapters have been reviewed and updated. Two new case studies have been added. Six chapters reflect significant revisions: Chapter 4, "Adhesive Materials"; Chapter 7, "Dental Cements"; Chapter 10, "Materials for Fixed Indirect Restorations and Prostheses"; Chapter 16, "Polishing Materials and Abrasion"; Chapter 19, "Instruments as Dental Materials"; and Chapter 31, "Vital Tooth Whitening Procedures."

Two appendices complete the text sections: Appendix 1 provides the Answers and Justifications to Review Questions and Case Studies, and Appendix 2 comprises the Skill Performance and Evaluation Sheets that correspond to Part II of the textbook, "Laboratory and Clinical Applications."

TEXTBOOK FEATURES

Objectives: All chapters list the information the student is expected to know by the end of the chapter subject matter.

Key Words and Phrases: These are listed alphabetically at the beginning of each chapter, appear in bold, and are defined as they occur within chapter content.

Summaries: At the end of each chapter, a distinct summary section reviews the major components presented.

Learning Activities: Part I, Chapters 1–22, includes a list of small group and classroom activities that promote understanding and application of the chapter content.

Review Questions: Multiple choice review questions in each chapter will reinforce student comprehension and aid in quiz and exam preparation.

Precautions and "Tips" Boxes: Part II, Chapters 23–39, of the text, "Laboratory and Clinical Applications." contains distinct text boxes labeled "Precautions" and "Tips for the Clinician."

The "Precautions" box promotes safety while working with the materials, and the "Tips for the Clinician" box offers advice so that the best results are achieved.

Answers and Justifications to the Review Questions: Appendix 1 includes the correct answers and justifications for the review questions in Chapters 1–36 and the Case Studies. This section will also aid in preparing for exams and quizzes.

Skill Performance Evaluations: Appendix 2 contains "lab sheets" that correspond to Part II, "Laboratory and Clinical Applications." These perforated, tear-out sheets allow for student self-assessment as well as instructor evaluation.

ANCILLARIES

The ancillaries for this textbook are available on the book's companion website "thePoint" at thePoint.lww.com. There are both "Student Resources" and "Instructor Resources." The Student Resources include learning objectives, assessments (chapter review questions), student aids, videos, appendices, case studies, and suggested readings. The Instructor Resources include PowerPoint presentations, image banks, and LMS course cartridges.

TO THE INSTRUCTOR

The textbook continues to be written in outline format. This provides a clear organization of the topic and facilitates the reading of both the theory and laboratory chapters. Some sections of many chapters continue to be labeled as optional. The instructor should feel free to designate other sections as optional as well.

The learning activities can serve as homework assignments, or individual or group activities in the lab or classroom. Certain activities could also serve as part of a laboratory practical exam.

The videos and image bank on "thePoint" Web site are available to make lectures and lab sessions less labor intensive and more time efficient.

The skills evaluation sheets in Appendix 2 are to serve as a criteria list for properly manipulating that particular material in a laboratory session. They are single-sided, perforated, and provide areas for both student and instructor evaluation. The chapters in Part II of the book can serve as a lab manual for these same selected materials.

With the review questions, the answers, and justifications (Appendix 1), we made an effort to not only explain why the answer is correct but to also explain why the other answers are incorrect. This section of the book is an additional learning opportunity. Please guide your students to it as they study for quizzes and exams.

It is hoped that Chapter 16, "Polishing Materials and Abrasion," is included in your topical outline for the course. This key chapter is pertinent to dental hygiene practice. It addresses the various polishing agents, the process of polishing as it relates to tooth abrasion and also presents air–powder polishing, specific abrasion rates, and dentifrices.

TO THE STUDENT

Despite the hopes of the authors and the reality of teaching dental materials, there may not be enough time in the academic term for the instructor to cover all the chapters in the text. The instructor chooses the chapters to be taught based on the dental materials curriculum set forth by your specific dental hygiene program. If that is the case, we hope that you will take it upon yourself to read over two specific chapters: Chapter 19, "Instruments as Dental Materials" (because you have paid a great deal of money for these) and Chapter 37, "Tips for the New Hygienist" (because it gives you a little insight on the "real world" of dental hygiene practice). These may not be assigned as required course reading but lend themselves to better preparing you to become part of the professional dental team.

In addition, if the case studies and review questions at the end of the chapters are not assigned or discussed, please use these on your own to prepare for quizzes, exams, and national, regional, or state board examinations. And, as mentioned above to the instructors, Appendix 1, "Answers and Justifications to Review Questions/Case Studies," provides not only the correct answer but also an explanation of why that answer is correct and the other choices are not. This can be considered as "extra" review material to help you to be better prepared.

SUMMARY

The authors have made a concerted effort to thoroughly edit and update not only our chapters but also have reviewed and made suggestions to improve those of the many contributors. We contacted two additional educators to revise content in existing chapters and to add new cases so the text is "that much better" as a teaching and learning tool.

We hope that the fifth edition of *Clinical Aspects of Dental Materials* is user-friendly, appropriately updated, and instrumental in helping students gain a basic understanding of dental materials. We wish all the instructors and students a very successful academic year!

Acknowledgments

The authors wish to express their thanks to the following individuals for their contributions to this edition:

To the eight contributing authors who provided their expertise for this edition, we appreciate your acceptance of our suggestions and editing. To those that are long-standing contributors, thank you for your ongoing cooperation and dedication to this project in the midst of busy schedules. To the two newest ones, Andrea and Ashlee, thank you for giving your time, effort, and knowledge to improve and expand the final manuscript.

A special thanks to a long-term contributor, Ms. Caren M. Barnes, RDH, MS, who has retired from the University of Nebraska Medical Center. In the arena of dental and dental hygiene education, she has made vast contributions to the professions with five editions of her own textbook, more than 30 additional textbook chapters and over 90 publications in refereed journals. She persevered through a serious, but temporary, illness to revise one of our more important chapters. We wish her the best in all future endeavors.

To the team, Jonathan, John, and Amy at Wolters Kluwer, Dharma at SPi, and all others behind the scenes, your guidance has been most appreciated.

And lastly, and by no means least, is Mrs. Karen Gierach, our friend and retired English educator, who has been our own personal editor. Her expertise with grammar, syntax, and diction has "saved" us on more than one occasion. A heartfelt thanks for all your time and effort.

Contents

Part III Case Studies

Theoretical Perspectives

Introduction

Objectives

After studying this chapter, the student will be able to do the following:

1. Summarize the reasons why a dental hygienist should be knowledgeable in the science of dental materials.
2. Explain the difference between biomaterials and dental materials.
3. Discuss some of the conditions that make the oral cavity a hostile environment.
4. Identify four characteristics or properties a dental material must possess to survive in the oral environment.
5. Explain how the following organizations evaluate and/or classify dental drugs, materials, instruments, and equipment:
   - American Dental Association (ADA)
   - U.S. Food and Drug Administration (FDA)
   - International Standards Organization (ISO)
6. Name three ways dental materials may be classified, and discuss each.
7. Specifically discuss the locations of all six cavity classifications and the appropriate restorative material to be used for each. Include the following in your discussion:
   - Anterior and/or posterior
   - Involvement of incisal angle
   - Involvement of proximal surface
   - Smooth surfaces versus pit and fissures

Key Words/Phrases

abutment
base
biocompatibility
biomaterials
bridge
cast
cavity preparation
dental implants
dental materials
denture
diagnostic cast
direct restorative materials
esthetic materials
fixed partial denture
impression
indirect restorative material
interim restoration
liner
luting agents
maxillofacial prosthesis
polishing
pontic
prosthesis
provisional restoration
removable partial denture
restorations
restorative materials
retainer
specifications
study model
temporary crown
temporary restoration

Introduction

What is "dental materials"? It is a subset of materials science, an applied science that combines chemistry, physics, and engineering with a little biology. Other important examples of materials science include food science, parts of pharmacology, and textiles. After all, we want our chips to be crunchy, our time-release medications to slowly dissolve, and our colored fabrics to stay bright. In dentistry, we do not want our fillings to break, our molars to dissolve, nor our incisors to "yellow." Understanding what makes one material strong and rigid while making another stretchy and snap back to its original shape will help us utilize the vast array of dental products to care for our patients.

I. Rationale for Studying Dental Materials

"Dental materials" is one of many required courses in the dental hygiene curriculum. It focuses on those items and products used in the prevention and treatment of oral disease and the promotion of health. The scope of practice of a dental hygienist includes the delivery of therapeutic, educational, and preventive patient services. Materials used in the practice of dental hygiene include instruments made from common industrial materials, therapeutic agents, and dental biomaterials used to prevent disease. At times, therapeutic dental products and preventive materials overlap.

The preventive aspects of dental hygiene include primary prevention, which attempts to reduce the occurrence of disease, and secondary prevention, which attempts to limit the destruction caused by disease. Both aspects of preventive dentistry involve the use of instruments (made from materials) and dental materials.

A dental hygienist should be knowledgeable in the science of dental materials for the following four reasons:

A. To Understand the Behavior of Materials

This will aid in the delivery of quality patient care. The dental hygienist must understand why specific materials behave as they do and why they are used for certain functions in certain locations to replace missing oral tissues. For example, the proper placement of sealants will prevent dental caries. The proper restoration of teeth and maintenance of restorations will limit the destructive effects of caries and periodontal disease. The proper care and maintenance of instruments (prevention of corrosion) are important when sterilizing and disinfecting. The proper use of dental materials is fundamental to the art and science of dentistry.

B. To Handle Materials Properly

Both preventive and restorative dentistry rely heavily on the proper use of biomaterials. While most of us can boil water, reheating pizza that does not result in a mushy crust requires the proper application of heat (try a low-temperature frying pan with a good dose of patience).

Biomaterials are man-made materials that are used to replace tissues or that function in intimate contact with living tissues. **Dental materials** are biomaterials used in or around the oral cavity. The hygienist may or may not be involved in the placement of restorations, but he or she plays a significant role in the placement of preventive materials and the maintenance of restorations. The proper handling of dental materials is important because improper handling will likely adversely affect their physical, chemical, and mechanical properties. In turn, this could affect the overall service to the patient.

Therefore, handling a dental material properly is a primary factor in the success or failure of its use. The goal of this text is to present dental materials and their manipulation from a clinical perspective. If materials are properly mixed and placed, improved patient care will result.

C. To Assess and Treat the Patient

The dental hygienist must be able to recognize all dental materials present in the mouth. These may be visible clinically and/or radiographically. Proper identification is important so that they are not mistaken for caries (radiographically) or improperly maintained. An example would be the clinical recognition of an all-ceramic crown. Acidulated phosphate fluoride (APF) gels can etch the surface of some ceramic materials. Using an APF gel is contraindicated for patients with ceramic restorations; instead, a neutral fluoride gel should be used.

D. To Educate the Patient

In many instances, patients may ask the dental hygienist to discuss the characteristics and properties of one dental material compared to another, both of which may be a reasonable option for the patient. Patients may also ask the hygienist to describe the steps involved in the fabrication of a certain type of restoration, or they may also inquire about home care regimens ("How will I take care of my new bridge?"). Knowledge of dental materials is critical so that the patient is given professional, complete, and correct answers.

II. Biomaterials and the Oral Environment

A. Oral Tissues as Biologic Materials

Whether a material is used for preventive or restorative purposes, the oral environment places great restrictions on which materials can be used and the manner in which those materials are used. When one realizes that oral tissues are themselves biologic materials, a variety of properties and functions are evident. All oral tissues must function in the hostile environment of the oral cavity.

1. Enamel

   Enamel is a hard, wear-resistant surface material. It is able to resist the compressive forces of biting, but it is weak in its resistance to bending and other forces that occur when food is ground by molars. Enamel is well supported by dentin. Enamel will dissolve in oral fluids if the pH is too acidic; dental caries is the result of such an acidic attack. Enamel is also responsible for the tooth's pleasing esthetic appearance.

2. Dentin

   Dentin makes up the bulk of the tooth. It acts as a cushion for the brittle enamel, and it provides strength to resist the complex forces that occur when biting. Dentin is more susceptible than enamel to acidic attack.

3. Pulp

   Pulp is connective tissue that contains nerves and blood vessels. It provides nutrients to the dentin and responds to stimuli with pain or sensitivity.

4. Periodontium

   Periodontium supports the tooth in a stable but dynamic position, and it provides feedback regarding the force placed on the tooth. Periodontium includes the periodontal ligament, cementum, and alveolar bone.

5. Gingival Tissue

   A very important function of gingival tissue is to seal out the many noxious agents of the oral cavity. Gingival tissue prevents chemicals and microbes from gaining access to the periodontium and deeper tissues in the body. Gingival tissues surround and attach to teeth, forming a barrier. Although the oral cavity is considered to be inside the body, in many ways it is more like the outside. Biomaterials placed in the oral cavity have very different requirements from those of devices implanted inside the body.

B. Replacement Materials for Oral Tissues

1. Restriction on Materials Use

   When oral tissue is lost, dental professionals attempt to replace it with a dental material. The replacement material mimics the function of the oral tissue, and it must withstand the same harsh environment. The biologic nature of the oral environment and the size of the oral cavity restrict the use of materials. These restrictions include the following:
   a. Biting forces that may fracture teeth and replacement material

   b. Degradation of:
      • Materials, such as corrosion of metal
      • Teeth, such as dental caries
   c. Temperature changes that cause restorations to contract and expand differently than teeth, causing leakage around the restoration as well as tooth sensitivity
   d. **Biocompatibility** (the lack of harmful effects to the patient)
   e. Esthetic demands of the patient

2. Effects of Dental Materials and the Oral Environment on Each Other

   The dental hygienist must understand the characteristics and properties of dental materials. This knowledge will provide insight regarding how a dental material may affect the oral environment. An orthodontic appliance makes oral hygiene difficult and increases the patient's susceptibility to gingival inflammation and caries. The oral environment affects the dental materials as well. Yeast or other microbes may colonize on a denture, causing it to become foul-smelling. These characteristics and properties may also limit the selection and use of a dental material.

III. History and Selection of Dental Materials

A. History

Why are certain materials chosen instead of others to serve as dental restorative materials? Actually, much has been learned throughout history by trial and error. Paraphrasing C.S. Lewis, "Experience is that most brutal of teachers." In ancient times, gold was used not only for its corrosion resistance but also for its "workability" or ease of processing. For centuries, humans have attempted to improve their appearance with adornments, such as jewelry and makeup. The replacement of lost teeth is an ancient practice. First, it was more likely for esthetics than for function. As dentistry developed throughout the ages, function became important. Some of the materials used included ivory, which was carved, and porcelain, which was fired into tooth shapes. By the 1800s, dentistry was becoming a scientifically based discipline. The pace of development of new materials quickened. Amalgam, a silver filling material, was frequently used. Porcelain could be crafted into inlays and crowns.

In the 20th century, dental materials science had developed into its own discipline. Numerous materials and techniques were developed. Precise casting techniques were developed for a variety of metals. Polymers and composites were adapted for nearly every dental material need. In the 21st century, new ceramic materials and processing technologies have been adapted by dentistry. Computer-aided design and manufacture are common along with other digital technologies. The pace of dental materials development is so fast that some of this text will be outdated before it is published.

Luckily, the basic concepts of materials science and their use do not change. Both the student and the practitioner need to understand the behavior of the materials they use. After all, they are the ones who must select a product from a rather long list of possibilities.

B. Selection of Dental Materials and Products

The knowledge gained in a dental materials course will aid in the selection of products. Manufacturers readily provide data regarding strength and a variety of other properties. At times, they also provide the results of short-term clinical trials. How reliable is that information? More importantly, how useful is that information? It has been a goal of dental materials scientists to predict the performance of a material from its strength and other mechanical properties. Unfortunately, success has been elusive. Clinical trials are the most reliable source of information for most products. The clinician must evaluate the product information, but he or she must also consider the source of that information.

IV. Standards for Dental Materials

Standards for dental materials have been developed in dentistry in the same manner as in other industries. Standards describe the properties of a product so that a user may select the proper material for a particular use. Standards are common in everyday life. Examples include the octane rating of gasoline, DVD formats, the size of nuts and bolts, computer communications protocols, and even the size of eggs. In the United States, standards are published and administered by the American National Standards Institute (ANSI). Many industries have organizations that work under the guidance of ANSI to develop and administer the standards for the products of that industry; the American Dental Association (ADA) is the institution that represents dentistry.

A. Council on Scientific Affairs of the American Dental Association

In the United States, standards and guidelines for evaluating dental products are developed and administered by the Council on Scientific Affairs of the ADA. The Council evaluates dental drugs, materials, instruments, and equipment. A successful evaluation culminates in awarding of the ADA's Seal of Acceptance. The applicant

(e.g., a toothpaste company or any manufacturer of a dentally related product) submits data for their product following the ADA guidelines. On approval of the product, the applicant is permitted to use the ADA's Seal of Acceptance. The Seal is illustrated in *Figure 1.1*. It is commonly seen on accepted brands of toothpaste and toothbrushes. The ADA Seal is awarded for a period of 3 years, after which the applicant must resubmit the product. In addition, advertising for products that have been awarded the ADA Seal is reviewed by the ADA.

Some of the ADA guidelines have very specific requirements for physical and mechanical properties that are measured in the laboratory and are called **specifications**. Specifications have been developed for many (but not all) dental materials. Unfortunately, researchers have not been able to develop a series of tests that adequately predict the clinical performance of many dental materials. As a result, the Acceptance Program relies on clinical data for the evaluation of many dental products. If a product is shown to be safe and effective, it can be given the Seal of Acceptance.

The Acceptance Program of the ADA is voluntary. Manufacturers are not required to have the Seal to market dental products in the United States. Although products might be approved for sale by the U.S. Food and Drug Administration (FDA), some products fail to meet the ADA

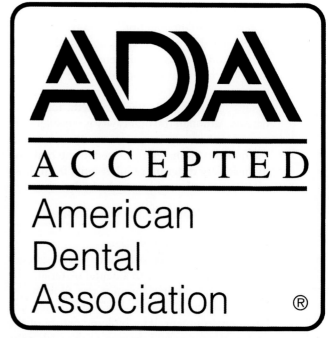

FIGURE 1.1. Seal of Acceptance of the American Dental Association. (Courtesy of the American Dental Association, Chicago, IL.)

specifications when tested. The ADA Professional Product Reviews are an excellent summary of dental materials and their properties.

B. Medical Device Amendments of 1976

The federal government, under the auspices of the U.S. FDA, has the authority under the Medical Device Amendments of 1976 to ensure the safety of all medical devices. The U.S. FDA considers dental materials to be medical devices. Medical devices are grouped into three categories:

1. Class I

These devices are the least regulated. Only good manufacturing practices are required. Prophy paste or brushes are two examples of such products.

2. Class II

Class II devices gain approval from the FDA after being shown to be equivalent to products currently in use. Equivalency is demonstrated by meeting performance standards, such as the ADA's Seal of Acceptance Program. Some dental products have been "grandfathered in," because they were marketed before 1976. Composite and amalgam restorative materials are two examples of Class II products.

3. Class III

These devices are the most regulated; they require premarket approval. Clinical data must be submitted to the U.S. FDA for evaluation before Class III devices are sold. If safety and efficacy of the device is supported by the data, the U.S. FDA then gives approval to market the product. Bone graft materials are common examples of such products.

C. International Standards Organization

Many other countries have dental specifications or standards and governmental regulations. To simplify the mass of regulations, the International Standards Organization (ISO) attempts to unify standards throughout its member countries. The ISO standards for many dental materials have been developed (and continue to be developed) under the guidance of the Fédération Dentaire Internationale, the international equivalent of the ADA.

Many dental products carry the "CE" marking symbol of the European Union on their packaging, as shown in *Figure 1.2*. CE stands for Conformité Européenne, and the marking is required for sales in most of Europe. The CE symbol indicates compliance with ISO standards and European Union marketing requirements for dental products.

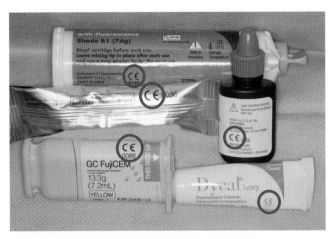

FIGURE 1.2. Photograph of dental products from several companies displaying the CE marking symbol.

D. Selecting Products

Dentists are fortunate because several products usually will meet the needs of a particular clinical situation. It is important to select and use materials that result in quality service to the patient. The same product may not do so for all practitioners. It is acceptable to select products based on handling characteristics, a company's reputation and service, or packaging. If two products have been shown to have excellent clinical performance, the ill-defined characteristics of "feel" or "handling" may be the final criteria that result in its selection. A product with the "right feel" will likely result in superior use and service to the patient. In the words of Dr. Karl Soderholm of the University of Florida, "the material must be your friend."

It is important to realize that most products require some time to learn to use them properly. If the clinician is always changing products to have the latest and greatest "widget bonder," he or she may be spending so much time learning to use new products that patient care may be affected. Of less consequence, that clinician will also have drawers, closets, and refrigerators filled with expensive, partially used dental products.

V. Classifications of Dental Materials

Like oral tissues, dental materials serve a variety of functions. Some materials replace lost tooth structure and restore the function of the teeth. These materials must withstand biting forces and therefore be strong and wear-resistant. Other materials are used to make impressions of oral tissues from which replicas are made. Many impression materials are soft and stretch a great deal when removed from the mouth. In dentistry, as in other disciplines, properties of a material must be matched to the use of that material. Dental materials can be classified in a number of ways but are typically classified by their use or function. Restorative materials are also classified by the location of fabrication or by the longevity of use.

A. Classification by Use

Materials used to replace lost oral tissues are called **restorative materials**. As mentioned earlier, those that replace lost tooth structure and restore the function of the teeth must be strong and hard (*Figs. 1.3–1.5*). Some restorative materials simulate the appearance of the tissues that are being replaced (see *Figs. 1.6 and 1.7*). Tissues simulated by restorative materials include the enamel of teeth (fillings and crowns), the mucosa of the periodontium

(dentures), and even the skin of the face (maxillofacial prostheses). Materials that are tooth-colored are often called **esthetic materials**.

1. Restorations

Depending on the degree of destruction of a tooth, different restorations or fillings are used to replace lost tooth structure. Some **restorations** replace a small to moderate amount of tooth structure and are supported by the remaining tooth structure. Such restorations are held in the tooth by undercuts (mechanical locks), adhesion, or both. An inlay is a restoration that is made outside the mouth, usually in a dental laboratory. Inlays do not have undercuts and are cemented or "luted" into the tooth (*Fig. 1.3*).

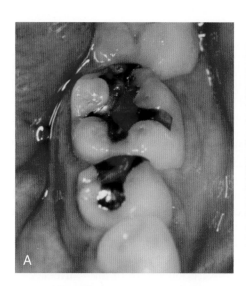
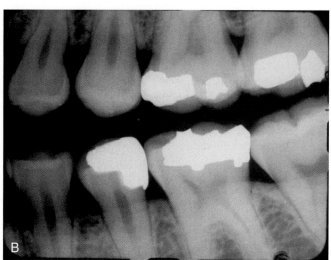
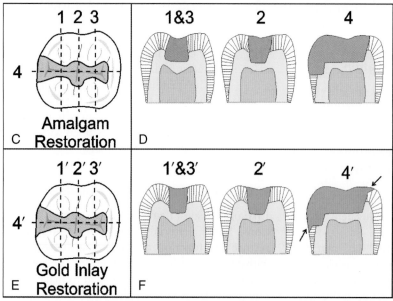

FIGURE 1.3. Photograph **A.** and radiograph **B.** of inlay (tooth #20) and amalgam (tooth #19) restorations. Drawings show the convergence and divergence of preparations for the two materials. The amalgam **C** and **D** has several convergent walls (undercuts) at 1 and 3. The inlay **E** and **F** has only divergent walls at 1′, 2′, and 3′. *Arrows* indicate bevels for a metallic inlay.

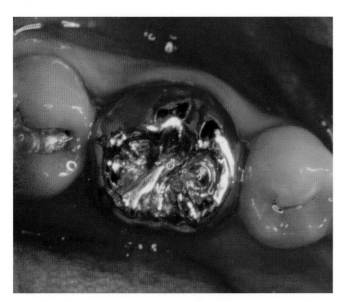

FIGURE 1.4. Photograph of a full gold crown.

Restorations are restricted to the physical size of the missing tooth structure. Excessively large restorations could affect speech or the patient's bite, or overwork the chewing muscles.

2. Crowns
Crowns are used to restore teeth when a substantial amount of tooth structure is missing.

Crowns encircle and support the remaining tooth structure (*Fig. 1.4*). Crowns are cemented in place similar to an inlay. If a crown or filling is too large or overcontoured, it will be detrimental to the health of the gingival tissues.

3. Bridges
A dental **bridge** replaces a lost tooth or teeth (*Fig. 1.5*). A typical dental bridge is much like a bridge over a river. At each end, the dental bridge is supported by an actual tooth called an **abutment**. Each abutment tooth is prepared and then restored with a crown called a **retainer**. The missing tooth is replaced with a false tooth called a **pontic**. A pontic is a replacement tooth, but only the crown portion of the tooth is replaced. The pontic and abutments are strongly joined together so that biting forces will not break the bridge. The dental bridge is cemented onto the prepared abutment teeth in the same manner as a crown or an inlay. Like all restorations, the physical size of a bridge is limited by the physiology and anatomy of the mouth.

4. Complete and Partial Dentures
Because of the ravages of caries or periodontal disease, some people lose many or all of their

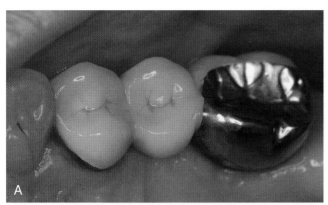

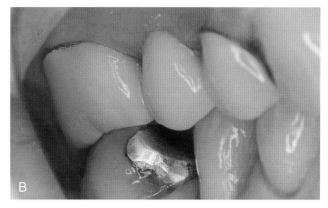

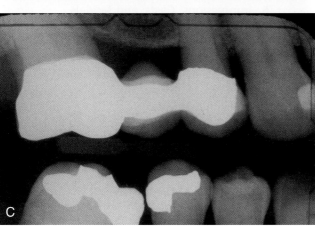

FIGURE 1.5. Photographs **A** and **B** and radiograph **C.** of a porcelain-bonded-to-metal bridge. Teeth #2 and #4 are retainers. #3 is a pontic.

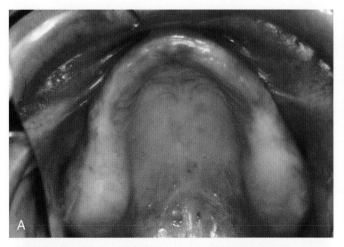

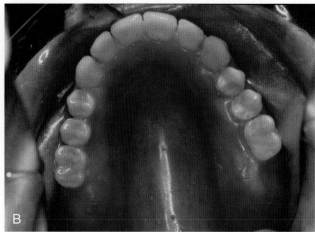

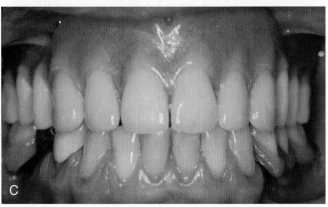

FIGURE 1.6. Photographs of **A.** an edentulous maxillary ridge and **B** and **C** denture in place. (Courtesy of Dr. Henry Miller, Greenburg, PA.)

teeth. If all the teeth of an arch are missing, the teeth are replaced by a prosthesis called a complete denture, as shown in *Figure 1.6*. A **prosthesis** is an artificial device that replaces a lost organ or tissues. A **denture** replaces missing teeth, bone, and gingiva after the teeth have been lost or extracted. A complete denture is supported by and precisely rests on the mucosal tissue covering the maxilla or mandible. The functions of a complete denture include chewing food (mastication), proper speech, and esthetics. Frequently, dentures improve a patient's self-esteem, appearance, and oral function.

If some teeth are present in an arch, the replacement prosthesis is called a partial denture. A bridge is often called a **fixed partial denture** because it is cemented into place (*Fig. 1.5*). A **removable partial denture** is sometimes referred to as a "partial" and replaces few or many teeth. A removable partial denture is placed and removed by the patient in the same manner as a full denture (*Fig. 1.7*). Typically, a removable partial denture has several metal clasps that are designed

to encircle several remaining teeth so that the prosthesis is stabilized, somewhat like the abutments of a fixed bridge. The replacement teeth of a removable partial denture are much like a section of a full denture. As with a complete denture, the teeth and gingival tissues are simulated to make an esthetically pleasing prosthesis for the patient. The remaining natural teeth greatly stabilize the partial denture and significantly improve function.

5. Impressions, Casts, and Models

When a restoration or prosthesis is constructed in a dental laboratory, a precise replica of the supporting tissues of the patient is required. To produce the replica (or positive copy), an impression is made of the prepared tooth or remaining alveolar ridge. The dental **impression** (or negative copy) is then filled with a material that solidifies to form the replica, as shown in *Figure 1.8*.

If a restoration is constructed on the replica, it is called a **cast**. If the resulting replica is used to study the size and position of the oral tissues,

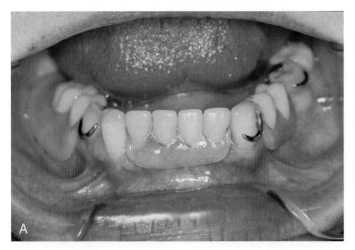
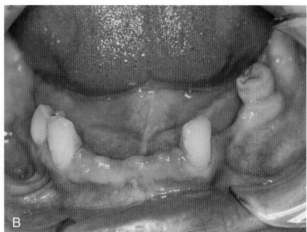
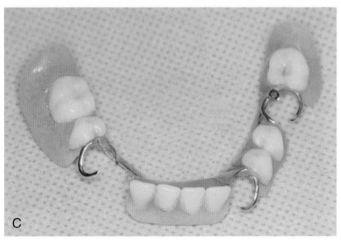

FIGURE 1.7. Photographs of a patient **A.** with and **B.** without a removable partial denture in place and **C.** the removable partial denture.

it is called a **study model** or **diagnostic cast**. A replica of the patient's oral tissues is frequently used for both functions. First, it is used to study the position of teeth and other oral tissues. Second, it serves as an opposing cast to aid in the construction of a restoration.

A variety of impression materials are used in dentistry. Most models and casts are made with gypsum materials, which are very similar to plaster of paris.

Intraoral optical scanners that can generate digital impressions are becoming popular, as shown in *Figure 1.8*. The digital impression can be used to make a restoration in the dental office via CAD/CAM technology or sent to a dental laboratory. Digital impressions can also be "interfaced" with 3D digital radiographs for treatment planning for orthodontics or implant placement.

6. Cements

   a. *As Luting Agents*

   After a crown has been made, it must be held in place (or "luted") to the prepared tooth. Luting is the same as gluing two objects together, and it is also called cementing. **Luting agents** are frequently called dental cements. The cement holds the crown onto the prepared tooth and fills in the microscopic gaps between the tooth and the crown. After mixing, cements must flow like a thin liquid so that a precisely made crown will fit properly. Several minutes after setting, the cement is expected to be strong and insoluble in oral fluids. Requirements of dental cements are quite rigorous. Proper handling of all materials, especially dental cements, is critical to successful patient care.

   b. *As Bases and Liners*

   Many of the materials used for luting crowns, bridges, or inlays may also serve other purposes. These include protecting the pulp from irritating materials, such as acids, or serving as insulating layers under metal restorations. Metals conduct hot and cold much more quickly than do dentin and enamel. Using a base or liner under a

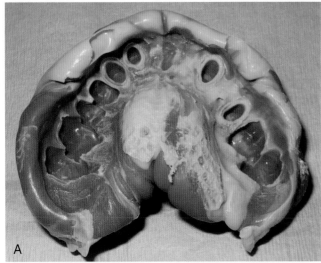

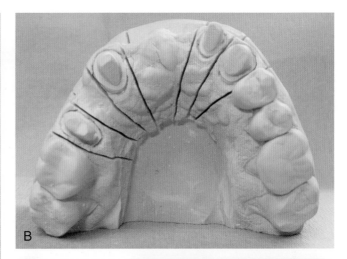

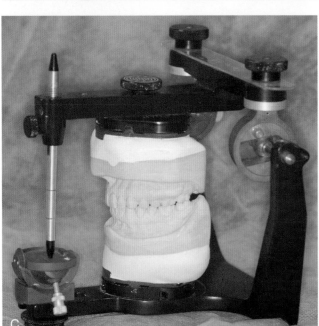

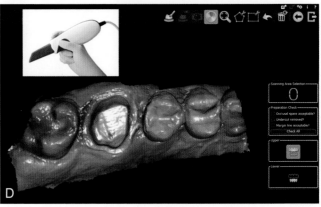

FIGURE 1.8. Photographs of **A.** an impression, **B.** a cast, **C.** casts mounted on an articulator, and **D.** an intraoral scanner and digital impression. (D, courtesy of Carestream Dental LLC—North America.)

metal restoration (between the pulp and the filling) can reduce or eliminate sensitivity to cold and hot foods and beverages (*Fig. 1.9*). The term **base** implies a degree of strength and thermal insulation, whereas the term **liner** does not. Historically, bases and liners were distinct groups, but now much overlap exists. The use of both terms best describes the function of these materials. A liner would be a relatively thin layer of material painted on to protect the underlying dentin from chemical irritation. A base has greater bulk, which serves to restore part of the missing tooth structure and to provide thermal insulation.

7. Temporary Materials

    a. *Temporary Crowns*

        When a crown is made in the dental laboratory, the dentist and patient must wait days or weeks before it can be cemented into place. What happens to the tooth that has been prepared for a crown? Such preparation requires that a surface layer be removed from the tooth. The thickness of the layer to be removed depends on the material that will be used to replace the missing tooth structure. Frequently, most of the enamel not already destroyed by decay is removed. If the tooth is vital (the pulp is alive), the patient will likely experience pain when eating, drinking, and, at times, breathing if the

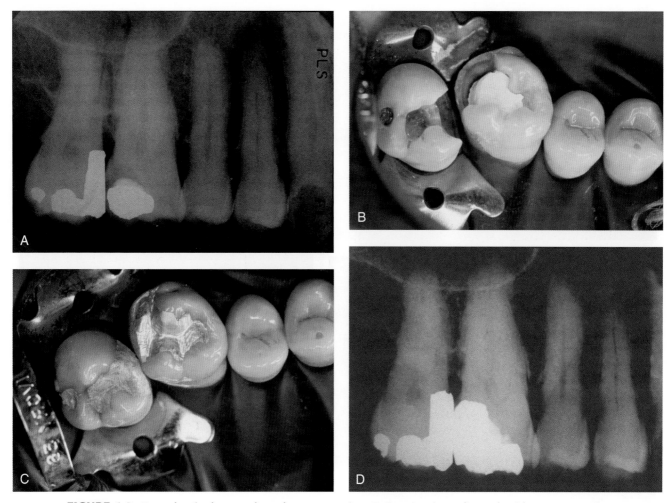

FIGURE 1.9. Example of a base and amalgam restoration. **A.** Preoperative radiograph with recurrent caries distal of #3. **B.** Photograph of cavity preparations in teeth #2 and #3. Tooth #3 has a base. **C.** Completed amalgam restorations. **D.** Postoperative radiograph. (Courtesy of Dr. Henry Miller, Greenburg, PA.)

crown preparation is not protected in some manner. Many times, the appearance of a front tooth that is prepared for a crown also is not esthetically acceptable. What is done to solve this problem? A temporary crown is made before the patient leaves the office (*Fig. 1.10*).

The **temporary crown** is constructed and luted during the same appointment in which the crown preparation is performed. Temporary crowns are not as strong or esthetically pleasing as permanent restorations, but they provide adequate service while the permanent crown is being made. Temporary crowns are typically made from plastics that are formed in the mouth. These replicate the missing tooth structure very closely. Other types of temporary crowns consist of metal or plastic shells (shaped like crowns of teeth) that are lined with the same plastic materials. Construction of temporary crowns is presented in Chapter 35.

Temporary crowns must be removed when it is time to cement the permanent crown. Temporary crowns are cemented with "weak" temporary cements so that they may be easily removed.

b. *Temporary Restorations*

At times, a dentist is unsure of the best treatment for a patient or a particular tooth. The exact condition of the pulp may not be obvious from the patient's symptoms. A dentist may remove all or part of the decay from a tooth and then place a **temporary restoration** to give the pulp time to heal before determining the specific treatment that is needed.

8. Preventive Materials

Several materials are used predominantly to prevent disease or trauma. These include the following:

a. Pit and fissure sealants, to prevent decay (*Fig. 1.11*).

b. Mouthguards, to prevent injury during athletic activities (*Fig. 1.12*).

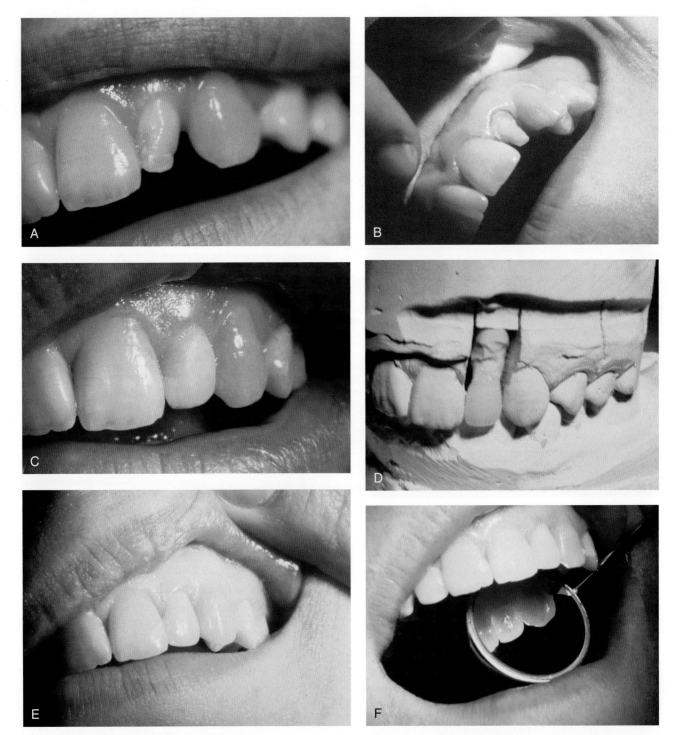

FIGURE 1.10. Restorative photographic series. **A.** Preoperative "peg-shaped" lateral incisor. **B.** Crown preparation. **C.** Temporary crown. **D.** Articulated casts with a permanent all-ceramic crown. **E** and **F.** Cemented crown in place.

c. Fluoride trays, custom and stock, which fit over the teeth to apply topical treatments. Custom fluoride trays look very much like custom mouthguards or bleaching trays (see *Fig. 1.12* and Chapter 18, Oral Appliances).

9. Polishing Materials

A tremendous amount of time in a dental practice is spent in polishing teeth, restorations, and appliances. Use of a rubber cup with an abrasive agent is termed **polishing**, but the predominant function is to remove stain, plaque, and debris

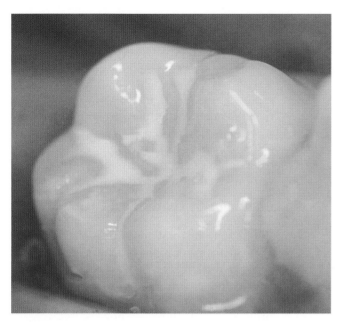

FIGURE 1.11. Photograph of tooth #19 with an opaque sealant.

from the tooth surface. True polishing involves moving an abrasive over the surface of an object to remove a thin layer of material. This action results in a surface that is clean, smooth, and lustrous. Dental professionals use many different devices and materials to polish teeth and restorations. Understanding the polishing process is important to achieving the desired result and is presented in Chapter 16.

10. Implants
Dental implants are considered to be part of restorative dentistry, but because of their specialized nature, they are segregated from other materials. **Dental implants** are typically screws or posts that are anchored into alveolar bone and protrude through the gingiva into the oral cavity. An illustration of a dental implant

is shown in Chapter 12. Implants are used to replace the root portion of lost teeth. Implants are unique in that they are both inside the body (in the alveolar bone) and outside the body (exposed in the oral cavity). Keeping the contents of the oral cavity from seeping along the surface of the implant into the supporting bone has been a very difficult problem. Luckily, this may be accomplished with the use of several materials if they are manufactured and handled properly.

Dental implants are used to support a great variety of restorations or prostheses. Single crowns, bridges, and dentures can be supported by dental implants. Often, a **maxillofacial prosthesis**, which is a combination intraoral and extraoral prosthesis such as an artificial nose/denture combination, is retained with intraoral and extraoral implants. Implants have had an extraordinary impact on patient care when traditional restorative treatments have failed to provide adequate function.

11. Specialty Materials
Many specialties in dentistry have products and materials unique to that field. At times, these products overlap (e.g., sutures), whereas others are limited strictly to that specialty (e.g., "rubber bands" or elastics used in orthodontics). Many times, the specialties of oral surgery and periodontics use the same (or very similar) materials for bone regeneration. These materials that are used in the dental specialties are discussed further in Chapter 13.

B. Classification by Location of Fabrication

1. Direct Restorative Materials
Some restorations are constructed directly in the oral cavity and are called **direct restorative**

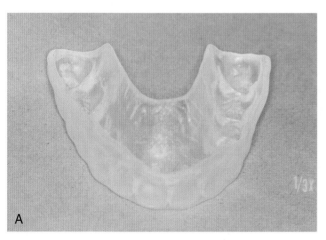

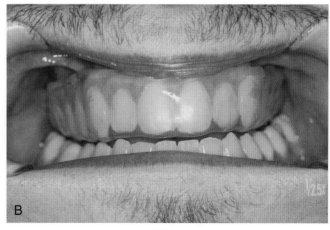

FIGURE 1.12. Photographs of **A.** a mouthguard and **B.** the mouthguard in place.

materials. A typical direct restorative material is placed in the **"cavity preparation"** that was "drilled" by the dentist when removing the decay (see *Fig. 1.9*).

Each material has its own requirements for the design of the cavity preparation. When initially placed, a direct material is a putty-like material that sets to become a hard, strong material. Direct restorative materials include the following:

a. Amalgam, a metallic material that is formed by combining liquid mercury with powdered metals. The freshly mixed amalgam is placed directly in the cavity preparation, is carved to resemble the missing tooth structure, and then hardens (see *Figs. 1.3 and 1.9*).

b. Composites, which are esthetic materials that polymerize in the mouth. These are supplied as pastes that are placed into the preparation and are set by a specific chemical reaction (*Fig. 1.13*).

c. Glass ionomers and other cements, which are mortar-like materials that set by an acid–base chemical reaction in the mouth (see *Fig. 1.13*) and resemble tooth material.

2. Indirect Restorative Materials

Other materials must be fabricated outside the mouth because the processing conditions of many materials would harm oral tissues. Such materials are called **indirect restorative materials** because they are made indirectly on a replica of the patient's oral tissues. Indirect materials include the following:

a. "Gold" crowns and inlays, which are restorations that are made by melting metals and pouring (forcing) them into molds of the exact size and shape needed for each patient (see *Figs. 1.3 and 1.4*).

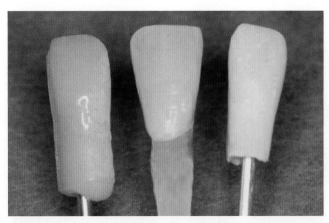

FIGURE 1.13. Photograph of, from *left* to *right,* a composite sample, an extracted tooth, and a glass ionomer sample.

b. Ceramic materials, which are processed by a number of techniques. Many times, a ceramic powder is fired at a very high temperature and becomes a solid object (just as a clay pot is fired). An example would be a porcelain crown (see *Fig. 1.10E and F*).

c. Indirect restorative polymers, which are plastics typically processed or cured at elevated temperatures and under high pressures. An example would be the pink "gingival" portion of a denture (see *Figs. 1.6 and 1.7*).

C. Classification by Longevity of Use

1. Permanent Restorations

Permanent restorations are those restorations that are not planned to be replaced in a particular time period. Although they are referred to as permanent, they are not. Fillings, crowns, bridges, and dentures do not last forever. All restorative dentistry wears out and fails! Quality restorative dentistry in a well-maintained oral cavity, however, will give the patient years and years of service. It is best to prevent the need for restoration and replacement of teeth by aggressive preventive dentistry. The cycle of restoration and re-restoration of teeth is becoming an important factor in the practice of dentistry. What is best for the patient for a lifetime of oral health must be considered along with the immediate dental needs of the patient.

2. Temporary Restorations

Temporary restorations are restorations that are planned to be replaced in a short time (e.g., a week or a month). As discussed earlier, temporary crowns are placed after the tooth is prepared for a permanent crown and are used to protect the tooth while the final restoration is being made at the dental laboratory (see *Fig. 1.10C*). Temporary restorations are sometimes called **provisional restorations**.

3. Interim Restoration

At times, dental treatment requires long-term temporary restorations or **interim restorations**. An example would be a patient who has a fractured front tooth and needs a crown but is presently undergoing orthodontic treatment. A large composite restoration may be adequate until orthodontic treatment is completed or the tooth is close to its final position, and a permanent crown may then be fabricated.

VI. Classification of Dental Caries and Restorations

Dental caries are not evenly distributed throughout the mouth. Certain surfaces of the teeth are particularly susceptible to carious lesions; others are nearly immune. In the late 1800s, Dr. G.V. Black classified the most common sites for dental caries. His classification system adequately describes most simple carious lesions. In high-caries patients, a single tooth may have more than one lesion. These lesions may be of the same class or of different classes. At times, extensive lesions could be described as being a combination of two classes.

A. Class I

The pits and fissures of teeth, particularly posterior teeth, are the most susceptible to dental caries. Pit and fissure caries are called Class I lesions, and the associated restorations are called Class I restorations. *Figures 1.14* and 5.10 show Class I caries and restorations in a molar.

B. Class II

The area of the tooth just below the interproximal contact is also susceptible to caries. If such a lesion occurs in a posterior tooth, it is called a Class II lesion. Dental radiographs are commonly used to diagnose Class II caries. *Figures 1.3*, *1.9*, *1.14*, 6.10, and 15.6 show Class II caries and restorations in molars and premolars.

C. Class III

If interproximal caries occur in an anterior tooth, it is called a Class III lesion. Dental radiographs and clinical examination are commonly used to

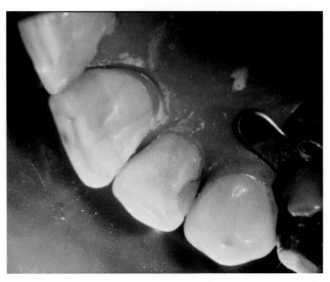

FIGURE 1.15. Photograph showing a Class III stained composite on the distal of tooth #7 and a Class III lesion (white chalky area) on the distal of tooth #8. (Courtesy of Dr. Birgitta Brown, Stockholm, SE.)

diagnose Class III lesions. *Figures 1.14 and 1.15* show Class III caries and restorations.

D. Class IV

If a Class III lesion is left untreated, it may progress and involve the incisal angle of an anterior tooth. A lesion that involves the incisal angle of an anterior tooth is called a Class IV lesion (see *Fig. 1.14*). Class IV restorations are also used to restore the incisal angle of an anterior tooth that has been fractured as the result of trauma, as shown in Figures 5.9 and 13.1B.

E. Class V

The gingival third of the facial and lingual surfaces of both anterior and posterior teeth is susceptible to caries when patients have poor oral hygiene or a high-sugar diet. Class V caries and restorations are shown in *Figures 1.14*, 5.12, and 6.13.

F. Class VI

The Class VI lesion was a later addition to Black's classification. As shown in *Figure 1.14*, a Class VI lesion involves the cusp tip or incisal edge of a tooth. Actually, a Class VI carious lesion is quite rare. For most people retaining a large number of teeth later in life, however, wear of cusp tips and incisal edges is not uncommon. When attrition causes dentin to become exposed, it wears much faster than the surrounding enamel because enamel is much harder than dentin. The result is a "dished-out" area of worn dentin (*Fig. 1.16*). Some clinicians call these restorations of such worn cusp tips and incisal edges Class VI restorations.

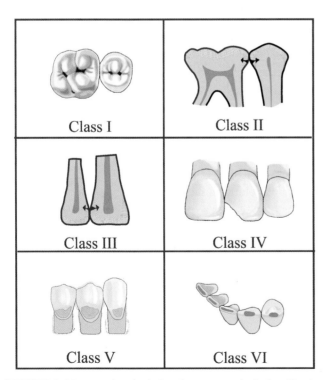

Class I	Class II
Class III	Class IV
Class V	Class VI

FIGURE 1.14. Drawing depicting the Dr. G.V. Black classification of caries.

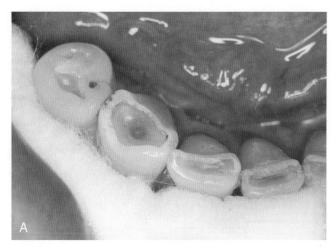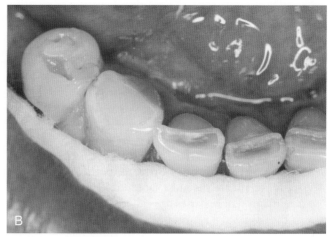

FIGURE 1.16. Photographs of **A.** severely worn teeth and **B.** a composite restoration protecting the dentin of tooth #27. (Courtesy of Dr. Birgitta Brown, Stockholm, SE.)

Summary

The dental hygienist should be knowledgeable in the science of dental materials for several reasons. It should be clear why a restorative material is prescribed for one restoration rather than for another. The best material is selected based on its behavior for providing function and service to the patient. Handling materials properly will enhance the function and longevity of the material that is placed into the patient's mouth. The hygienist must be able to recognize all dental materials so that they can be maintained in the proper manner. The ability to educate patients and answer their questions about the characteristics and properties of dental materials is yet another reason.

Dental professionals must remember that oral tissues, such as enamel, dentin, pulp, periodontium, and gingival tissues, are biologic materials and that they function in the hostile environment of the oral cavity. This environment places restrictions on which materials may be used to replace oral tissue. These restrictions include biting forces, degradation of teeth and materials, temperature changes, biocompatibility, and esthetics.

In the United States, standards are published and administered by ANSI. Other organizations work under their guidance to develop and administer standards for products of their industry. The ADA's Council on Scientific Affairs is one such organization that sets the standards and guidelines for evaluating dental products. The Medical Device Amendment of 1976 ensures the safety of all medical devices. The U.S. FDA considers dental materials to be devices, of which there are three classes. The ISO attempts to unify the standards of its member countries throughout the world.

Dental materials can be classified in three ways: by use, by location of fabrication, or by longevity. When classifying by use, a dental material would be listed under one of the following categories: restorations, crowns, bridges, and complete and partial dentures; impressions, casts and models, and cements; temporary materials; preventive materials; polishing materials; implants; and specialty materials. When classifying by location of fabrication, a dental material would be listed under one of the two categories: direct restorative materials, which are fabricated directly in the mouth and include materials such as amalgam, composites, and glass ionomer; and indirect restorative materials, which are fabricated outside the mouth and include materials such as gold, ceramics, and special polymers. When classifying by longevity of use, a dental material would be listed under one of the three categories: permanent, temporary, and interim restorations.

Dental caries and restorations are also classified into six categories. These categories were developed by Dr. G.V. Black during the late 1800s and are still used today.

Learning Activities

1. Discuss other examples of products used in everyday life that have standards on which we rely for their safety and effectiveness.

2. In the clinic, divide into pairs and, with the use of hand and/or mouth mirrors, look for different kinds of dental materials, such as restorations, sealants, orthodontic retainers, and temporary restorations.

3. Classify the restorations that you found in activity 2 using Black's classification system.

4. Using a large selection of extracted teeth, attempt to identify caries or restorations of each of Black's classifications (I–VI).

5. Classify five of the restorations found in activity 2 by the location of fabrication (direct or indirect).

6. Use de-identified patient charts and radiographs to look for restorations and other dental materials.

7. In a drugstore, see how many different kinds of over-the-counter dental products are available that carry the ADA Seal of Acceptance.

8. Referring to the following list of restorations, briefly discuss the specific home care instructions that would be necessary for your patient to maintain optimal oral health:
   • A four-unit, fixed partial denture
   • An implant
   • A removable partial denture
   • A porcelain-fused-to-metal crown.

 ## Review Questions

Question 1. **In the United States, standards for dental materials are developed and administered by the:**

a. FDA (Food and Drug Administration)
b. ADA (American Dental Association)
c. AADR (American Association for Dental Research)
d. OSHA (Occupational Safety and Health Administration)

Question 2. **All of the following are reasons for a dental hygienist to have knowledge and understanding of dental materials EXCEPT:**

a. Explaining the different types of restorative materials available to the patient
b. Assessing the patient's oral condition
c. Deciding which material is best for the patient's restoration
d. Understanding the behavior of dental materials

Question 3. **An amalgam restoration located on the gingival third of tooth #3 would be a Class _____ restoration.**

a. I
b. II
c. III
d. IV
e. V
f. VI

Question 4. **The biologic nature of the oral environment and the size of the oral cavity restrict the use of dental materials. One restriction is the degradation of restorations.**

a. The first statement is true; the second statement is false.
b. The first statement is false; the second statement is true.
c. Both statements are true.
d. Both statements are false.

Question 5. **When the temperature changes in the mouth, the teeth and most restorative materials expand and contract by the same amount. No leakage occurs around the restoration.**

a. The first statement is true; the second statement is false.
b. The first statement is false; the second statement is true.
c. Both statements are true.
d. Both statements are false.

Question 6. **Which of the following oral tissues provides feedback to the individual regarding the forces placed on the tooth?**

a. Pulp
b. Dentin
c. Periodontium
d. Gingival tissue

Question 7. **Which of the following restorations is utilized when a substantial amount of a tooth is missing?**

a. Crown

b. Pontic

c. Implant

d. Fixed partial denture

Question 8. **The design of a cavity preparation aids in the retention of a restoration. The walls of an amalgam preparation diverge while the walls of an inlay converge.**

a. The first statement is true; the second statement is false.

b. The first statement is false; the second statement is true.

c. Both statements are true.

d. Both statements are false.

Question 9. **If a restoration is fabricated on a replica (positive reproduction) of a patient's teeth, it is referred to as a:**

a. Student model

b. Cast

c. Diagnostic cast

d. Any of the above terms may be used

Question 10. **An example of an indirect restorative material would be:**

a. Amalgam

b. Glass ionomer cement

c. Composite

d. Ceramic (porcelain)

Question 11. **Medical devices are grouped into three categories according to Medical Device Amendment of 1976. Which class of devices is most regulated?**

a. I

b. II

c. III

d. IV

Question 12. **Using *Figure 1.9A and D*, which of the following best describes the roots of the teeth?**

a. Calculus is visible on the distal of tooth #2.

b. Calculus is visible on several roots.

c. The roots are radiographically foreshortened.

d. The roots are radiographically elongated.

Materials Science and Dentistry

Objectives

After studying this chapter, the student will be able to do the following:

1. List the phases into which materials are classified. Discuss the varying amounts of attraction between the molecules and atoms of each phase. Recall the differentiating characteristics of each phase.
2. Explain the basic difference between primary and secondary bonds.
3. Name the three types of primary bonds and describe the differences between them.
4. Summarize the similarities and differences of secondary bonds, which include permanent dipoles, hydrogen bonds, and fluctuating dipoles.
5. Contrast the bonding characteristics of metals, ceramics, plastics, and composites.
6. Compare any similarities and differences of colloids and emulsions.

Key Words/Phrases

amorphous
ceramic
colloids
composites
covalent bonds
cross-linking
crystalline
dental materials
emulsions
fluctuating dipole
hydrogen bonds
ionic bonds
long-range order
materials science
metallic bonds
metals
permanent dipole
polymers
primary bonds
secondary bonds
short-range order
valence electrons

Introduction

Many different kinds of materials are used to make the products we use in everyday life and in the profession of dentistry. Understanding the behavior of materials is important in the selection, placement, and maintenance of dental materials. The behavior of any given material is based on the atoms and the atomic bonds in that material. Many will think the material covered in this chapter is too theoretical for dental hygiene students. If so, the authors urge you to skip this chapter and read only the summary at the end.

I. Materials Science

Materials science is the part of the physical sciences that seeks to explain the properties and performance of materials by examining their internal structure. Materials science is a combination of chemistry, physics, and engineering rather than a separate scientific domain. Materials science tries to explain why materials behave as they do, based on the atoms and molecules in materials and the bonds that exist between these atoms and molecules. Materials science also tries to understand the effects of manufacturing processes on materials and any changes in materials that may occur during the useful life of a product. In dentistry, a subgroup of materials science has developed. This subgroup, called **dental materials**, is part of the larger field of biomaterials and, at times, is called dental biomaterials. Whatever term we use, however, the goal is to understand why materials behave the way they do and how the clinician can maximize the performance of these materials.

In this book, the handling (processing) of dental materials will be stressed, and a discussion of the underlying materials science will be included as well. At times, simply memorizing step-by-step procedures will seem to be much easier, but understanding their nature will simplify the use of the vast number of materials currently on the market. No other branch of scientific inquiry has a greater impact on our day-to-day lives than the development of new materials and the innovative ways in which these materials are being used.

Another branch of materials science, food science, is important to our everyday lives. The same laws of nature that govern dental materials also make ice cream creamy, fudge chewy, and Jell-O jiggle. Whenever possible, everyday examples of these concepts are included in this text.

II. Atomic Bonding

How do teeth withstand the forces that occur when we bite and grind food? To understand the strength of teeth, we need to understand the nature of atomic bonds. Teeth and restorative materials need to be stronger—and to have stronger atomic bonds—than the food we eat.

A. Phases

We commonly classify materials into one of the three phases: solid, liquid, or gas. Familiarity with these phases will provide a foundation for understanding the nature of the forces that hold atoms together in materials. Later in this chapter, we discuss colloids, which are a mixture of two of these phases.

1. Gases

The atomic bonds between gas molecules are very weak. These bonds are easily broken by the normal microscopic vibrations of atoms at room temperature. These atomic vibrations are the result of the thermal energy of the material. Gases have no molecular organization and will take on the three-dimensional shape of the container that they fill. If thermal energy is removed by cooling, gases condense into liquids. An example is the condensation of water vapor on the outside of a mug of ice-cold root beer on a hot, humid day.

2. Liquids

Liquids have stronger attraction between molecules than gases do, but this attraction is not strong enough to carry a load or to maintain a shape without support. The attraction between molecules results in short-range order. **Short-range order** is a consistent spatial relationship among atoms or molecules 5 to 10 neighbors apart. Liquids lack long-range order. Molecular attraction keeps liquids from boiling, but not always from evaporating. Other characteristics of a liquid are vapor pressure, boiling temperature, viscosity, and surface tension.

3. Solids

Solids exhibit the strongest attraction between atoms and molecules. The atomic bonds of solids maintain the shape of objects and resist external forces placed on them. Solids can be classified as crystalline or amorphous. **Crystalline** solids have a consistent spatial relationship of atoms or molecules repeated hundreds to thousands to millions of times that is called **long-range order** (*Fig. 2.1A*). The distances and angles among such atoms or molecules are uniform, much like rooms in a dormitory or hotel. Table salt, diamonds, and the hydroxyapatite of teeth are crystalline solids. Crystalline solids have both short-range and long-range order of their atoms or molecules.

Amorphous solids (*Fig. 2.1B*) have the same strong atomic bonds present in crystalline

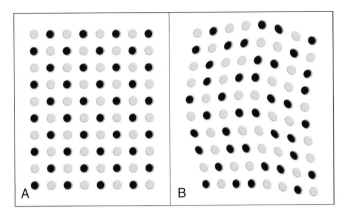

FIGURE 2.1. A two-dimensional depiction of the arrangement of atoms in a crystal **A.** and an amorphous solid **B.**

materials, but have only short-range order, much like liquids. The long-range order of an amorphous solid is more irregular or disorganized. The glass in a window or a dental mirror is an amorphous solid.

Some solid objects are strong, while others are weak. The difference is determined by the type of atoms that make up the material and the strength of the atomic bonds that hold the material together.

B. Atomic Bonds in Solids

How does a strong solid object know how much force it needs to resist the load of an object resting on its surface? If you place a 2-lb book on a table, the table pushes up with 2 lb of force, just enough to support the book—not too little and not too much. How does the table know to push up with 2 lb of force? This "smart" behavior is a characteristic of solid objects and a function of the nature of atomic bonds in materials.

Atomic bonds are a result of electromagnetic (EM) force. For this discussion, we will focus on the electronic part of the EM force. The electronic force causes positive charges to attract negative charges and negative charges to attract positive charges. Positive charges are repelled by positive charges, and negative charges are repelled by negative charges. The magnetic force exhibits similar attraction and repulsion and is easily demonstrated with two magnets. We will use the familiar magnetic force to help us understand attraction and repulsion. The north pole of a magnet attracts the south pole and repels the north pole. It takes force to bring the north poles of two magnets into proximity. The closer they get, the harder you have to push, much like a spring. In fact, the atomic bonds between atoms act much like the springs of a mattress or a car.

To compress a spring, it must be pushed. To stretch a spring, it must be pulled. When no force is applied to a spring, it is said to be unloaded and has an equilibrium length. When force is applied, the spring changes length and resists the applied force by developing an equal and opposite force. Solids can be thought of as a collection of millions and millions of springs or atomic bonds. When you place a book on a table, the atomic bonds of the table are compressed and oppose the force of the book. The heavier the book, the more the bonds are compressed and the greater the force that is developed in the table. Is this really true? We do not see the table change height when we put the book on it. We must remember that the table has millions and millions of atoms and, therefore, millions and millions of atomic bonds. Each bond is compressed a submicroscopic distance. The total of the change in length of these bonds is still microscopic, too small to be seen by the unaided eye, but the change in height of the table can be measured with specialized equipment. Again, the atomic bonds of the table are compressed when a book is placed on it, and these bonds act like springs. When one stretches a rubber band, the same phenomenon occurs, but it can be seen by the unaided eye. Different kinds of internal atomic bonds respond to external forces in different manners.

The change in the height of the table when a book is placed on it is an example of something that happens we cannot see. These changes may be microscopic, or they may occur very slowly and, thus, may not be noticed. Such changes occur in dentistry: teeth compress when biting, erupt into the mouth, change color during a person's lifetime, wear, or dissolve in acid, forming caries.

C. Primary Bonds—Optional

Primary bonds are the strong bonds between atoms that involve the transfer or sharing of electrons between atoms. In high school and college chemistry classes, the ionic and covalent bonds are presented. Another bond that is important to the understanding of certain materials is the metallic bond. All bonds are a result of the EM force and the distribution of positive and negative charges of atoms and molecules.

The atom is made of protons, neutrons, and electrons. The protons and the neutrons make up the nucleus; the electrons move around the nucleus in shells. Electrons in the outer shell of atoms are involved in chemical reactions and atomic bonding. They are called **valence electrons**. When discussing atomic bonding, it is easier to group the nucleus with the nonvalence electrons into what is called the "positive core." The remaining valence electrons are those that are principally involved in atomic bonds. We can therefore restrict our discussion to the positive core of the atom and the valence electrons. Explaining why some elements form metallic bonds and others form covalent bonds is beyond the scope of this text (and its authors' understanding of the subject). However, understanding how atoms fill up their outer shell with electrons from other atoms will help us to understand the nature of atomic bonds and give us some insight regarding why materials behave as they do.

1. Ionic Bonds

Ionic bonds are the result of an electron being given up by one atom and being accepted by another. Why does an atom give up or accept an electron? Atoms are "content" when their outer shell of electrons is full; in this situation, they have a lower state of energy. An element like sodium has one valence electron in its outer shell, and it will readily give up this valence electron. If a sodium atom gives up this valence electron, the next inner shell becomes the outer shell and is a full shell. The atom then becomes an ion with a charge of +1. An element such as chlorine, however, is one electron short of filling its outer shell. Therefore, chlorine readily accepts an electron and becomes an ion with a charge of –1. When sodium and chlorine atoms have full outer shells, the opposite electrical charges of these ions attract each other and form atomic bonds. The result is NaCl or sodium chloride (table salt).

Chemical reactions, in which atoms fill their outer shells with electrons and form bonds, are examples of nature lowering the energy of a system. Other examples of systems lowering their energy include a ball rolling downhill, water flowing over a waterfall, a candle burning, and a battery powering a flashlight. The conversion of energy from one form to another (whether chemical, electrical, mechanical, or thermal) is governed by the laws of thermodynamics. Again, such forbidding subjects are beyond the scope of this text.

Let's get back to the ionic bond. A grain of table salt (sodium chloride) has billions and billions of sodium and chloride ions. Ionic bonds hold the ions together. Oppositely charged ions attract each other (negative chloride ion and positive sodium ion). Ions with like charges repulse each other. The strength of the salt grain is the sum of the attraction of opposite charges minus the repulsion of like charges.

The distance between ions has an important effect on the strength of the attraction or repulsion. The strength of both is inversely proportional to the square of the distance between the ions. Thus, the force between the ions falls rapidly as the distance between the pair increases.

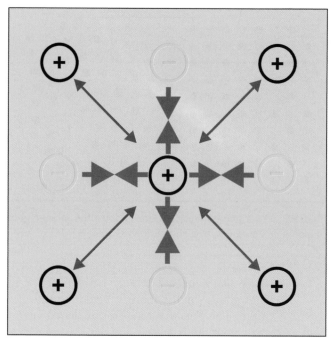

FIGURE 2.2. A two-dimensional depiction of an ionic material. The *green arrows* pointing toward each other represent the attraction of unlike-charged ions. These ions are closer; therefore, the force is stronger. The *red arrows* pointing away represent repulsion of like-charged ions. The like-charged ions are farther apart; therefore, the force is weaker.

The arrangement of ions in sodium chloride results in the negatively charged chloride ions surrounding each positively charged sodium ion. Likewise, each negative ion is surrounded by positive ions. The familiar checkerboard pattern is a two-dimensional example of such an arrangement. As a result, the attraction between oppositely charged "next-door neighbors" is strong because they are close together. The repulsion of similarly charged ion pairs is weaker because they are farther apart (*Fig. 2.2*). The attraction forces overpower the repulsive forces, and the result is a strong material.

2. Covalent Bonds

Covalent bonds between two atoms are the result of two atoms sharing a pair of electrons (*Fig. 2.3*). Sharing electrons with other atoms allows an atom to fill its outer shell with electrons and, thus, to lower its energy. How does sharing a pair of electrons bond two atoms together?

The physical space that an electron occupies around the nucleus is called an orbital, and it is centered around the nucleus when not involved in an atomic bond. When two atoms share an electron, the shape of the orbital changes. When a pair of electrons is shared and forms a covalent bond, the orbital surrounds both

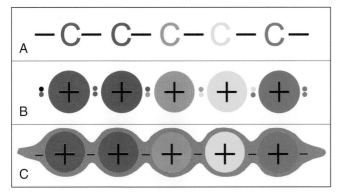

FIGURE 2.3. Three representations of covalent bonds between carbon atoms. In **A.** *lines* represent the bonds. In **B.** pairs of shared electrons represent the bonds. In **C.** the distribution of the electrons is shown. Note in **C** the alternating negative charges of the electrons and positive charges of the cores.

atoms. Now the electrons spend some time in the physical space between the two atoms. By spending time between the two atoms, bonding of the two atoms occurs. A partial negative charge is created by the presence of the electron pair between the two atoms. The partial negative charge of the bond is attracted to the positive cores of the two atoms that are sharing the electron pair. The positive core of the first atom is attracted to the relatively close partial negative charge (because of the electron pair spending time there) between the atoms. The same is true for the second atom that shares the electron pair.

The attraction of the partial negative charge to the two positive cores is greater than the repulsion between the positive cores because the distance between the two positive cores is greater. We have probably set organic chemistry back a century with this simplistic description of the covalent bond, but it will serve our purposes and help to explain the behavior of polymers (and it's the best the authors can do).

Covalent bonds between the two atoms sharing the electron pair are strong and very directional. However, few materials are bonded with only covalent bonds. One well-known material that is covalently bonded is diamond. Each carbon atom is bonded to four other carbon atoms by a covalent bond. One of the hardest materials known results from this bonding. Many materials are the result of long chains of covalently bonded atoms. The chains are strong, but the materials are not always strong. This is because their properties are determined by the manner in which the long chains are bonded to each other. Polymers are long chains of covalently bonded carbon atoms. Examples of polymers

include man-made plastics and rubbers as well as many biologic macromolecules, such as proteins and DNA. The varied properties of polymers and plastics will be better explained in the discussion of secondary bonds.

3. Metallic Bonds

Metals have characteristic properties that allow us to easily identify a material as being a metal. Metals are typically dense, heavy materials. They are good conductors of both electricity and heat, are cold to the touch at room temperature, and, if shaped properly, will ring like a bell if struck. All these properties of metals are a result of metallic bonds. **Metallic bonds** are similar to covalent bonds in that valence electrons are shared between atoms. The difference is that the electrons in a metal object are not shared by two atoms; instead, they are shared by all the atoms that make up that object (*Fig. 2.4*). We can illustrate this difference by comparing a marriage to students in a school. In a marriage, the relationship is between two people, and the sharing is between those two. Within a school, however, all students are part of the student body. They have a less intense relationship, but they all share the feeling of being part of the school.

Metals can be thought of as positive cores in a cloud of negative mobile valence electrons, much like chocolate chips in ice cream. The chocolate chips are the positive cores, and the ice

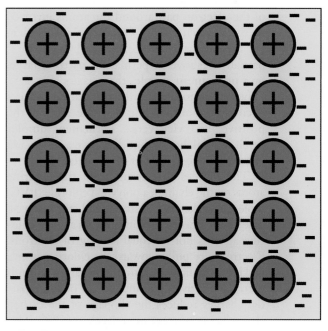

FIGURE 2.4. A two-dimensional representation of the metallic bond. Note that the positive cores (nuclei and nonvalence electrons) are surrounded by an electron "cloud."

cream is the electron cloud. Because the positive cores (the chips) are surrounded by electrons (the ice cream), the negative–positive electric charges cause the electrons to be attracted to the positive cores. Again, the positive cores are repelled by each other, and the negative electrons are repelled by each other. And again, the electrons are closer to the positive cores than the positive cores are to each other, so the attraction is greater than the repulsion. This results in a weak primary bond in all directions. The enormous number of bonds in a metal results in a strong material. Later, we will see that the nondirectional nature of metallic bonds has an important effect on the properties and use of metals.

D. Secondary Bonds—Optional

Secondary bonds, or van der Waals forces, are the result of partial charges from an uneven distribution of electrons around an atom or a molecule. The partial charges can be temporary or permanent, very weak or somewhat strong. Secondary bonds are important in determining the properties of polymers because they determine the interaction of the polymer chains and, thus, the properties of the polymer itself.

1. Permanent Dipoles

Depending on the type of atoms bonded by a covalent bond, the shared electrons may not be shared equally. Some atoms are "greedy" and pull the shared electrons more strongly toward themselves. The result is an uneven distribution of the electron pair around the atoms involved in the covalent bond. One atom involved in the bond is partially positive, and the other is partially negative. A permanent partial charge, or a **permanent dipole**, thus occurs (*Fig. 2.5*). When one molecule with such partial charges encounters another, the negative attracts the positive, and vice versa. Permanent dipoles result in weak bonds, but they have a significant effect on the behavior of many materials.

The dipoles that result from the chlorine atoms on the chain of a polyvinyl chloride (PVC) molecule make PVC a strong and stiff material. The bond between the carbon atom and the chlorine atom is not an equal sharing of electrons. Electrons are pulled toward the chlorine atoms, making it partially negative. The carbon atom is partially positive. The interaction of these partial charges reduces the slippage of the carbon chains by one another in molecules of PVC. This results in a strong, stiff plastic (commonly used for drainpipes in houses). When electrons are more evenly distributed, the dipoles are much

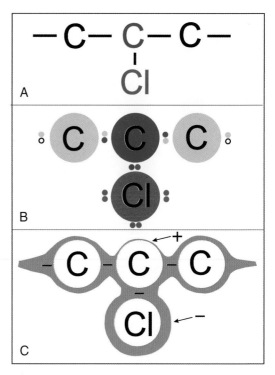

FIGURE 2.5. Three representations of a permanent dipole. In **A.** *lines* represent the bonds. In **B.** pairs of shared electrons are shown. In **C.** the distribution of the electrons is seen. The electron density is greater around the chlorine atom and less around the middle carbon atom. Note in **C** the uneven distribution of the electron density that results in partial charges or dipoles.

smaller, and the material is much weaker and much less stiff. An example of such a material is polyethylene, which is commonly used as a plastic wrap for food.

2. Hydrogen Bonds

Hydrogen bonds are a special case of a permanent dipole. The hydrogen atom contains only one electron. When this single electron is pulled away from the hydrogen nucleus by a "greedy" atom, such as oxygen, the nucleus is left partially unshielded, but to a much greater extent than in other elements with multiple electrons. The resulting interaction between molecules results in a bond that is much stronger than other secondary bonds.

We can understand the significance of unshielding the hydrogen nucleus if we consider four children in two beds during the cold of winter. Two children in one bed have one blanket, and the other two children have three blankets. If the blankets of both pairs of children were shared equally, then the partners in each pair would be equally comfortable. Each pair of children in a bed would have two blankets. However, our story has one bed with one blanket and one bed with three blankets. What happens if one child of the pair with three blankets gets cold and pulls one of the blankets completely over to his or her side of the bed? The other child is left with two shared blankets and might not notice much difference. What if the same thing happens with the other pair of children, the two with only one blanket? When the single blanket is pulled away, one child will get cold while the other child stays warm.

So is the case of the hydrogen atom: when its partner pulls away its only electron, its nucleus is more unshielded than the nucleus of other elements with multiple electrons in the same situation. A strong dipole occurs, and significant bonding between molecules results. Hydrogen bonding is important in biologic polymers, such as proteins and DNA. The three-dimensional structure of enzymes is determined by hydrogen bonding as the protein chain folds back on itself. In DNA, it is the hydrogen bonds that pair thymine with adenine and cytosine with guanine in the cross-links of the double helix.

3. Fluctuating Dipole

What about atoms or molecules without a permanent dipole (partial charges)? How do they stay together as solids or liquids? The noble gases, such as helium (He), have a symmetrical charge distribution; they have no dipole. Molecules of two of the same atoms, such as nitrogen gas, theoretically have a symmetrical charge distribution. Such atoms and molecules with a symmetrical charge distribution have very weak bonds between molecules. These gases need to be cooled to very low temperatures to liquefy. Their bonds are the result of an intermittent, uneven distribution of electrons around the atoms or molecules. These weak bonds are called a **fluctuating dipole**. Although this uneven distribution lasts only for an extremely short time and is always changing, positive and negative charges result, as does a very weak attraction between these atoms or molecules.

If one thinks of an outside light at night during the summer, one can get a feeling for this ever-changing distribution. The insects flying around the light can be thought of as electrons, and the light is the positive core. The insects seem to fly around the light as if attracted by some unseen force. They are unable to escape the close proximity of the light, similar to the relationship of an electron and a positive core. If one observes the insects and the light for a few seconds, one sees that the insects are not always evenly spread out around the light. Sometimes, for a just a second or so, they congregate more

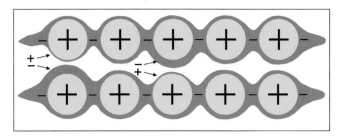

FIGURE 2.6. A fluctuating dipole. The intermittent, uneven distribution of the electron density (*purple area*) results in a constantly changing, or fluctuating, dipole.

to one side than to the other. The unevenness then quickly changes.

Electrons around uncharged atoms and molecules behave in the same way. (Of course, the physical size of their orbits and the duration of the unevenness are millions and millions of times smaller than those of the insects and the light.) The result is a constantly changing, very weak attraction that allows uncharged atoms and small molecules to be cooled down and liquefied, but only at very low temperatures. The fluctuating dipoles of large uncharged molecules, such as some polymers, result in weak materials at room temperature (*Fig. 2.6*).

4. Summary

Secondary bonds are the result of uneven electron distribution around atoms and molecules. The more uneven the distribution is, the stronger the charge, the greater the attraction, and the stronger the bond. Secondary bonding in materials is most important when combined with covalent bonding, as in polymers.

III. Materials and Their Atomic Bonds

The atoms that make up a material and how these atoms are bonded determine the properties of that material. Weak bonds make for weak materials, and vice versa. Materials can be classified into three categories based on their primary atomic bonds: metals, ceramics, and polymers. A fourth category is composites. Composites are "mixtures" of two materials from two different categories. Dental composites are a combination of a ceramic and a polymeric material.

A. Metals

Metals are held together with metallic bonds. Few metals, however, have pure metallic bonds. Most metals have bonds that are predominantly metallic but that also show some covalent or ionic tendency. The broad range of mixtures of metallic and other primary bonds results in metallic materials with a range of properties. In this chapter, we focus on metals in which the metallic bond predominates. A good example is 24-carat gold, which is pure gold. Gold is ductile, meaning that it can easily be bent without breaking yet retains its strength. Gold behaves differently than a ceramic material, such as porcelain, or a plastic material. This mechanical behavior is a result of the metallic bond.

What happens when an object is bent? Some atoms are pushed together. Others are pulled apart. Still others slide past one another. We will focus on the atoms' ability to slide by one another because this is an important determinant of mechanical properties. In a metal, each atom (positive core) is surrounded by an electron cloud. The positive core "feels" the attraction and repulsion of all the charges that make up the object, but what the core feels is dominated by the outer electron cloud. What happens if an atom slides by another atom? Does the atom feel any difference in its surroundings? The electron cloud is still there and has not changed. Thus, the atom feels little (if any) difference. The surroundings (or the atomic bonding) have not changed, so the properties do not change. The ease with which metals can be bent and shaped enabled early humans to make strong tools that were tough and resisted fracture. What would happen if you tried to make a hammer out of a ceramic or a polymeric material rather than a metal?

In dentistry, we bend orthodontic wires and clasps of partial dentures. We also use instruments to adapt (marginate) the edges of a gold restoration closely to the tooth. All are examples of bending metals, a process that forces the atoms to slide against each other. It is the metallic bond that enables metals to have such useful properties.

B. Ceramics

The atoms of a **ceramic** material are bonded with ionic bonds. Table salt (NaCl) is a good example. Salt is strong but brittle. If enough force is applied to a grain of salt, it can be crushed. Why is salt so brittle? What happens if a Na ion slides away from its original position next to a Cl ion? Each Na ion is surrounded by Cl ions and vice versa. The nearest neighbors have opposite charges and the result is attraction. Therefore, as a Na ion slides past a Cl ion, it approaches another Na ion with the same charge, and now, there is repulsion where there once was attraction. The Na ions push away from each other, and the material breaks or fractures.

Many ceramic materials used in everyday life, such as dishes, concrete, china, and bricks, are bonded by both ionic and covalent bonds. The ionic bond dominates the behavior of the material, resulting in strong, brittle materials. The strong

nature of the bonds of these materials is reflected in the high temperatures needed to process many ceramic materials and their chemical stability.

In dentistry, the notable advantage of ceramic materials is the range of esthetics that can be produced. Crowns made of ceramic materials are colored to match the appearance of the patient's natural teeth. These materials are also translucent, meaning that some light passes through, as in natural teeth. This translucency gives the ceramic crown a more natural appearance that other materials cannot provide (see Fig. 1.10F).

In summary, ceramic materials are strong when compressed, because the atoms are forced together. However, ceramic materials are weak and brittle when pulled or bent.

C. Polymers or Plastics

Polymers are composed of long chains of covalently bonded, repeating units. The chains are thousands of units long and consist of carbon, hydrogen, and other elements. A wide variety of polymers are used in everyday life. Some are soft, weak, and flexible; these are called "plastics." They make good toys, garbage bags, and fabrics. Others are hard, stiff, and fairly strong; these are called glassy polymers or resins. Such polymers are used to make parts for cars, outdoor furniture, plumbing pipes, and dishes. Another important group can be stretched out a great deal and still return to their original shape; these are called rubber materials. Where would we be without elastic waistbands or rubber gloves?

Why do polymers exhibit such a wide range of properties? Some properties of polymers are dependent on the covalent bonds between the carbon atoms that make up the backbone of the polymer molecule or chain. However, it is the variety of bonds between polymer chains that results in such a wide variety of polymeric materials.

The weakest bond between chains is the fluctuating dipole (rapidly changing partial charges). It occurs in polymers that do not have significant permanent charges in the backbone of the chain or side groups (*Figs. 2.6 and 2.7A*). Fluctuating dipole bonds are easily broken, and the chains readily slide by one another at room temperature. At room temperature, these polymer chains tend to resemble a plate of spaghetti. The polymer chain or piece of spaghetti is twisted and winds its way through the mass, which can easily be bent and pushed about. Plastic bags are made of such materials. If they are bent or stretched, the chains readily slide against one another. Such linear polymers are processed by heating (melting), which increases chain slippage; they are then molded or extruded. In dentistry,

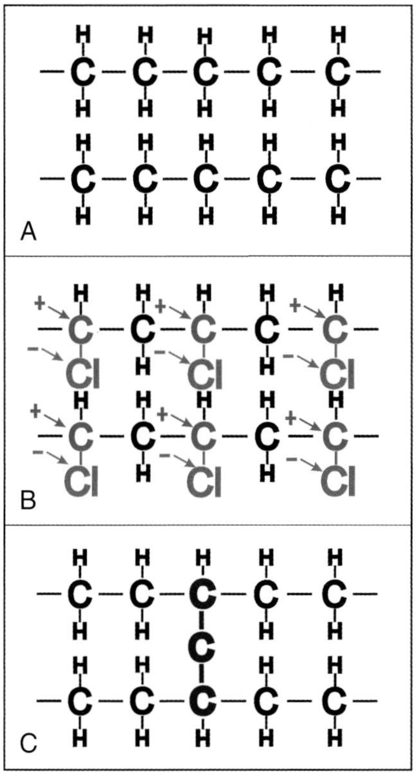

FIGURE 2.7. Three kinds of chain-to-chain interactions in a polymer. **A.** Linear polymer has weak secondary forces, as in *Figure 2.6*. **B.** Polymer with a permanent dipole is stronger. **C.** Cross-linking covalent bonds result in an even stronger polymeric material.

moldable polymers are used to make bleaching trays and fluoride trays; see Chapter 18, Oral Appliances, and Chapter 31, Vital Tooth Whitening.

If the polymer chain has a side group or atom that results in an uneven distribution of electrons, a partial charge will result. This is illustrated in *Figure 2.7B*. A greedy atom, such as chloride of PVC, will pull electrons away from some carbon atoms and cause the chain-to-chain interaction to greatly increase. In our pasta example, the spaghetti sticks to itself to a small extent. Now our polymer chains are much more "sticky" and the material is stiffer and stronger. As the number and intensity of the charges increase, the strength and stiffness of the polymer increase. Also, higher temperatures are required to melt these polymers when they are processed. Some dental instruments are made from these stiff, plastic materials.

Polymers have been developed that go beyond the weak bonding of secondary bonds and incorporate primary atomic bonds between the chains in their polymeric structure. These polymers have cross-links between the chains (*Fig. 2.7C*). The chains are linked by covalently bonded atoms to form a three-dimensional structure and can no longer slide past each other, resulting in stiff, strong

material. The structural biologic polymers, such as collagen fiber in animals and wood fiber in plants, fit into this group. Dental composite filling materials use cross-linked polymeric materials. Heat will not melt these polymers; the chains cannot slip by each other. If these materials are heated to a high-enough temperature, however, decomposition results, such as the burning of wood or Mike's "blackened mystery meat."

A few man-made polymers have charged groups hanging off the polymer backbone that result in ionic bonds between chains. Such polymers are not widely used in everyday life, but one is used in dentistry: polyacrylic acid, which will be discussed later. In biology, several amino acids have groups that ionize. These charged groups are the part of a protein that greatly affects its three-dimensional structure and function. The three-dimensional structure of protein is critical if an enzyme is to function properly.

Why do we keep using examples from biochemistry? The typical dental hygiene student has a good background in biology. Man-made polymers follow the same "rules" as those of the biologic polymers with which the student is familiar. Biologic polymers, such as collagen and DNA, form helical structures. It is the stretching of these helixes (coils) that enables biologic polymers to stretch when we bend our joints. Man-made polymers have the same coiled three-dimensional structures. However, what keeps the coils from sliding by each other when they are stretched? A few covalent cross-links along the polymer chain keep the coils in place and prevent their movement. Depending on the interaction of the coils, some man-made polymeric materials can also stretch and return to their original shape.

Just like biologic rubbery materials, man-made rubber materials have polymeric coils that stretch out and recoil, similar to the springlike toy called a "Slinky." Rubber bands and polymeric impression materials are examples of materials that stretch and return to their original shape. A better description of a rubber material is a pile of Slinkies tangled together, with a few wired together. The linking of one coil (or polymer chain) across to another with wire (or a covalent bond) is called **cross-linking**. The mass can be stretched, but it cannot be untangled. The more cross-links that a rubber material has, the stiffer it will be. If too many cross-links are present, the rubber is too strong and hard, and it behaves more like a stiff plastic.

D. Composites

Composites are materials that are made of two or more different materials. Common composites are mixtures of a polymer and a ceramic, such as fiberglass. Each material that makes up a composite is called a phase. Materials or phases are chosen and combined so that the resulting composite has properties better than those of either component material. A composite is a kind of "team" of materials and is usually best appreciated on a microscopic level. The properties lacking in one material are compensated for by those of the other material. Strong, lightweight materials and products result. Sporting goods, such as skis, rackets, and golf clubs, are made from composite materials to minimize weight while retaining strength and flexibility. In dentistry, composites were first used as an esthetic restorative material, but today, they are commonly used for a variety of purposes. Enamel is a composite of apatite (a ceramic material) and protein (a polymer).

E. Colloids

Colloids are also two-phase materials. Colloids are mixtures of gases, liquids, or solids at the microscopic level. Colloids are not true solutions of one material dissolved in another, such as salt-water. Colloids are suspensions of one material in another, such as fog (a suspension of water droplets in air). Properties of composite materials are a result of the properties of the component materials. Properties of colloids, however, are a result of the properties of the components but are also greatly affected by the properties of the surfaces of the component phases. It is the large amount of surface area around the small particles that gives colloids their properties. When we discuss adhesion and bonding, we will again discuss the subject of surface science. Common colloids are Jell-O, foam, milk, smoke, and emulsions. Several dental impression materials are also colloids, as are fluoride foams.

Emulsions are a type of colloid composed of two liquids that do not blend together to form one liquid. When the two liquids are vigorously mixed, tiny droplets of each liquid are formed and dispersed among droplets of the other liquid. Oil-and-vinegar salad dressing is a good example. The oil and vinegar do not blend, but when they are vigorously shaken, a new liquid seemingly results. This new liquid is an emulsion of oil and vinegar. The surfaces of the two liquids are temporarily stable, and the dressing is neither vinegar nor oil. The resulting dressing, however, combines the taste of both and the spices dissolved in each. Milk as well as liquid soaps and lotions are emulsions.

The transformation from a liquid to a gel is the important feature of other colloid materials. Jell-O and jellies are good examples. If warmed, these materials become liquid. If cooled, they become a semisolid gel. In dentistry, hydrocolloid impression material behaves in this manner.

F. Teeth and Food

One of the main functions of teeth is to start the digestion of food. Food varies a great deal in texture, from mashed potatoes to rock candy. Teeth chop, tear, and grind a variety of materials to allow the digestive fluids to access the greater surface area that is inherent in smaller pieces of food. Teeth, jaws, and muscles are able to apply a great amount of force to food to crush it. The teeth must withstand these forces for a lifetime. Luckily, teeth are made from materials that are able to resist these forces. Teeth are stronger than the food we eat. The dental restorative materials that are used to replace tooth structure must have these same characteristics. In the next chapter, we discuss the mechanical and physical properties of materials. We will compare dentin and enamel to restorative and other materials used in dentistry.

Summary

Properties of materials are a result of their atomic bonds. Materials can be classified into one of the three phases: solid, liquid, or gas. A solid object exhibits the ability to support itself and other objects because solids have the strongest atomic bonds. Liquids have weaker bonds and need to be confined on most sides by a container. Gases have the weakest of all bonds and their atoms need to be contained in all the three dimensions.

Atoms of materials are held together by two types of atomic bonds: primary and secondary. Primary bonds are those that involve the transfer or sharing of electrons between atoms. There are three kinds of primary bonds: ionic, covalent, and metallic. Ionic bonds result when an electron is given up by an atom and accepted by another. The atom that gives up the electron becomes a positive ion, while the atom that receives the electron becomes a negative ion. The positive and negative ions attract each other by the electromagnetic force and form an ionic bond. When two atoms share a pair of electrons, a covalent bond is formed. A metallic bond involves sharing many electrons by all the atoms in the material. Covalent and metallic bonds are also the result of positive and negative electromagnetic attraction of atoms and their electrons.

Secondary bonds occur when a partial charge is created from an uneven distribution of electrons. The three types of secondary bonds are hydrogen bonds, permanent dipoles, and the fluctuating dipole. Of the three, the hydrogen bond is the strongest, and the fluctuating dipole is the weakest. The hydrogen bond is important in biologic molecules such as DNA and proteins, and biologic materials such as ligaments and cartilage.

Materials can be classified into three categories based on their primary atomic bonds: metals, ceramics, and polymers. Composites are a combination of two solid materials and may be considered a fourth category. Metals are ductile, yet retain strength when bent because the metallic bond allows atoms to slide by one another and not disrupt the bonds in the metal. Ceramic materials are strong when compressed, but weak and brittle when pulled or bent. When the arrangement of the positive and negative ions in a ceramic material is changed, attraction may change to repulsion and a break or fracture is likely. Polymers or plastics have a range of properties because they have covalent bonds and a range of secondary bonds in their atomic structure. Many different polymers are used to make everyday products. Those that are soft, weak, and flexible are termed plastics or rubber. Those that are hard, stiff, and strong are called resins or glassy polymers. Composites are a mixture of two or more distinct materials. An example is fiberglass, made of both a polymer and a ceramic.

Learning Activities

1. Pick out several objects in the room. Discuss the type of materials used to manufacture those objects, the kind of atomic bonds in the materials used, and the properties that result.

2. Describe the advantages and disadvantages of using a metal, a ceramic, or a polymer as a restorative material.

3. Using the Internet, search for "colloid." Visit several sites that list everyday examples of colloids. Which of these colloids have you seen? Touched? Eaten?

Review Questions

Question 1. **The molecules found in a pane of glass can be best described as:**

a. Crystalline solid, having short-range order only

b. Crystalline solid, having both short-range and long-range order

c. Amorphous solid, having long-range order

d. Amorphous solid, having short-range order

Question 2. **A partial charge resulting from an uneven distribution of electrons around an atom forms a bond known as:**

a. Metallic

b. Secondary

c. Covalent

d. Ionic

Question 3. **What type of bond is formed when the electrons are shared by all the atoms that make up that object and may be thought of as "positive cores" in a "cloud of negative mobile valence electrons"?**

a. Metallic

b. Secondary

c. Covalent

d. Ionic

Question 4. **A notable advantage of using ceramic materials in dentistry is the property of:**

a. Transparency

b. Translucency

c. Opacity

d. Brittleness

Question 5. A dental polymer with many cross-links as compared to one with no cross-links would be a dental material that is:

a. Flexible but strong

b. Flexible and weak

c. Stiff and strong

d. Stiff but weak

Question 6. All of the following are examples of a composite except:

a. Set Jell-O with sliced peaches

b. Enamel

c. Fiberglass

d. Tin foil

Question 7. When the shared electrons of a covalent bond are not shared equally, and one of the bonded atoms is partially positive and the other is partially negative, a _____ is formed.

a. Permanent dipole

b. Fluctuating dipole

c. Hydrogen bond

d. Primary bond

Question 8. The sliding of atoms past each other allows this material to bend, not fracture, and maintain its strength. This material is an example of a:

a. Metal

b. Ceramic

c. Polymer

Question 9. A mixture of two liquids that do not blend together to form one liquid is termed a (an):

a. Composite

b. Emulsion

c. Colloid

d. Solution

Question 10. When two atoms share a pair of electrons, the resulting atomic bond is termed a (an) _____ bond.

a. Secondary

b. Ionic

c. Covalent

d. Metallic

Physical and Mechanical Properties of Dental Materials

Objectives

After studying this chapter, the student will be able to do the following:

1. Describe or define the key words and phrases.
2. Relate the physical properties of materials discussed in this chapter to their use in dentistry.
3. Define wetting. Include in the definition a drop of liquid and the contact angle formed with the surface.
4. Name the units of measure for the following properties:
   - Density
   - Heat capacity
   - Stress
   - Strain
   - Modulus of elasticity
5. Define "proportional limit," and name two other nearly equivalent terms.
6. Name the four types of stress, and provide an example of each found in everyday life.
7. Describe two situations in which dental materials are subjected to bending stresses when in function.
8. Compare the properties of "toughness" and "hardness," and provide examples.
9. Explain the difference between stress relaxation and creep.
10. Discuss the phenomenon of stress concentration, and compare its effects on a poorly placed amalgam restoration as well as on a properly placed one.

Key Words/Phrases

abrasion resistance
bending
biologic properties
chemical properties
coefficient of thermal expansion
color
compression
creep
density
elastic deformation
elastic limit
elasticity
fatigue
force
fracture toughness
galvanic shock
Goldilocks principle
hardness
heat capacity
heat of fusion
heat of vaporization
load
mechanical properties
modulus of elasticity
percolation
permanent deformation
physical properties
plastic deformation
Poisson's ratio
proportional limit
resilience
shade guide

(continued)

Key Words/Phrases (*continued*)

shear	tension	vapor pressure
solubility	thermal conductivity	viscosity
specific heat capacity	torsion	water sorption
strain	toughness	wetting
stress	ultimate compressive strength	yield point
stress concentration	ultimate strength	
stress relaxation	ultimate tensile strength	

Introduction

When substituting one material for another, as in the restoration of teeth, we must be aware of the requirements for the new material. It seems obvious that the replacement material should have the same characteristics as enamel, which is very hard and strong. Should dentists restore teeth with the strongest and hardest material? In certain situations, the replacement material should have the same appearance as teeth for proper esthetics. Several other questions also need to be addressed: Is the material as good a thermal insulator as enamel and dentin are? Is the material "kind" to the pulp of the tooth? Does the material break down and release toxic chemicals?

We should also consider the cost of materials and labor when selecting restorative materials. As the list of requirements grows, we begin to realize that the criteria for an ideal restorative material are many and varied. Unfortunately, no ideal material exists, so we are always compromising in one way or another. The only sure way to eliminate this difficult dilemma is through prevention.

The important question is: what are the requirements for a particular restoration for a particular tooth and patient? Determining what is required and what will best meet the clinical situation are complex questions. Typically, a compromise is made among the many factors being considered. This chapter discusses many of these factors or properties of materials. In addition, this chapter describes the relationship between these properties and the materials science concepts previously discussed.

In everyday life, we notice that different materials have different properties. When we pick up an object, we feel its weight, which is an indication of its density. We also feel its temperature, which is an indication of its thermal "content" and its ability to transmit heat. Some objects feel strong and hard; others feel weak and flexible. Engineers have devised a variety of laboratory tests to quantify the properties of materials. Dental materials scientists use the same tests (as well as several others) to describe the physical properties of materials used in dentistry.

I. Properties of Materials

Properties of materials can be divided into three categories: physical, chemical, and biologic. **Physical properties** are based on the laws of physics that describe mass, energy, force, light, heat, electricity, and other physical phenomena. Color, density, and thermal conductivity are examples of physical properties. **Mechanical properties** are a subgroup of physical properties. Mechanical properties describe a material's ability to resist forces. Mechanical properties are dependent on the amount of material and on the size and shape of the object. Examples are strength and stiffness. **Chemical properties** describe the setting reactions as well as the decay or degradation of materials. For example, gypsum products (used to make study models) set by a precipitation process, whereas dental composites polymerize. **Biologic properties** of materials are the effects the materials have on living tissue. For example, a crown should not irritate the gingiva, tongue, or buccal mucosa.

The chemical and biologic properties of dental materials are discussed with each group of materials presented in the chapters that follow. This chapter focuses on the physical and mechanical properties.

II. Physical Properties

A. Density

The amount or mass of a material in a given volume is the **density** of the material. A common unit of density is g/cm^3. Density depends on the type of atoms that are present (as the atomic number increases, so does the density), the packing together of atoms and molecules, and the voids in the material. The high density of most metal objects makes them feel heavy. Most metals have high atomic numbers, and their atoms are packed closely together into solids. A metal maxillary partial denture will feel heavy and have a tendency to become "unseated" if it is not designed to adapt to the remaining teeth.

B. Boiling and Melting Points

Boiling and melting points are physical properties of materials. In analytical laboratories, they can be used to help identify chemicals. Mixtures often have a melting or boiling range rather than a specific melting or boiling point. Dental waxes are an example of mixtures with a melting range. When an object melts or boils, the atomic bonds between the atoms or molecules are broken by the thermal energy of the material. Some dental metals melt at very high temperatures and are very difficult to work with. Other materials do not boil or melt; instead, they decompose if heated sufficiently. Wood and cookie dough are common examples of materials that decompose.

C. Vapor Pressure

Vapor pressure is a measure of a liquid's tendency to evaporate and become a gas. As the temperature of a liquid increases, the vapor pressure also increases. We notice that steam rises from a pot of water more and more as it is heated because the increased thermal energy allows more atoms or molecules to escape from the liquid and become vapor. Materials with a low vapor pressure, such as cooking oil, do not evaporate quickly. Materials with a high vapor pressure, such as rubbing alcohol, evaporate readily at room temperature.

Materials with a high vapor pressure are very useful as solvents in the application of viscous (syrupy) liquids, such as glue or paint. The viscous liquid is "thinned" by mixing it with a solvent. This "more runny" mixture is then applied to a surface. As the solvent evaporates, it leaves behind a thin layer of the viscous liquid. In dentistry, we use solvents to apply a thin layer of a thick liquid, such as copal varnish or a dentinal adhesive. Rubber cement, oil-based paints, and perfumes use the same process: a mixture is applied and the solvent evaporates, leaving behind a thin film of the desired substance.

Methyl methacrylate, a component of dental acrylic resins (plastics), has a high vapor pressure and can evaporate easily when a denture is processed. Porosity may result, weakening the denture. Denture-processing techniques are designed to minimize the evaporation of methyl methacrylate and the resulting porosity (see Fig. 11.3).

D. Thermal Conductivity

In the kitchen, we use a wooden spoon to stir hot liquids. We do not use a metal spoon because it conducts heat well and would quickly become too hot to hold. In dentistry, we are also interested in the thermal conductivity of materials. **Thermal conductivity** is the rate of heat flow through a material. Measurement of thermal conductivity depends on the distance the heat travels, the area in which the heat travels (much like the size of the pipe through which water travels), and the difference in temperature between the source and destination. Because thermal conductivity is a rate, it is measured as heat flow over time. Thermal conductivity is measured as calories/second·meter·degree. Pulpal sensitivity is likely if conductive materials, such as metals, are placed in close proximity to the pulp. If caries are deep and a metal restoration is planned, an insulating base is placed beneath the metal restoration to insulate the pulp from hot and cold stimuli (see Fig. 1.9).

E. Heat Capacity

Some objects, such as a "microwave warming trivet," can store a lot of heat. The **heat capacity** of a material is a measure of the amount of thermal energy that a material can hoard. Some materials require more energy than others to heat. The **specific heat capacity** of a material is the amount of energy needed to raise the temperature of one unit of mass of that material by 1°C. Specific heat capacity is measured as cal/g·deg. The heat capacity of water is 1 cal/g·deg.

F. Heat of Fusion and Vaporization

The **heat of fusion** is the amount of energy required to melt a material. Conversely, the **heat of vaporization** is the amount of energy required to boil a material. Both are typically large in relation to the heat capacity. It requires 80 times more energy to melt a given quantity of ice than to increase the temperature of the same amount of water by 1°C. It takes 540 times more energy to boil that same quantity of water. The high heat of fusion allows a small amount of ice to effectively cool a much larger amount of beverage without excessive dilution as it melts. We shall see that the heat of fusion of metals must be overcome when melting gold for casting a crown. The solid metal must be heated to the melting temperature, and then, a significant amount of energy must be added to melt the metal.

G. Coefficient of Thermal Expansion

If a balloon filled with room temperature air is brought outside on a cold January day in West Virginia, the balloon shrinks. This is a visible example of what happens to nearly all materials when cooled: they shrink or contract. On the other hand, most materials expand when heated. The **coefficient of thermal expansion** is a measure of this change in volume in relation to the change in temperature. This concept, however, is slightly more complicated than that explanation suggests.

The coefficient of thermal expansion is a fractional change in volume or length. In *Figure 3.1*, several examples of expansion are illustrated. In *Figure 3.1A*, the 10-unit-long bar is extended by

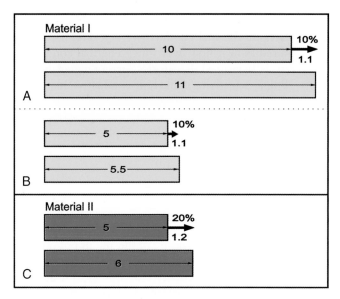

FIGURE 3.1. Three examples of expansion of a material in terms of percentage or fractional change in length.

1 unit (or 10%). The new bar is now 1.1 times the original length. In *Figure 3.1B*, the 5-unit-long bar is extended by 0.5 unit, becoming 5.5 units long. It is also 10% longer (or 1.1 times the original length). Therefore, larger objects of the same material expand more in quantity than smaller objects do, but larger objects expand by an equal amount in terms of the percentage or fractional change. In *Figure 3.1C*, a different material expands more, and the result is a 20% change in length. We look at fractional change of length again later in this chapter, when strain is discussed.

Our interest in the coefficient of thermal expansion of dental materials is in relationship to those of enamel and dentin. A polymeric material, such as polymethyl methacrylate (an early tooth-colored restorative material of the 1950s), shrinks and expands seven times more than tooth structures. Compared with that filling material, the restorative materials of today more closely match the coefficient of thermal expansion of teeth. When the mismatch is great, the restoration will shrink with cold beverages, opening gaps between the restoration and the tooth. When the tooth heats up again and expands, the gap is closed. The process of heating and cooling, and the accompanying opening and closing of the gap, is called **percolation**. Percolation results in microleakage, tooth sensitivity, and recurrent decay. Microleakage is discussed in Adhesive Materials.

H. Electrical Conductivity

Electrical conductivity is not typically thought of as an important property, but we should know which materials are conductive. Metals are good electrical conductors. Polymers and ceramics are poor conductors and are termed insulators. During electrosurgery or electronic pulp testing, it is important to know which restorations are conductive and which are not. Electrical conductivity also affects corrosion, which will be discussed in the section on instruments. Occasionally, a new amalgam filling will hurt when it is touched with a metal fork. This **galvanic shock** is the result of electricity flowing from the fork to the amalgam and through the pulp.

I. Viscosity

When placing materials, the handling characteristics of those materials are important. Some materials should flow easily and wet the surface. Other materials need to be more like putty, which can be adapted or formed into a desired shape. The **viscosity** of a material is its ability to flow. Thick or viscous liquids flow poorly, whereas thin liquids flow easily. Viscosity is a temperature-dependent property. For example, pancake syrup pours much more easily when it is warmed. Viscosity is measured as g/m·s, or as poise (P). Water at 20°C has a viscosity of 0.01 P, or 1 centipoise (cP). Impression materials have viscosities between 100,000 and 1,000,000 cP.

A low viscosity and the ability to wet a surface are important in the use of many dental materials. **Wetting** a surface with an adhesive material, such as a sealant, brings the material into intimate association with the surface so that chemical and micromechanical bonding can occur. Wetting is measured by determining the contact angle of a liquid on a solid, as shown in *Figure 3.2*. A low-contact angle, such as that of a drop of water on a piece of ice, indicates good wetting. A high-contact angle, such as that of a drop of water on most plastics, indicates poor wetting. Another example of wetting in dentistry occurs when a gypsum product (plaster) is poured into an impression. If the mixed material wets the surface of the impression

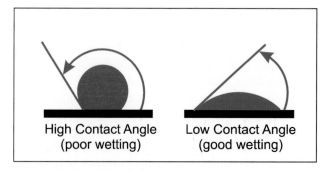

FIGURE 3.2. Contact angle measurements demonstrate a liquid's ability to wet a surface.

material, the fine details of the impression will be reproduced in the cast. If poor wetting occurs, bubbles will likely result in insufficient detail and an unusable cast.

J. Hardness

Enamel is the hardest biologic tissue in the human body. Hard materials resist scratching and indenting by soft materials. **Hardness** is a property that is measured by scientific instruments that press a special tip into the surface of the test material. The tip has a characteristic shape made of a very hard material, such as steel or diamond, as shown in *Figure 3.3*. The size of the indentation created is then measured. Hardness is calculated based on the size of this indentation. Several different methods can be used to measure hardness. The Brinell and Knoop methods are illustrated in *Figure 3.3*. Two other methods are called the Rockwell and Vickers hardness tests. The Knoop hardness number (KHN) of enamel is 350, whereas the KHN of dentin is 70. Some dental materials are harder than enamel. Porcelain has a KHN of 400 to 500. Other materials are not as hard as enamel. For example, acrylic denture teeth have a KHN of 20.

K. Durometer Measurements

Some materials are soft and even spongy. One example would be the rubber grip sometimes used on an instrument's shaft. A different kind of hardness test is used for these materials because a surface hardness indentation will not occur. A durometer measures how deep a steel ball will

sink when pressed into the surface of a soft material. Durometers are used to measure the hardness of impression materials and other elastic polymers.

L. Abrasion Resistance

Harder materials tend to be more resistant to abrasion than softer materials. In dentistry, we are interested in the **abrasion resistance** (wear resistance) of dental restorations to food, opposing teeth, and other dental materials such as ceramic crowns or porcelain denture teeth. We are also interested in the wear of natural teeth opposing dental restorations. If a restorative material is too hard, it will wear the opposing teeth at an unacceptably accelerated pace. An example is the excessive wear of natural teeth that oppose a denture with porcelain teeth. Therefore, a restoration must be hard enough so that the restoration does not wear away, but not so hard as to excessively wear away the opposing teeth. This is a good example of what has been called the **Goldilocks principle**: not too hard, not too soft, just right. More often than not, a material's properties need to fit within a particular range of values, not the maximum value, to be the material of choice.

M. Solubility

Materials placed in the oral cavity are exposed to various aqueous fluids. The solubility of materials in water is an important consideration. **Solubility** is the amount of a material that dissolves in a liquid, such as water. Sugar is a highly soluble material, but enamel is not. Restorative materials should not appreciably dissolve in the mouth. Additionally, some materials tend to dissolve faster in acidic environments. To measure solubility, a test sample is immersed in water. The weight of the material dissolved into the water is the solubility of that material. The solubility of some dental cements is measurable and clinically significant. Excessive solubility leads to loss of material and increases the risk of recurrent decay.

N. Water Sorption

Some materials absorb water. This property is termed **water sorption**. Water sorption is measured much like solubility. A test sample is immersed in water, and the weight that is gained by that sample is the water sorption. A cookie dunked in milk is an example of milk sorption. When materials absorb water, they tend to swell. Some materials both dissolve and absorb water at the same time, making measurement of one of these properties difficult. Many polymers absorb a small amount of water over time and slightly swell as a result.

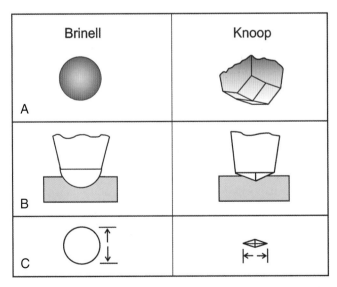

FIGURE 3.3. Comparison of two hardness indenter tips, the Brinell and the Knoop. **A.** Perspective views of the two tips. **B.** Cross-section of the tips in contact with test samples. **C.** Test material showing the indentation that is measured to calculate hardness.

O. Color

The appearance of a restoration for an anterior tooth can be a factor when choosing materials. The color and surface luster of the restoration are important. In addition, the shape and health of gingival tissues adjacent to a restoration are also noticed.

Color is a complex phenomenon that is a psychological response to a physical stimulus. The physical stimulus is the light reaching the rods and cones of the eye. Because processing of that stimulus by the brain is a psychological phenomenon, the perception of color varies between individuals. Two people may agree that two objects match in color, while a third person disagrees. In addition, the color of an object depends on the light in which the object is viewed. For all these reasons, matching restorative materials to a patient's teeth can be difficult.

Two types of systems are used to measure color. Both use three numbers to describe a color. One system involves matching the test object to color tabs resembling those available in a paint store. It is called the Munsell color system. Each tab has hue, chroma, and value numbers assigned. Hue is the fundamental color of an object, as in red, green, or blue. Chroma is the strength or color saturation of the hue, as in pink versus red. Value is the light or darkness of the color, as in shades of gray. In dentistry, esthetic materials have their own set of color tabs or shades, called a **shade guide**. Some manufacturers use a standard set, such as the VITA shade guide, which is shown in *Figure 3.4*. Recently, handheld devices have been developed that measure the color of teeth through a digital camera. These devices provide maps of the various shades of a tooth.

The other system involves measurement of color with a spectrophotometer or a colorimeter. A spectrophotometer measures the intensity of light that is reflected by an object at numerous wavelengths of visible light. The colorimeter measures light at several wavelengths, much like the human eye. For both devices, the data are mathematically manipulated by a computer to reduce the information to three numbers: L*, a*, and b*. The number L* is very similar to value. The number a* is a measure of the red–green character of a color. The number b* is a measure of the blue–yellow character of a color. The measurement of color with spectrophotometers is common in dental research. Several colorimeters and other digital devices are available for clinical use (see Fig. 31.2).

The interaction of teeth and dental materials with ultraviolet light causes fluorescence and affects their appearance. Fluorescence of restorations is important when fluorescent lighting or "black" lights are present. Inadequate fluorescence will make a crown or a filling appear dark in certain lighting, but excess fluorescence will make a tooth "glow" in the same lighting.

P. Interaction of Materials with X-Rays

When interpreting radiographs, the dental hygienist must be aware of the appearance of the radiographic image of dental materials. Some materials are radiolucent and are not seen on radiographs. Examples are some ceramic materials and denture acrylic resin. Other materials, such as metal restorations, are radiopaque and are evident on radiographs. Some dental restorative materials have been formulated by the manufacturer to match the radiopacity of enamel to facilitate the diagnosis of recurrent decay. Dental materials and their radiographic appearance are discussed further in Chapter 15.

III. Mechanical Properties

Because teeth are used to tear and grind food, they must be strong, and so must the materials that are used to replace missing tooth structure. Luckily, engineers and materials scientists have studied materials and their use for centuries. Dentistry has used this information along with trial and error.

What happens to a tooth or restoration when we bite on it? An external force (biting) is placed on the tooth. A **force** is a weight or **load** applied to an object. Inside the tooth, an internal stress develops to resist the applied external force. This **stress** is the force divided by the area on which the force has been applied. The internal stress that develops in the tooth is equal to the external force applied; however, they are opposite in direction.

Why don't teeth break when we use them to grind our food? Teeth are composed of strong materials with strong atomic bonds. Teeth and their atomic bonds are stronger

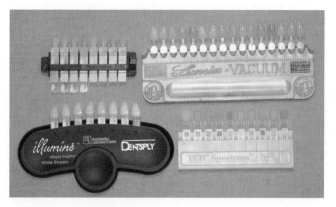

FIGURE 3.4. Photograph of several shade guides, including a VITA shade guide (*top right*).

than the stresses that develop as a result of biting. On the other hand, food cannot resist these forces and breaks because the strength of the weak atomic bonds of the food morsel is exceeded.

A. Elasticity

Just like the atoms of the table on which we placed a book in Chapter 2, Materials Science and Dentistry, the atomic bonds of teeth can be thought of as microscopic springs. These springs are compressed each time we bite. When we relax our bite and our teeth are no longer in contact, the springs return to their original length.

Let's use the example of a common spring to help us understand how atomic bonds and materials respond to forces. If we take a typical spring from a hardware store and hang an object, such as a monkey charm, from it, we can see the coils separate as the spring stretches out (*Fig. 3.5*). As we increase the number of charms hanging from the spring, the length of the spring increases. If the weight of charms is not too great, we find that the length increases by the same amount with each additional charm. Fishermen use this same concept when they use a fisherman's scale to weigh fish (so they know how big a lie to tell). As the size of the fish increases, the spring is stretched out more, and a greater weight is read on the scale. This is how atomic bonds are stretched when we use our teeth. If the charms are removed from the spring, the spring returns to its original length. In other words, the atomic bonds that were stretched return to their original length.

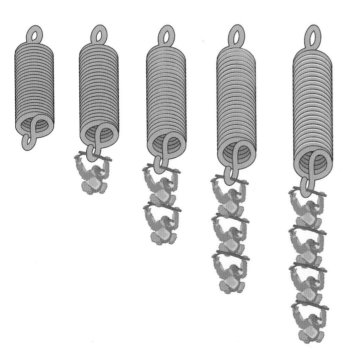

FIGURE 3.5. An illustration of elasticity: as the load increases, so does the elongation.

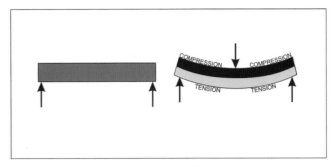

FIGURE 3.6. Bending is a combination of tension and compression.

In everyday life, we tend to see more examples of objects that are bent than we do of objects that are stretched. When an object is bent, the same stretching of atomic bonds occurs in some parts of that object. In other parts, however, compression of atomic bonds occurs, as shown in *Figure 3.6*. When the force is removed, the object returns to its original shape because the atoms return to their original position. Scientists and engineers have extensively investigated this phenomenon of change in shape and return to the original shape. This phenomenon is called **elasticity**. Force (a measure of push or pull), stress, and change in shape have been quantified, and their relationships have been extensively studied.

B. Strain

When an object, such as a book, is placed on a table, force is placed on that table. The force affects the table. Again, inside the table, an equal and opposite force or stress develops that resists the load of the book. The force or stress that develops in the table is caused by the stretching (or compression) of atomic bonds. The more books that are placed on the table, the greater the load becomes, the more the bonds are stretched, and the greater the stress that occurs in the table.

The compression or elongation of a loaded object is typically very small. It is measured in terms of the fractional change in length, as previously discussed. **Strain** is the change in length divided by the original length. Strain is measured as a fraction (such as 0.02) or as a percentage (such as 2%). The longer the object is, the more it must be stretched to have the same strain (compare *Fig. 3.1A and B*).

C. Stress

As mentioned earlier, the force that develops in a loaded object is called stress, and stress is proportional to the applied force or load. Stress is also related to the size of the object. In *Figure 3.7*, the number of charms hanging from a spring is increased, but the size of the spring is increased

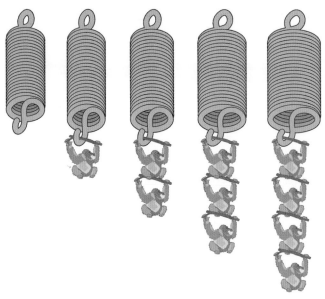

FIGURE 3.7. Larger springs can support larger loads without additional elongation.

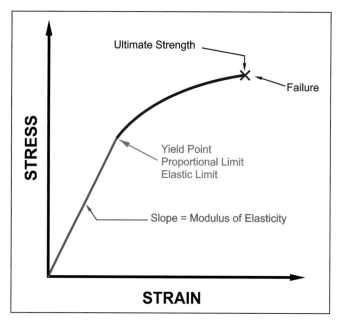

FIGURE 3.8. Typical stress–strain plot.

at the same time. The change in length or strain remains constant, as does the stress in the spring. **Stress** is the load (force) divided by the cross-sectional area of the object:

stress = load/area

When a load or a force is applied to an object, the stress occurs throughout the object's entire length. The expression "a chain is only as strong as its weakest link" is based on this principle. Each link of the chain must bear the load.

Stress is measured as pounds per square inch (psi). In the metric system, stress is measured as pascals. Typical stresses are large, and the mega-pascal unit is used to reduce the number of zeros (nonsignificant figures).

D. Relationship of Stress and Strain

The load (stress) and the change in length (strain) are proportional. They always occur together; you cannot have one without the other (like love and marriage?). If the load is small, the change in length may be difficult to measure. The proportionality constant, or the slope of a graph of stress versus strain, is called the **modulus of elasticity**, or Young's modulus:

modulus of elasticity = stress/strain

The stress–strain relationship is graphed in *Figure 3.8*. The modulus of elasticity (or, more simply, the modulus) is characteristic of a material and its atomic bonds. It is the scientific term for the stiffness of a material. The higher the modulus of elasticity is, the stiffer the material. Enamel

has a high modulus of elasticity. A rubber band has a low modulus of elasticity. As with stress, the modulus is measured as psi or pascals; however, the numbers are much larger. When a large number (a stress) is divided by a small number (a strain), a very large number results. Thus, the modulus of a material is often given in kpsi (thousands of pounds per square inch), or gigapascals.

E. Stress–Strain Plot

If we were to continue adding charms to the spring of *Figure 3.5*, we could graph the number of charms and the length of the spring (or the change in length of the spring). Initially, we would get a straight line, as shown in *Figure 3.8*, with the slope being equal to the modulus of elasticity. Also, if we take all the charms off the spring, the spring should return to its original length. When a stress is removed and the object returns to its original length, the initial change in length is called **elastic deformation**. If we continue adding charms, however, at some point the line on the graph begins to curve, which means stress is no longer proportional to strain. At this point, if we take all the charms off the spring, the spring does not return to its original length. It has become permanently stretched out. This condition is termed **plastic deformation** or **permanent deformation**. Plastic deformation occurs when an orthodontic wire is bent to fit a patient's arch. Force is placed on the wire and it bends. If the force is great enough, the wire will not return to its original shape; it has been plastically deformed. The point on the stress–strain plot at which the line starts to curve and plastic deformation begins is called the **elastic limit**, the **proportional limit**, or the **yield point**, as shown in *Figure 3.8*. These three terms are different mostly in the method of measurement, not in concept.

If we could keep loading on more and more charms, at some point the spring breaks (or failure occurs). We have exceeded the strength of the spring. The stress at that point is called the **ultimate strength**. If the test is a tensile test, it is then called the **ultimate tensile strength**. Likewise, if the test is a compressive test, it is then called the **ultimate compressive strength**. The load (charms) on the spring has caused a stress (force) to develop in the spring that is greater than the strength of the atomic bonds that hold the material together; as a result, the object breaks. This is bad for bridges, whether they are in someone's mouth or underneath someone's car.

F. Types of Stress

We have discussed compression and tension, but other types of stress exist. It is important to remember that in the real world, a single kind of stress rarely occurs. Combinations of several kinds of stresses are most common.

1. **Compression** is a pushing or crushing stress.
2. **Tension** is a pulling stress.
3. **Shear** (slip) stress occurs when parts of an object slide by one another. For example, if the front and back covers of a book are pushed in opposite directions, the pages slide or "shear" by each other.
4. **Torsion** stress is a twisting force. Turning a doorknob is an example of a torsional stress.
5. **Bending** is a common stress and is actually a combination of several types of stresses, as illustrated in *Figure 3.6*. When an object is bent, one side is compressed, but the opposite side is stretched. In addition to these compressive and tensile forces, shear forces also occur inside the object. A variety of bending tests are used to examine the ability of materials to resist bending.

G. Mechanical Properties of Dental Materials

Each use of a dental material has its own set of physical and mechanical requirements (*Fig. 3.9*). These requirements are discussed along with each category of dental materials in the chapters that follow. In restorative dentistry, the materials that we use for fillings and crowns need to be stiff and strong. The materials that we use for taking impressions are much less stiff than restorative materials. Some impression materials are quite flexible and stretch a great deal.

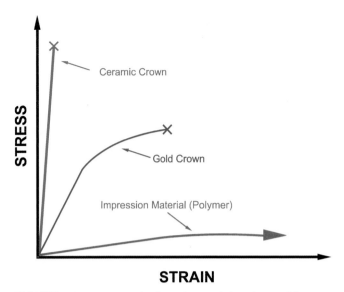

FIGURE 3.9. Stress–strain plots of several dental materials. Note that the *x*-axis for the impression material has been compressed.

To function properly, a restoration must be hard (hardness), strong (yield strength), and stiff (modulus) enough to withstand the forces of mastication. For many uses of materials, the yield strength is more important than the ultimate strength. If a gold crown yields or plastically deforms (changes shape) when one bites down, it is no longer the same shape and is not likely to fit the tooth preparation precisely. Recurrent caries is then likely. Thus, we are much more concerned with the fit of a restoration in service (not exceeding the yield strength) than we are with a restoration breaking (ultimate strength). For brittle materials, such as a ceramic crown (see Fig. 1.10E and F), yield strength and ultimate strength are essentially one and the same (*Fig. 3.9*).

The concept of plastic and elastic deformation needs a little more attention. Elastic deformation occurs whenever force is applied to an object. As the force increases, plastic deformation may occur. However, plastic deformation may or may not be a bad thing. Most of the time, we do not want a restoration or an impression to be plastically deformed (permanently distorted) when force is applied. We want the restoration and the teeth to be elastically deformed and return to their original shape when the biting force is removed. The same is true for impressions. Impressions should return to their original shape after they have been removed from the mouth. If not, the resulting stone cast will not be the same size as the teeth or cavity preparation. For most uses of materials, plastic deformation is not a good thing, but exceptions do exist. One is the bending of an orthodontic wire.

H. Other Mechanical Properties of Interest—Optional

1. Poisson's Ratio

Solid objects deform a little differently than our spring with the monkey charms. Stretch a rubber band and notice how the width of the rubber band narrows as it is stretched, as shown in *Figure 3.10*. All materials change shape in three dimensions, even if the stress is only in one direction. **Poisson's ratio** is a mechanical property that is the ratio of the strain in the direction of the stress to the strain in a direction perpendicular to the stress. So, when we bite on a filling and apply compressive force in the occlusal apical direction, the filling becomes wider in the mesial–distal and the buccal–lingual directions (but only to a microscopic degree). If a dental restoration is distorted in one direction, it will likely be distorted in the other two directions as well.

2. Resilience and Toughness

Anyone watching televised college football games sees the players wearing brightly colored mouth guards. The plastic mouth guard material is chosen for its ability to absorb energy. The energy of a blow to the mouth will not cause trauma if the energy is absorbed by the mouth guard rather than by the teeth and the other facial structures. Such an ability to absorb energy and not become deformed is called **resilience**. Resilience is measured as

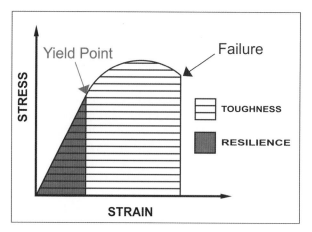

FIGURE 3.11. Resilience and toughness are measured from different areas on the stress–strain plot.

the area under the stress–strain curve up to the yield point.

Other safety devices are designed to absorb energy while distorting or fracturing. A crash helmet is successful if the wearer is not injured; whether the helmet is broken does not matter. The energy absorbed (as by the helmet) up to the failure point on the stress–strain diagram is the **toughness** of the material. The helmet can be replaced; a person's head cannot (except in Frankenstein movies).

Both resilience and toughness are illustrated in *Figure 3.11*. Plastics in general have high resilience and toughness values.

3. Fracture Toughness

Some materials do not plastically deform easily. They just fracture. Such materials are susceptible to cracks and defects. **Fracture toughness** is a measure of the energy required to fracture a material when a crack is present. Fracture toughness is measured in units that are quite odd: megapascals times the square root of meters ($MPa \cdot \sqrt{m}$). Glass and dental porcelain have a low fracture toughness value, whereas metals have high fracture toughness values. Many researchers have sought to better dental composites by improving their fracture toughness, as this property is the best predictor of clinical success.

4. Fatigue

We use our teeth over and over again to grind food. The mechanical properties that we have discussed in this chapter are tested by compressing or pulling materials until the specimen breaks during a one-time test. This type of testing may be good for disposable items, such as baby diapers and patient napkins, but most things used in dentistry are used multiple

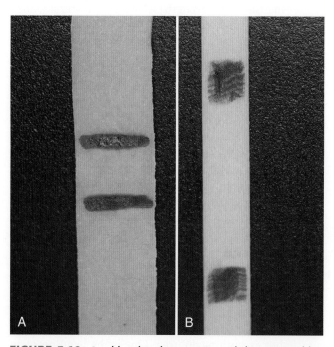

FIGURE 3.10. A rubber band at rest **A.** and the same rubber band stretched approximately 200% **B.**

times, such as restorations, scalers, and perio probes. Many things fail after being stressed repetitively for a long time, and such failure is called **fatigue**. An example of fatigue is when a scaler breaks. Fatigue testing more closely replicates such real-world use. A test specimen is repeatedly compressed, pulled, or bent with a given amount of force, and the number of cycles needed to break the specimen is recorded. Increasing levels of force are plotted against the number of cycles that it takes to break the test specimen. Based on these data, researchers can predict the amount of stress (the fatigue strength) that the material can endure without breaking. Isn't it good to know that you can drive over that bridge forever and it will not collapse (assuming the metal reinforcements do not corrode and the concrete does not deteriorate)?

I. Time-Dependent Properties—Optional

Changes that occur too slowly to be easily observed were discussed in Chapter 2, Materials Science and Dentistry. Some slow changes reflect mechanical properties of interest. Just as glaciers flow and continents drift, certain dental materials change too slowly to be easily observed but fast enough to affect the use of the material and the resulting patient care. Two of these changes follow:

1. **Creep** is the small change in shape that results when an object is under continuous compression. It can be thought of as very slow flow. Creep was once considered to be an important factor in the selection of an amalgam. However, it only grossly differentiates between products. Amalgam and composite restorations can slowly change shape (creep) as the result of continuous stress. It is important to note that although we typically think of viscosity and flow only as properties of liquids, solids also flow. We cannot observe this slow flow, however, because it takes

place over a long period of time (the same way that bureaucracies change).

2. **Stress relaxation** is similar to creep. Both occur slowly, over time. Creep is a slow change in shape, but stress relaxation is a slow decrease in force over time. If a rubber band is stretched to a constant length, the pull of the rubber decreases (or relaxes) over time. The loss of pull (decrease in stress or force) by the rubber band over time is called stress relaxation. The same loss of force or stress relaxation occurs with orthodontic elastics or rubber bands. As a result, orthodontic patients must frequently change their rubber bands to apply the proper force to their teeth. Both creep and stress relaxation increase as temperature increases.

J. Stress Concentration

Previously in this chapter, it was stated that loads applied in one direction result in stress in all three dimensions. The real world is even more complex. It is difficult to make objects without holes, scratches, cracks, bubbles (voids), or other defects, but defects do not simply require the rest of the object to carry a greater load. Stress increases around defects. This phenomenon is called **stress concentration**. Fracture becomes more likely because cracks can develop around a defect and spread throughout the object. A glass cutter makes a scratch that concentrates stress at a single location. When a bending stress is applied to the glass, fracture occurs along the scratch, where stress is concentrated, resulting in the shape the cutter desired. Controlling defects in objects is important to reduce stress concentration and produce stronger products. In dentistry, it is important to mix and handle materials properly to reduce the occurrence of voids (bubbles) and defects. Designing restorations properly, polishing surfaces, and glazing porcelain can remove surface defects that concentrate stress. The result is longer-lasting restorations and improved patient care.

Summary

The dental materials used to replace tooth structure will vary depending on the type of restoration and the specific tooth. No restorative material has all the characteristics identical to those of natural tooth structure. Usually, a compromise regarding one or more of the properties must be made. This chapter discussed these properties and the extent to which these properties can be compromised. Properties of materials may be divided into three categories: physical, chemical, and biologic. Mechanical properties are a subgroup of physical properties. Examples of physical properties include density, boiling/melting points, vapor pressure, thermal conductivity, heat capacity, heat of fusion, heat of vaporization, and coefficient of thermal expansion, to name a few. Mechanical properties include elasticity, stress, strain, modulus of elasticity, and yield strength. Types of stresses include compression, tension, shear, torsion, and bending. Resilience, toughness, fatigue, creep, stress relaxation, and stress concentration are other mechanical properties that affect the practice of dentistry.

Learning Activities

1. In the library or online, look up the specific heat and the heat of fusion for gold. Calculate the energy required to melt 1 kg of gold, and compare this with the energy required to raise the temperature of 1 kg of gold by 1°C.

2. Bring several objects that are an off-white color to a paint store or the paint section of a hardware store. Have different people match the color of the objects with the store's "paint tabs." Compare the results. Most paint stores have color-measuring devices. Compare your results to the results of the device (if available).

3. Compare the color of several students' teeth to a shade guide. Did each student pick the same shade for each test tooth?

4. Using a spring and several metal pipe fittings purchased at a hardware store, plot the length of the spring versus the number of fittings hanging from the spring. Calculate the spring constant in terms of fittings per meter of stretch.

5. Stretch a rubber band while noting the change in its width and length. Are there other objects that show the same changes?

6. Bend a wire or twist tie until it breaks as an example of fatigue.

7. Support the ends of a piece of licorice. Observe the amount of sag for each day of the week. What mechanical property does this exemplify?

Review Questions

Question 1. A drop of water on a Popsicle is an example of:

a. Poor wetting (low-contact angle)

b. Good wetting (high-contact angle)

c. Good wetting (low-contact angle)

d. Poor wetting (high-contact angle)

Question 2. The tightening of a guitar string is an example of which of the following stresses?

a. Compression

b. Torsion

c. Shear

d. Tension

Question 3. The modulus of elasticity is an indication of what property of a material?

a. Resilience

b. Strength

c. Stiffness

d. Tension

Question 4. Cooled materials will contract, and heated materials will expand. A measurement of this change in volume in relation to change in temperature is called the coefficient of thermal expansion.

a. The first statement is true; the second statement is false

b. The first statement is false; the second statement is true

c. Both statements are true

d. Both statements are false

Question 5. When a stress is induced in a material that is greater than the material's yield strength, the stress is _____ proportional to the strain, and the material does not return to its original shape.

a. Always

b. No longer

c. Equally

d. None of the above

Question 6. Which formula defines the modulus of elasticity?

a. Stress/strain

b. Stress^2/strain

c. Strain/stress

d. 2 × stress/strain

Question 7. An example of a physical property is:

a. Density

b. Strength

c. Stiffness

d. Setting reaction

Question 8. A twisting force is termed:

a. Compression

b. Shear

c. Tension

d. Torsion

e. Bending

Question 9. The ability of a material to dissolve in liquid is termed:

a. Viscosity
b. Water sorption
c. Solubility
d. Wetting

Question 10. Elasticity is an example of which of the following properties?

a. Physical
b. Mechanical
c. Chemical
d. Biologic

Question 11. The rate of heat flow through a material is referred to as:

a. Heat of fusion
b. Coefficient of thermal expansion
c. Heat capacity
d. Thermal conductivity

Question 12. Jennifer is a practicing hygienist who goes to a nearby restaurant each day for lunch. She often orders a cola with ice and a bowl of homemade soup. As she eats and drinks, her composite restorations (tooth-colored) and tooth structure are expanding and contracting at different rates. This change in volume or length of these materials due to the hot food and cold drink is referred to as:

a. Heat of fusion
b. Coefficient of thermal expansion
c. Heat capacity
d. Thermal conductivity

Question 13. Fingernail polish remover has "solvent" properties, as it will remove the polish from our fingernails. Another property polish remover has is its tendency to evaporate. Fingernail polish remover can be said to have:

a. A high vapor pressure
b. A low vapor pressure
c. No vapor pressure
d. An intermittent vapor pressure

Questions 14–16. Match the properties listed below with the procedures or situations in questions 14, 15, and 16.

a. Solubility
b. Compression
c. Stress concentration
d. Viscosity

Question 14. _____ is the force used to condense an amalgam in a preparation.

Question 15. A hardened cement having "low"_____ can firmly hold a patient's gold crown in place for years in a wet environment.

Question 16. _____ is the term given to the increase of stress around defects within an object.

Adhesive Materials

Objectives

After studying this chapter, the student will be able to do the following:

1. Describe an "adhesive."
2. Explain the difference between micromechanical bonding and macromechanical bonding and provide an example of each type.
3. Recall three benefits the patient receives from restorations that are bonded to tooth structure.
4. Compare the differences between the microanatomy of enamel and dentin regarding etching and bonding. The comparison should include the following terms:
   - Orthophosphoric acid
   - Enamel tags
   - Smear layer
   - Hybrid layer
   - Primer
   - Adhesive
5. Discuss two of the earlier fallacies about dentinal bonding and how research has changed current practice.
6. Summarize the main differences between glass ionomer cements and dentinal bonding.

Key Words/Phrases

acid etching
adherend
adhesive
adhesive failure
biofilm
cohesive failure
dentinal bonding
enamel bonding resin
enamel tags
glass ionomer cements
hybrid layer
hydrophilic
hydrophobic
interface
macromechanical bonding
margins
microleakage
micromechanical bonding
micropores
orthophosphoric acid
percolation
polycarboxylate cements
postoperative sensitivity
primers
resin tags
smear layer

Introduction

Adhesion, or bonding, is the joining together of two objects, using a glue or cement. It is common in everyday life; it is used in manufacturing, repairs, and dentistry. It is also important when a protective layer is applied to an object, such as when a metal surface is painted to prevent rust or when a pit and fissure sealant is applied to prevent decay.

The definition of adhesion or bonding in dentistry is not concise. A material that can stick to a flat surface or bond two flat surfaces together is typically called an "**adhesive**." Most dental materials that are adhesive involve micromechanical adhesion or bonding. Remember that all dental materials must function in a wet, hostile environment for an extended period of time to be useful. Therefore, the oral environment limits the types of adhesives used in dentistry.

True adhesion involves chemical bonds between the materials being joined, but not all bonding to tooth structures is truly adhesive. In this text, the terms "adhesion" and "bonding" will be used interchangeably, but neither will signify chemical bonding (unless specifically stated).

Micromechanical bonding of dental materials to tooth structure is common. Micromechanical bonding also occurs in everyday life, when materials such as superglue are used. We will define **micromechanical bonding** as bonding using surface irregularities smaller than can be seen with the naked eye or felt with a dental explorer. The result of micromechanical bonding can be difficult to distinguish from true adhesion.

Macromechanical bonding is also common in everyday life and in dentistry. With this type of bonding, surface roughness can be seen and/or felt. **Macromechanical bonding** is the mechanism by which most glues join two pieces of wood, repair broken toys, and do many other things.

The mechanisms for micromechanical and macromechanical bonding are much the same. The difference is that they occur at a different scale or physical size. The glue or cement flows into surface irregularities and fills them. The glue then sets or hardens and is locked into the surface irregularities of the objects being joined. If the glue is strong, the objects are now joined together. The main advantage of micromechanical bonding is that a greater number of small surface irregularities are used compared to macromechanical bonding. In addition, force is more evenly distributed on the joint with micromechanical bonding, making it stronger than macromechanical bonding. Screws, nails, nuts, bolts, and other fasteners are examples of macromechanical joining of objects at an even larger scale. With this type of joining, stress is greatly concentrated in the vicinity of the fastener.

In dentistry, macromechanical bonding is used for cementing or luting crowns and bridges to teeth with "nonadhesive" cements. Dental cements fill in the roughness on the surface of the tooth and on the inside of the crown. The crown is luted or glued in place in the same manner as two pieces of wood are glued together. A crown is shown in Figure 1.4.

I. Adhesive Materials in Dentistry

A. Use of Adhesion/Bonding in Dentistry

1. **Retention of Restorations**
   Adhesion is commonly used to keep restorations in place. Undercuts (as illustrated in Fig. 1.3) and other mechanical locks are not necessary when adhesive materials are used. Sometimes, adhesion is used to bond a weak esthetic restorative material, such as a porcelain veneer, to the stronger remaining tooth structure so that the tooth supports the weak restorative material. Adhesion is also used to attach orthodontic brackets and other appliances to teeth.

2. **Reduction of Microleakage**
   Adhesion reduces or eliminates microleakage of restorations (*Fig. 4.1*). It also reduces postoperative sensitivity. **Microleakage** is the seeping and leaking of fluids and bacteria between the tooth/restoration junction or **interface**. Microleakage increases the likelihood of recurrent caries and postoperative sensitivity. **Postoperative sensitivity** is caused by fluids and bacteria moving in and out of the interface between the restoration and the tooth. If the pulp is irritated by fluid movement or bacterial metabolic wastes (acids), pain occurs.

   When teeth are heated and cooled by the ingestion of hot and cold foods, expansion and contraction occur. If the coefficient of thermal expansion for a restorative material does not match that of the tooth, they expand and contract at different rates. Repeated expansion and contraction of teeth and restorations at different rates result in fluids being sucked in and pushed out at the margins of a restoration. This phenomenon is called **percolation** and is illustrated in *Figure 4.1*.

   Adhesion also reduces staining of the margins of esthetic materials. **Margins** are the junction of the tooth and the restoration. Margins that leak frequently become dark, stained, and unesthetic (see *Fig. 4.2*). Sealing the margins of restorations reduces or eliminates microleakage and reduces postoperative sensitivity and staining.

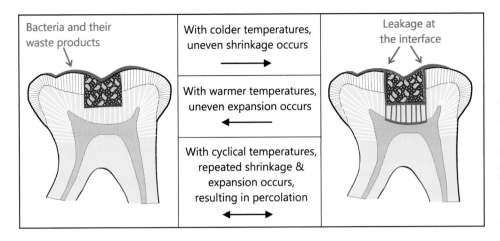

FIGURE 4.1. Illustration of the effects of temperature changes and microleakage. When the coefficient of thermal expansion of a restorative material does not match that of the tooth structure, uneven expansion and contraction occur. In turn, gaps, leakage and percolation occur at the interface of the restoration and the tooth.

3. Reduction of Recurrent Caries

The most important reason to reduce microleakage is to minimize the likelihood of recurrent caries (secondary decay). Recurrent caries is decay that occurs at the margin of a restoration. If no space exists between the restoration and the tooth, bacteria do not have a well-protected niche in which to colonize and proliferate. Smooth surfaces of teeth and sealed margins are much more resistant to decay than are pits, fissures, and gaps at the margins of restorations.

B. Development of Dental Adhesives

1. Historical Perspective

Acid etching was initially conceived by Dr. Michael Buonocore in the 1950s to seal pits and fissures. An acid is applied to enamel to etch the surface. The etched surface is rough, allowing a low-viscosity adhesive (resin system) to flow into the irregularities and then cure (or set). **Acid etching** is a micromechanical bonding technique that was first used to retain pit and fissure sealants. Later, when dental composite

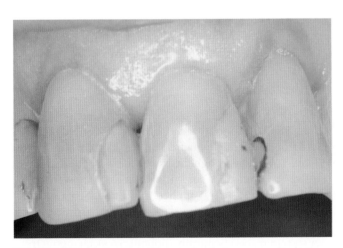

FIGURE 4.2. Photograph of several anterior composite restorations. Note the significant staining of the margin of tooth #10.

restorations were developed in the 1960s, acid-etching techniques were used during placement. This reduced leakage and staining of margins.

Many other uses for acid etching and composite materials were developed in the 1970s and 1980s. With composite materials and acid-etching techniques, orthodontic brackets could be bonded to the labial surface of teeth rather than needing to be welded onto a metal band for every tooth. Soon, researchers learned that the enamel of the tooth and the metal of the fixed bridge could be both etched and then bonded together. Plastic, composite, and porcelain veneers were developed that could be bonded to the labial surface of anterior teeth to hide discolored enamel, to close spaces, and to change the shape of teeth. Dentists used etched composites to bond together mobile, periodontally involved teeth; to stabilize replanted, avulsed teeth; and to stabilize segments of fractured jaws. The acid-etched composite is the "gold standard" of adhesion in dentistry, against which all other materials and techniques are compared to judge strength of bond, utility of use, and longevity.

2. Chemical Adhesion in Dentistry

Acid etching solved the problem of bonding dental materials to enamel, but bonding dental materials to dentin was more difficult. In the 1970s, Dennis Smith developed the first chemically adhesive dental cement, called polycarboxylate cement. **Polycarboxylate cements** use polyacrylic acid and zinc oxide. Later, Wilson, Crisp, and McLean developed glass ionomer cement. **Glass ionomer cements** also use polyacrylic acid, but they include glass powder instead of zinc oxide. Both materials are based on polyacrylic acid, and both chemically bond to dentin and enamel. They are discussed later in this chapter.

A number of glass ionomer materials were developed for various uses, with luting and restorative materials being the most popular. However, glass ionomer materials lack the esthetic appearance and mechanical toughness of dental composites.

3. Dentinal Bonding Agents

In the 1970s and 1980s, products were developed that supposedly bonded composite materials to dentin. By the 1990s, dentinal bonding of composites had become a clinically proven reality. Because dentinal bonding incorporates acid etching, it should be thought of as an extension of the acid-etching process rather than as a replacement for it. Dentinal bonding systems continue to be developed and are now used to bond amalgam and ceramic and cast metallic restorations to dentin and enamel. In fact, nearly every restorative material can now be bonded to dentin or enamel with the use of some product and technique. However, the longevity and efficacy of some of these bonding techniques continue to be evaluated by clinical research.

C. Surface Factors

1. Cleanliness

When applying an adhesive to an object, the surface must be clean. Otherwise, the adhesive will bond to the dirt and debris on the surface rather than to the surface itself. This would be like putting a Band-Aid on Pig-Pen of the "Peanuts" comic strip. (Pig-Pen is the character who is so dirty that a dust cloud follows him wherever he goes.) The Band-Aid would bond to the dirt rather than to Pig-Pen. Adhesives will not bond to any surface irregularities that are filled or covered by debris. If the surface and the adhesive are not somewhat chemically compatible, the adhesive will not wet the surface adequately, the adhesive will not flow into the irregularities, and the bonding will be poor. Whether the adhesive bonding is macromechanical, micromechanical, or truly adhesive (chemical), the surface must be clean to allow intimate association of the adhesive (bonding material) and the **adherend** (the surface).

2. Biofilms

In the oral cavity, it can be difficult to keep surfaces clean. A clean surface is one that is uncontaminated by oral fluids, such as saliva, blood, or crevicular fluid. Once a surface is contaminated by any oral fluid, it immediately becomes covered by a layer of biofilm. A **biofilm** is a coating that derives from organisms, both large and small. Biofilms in the mouth start as molecular coatings (the enamel pellicle) and grow into a community of microorganisms (plaque).

For bonding purposes, the surface is no longer amalgam, enamel, or composite; the surface the adhesive "sees" or "feels" is biofilm. Biofilms reduce (or even prevent) bonding of many dental adhesives. To remedy this, use of a dental rubber dam is recommended when working with adhesive materials. The biofilm from saliva helps to lubricate the food bolus for swallowing, so it should not be surprising that biofilms are readily soluble in stomach acid and, therefore, do not inhibit the digestion of food. Luckily, the enamel pellicle is easily removed when acids are used to etch enamel and dentin.

D. Testing Adhesion: Optional

Much work has been done to measure the bond strength of various materials that are bonded to dentin and enamel. Usually, a small portion of material is bonded to a tooth and then pushed or pulled in an attempt to remove it. The force necessary to push or pull the bonded material off the tooth is measured in megapascals (mPa). One megapascal is equal to 145 pounds per square inch (psi). The resulting numbers are used to compare the effectiveness of the adhesive. A bond strength of 20 to 25 mPa (2,900–3,400 psi) is necessary for clinical success in high-stress areas of the mouth. Such numbers are useful only for general comparisons, however. In addition, one must know how the material broke off the tooth (where the fracture occurred). If the adhesive came off cleanly, then the break occurred at the interface. This type of break is called an **adhesive failure**. This is a test of bond strength. If the failure occurred inside the bonding material, the break is called a **cohesive failure**. This is a measure of the strength of the bonding material, not of the bond itself. If, during the testing procedure, the adhesive breaks the tooth, this is also a cohesive failure, and it signals that the strength of the bond is greater than the strength of the teeth. A bond that is stronger than tooth structure provides no advantage because the teeth, rather than the restoration, will break during failure.

II. Acid Etching

Acid etching was the first successful technique for bonding dental materials to tooth structure (*Fig. 4.3*). Acid creates a microscopically rough enamel surface, as shown in *Figures 4.3 and 4.4A*. This roughened surface has sometimes been termed "**enamel tags**" or "**micropores**." A low-viscosity liquid polymer system is applied to the roughened surface. This liquid must wet the surface adequately so that it will flow into the micropores created by the etchant. The polymer system reacts chemically (polymerizes), changing from a liquid into a solid. The new solid is now bonded to the micromechanically roughened enamel surface. A variety of acids and polymer systems are possible, but because of time restrictions and oral conditions, only a few are suitable for dental use.

A. The Acid-Etching Process

First, the enamel surface is cleaned with pumice or a similar abrasive. The debris and pumice are then rinsed away with water, and the area is dried with compressed air (*Fig. 4.3A*). The acid or etchant, which is typically 37% **orthophosphoric acid**, is applied for 15 to 30 seconds to permanent teeth. The acid is rinsed away with water, and the surface is completely dried again with suction and compressed air (*Fig. 4.3B*). Next, the liquid bonding resin (polymer system) is applied. The polymer system chemically reacts or "cures" (*Fig. 4.3C*). Finally, layers of restorative materials are chemically bonded to this initial layer of bonding resin (*Fig. 4.3D*).

The term "etchant" is preferred in front of a patient rather than any word or words that use the term "acid." Sometimes, the etchant is called a "conditioner." However, that term can be confusing because other different dental materials are also called conditioners.

B. Enamel

1. The acid-etching technique is used to bond materials to enamel, but not to dentin. The technique is simple and micromechanical, and it has not changed appreciably over the years.
2. It is more effective to bond the polymer resin to the ends of enamel rods than to the long axis of the rods.

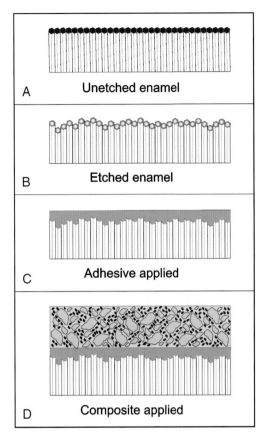

FIGURE 4.3. Schematic representation of the acid-etching process for enamel. **A.** Vertical bars represent a clean surface composed of enamel rods. **B.** Etching dissolves some of the enamel rods, creating a rough surface. **C.** Adhesive flows into the irregularities between and within the rods. The adhesive then sets and covers the surface with a layer of resin. The adhesive is micromechanically locked into the spaces between the enamel rods. **D.** The composite restorative material is applied and bonds to the underlying resin.

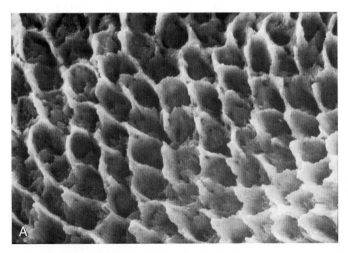
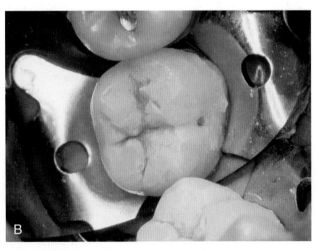

FIGURE 4.4. **A.** Scanning electron micrograph of etched enamel. (Reproduced from Hormati AA, Fuller JL, Denehy GE. Effects of contamination and mechanical disturbance on the quality of acid-etched enamel. *J Am Dent Assoc.* 1980;100(1):34–38, with permission) **B.** Photograph of etched enamel on the second molar (taken in a mirror). Note the chalky or frosty appearance of the surface, and compare this with the glossy surface of the unetched first molar. (Courtesy of Dr. Ronald House, Bethesda, MD.)

3. The acid-etching technique has a "built-in" quality control check. If the enamel is properly etched and dried, it appears chalky or frosty white, as shown in *Figure 4.4B*.

4. Years of clinical data demonstrate the advantages of using acid-etching techniques for bonding to enamel. Pit and fissure sealants prevent caries, and the margins of composite restorations stain less frequently. Composites can be bonded to teeth to correct fractures, rotations, or other defects.

C. Acids

Many acids have been used to etch enamel. Orthophosphoric acid at 37% (or 3/8) concentration is the most commonly used today. Etching removes part of the enamel rod, leaving a microscopically rough surface, as shown in *Figure 4.4A*. Etching may dissolve the periphery of enamel rods, the core of the rods, or both in different areas. One can overetch, however, and crystals can form (precipitate) from the calcium and phosphate ions initially dissolved. Such precipitated crystals can inhibit bonding.

D. Time

The recommended time for etching enamel is typically 15 to 30 seconds depending on the manufacturer or product. Deciduous teeth need to be etched for a longer time than permanent teeth. The enamel rods of deciduous teeth are less regularly arranged, so a longer etching time (30–40 seconds) is required to obtain a surface with sufficient roughness for bonding. The results of acid etching of deciduous teeth are less reliable than those of permanent teeth. Should etched enamel become contaminated by saliva, it should be re-etched with the same acid, but only a 5-second etch is necessary.

E. The Surface

Although the technique is simple, one must keep the surface clean and dry. The surface is very sensitive to contamination after etching. Reasons for a clean surface were explained previously.

F. Resin Systems (Materials Used with Acid Etching)

1. Low-Viscosity Resin

The first low-viscosity resin system to be used was polymethyl methacrylate. Resin systems, later developed for use as restorative dental composites, were used in conjunction with acid-etching techniques. All resins used today wet the etched surface well and flow into the

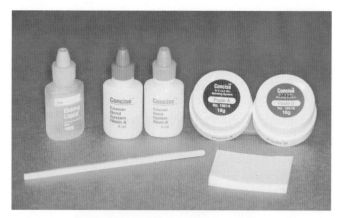

FIGURE 4.5. An enamel bonding and composite system. The acid etchant is on the *left*, two chemically activated resin bottles are in the *center*, and two jars of the chemically activated composite restorative materials are on the *right*.

microscopic irregularities. The low-viscosity resin system is also called **enamel bonding resin** (or, simply, "the adhesive"). All resin systems used today set by addition polymerization. (Addition polymerization is presented in Direct Polymeric Restorative Materials, Chapter 5.) Polymerization, or the setting process of the resin, can be activated (started) with light or a chemical reaction.

2. Composite Material

After the bonding resin is set, a composite restorative material is placed. The composite material sets by the same chemistry as low-viscosity resin and chemically bonds to the resin. A chemically activated acid-etched composite kit is shown in *Figure 4.5*.

III. Dentinal Bonding

Once acid etching was shown to be an effective clinical procedure, the focus turned to the development of techniques for bonding to dentin. The typical cavity preparation has more dentin than enamel available for bonding. A number of assorted complex chemical systems were developed. These systems were designed to chemically bond to collagen and other components of tooth structure. The intimate association of adhesive and tooth structure that is required for chemical bonding requires good wetting of the tooth surface. Chemical bonding was the intent, but micromechanical bonding was the result. Current **dentinal bonding** systems function by way of micromechanical bonding and secondary atomic bonds. It is doubtful that any of these systems bond to tooth structure principally by primary atomic bonds. In reality, dentinal bonding systems are an extension of the acid-etch technique.

A. Dentinal Bonding Systems

1. Tooth Tissues

Dentinal bonding systems bond to both enamel and dentin. Because enamel is the outer layer of tissue, it is important that these systems bond to enamel. Without a strong bond to enamel, microleakage at the enamel–composite interface would increase the likelihood of recurrent caries even if a sufficient bond to dentin prevented deeper penetration of bacteria.

2. Structure of Dentin

Dentin is composed of intratubular dentin, intertubular dentin, and dentinal tubules. The tubules are filled with odontoblastic processes. Intratubular dentin and intertubular dentin are highly mineralized, but the odontoblastic processes are mostly water. In addition, different types of dentin exist: primary, secondary, reparative, sclerotic, and dead tracts. As one can see, dentin is much more variable and complex than enamel. Bonding to dentin has been a difficult problem for scientists to solve.

3. Smear Layer

When dentin is cut or prepared by dental instruments, a layer of debris called the **smear layer** is produced on the surface (*Fig. 4.6A*). It is similar to sawing green, sap-filled, sticky pine wood; the sawdust and sap stick to the newly cut surface. The smear layer on dentin also extends a short distance into the dentinal tubules. It is made of ground dentin that weakly adheres to the cut dentin surface. Enamel, on the other hand, cuts more cleanly because it is a harder more highly calcified tissue.

4. Historical Fallacies and Dentinal Bonding

The historical development of dentinal bonding systems in the United States is interesting in that several erroneous beliefs needed to be changed. First, it was believed that composites irritate the pulp and so should not be placed directly on dentin. In fact, it is the microleakage of composites or other dental materials that causes pulpal irritation. Second, it was believed that etching dentin would irritate pulp tissue, remove the smear layer that protects the pulp, and cause postoperative problems. In the 1990s, the "total etch technique" was accepted. Etching dentin and enamel at the same time is now accepted.

In summary, current research supports the etching of dentin and the use of dentinal bonding systems to reduce microleakage. While some believe that any and all dentin should be etched, more conservative clinicians will, on rare occasions, place a protective material in deep cavity preparations to protect the pulp from irritation by the acid. Etching dentin close to the pulp is thought to be like rubbing salt in an open wound, with the deeply prepared dentin being the open wound.

5. History of Dentinal Bonding Systems

Dentinal bonding systems started out quite complex, requiring as many as six materials to be applied to the cavity preparation. Enamel and dentin were treated differently. Enamel only (not the dentin) was first etched, rinsed, and

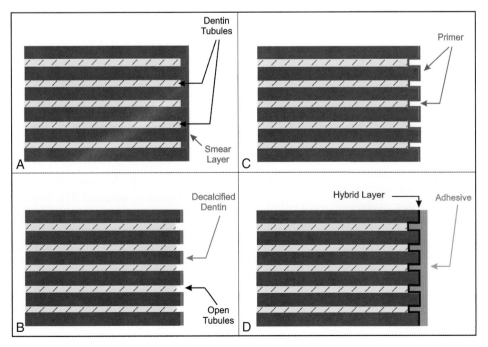

FIGURE 4.6. Schematic representation of a three-step dentinal bonding system. **A.** Prepared dentin is covered by a smear layer. **B.** When the enamel and dentin are etched, the smear layer is removed, the surface of the dentin is decalcified, and the dentinal tubules are opened. **C.** Primer flows into the open tubules and the decalcified dentin. **D.** Adhesive covers the primer and the hybrid layer.

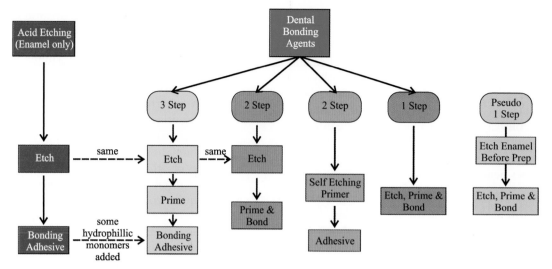

FIGURE 4.7. Diagram of the relationship of the various steps in acid etching for enamel bonding and a variety of dental bonding systems.

dried. Next, the dentin was "conditioned" with a weaker acid or a chelating agent. Chelating agents form molecular complexes with calcium and other ions, and they are used to remove the smear layer and to decalcify the dentin surface. Application of a dentin primer was next, and that was followed by the resin adhesive. With many products, two liquid components were mixed to obtain the primer or the adhesive materials before they were applied to the tooth. Primers were air-dried or cured or both, depending on the system. Adhesive resins were cured before the composite material was placed.

Today, a variety of relatively simple dentinal bonding systems abound, as illustrated by *Figure 4.7.* Three-step systems, not much different than the two-step acid-etching technique (etch and apply bonding resin), have demonstrated long-term clinical success. Simpler two-step systems have been become quite popular. Recently, one-step systems that use self-etching primers and adhesives were introduced. In general, as the number of steps was reduced, the system may be easier to use but not always better. A generic three-step dentinal bonding system is described in detail in the following section to provide a theoretical understanding of the clinical process. Please note it is important to understand and follow the manufacturer's directions for each product used.

B. Three-Step Dentinal Bonding System

1. Etch Dentin and Enamel
The first step is the etching of both dentin and enamel as in the acid-etch technique, as shown in *Figure 4.6B.* Typically, 37% orthophosphoric

acid is used on the enamel and dentin. This is called the "total etch" technique. Etching dentin removes the smear layer from the surface of the dentin as well as the plugs of material forced into the dentinal tubules during cavity preparation. Some etchants have small amounts of additives that are supposed to disinfect the tooth surface. These additives may also reduce the fluid that oozes from the cut odontoblastic processes and the opened tubules. Reducing this fluid makes the surface less wet and aids in application of the resin. Etching also decalcifies a layer of dentin several microns thick. Collagen fibers, a major organic component of dentin, are left on this decalcified surface. After etching, the surface is rinsed with water (as with acid etching), but the surface is only slightly dried (not desiccated), either with a gentle stream of air or by blotting. This is called "wet bonding." Overdrying etched dentin can cause the decalcified collagen fibers to "collapse" into a dense mat. Penetration of the mat by the primer is less effective; therefore, the bond to dentin is weaker.

2. Apply Primer
The second step is the application of the primer. **Primers** are similar to the low-viscosity resins used in enamel bonding systems. The important difference between primers and those resins is that primers have a lower viscosity and are much more tolerant of a wet surface (**hydrophilic**). The primer contains a volatile solvent, such as acetone or ethanol, to thin the organic chemicals and improve flow and wetting of the etched surface. These hydrophilic chemicals wet the etched enamel and dentin surfaces well.

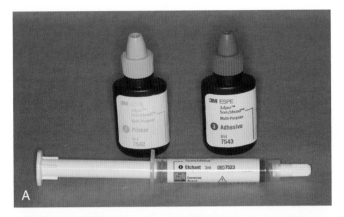

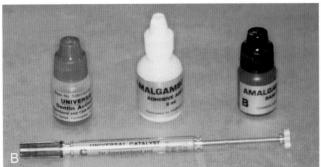

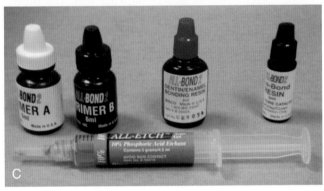

FIGURE 4.8. Photographs of three three-step dentinal bonding systems. **A.** Light-activated Scotchbond MultiPurpose. **B.** Chemically activated Amalgambond. **C.** All-Bond2. Use of the bottle on the far right results in a dual-cure system.

The primer flows into the surface irregularities of etched enamel, much as the enamel bonding resin did. In fact, the hydrophilic primer is more tolerant of a moist (or even a contaminated) surface. In addition, the primer flows into the open tubules of etched dentin. More importantly, the primer also flows around the collagen fibers that were exposed when the dentin was etched, as shown in *Figure 4.6C*. Most primers do not set on their own; rather, they set when a third material is applied. The primer is a wetting agent that aids flow of the adhesive into the tubules and around the collagen fibers. The surface should appear slightly "shiny" or wet if the primer is properly applied.

3. Apply Adhesive
   The third step is the application of the "adhesive" material, as shown in *Figure 4.6D*. The adhesive material is a low-viscosity resin, much like that used in enamel bonding resin systems. While the dentinal bonding adhesive may contain some hydrophilic chemicals as in the primer, the adhesive is **hydrophobic**; it does not like a wet surface. The dentinal bonding adhesive sets, or polymerizes, in the same manner as the enamel bonding resin.

4. Composite Placement
   After the dentinal bonding system has been placed and polymerized, the composite material is applied. The composite material bonds to

the dentinal bonding material as in an enamel bonding system. The result is retention of the restoration and reduced microleakage. Several three-step dentinal bonding systems are shown in *Figure 4.8*.

5. Dentinal Bonding Adhesive Mechanisms
   Dentinal bonding systems use two adhesive mechanisms, as shown in *Figures 4.6 and 4.9*. The first is micromechanical bonding; resin

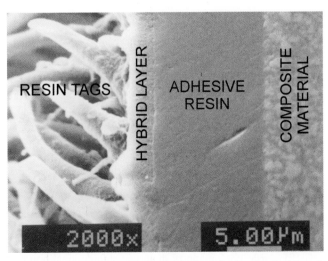

FIGURE 4.9. Scanning electron micrograph of a dentinal bonding system. A dentinal bonding system and composite were applied to the dentin. The dentin was removed by etching with an acid. The micrograph shows material that was in dentinal tubules (resin tags) and the hybrid layer. (Courtesy of BISCO, Inc.)

material is locked in the dentinal tubules as **resin tags**, much like in the acid-etching technique. The second is the formation of a **hybrid layer** composed of resin and decalcified dentin (collagen). Both mechanisms occur at the same time. Certain products form some primary atomic bonds. The significance of these primary bonds is tentative. The hybrid layer mostly involves secondary bonding because both collagen and primers have polar groups attached to the main polymer chains. Chemicals developed for dentinal bonding have the potential to react with collagen, but evidence of such primary bonds is lacking. The hydrophilic nature of the primer, which allows it to wet the etched dentin surface, is the important characteristic of these materials.

6. Clinical Research

Several products have more than 25 years of clinical data to support their effectiveness. The problem is that most dentinal bonding products on the market are "new and improved." Dental bonding systems continuously change. Only short-term, 6- or 12-month data are available for many new products. Surprisingly, the clinical performance of several "old" three-step systems is as good as or better than many of the new easier products.

C. Two-Step Dentinal Bonding Systems

Newer dentinal bonding systems have reduced the number of steps to two. Several products are shown in *Figure 4.10*. While they would seem to be more convenient, some two-step systems have

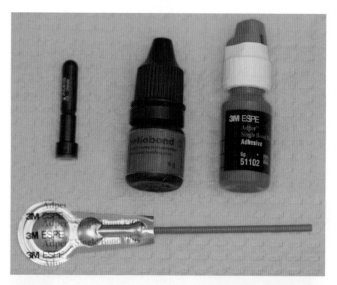

FIGURE 4.10. Photograph of three two-step dentinal bonding systems; *top, left to right*: Prime & Bond NT (unidose), Heliobond, Single Bond, and *bottom* Single Bond (unidose). Note: The acid etchant utilized for two-step dentinal bonding systems is not pictured.

little advantage in terms of time needed to apply materials. A few two-step products actually take longer than some three-step products. Some advocate the use of these systems when placing sealants or orthodontic brackets because the adhesive is more tolerant of contamination by saliva or other oral fluids.

1. Etch

Dentin and enamel are etched the same as three-step systems using the same products. The smear layer is removed and surface dentin is decalcified. The rinse water is carefully removed by gently blowing with compressed air or blotting because desiccation of the dentin must be avoided.

2. Apply Adhesive

The adhesive of a two-step system is a combination of the primer and adhesive of the three-step system. The resin system is more hydrophilic than three-step systems. Solvents are present and aid in the wetting of the etched surface. Solvents are evaporated by gently blowing with air. For many products, two layers of the adhesive are required. The adhesive is light cured and the composite restorative material placed.

D. Two-Step Systems with Self-Etching Primers

In these two-step systems, the etch and primer are combined into one step (bottle) while the adhesive is applied as a second step. Etching of uncut enamel is questionable for some products. Some clinicians etch the enamel with phosphoric acid to ensure a proper etch. Thus, this procedure becomes a three-step process. Most manufacturers recommend scrubbing the dentin with these self-etching primers for 20 seconds.

E. One-Step Self-Etching Adhesives

One-step systems that use self-etching adhesives seem to be the ultimate simplification of dentinal bonding. Several products are shown in *Figure 4.11*. The self-etching adhesives are very acidic organic chemicals that etch the enamel and dentin. Solvents are included to aid in surface wetting and evaporation of water. Hydrophilic resins are also included. Several problems can occur with some of these new products. Several do not etch uncut enamel well. Shelf life may also be a problem for one bottle systems. The acidic adhesive may deteriorate over time resulting in incomplete polymerization. Complete polymerization of the resin is very important as any uncured resin components will irritate the pulp. There is one advantage of using self-etching adhesives. Any part of the tooth etched by the adhesive will be covered

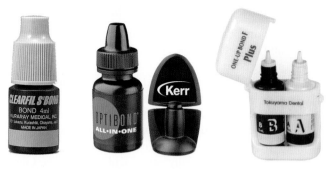

FIGURE 4.11. One-step dentinal bonding systems; *left to right*: Clearfil S³ Bond, OptiBond All-In-One (bulk and unidose), and One-Up Bond F Plus. Note: One-Up Bond is a two-component, one-step system.

and protected by the adhesive. Laboratory and clinical results for some of these one-step systems are promising. After applying the adhesive following the manufacturer's directions, the adhesive is light cured and the composite restorative material placed. One-step self-etching systems have largely evolved into "universal adhesives."

F. Universal Adhesives

Recently, dental manufacturers have gone a step further. We now have adhesives that are called "universal adhesives" shown in *Figure 4.12*; they bond to everything and can be used with several different techniques. The clinician can etch both enamel and dentin and apply the universal adhesive to dentin and enamel as with the two-step systems. The clinician can etch only enamel and apply the universal adhesive to dentin and enamel as with a pseudo one-step system. This technique is called selective etching and was first used with one-step systems that were not effective on uncut enamel. A small blunt needle is used to apply etchant only to the enamel margins, as shown in Figure 25.6.

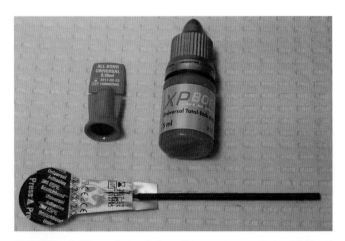

FIGURE 4.12. Universal bonding systems. *Top*: All-Bond Universal (unidose) and XP BOND (bulk). *Bottom*: Scotchbond Universal.

Another technique is to apply the adhesive to both enamel and dentin as a one-step self-etching adhesive. It gets even better; manufacturers claim these adhesives bond not only to enamel and dentin but also to ceramic and metallic materials. Thus, they are described as universal adhesives. Research has shown they do bond to a variety of restorative materials but not as effectively as the more complex "tried and true" procedures.

G. Dual-Cure Adhesives

Composite cements (see Chapter 5, Direct Polymeric Restorative Materials) are used with dental bonding systems. If a crown is metal or porcelain bonded to metal, a chemically activated cement and bonding system is used. (Light cannot get through the metal.) Most dentinal bonding systems have an additional component (bottle), which can be mixed with the adhesive to form a dual-cure adhesive (*Fig. 4.8C*). Dual-cure materials are discussed in Direct Polymeric Restorative Materials.

H. Future Expectations or Thou Shall Not Covet the Future's Dental Materials

One is likely to say adhesive dentistry is more complicated than quantum mechanics; whatever that is, the fact is it keeps getting better but we need to be aware not all products deliver on marketing claims. Remember what Epicurus said thousands of years ago, "Do not spoil what you have by desiring what you have not; remember that what you now have was once among the things you only hoped for."

IV. Glass Ionomers

A. Materials Based on Polyacrylic Acid

Glass ionomers are one of the two adhesive materials that are based on polyacrylic acid. The other is polycarboxylate cement, which is covered in greater detail in Chapter 7. Glass ionomers started as a separate category of dental materials. They have evolved to become one end of a continuum of products, with dentinal bonding systems/composites at the other end. This is discussed more in Direct Polymeric Restorative Materials and is illustrated in Figure 5.13.

B. Polycarboxylate and Glass Ionomer Cements

Polycarboxylate cement was developed by Dennis Smith in London in the 1970s. He combined the common dental cement powder, zinc oxide, with a new liquid, polyacrylic acid, dissolved in water (yes, a polymer dissolved in water). Wilson and Crisp combined Smith's new liquid with the other common dental cement powder, which was finely ground or powdered glass. Their new material was

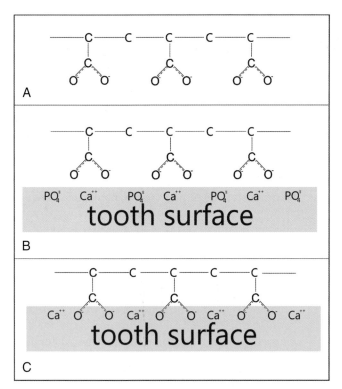

FIGURE 4.13. Schematic representation of **A.** the polyacrylic acid molecule in solution. Note that the carboxylic acid groups have ionized, **B.** bonding between carboxylic acid groups and calcium ions in tooth structure and **C.** bonding carboxylic acid groups substituting for phosphate ions in tooth structure.

named glass ionomer cement. Polyacrylic acid is a long-chain molecule with acid (carboxyl) groups hanging off the side, as shown in *Figure 4.13A*. The acid groups react with the powder when the material sets to form a solid mass. The acid groups can also react with tooth structure and chemically bond to dentin and enamel (see *Fig. 4.13B and C*).

C. Bonding Mechanisms of Glass Ionomers

Bonding "true" glass ionomer materials to enamel and dentin is simple compared to dentinal bonding systems and composites. No separate adhesive is placed and then followed by the restorative material. Instead, the glass ionomer material itself is the adhesive and the restorative material. In addition to chemical adhesion, micromechanical retention is possible if the surface has microscopic irregularities, such as partially open dentinal tubules. Glass ionomer materials are covered in more detail in Chapter 7, Dental Cements.

At first, glass ionomer materials were directly applied to dentin and enamel. Later, dentin surfaces were cleaned or "conditioned" with an aqueous solution of polyacrylic acid before placement of the glass ionomer material. The result is a cleaner surface (with the smear layer removed) and better bonding. The dentin tubules are not opened, as when dentin is acid-etched, and dentin is not decalcified to produce a hybrid layer.

V. Uses of Bonding in Dentistry

Depending on the clinical situation, the dentist will choose among a variety of adhesive materials. Acid etching of enamel is still used to place pit and fissure sealants and to bond orthodontic brackets. Dentinal bonding systems are the norm when composite restorations are placed and are used to reduce the sensitivity of exposed root surfaces of teeth. Glass ionomer materials are the materials of choice for many clinicians when a cervical lesion has margins in both enamel and dentin or the patient has a high risk for caries. Note that all adhesive materials require proper handling and a clean surface for maximum bonding.

Summary

Many materials in dentistry rely on the property of adhesive bonding for success. This type of bonding is usually considered to be micromechanical because the bonding occurs at a level too small to be seen by the naked eye. An example of macromechanical bonding in dentistry is the cementing of crowns and bridges to teeth, similar to the manner in which two pieces of wood are glued together.

Uses of adhesive materials in dentistry include retention of restorations, reduction of microleakage, and reduction of recurrent decay. Cleanliness and biofilms are important factors to consider before using adhesive materials. For bonding success, the surface must be clean to allow intimate association of the adhesive (bonding material) and adherend (the surface).

Today, the acid-etching process is used to micromechanically bond dental materials to enamel. A microscopic rough surface is created, which allows a low-viscosity polymer resin to flow into the rough "enamel tags" or "micropores." The procedure requires that the surface be cleaned with an abrasive, etched with orthophosphoric acid, and coated with a bonding resin before the restorative material can be applied. Between these steps, the enamel surface is thoroughly rinsed and dried.

To bond to the dentin, an extension of the acid-etch technique is used. Cut or prepared dentin differs from enamel in that it is covered by a "smear layer." The traditional, three-step dentinal bonding process consists of etching dentin and enamel, applying primer, and then applying adhesive. Next, the tooth is restored with a composite material. Dentinal bonding systems utilize two adhesive mechanisms: micromechanical bonding and the formation of a hybrid layer. The hybrid layer is composed of resin and decalcified dentin. Both mechanisms occur at the same time, and neither relies on primary atomic bonds.

Two- and single-step systems simplify the dentin bonding process. They combine two or all of the three etch, prime and bond steps.

Another adhesive dental material is glass ionomer cement, which is composed of polyacrylic acid and finely ground or powdered glass. No separate adhesive is placed and then followed by the restorative material because the glass ionomer itself is chemically adhesive to tooth structure. The glass ionomer can serve as both the bonding agent and the restoration.

Depending on the patient's needs, the dentist will choose among the available adhesive materials. All adhesive materials must be handled properly to ensure maximum bonding.

Learning Activities

1. Obtain several extracted teeth, and place composite material on both etched and unetched enamel. Push off the composite material with an instrument. Is there a difference in the force needed to remove the composite from the prepared surfaces?

2. Place a drop of adhesive from a dentinal bonding system on enamel that has been etched and on enamel that has been etched and then contaminated with saliva. Is there a difference in the contact angles formed by the adhesive on the two surfaces?

3. Make 1-mm-thick specimens of a hybrid composite (or any composite material on hand) and a glass ionomer restorative material. Compare the appearance (surface texture, color, and opacity) of these materials.

Review Questions

Question 1. Postage stamps are now self-adhesive. The paper (actual stamp) is referred to as the _____, and the sticky material on the back of the stamp is termed the _____.

a. Adherend, adhesive
b. Adhesive, adherend
c. Adhesive, bonding agent
d. Adherend, biofilm

Question 2. Kristin has orthodontic appliances, commonly known as "braces." These include metal brackets directly bonded to the facial surface with a bonding material. One bracket breaks off, and the "failure" occurs within the bonding material. This type of failure is considered to be:

a. Adhesive
b. Adherend
c. Cohesive
d. Macromechanical

Question 3. On the lines below, use the numbers 1 through 8 to place the steps of the acid-etching process and restoration placement in correct sequence.

_____ Clean surface is rinsed with water.
_____ Etched surface is rinsed with water.
_____ Bonding resin is applied.
_____ Enamel is cleaned with pumice.
_____ Cleaned surface is dried with air.
_____ Etched surface is dried with air.
_____ Restorative material is applied.
_____ Etchant is applied.

Question 4. Orthophosphoric acid (enamel etchant) is commonly used in a _____ concentration.

a. 27%
b. 30%
c. 37%
d. 47%
e. None of the above

Question 5. **Why do primary teeth need to be etched longer than permanent teeth?**

a. It compensates for potential behavioral management problems
b. The enamel is denser on primary teeth
c. The enamel rods are more regularly arranged than on permanent teeth
d. The enamel rods are less regularly arranged than on permanent teeth

Question 6. **Dentinal bonding systems function by way of:**

a. Micromechanical bonding and secondary atomic bonds
b. Macromechanical bonding and secondary atomic bonds
c. Micromechanical bonding and primary atomic bonds
d. Macromechanical bonding and primary atomic bonding

Question 7. **The "dentin debris" that is created when dentin is cut or prepared by dental instruments is called:**

a. Adhesive layer
b. Smear layer
c. Primer layer
d. Chelating agent

Question 8. **The use of bonding in dentistry serves all of the following functions EXCEPT:**

a. Reduction of recurrent caries
b. Retention of color in the restoration
c. Reduction of microleakage
d. Retention of restorations

Question 9. **An adhesive mechanism of a dentinal bonding system is a hybrid layer. It is composed of:**

a. The smear layer and resin
b. Dentin primer and decalcified enamel
c. Resin and decalcified enamel
d. Resin and decalcified dentin

Question 10. **The following are all historical fallacies about dentinal bonding except one. Which one is the EXCEPTION?**

a. Composites irritate the pulp
b. Dentin should not be etched
c. The smear layer is "dentinal debris"
d. The smear layer should be left to protect the pulp

Direct Polymeric Restorative Materials

Objectives

After studying this chapter, the student will be able to do the following:

1. Name the two types of polymerization reactions commonly seen in dental materials, and explain the meaning of "addition" in "addition polymerization."
2. Discuss the following properties of restorative resins:
   - Polymerization shrinkage
   - Coefficient of thermal expansion
   - Abrasion resistance
3. Summarize the relationship between a filler particle, the matrix, and the coupling agent of a composite restorative material.
4. Compare the advantages and disadvantages of light-activated and chemically activated composite materials.
5. Explain the importance of proper eye protection when light-curing dental materials.
6. Relate the importance of the following procedures and/or characteristics of dental composites:
   - Depth of cure
   - Addition of material in increments
   - Inhibition by air
   - Unreacted C=C bonds
   - Shades
   - Shortcomings of the matrix
7. For filler particles found in dental composites, summarize the importance of the following properties:
   - Composition
   - Size
   - Amount (percentage)
   - Abrasion resistance
   - Refractive index
   - Clinical detection
8. Choose one of the three types of dental composites, and justify its use in the following dental situations:
   - Bonding orthodontic brackets to enamel
   - Class V "gingival notch" restoration
   - Small class I or II restoration
9. Briefly explain the reason(s) for the development of flowable and condensable composites.

(continued)

Key Words/Phrases

activation
addition polymerization
compomer
condensable composites
crazing
depth of cure
diluent
dual cure
filler particles
flowable composites
free radical
hybrid composite
incremental addition
inhibitor
initiation
macrofilled composite
matrix
microfilled composite
monomers
oligomer
percolation
pit and fissure sealants
polymerization
polymers
preventive resin restoration
propagation
silane coupling agent
termination
thermoplastic polymers
thermoset polymers

Objectives (continued)

10. Discuss the role the dental hygienist should play in the placement and maintenance of pit and fissure sealants.
11. Discuss the use of a primer with pit and fissure sealants.
12. Briefly describe "preventive resin restoration" and "composite cement."
13. Assess the positive and negative characteristics of light-cure and chemical-cure glass ionomer cements.
14. Discuss the similarities between compomers, glass ionomers, and composites.

Introduction

Polymers are materials that are made of large, long molecules formed by chemically reacting molecular building blocks called monomers. A variety of polymers exist, and they exhibit a variety of properties. The chemical reaction that links the monomers together to produce a polymer (macromolecule) is called **polymerization**. Common polymers or "plastics," such as polyethylene and Plexiglas (an acrylic resin), are made by addition polymerization and are used to make soda and milk bottles and many other everyday objects. Polyethylene materials have long, linear chains that are easily recycled because they can be remelted and reprocessed. These materials are called **thermoplastic polymers** because they can be heated (thermo) and molded or shaped (plastic) after the polymerization reaction, similar to wax.

Polymers with a cross-linked rather than a linear structure tend not to melt. Rather, they decompose. These materials are called **thermoset polymers**. They cannot be heated and molded, so their use requires them to be in the final shape when the polymerization reaction occurs. They tend to be stronger and tougher than thermoplastic materials. Most dental resins are cross-linked and are therefore thermoset.

Polymers were introduced in Chapter 2, Materials Science and Dentistry. In this chapter, we discuss acrylic resins and dental composites used to replace and restore teeth.

I. Acrylic Resins

Acrylic resins were first used in dentistry for denture bases (see Figs. 1.6 and 1.7). A denture base is the pink plastic part of a denture that simulates the gingiva and the lost alveolar bone. Denture teeth are bonded to the base to

form the denture. Dental acrylic resin is the same polymer used in Plexiglas, a tough plastic that serves as a glass substitute in windows. Acrylic resins have been adapted for many uses in dentistry and are covered in greater detail in later chapters. The chemistry of acrylic resins is presented in this chapter because it is the same chemistry as that of most direct polymeric restorative materials. Acrylic resins were once used for anterior restorations but were very susceptible to recurrent decay. When dental composites became available, direct acrylic restorative materials were made obsolete. The shortcomings of acrylic resins and the improved performance of composite materials are discussed in this chapter.

A. Addition Polymerization—Optional

The polymerization reaction of acrylic resins, called addition polymerization, is very common in dental materials. The other common polymerization reaction, condensation polymerization, will be covered when impression materials are discussed. Acrylic resins and composite materials, such as restorative materials, cements, sealants, and adhesives, all set by addition polymerization. The common factor relating all these materials to each other is the same chemical structure of the reactive or functional group. The functional group is the part of the molecule responsible for its important chemical properties.

1. Functional Groups

Monomers are molecules with a reactive group that participates in the polymerization reaction. This reactive group is called the functional group. The functional group of acrylic resin monomers is the carbon–carbon double bond. We will denote this bond as $C{=}C$. The "double bond" has two pairs of electrons shared by the two carbon atoms, so four electrons are involved in the double bond. Although $C{=}C$ is the reactive part of the monomer, other atoms and side groups (besides hydrogen) can be bonded to either or both of the carbon atoms of the $C{=}C$.

The side groups become pendants (like a charm on a charm bracelet) on the polymer chain, and they determine the chemical and physical properties of the resulting polymer.

2. Free Radicals

The chemical (polymerization) reaction of acrylic resins is called free radical or addition polymerization. The first name, free radical polymerization, is used because a free radical, an unpaired electron, is involved in the reaction. The other name, **addition polymerization**, is used because one monomer at a time is added to the polymer chain as the reaction proceeds. Addition polymerization is a very common polymerization reaction used to make a variety of polymers or plastics.

B. Steps in Addition Polymerization—Optional

1. Initiation

The first step in addition polymerization reaction is called **initiation**. Actually, initiation can be thought of as two reactions. The first involves several **activation** methods to form a **free radical**, which is a molecule with an unpaired electron (*Fig. 5.1A*). In the second reaction, the free radical reacts with a monomer molecule to start a growing chain (*Fig. 5.1B*).

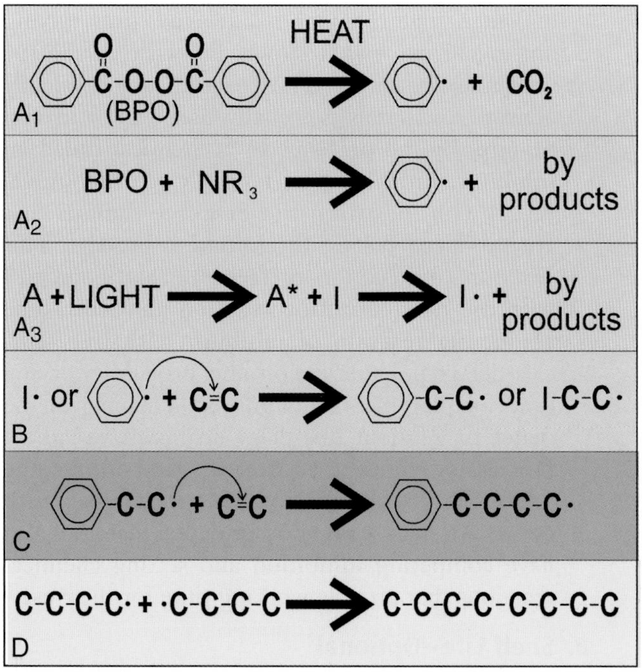

FIGURE 5.1. Initiator molecules are activated by **A₁.** heat, **A₂.** chemical reaction, and **A₃.** light to form free radicals. **B.** Initiation of chain growth, **C.** propagation of chain growth, and one example of **D.** chain termination are also illustrated. *A*, activator; *I*, initiator; *BPO*, benzoyl peroxide; *NR₃*, tertiary amine; •, unpaired electron, a free radical; *, an excited molecule.

a. *Formation of Free Radicals (Polymerization Activation)*

An initiator molecule can become activated (changed into a free radical) by heat, light, or a chemical reaction. Several types of chemical reactions are used in dentistry to form free radicals. One is a chemical reaction that begins when chemicals are mixed together. The other is a chemical reaction that is started by light (*Fig. 5.1A*).

As a result of the various activation methods, materials are classified as heat activated (also known as heat cure), chemically activated (also known as cold cure or chemical cure), or light activated (also known as photo cure or light cure). In this text, heat and chemical activation will be presented in detail, whereas light activation will be described only in general terms.

b. *Reaction of Free Radical and Monomer*

Regardless of the method by which the free radical is formed, the second reaction during initiation of polymerization is for the free radical to react with the C=C of the monomer. As previously mentioned, a free radical is an unpaired electron. An unpaired electron is "unhappy" (high-energy state) and wants to form an atomic bond by pairing with another electron (forming a lower-energy state). In addition polymerization, it does so by reacting with one of the electron pairs of the C=C of the monomer. A group of three electrons, however, is not the result. Rather, a single C–C bond and another free radical on the end of the growing chain are formed, as illustrated in *Figure 5.1B*. The first "link" in the growing chain has been added.

2. Propagation

Figure 5.1C illustrates the second step in addition polymerization, which is the growth or lengthening of the chain. This step is called **propagation**. The free radical of the "initiated chain" reacts with a monomer, and the chain is one monomer longer. The process is similar to initiation. Propagation involves adding the second, third, fourth, and later monomers to the growing chain until that chain is hundreds or even thousands of monomers long. Polymerization continues as long as monomers are available to react with the free radical at the end of the growing chain. Polymerization reactions result in a long chain of monomers. Such addition polymerization reactions are also called chain-lengthening reactions.

3. **Termination**

Two free radicals at the ends of two growing chains may react. If they do, they will form a carbon–carbon bond, as illustrated in *Figure 5.1D*. At this point, no free radicals are left to continue growth of the chain. **Termination** of polymerization of both chains is the result; thus, termination is the name given to this step. Free radicals also react with contaminants, which may also cause termination of polymerization.

C. Activation of Addition Polymerization

1. Heat Activated

Heat-activated acrylic resins typically use benzoyl peroxide (BPO) as the initiator. Heat is the activator. When heated to 60°C, BPO breaks down into CO_2 and free radical molecules, as illustrated in *Figure 5.1A$_1$*. Heat-activated acrylic resins are manufactured as a powder/liquid systems. The powder and liquid are mixed to form a dough for molding into the desired shape. The polymerization reaction does not start until the material is heated, typically in a hot water bath. Most complete and partial dentures use heat-activated acrylic resins for the denture base.

2. Chemically Activated

Chemically activated acrylic resins, as well as composite materials, commonly use BPO as the initiator. A variety of chemicals is used as the activator. Activators used in dental polymers belong to a group of chemicals called tertiary amines. We will use NR_3 to denote a tertiary amine, which is an organic molecule with a nitrogen atom bonded to a three carbon-containing groups. *Figure 5.1A$_2$* shows the reaction of the tertiary amine with BPO and the formation of free radical molecules. Chemically activated materials are typically a powder and a liquid that are mixed together to start the polymerization process. Chemically activated acrylic resins are used to make temporary crowns, custom impressions trays, orthodontic retainers, and many other dental devices.

3. Light Activated

Light-activated dental materials use several activator and initiator chemicals. The activator absorbs light and then reacts with the initiator. *Figure 5.1A$_3$* represents the formation of free radical–containing molecules by light activation. Light-activated materials are supplied as a single paste; no mixing is required. The polymerization process does not begin until the material is exposed to a very bright light source. The "set on demand" nature of light-activated

materials has made them very popular. The most common light-activated dental materials are composite restorative materials, but a few light-activated acrylic products exist.

4. Dual-Cure Materials

Several dental materials have both chemical and light-activated capabilities. These materials are called **dual-cure** materials. Polymerization is started with a curing light, but material that cannot be reached by the intense light sets by the chemical activation mechanism.

D. Addition Polymerization Is an Exothermic Reaction

In chemical factories, the heat of this rapid exothermic polymerization reaction must be removed, or the rise in temperature can become dangerous. Dental acrylic resins react by addition polymerization and are also quite exothermic. In a later chapter, we see that controlling the rise in temperature is important for the proper processing of an acrylic denture.

II. Inhibitors and Competing Reactions

A. Working Time

Polymerization reactions can occur very rapidly. For a dental material to be useful, the reaction must either occur when desired (as with light-activated materials) or be delayed after mixing and occur somewhat slowly (as with chemically activated products). The reaction of chemically activated materials is initially delayed for several minutes by the presence of a chemical called an inhibitor. An **inhibitor**, typically hydroquinone, reacts with (destroys) the first free radicals that are produced during the initiation process. This reaction (destruction of free radicals) competes with the polymerization reaction and wins. The competing reaction of inhibitor with free radicals delays polymerization and provides working time for placement, molding, and shaping of the material. Without this delay, materials would set too fast for clinical use. After a period of time, the inhibitor is used up, and polymerization begins to occur. We shall see that other dental materials also have competing inhibition and setting chemical reactions that provide working time for their use.

B. Shelf Life—Optional

The liquid component of an acrylic resin product is almost entirely composed of monomer. In theory, one free radical could polymerize an entire container of monomer. This can happen when acrylic resin products are stored for several years. To prevent this and provide a reasonable shelf life for their products, manufacturers add a small amount of inhibitor to materials that contain monomer. Inhibitors are present at a much smaller concentration in light-activated and heat-activated products than they are in chemical-activated systems. Inhibitors provide shelf life for monomer-containing mixtures of materials. Without an inhibitor, what was once a liquid or a paste would become a solid chunk of polymer over time.

III. Problems with Unfilled Resins

Polymers without filler additives are not suitable for use as restorative materials. A discussion of several problems will aid our understanding of the importance of fillers.

A. Polymerization Shrinkage

Polymerization reactions make a few very large polymer molecules from many small monomer molecules. Atoms and molecules become packed much closer together when polymerized, and the resulting material is smaller in volume than the starting components. Polymerization shrinkage is an important problem with the use of polymers. In dentistry, polymeric restorative materials shrink when they set; thus, they have the potential to open gaps at the margins of these restorations. Bonding materials to tooth structure reduces the potential for these gaps and the resulting microleakage.

B. Coefficient of Thermal Expansion

Polymeric materials have high coefficients of thermal expansion compared to tooth structure. In fact, these coefficients can be from 2 to 10 times greater. Repeated expansion and contraction of polymeric restorative materials can open and close gaps at the margin of a restoration. This phenomenon is called **percolation** and is illustrated in Figure 4.1. As a result, leakage increases, and recurrent caries are much more likely.

C. Strength and Abrasion Resistance of Polymeric Materials

Even the best polymers are unable to withstand occlusal forces in the oral environment. They lack strength and abrasion resistance. Polymeric materials are useful in dentistry, however, because they can be placed into a cavity preparation as a plastic mass and then molded and shaped. Next, they are polymerized in the mouth, forming a replacement for lost tooth structure. Forming a restoration directly in the mouth is very useful, but time and temperature limit which polymers can be used.

IV. Improvements to Dental Resins

Several techniques have been used to improve dental resins. These techniques originated in nondental industries, but they have greatly improved polymeric restorative materials. The most successful and notable individual in this process was Dr. Raphael Bowen, who developed the first dental composites.

A. Fillers and Silane Coupling Agents

Industrial uses of polymers greatly expanded when strong, hard fillers were added to strengthen plastics to form composites. Fiberglass is one such material. It combines a polymer with glass fibers and is much stronger and more useful compared to the polymer alone. Composite materials were introduced in Chapter 2, Materials Science and Dentistry. **Filler particles** are typically inexpensive, strong, hard ceramic materials. Many fillers are naturally occurring silica (SiO) minerals, but others are specially prepared glass materials (also silica based).

Dr. Bowen incorporated a strong ceramic filler particle into his polymer system to form a much stronger dental restorative material. Two examples of dental composites are shown in *Figure 5.2*. To obtain the maximum benefit from the addition

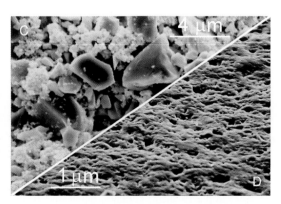

FIGURE 5.2. Scanning electron micrographs of two dental composites **B** and **D** and their filler particles **A** and **C**. The smaller filler particles result in composite restorations with a smoother surface. (Courtesy of BISCO, Inc.)

of these particles, the polymer (or matrix, as it is called in a composite system) is bonded to the filler particle with a coupling agent. The coupling agent couples, or transfers, stress from the relatively weak matrix to the relatively strong filler. Dental composites use ceramic filler particles coated with silane coupling agents. Silane coupling agents work a bit-like soap; they have a different chemical group at each end of the molecule. **Silane coupling agents** are molecules that react with the polymer matrix at one end and with the ceramic filler at the other end, as illustrated in *Figure 5.3*. The end that reacts with the polymer matrix has a C=C that participates in the addition polymerization reaction. The other end has a silane group, hence the name silane coupling agent. The silane group has silicon and oxygen atoms that react with the silicon and oxygen on the surface of the ceramic filler particle.

Fillers are selected for their physical properties. Luckily, the strong, hard ceramic materials that are chosen also have a low coefficient of thermal expansion. When mixed with polymers, the resulting dental composites have coefficients closer to that of tooth structure than the polymers on which they are based. Because a composite has less polymer in the system, polymerization shrinkage is reduced when the material sets.

Manufacturers try to maximize the filler content of their dental composites because adding more filler increases strength, decreases polymerization shrinkage, and decreases thermal expansion to

nearer that of tooth structure. However, there is a limit to the amount of filler that can be added. When mixing dough for bread, excess flour results in a defective product; the same is true for filler in dental composites. If all filler particles are not properly wetted by the liquid monomers, voids and gaps between the filler particles result. As previously mentioned, voids do not resist any stress placed on a material; they also concentrate stress in the material in the vicinity of the void.

B. Bowen's Resin—Optional

In addition to adding fillers to form composites, Dr. Bowen also developed a polymer for dental composites. This molecule is actually a combination of several monomer molecules to form what is called an **oligomer**. The notable features of Dr. Bowen's oligomer are polar side groups that increase chain-to-chain hydrogen bonding and two reactive C=C groups. Because each C=C group can participate in the formation of a growing polymer chain, the oligomer is called bifunctional. Bifunctional monomers and oligomers result in cross-linking and greatly improve the strength of the resulting polymer. Dr. Bowen's oligomer is called bis-GMA and is illustrated in *Figure 5.4* along with methyl methacrylate, the monomer most commonly found in dental acrylic systems, and triethylene glycol dimethacrylate. The bis-GMA is a very viscous material and needs to be diluted and thinned with other bifunctional monomers, such as triethylene glycol dimethacrylate, when dental composites are formulated. Although bis-GMA is more properly called an oligomer, we shall use the term monomer when referring to it.

V. Composite Materials

Composite materials are the combination of two materials. The result is a material that is superior to either component alone.

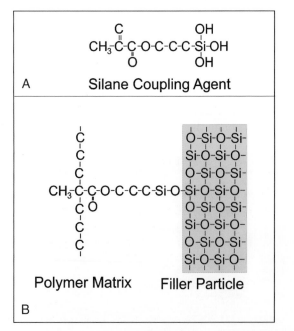

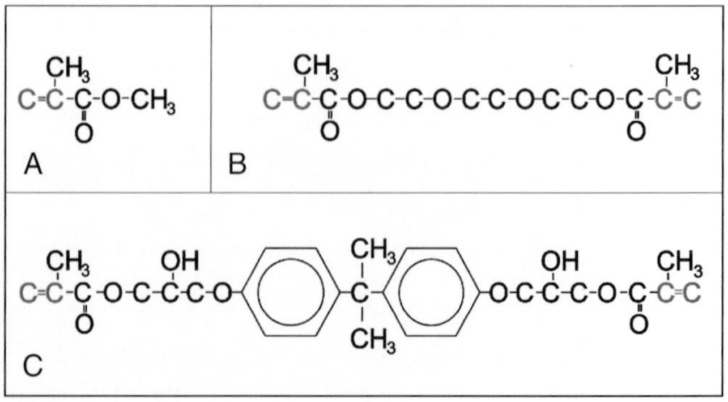

FIGURE 5.3. A. Example of silane coupling agent and **B.** its reaction with the polymer matrix on the *left* and the filler particle on the *right*.

FIGURE 5.4. Structure of **A.** methyl methacrylate, **B.** triethylene glycol dimethacrylate, and **C.** bis-GMA.

A. Dental Composites

Dental composites are supplied in a variety of shades (colors) and handling characteristics. Their use continues to expand and replace other materials. Before dental composites were introduced, other esthetic materials were used, such as acrylic resins, but they lacked clinical efficacy. Acrylic resin materials had a high coefficient of thermal expansion, and polymerization shrinkage was excessive. Recurrent caries around and under acrylic resin restorations was typical. Silicate cements were also used as an esthetic material, but they dissolved too quickly and required frequent replacement. In the 1960s, when dental composites were developed, they quickly replaced acrylic resin and silicate restorative materials.

B. Components of a Dental Composite

Dental composites are composed of two phases: matrix and filler. The matrix is soft, weak, flexible, and prone to wear compared to the filler. In addition, two "molecular components" are present: a silane coupling agent and a polymerization system.

1. Matrix

The **matrix** of a dental composite is a polymer, typically bis-GMA or a similar monomer. An organic chemical called a **diluent** is added to control the viscosity of the final product. For both bis-GMA and the diluent, C=C is the functional group. The matrix of a dental composite polymerizes by a chemical reaction (addition polymerization). Polymerization is activated by a chemical reaction (chemical activation) or light energy (light activation). Light-activated materials are the most commonly used dental composites, but chemically activated materials have their uses.

The polymer matrix of dental composites is chemically similar to enamel and dentin adhesives. Composites chemically bond to primers and adhesives of dental bonding systems because both have C=C functional groups and both set by addition polymerization, as discussed earlier. Adhesives of enamel bonding systems and dentinal bonding systems are typically bis-GMA and diluents formulated to have the proper viscosity. The currently used dentinal bonding systems, composite restorative materials, and resin cements are very compatible with each other. It is common to use a dental bonding system from one manufacturer and composite restorative material from another.

The matrix of a dental composite has several important functions. The matrix is the phase that polymerizes to form a solid mass and bonds to tooth structure. However, the matrix has several shortcomings. It is the weakest and the least wear-resistant phase of a dental composite

material. It also absorbs water and can stain and discolor. Therefore, manufacturers minimize the matrix content of composite materials by maximizing the filler content. Stronger composite materials result.

2. Fillers

In the beginning, fillers in dental composites were naturally occurring quartz materials (sand). Quartz materials are strong, hard, and chemically stable in the oral environment. Recently, manufacturers have "engineered" glass materials for dental composites. These engineered glass materials are formulated to have the proper strength, hardness, and chemical properties as well as optical properties for use in dental composites. The glass is ground to have the proper-size particles. These particles are coated with a silane coupling agent. The silanated filler is mixed with monomers, diluents, coloring agents, and other chemicals to form the paste that is purchased from the manufacturer.

a. Filler Size

The size of the filler in a dental composite determines the surface smoothness of the resulting restoration. Larger particles result in a rougher surface (see *Fig. 5.2*). Composites are most often classified by the size of their filler particles. This text will discuss three categories of dental composites: macrofill, microfill, and hybrid (blends). In reality, each category of composite has some range of particle size. It would be needlessly expensive for manufacturers to select a narrow range of particle size.

b. Evolution of Fillers

Filler particles have evolved from the strongest, most abrasion-resistant materials to somewhat softer, less abrasion-resistant materials. A softer particle is more likely to wear down rather than to be pulled out of the matrix when abrasion occurs. If a particle is pulled out, the surface is now soft resin that will wear away quickly. If the particle wears and stays partially embedded in the matrix, however, the surface has an overall greater abrasion resistance and wears at a slower rate.

c. Filler Content (Amount of Filler)

With the exception of proper handling, the percentage of filler is the most important determinant of the physical properties of dental composites. As the filler content increases, the resin content decreases. Therefore, polymerization shrinkage decreases, and the coefficient of thermal expansion becomes more like that of tooth structure. Hardness and abrasion resistance increase as well.

3. Silane Coupling Agents

Although not a true phase in a dental composite, the silane coupler is a very important component of the material. The silane coupler must be chemically compatible with both the filler and the resin phases. Manufacturers have accomplished this, and the stress placed on a restoration is thus transferred from the weaker resin phase to the stronger filler phase. Dentistry has recognized the effectiveness of silane couplers and now uses them to silanate ceramic restorations, such as a crown, in the dental lab or at chairside. The silane coupling agent enables adhesive materials to bond ceramic restorations to tooth structure.

One theory of composite wear proposes that the bond between the silane coupler and the filler particle is slightly soluble in the oral environment. As the bond is broken, the filler particles are pulled out of the resin matrix, exposing the soft resin. The resin is then worn away, exposing more filler particles to the oral environment, and the cycle continues.

4. Polymerization Systems

Two polymerization systems are used to convert the matrix–filler paste to a solid composite material. All dental composites use addition polymerization.

a. *Chemically Activated Materials*

Chemically activated materials are two-paste systems, as shown in *Figure 5.5*. One paste contains the tertiary amine, and the other contains the BPO initiator. The pastes have different colors and are mixed at chairside until the two colors blend into one. The pastes are supplied in small plastic jars or screw-type syringes. When the two pastes are mixed, the inhibitor destroys the free radicals that are produced for a short period

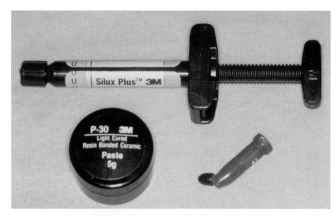

FIGURE 5.6. Light-cure composites are supplied as a jar (or tub), screw-type syringe, and compule (unit dose).

of time, as previously described. This results in a limited amount of working time to place and contour the material. When the inhibitor has reacted completely, polymerization begins. Because two pastes are mixed, air bubbles are unavoidably incorporated during mixing. Any porosity, such as these air bubbles, weakens the set material and increases staining. Care must be taken to minimize these defects in the final product.

b. *Light-Activated Materials*

Light-activated materials are single-paste materials that are mixed by the manufacturer, as shown in *Figure 5.6*. Because no chairside mixing occurs, manufacturers can make the paste thicker, with less matrix and more filler particles. In addition, voids are minimized by the manufacturing process; a stronger restoration is the result.

Light-activated materials set when exposed to a very bright light. As a result, the working time is variable and can be quite long if the operator desires. The setting time is short. The wavelength of the light source is matched to the activator chemical in the material. The intensity of the light source is greatest around 470 nm. Light absorption of the activator is also greatest at 470 nm. Light with a wavelength of 470 nm is blue light that is visible to the human eye. Because the light is very bright, direct viewing of the light source will damage the eye. Even indirect (reflected) observation of the curing light is contraindicated. Light shields have been incorporated into current curing lights to protect the operator's eyes, as shown in *Figure 5.7A*.

Light sources include halogen lights (*Fig. 5.7A*), plasma arc lights, argon lasers, and blue light-emitting diodes (*Fig. 5.7B and C*). Halogen lights are similar to slide projector bulbs. Plasma arc lights are similar to some

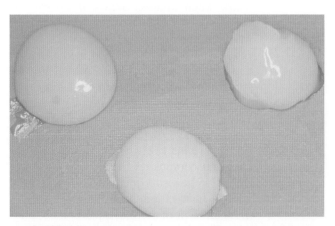

FIGURE 5.5. Photograph of the base and catalyst pastes (*top*) of the Concise system shown in Figure 4.4 and the mixed composite material (*bottom*).

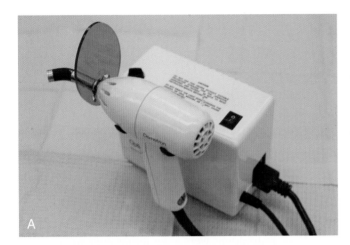
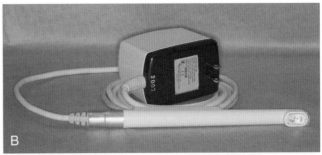
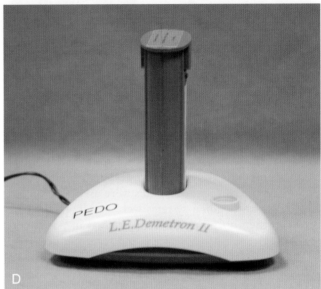
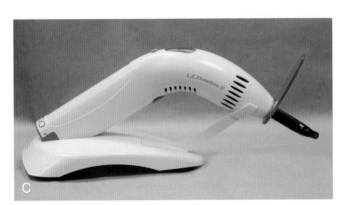

FIGURE 5.7. Photograph of dental curing lights. **A.** A conventional halogen curing light with a shield designed to protect the operator's eyes from the intense light. **B.** A light-emitting diode curing light with a power cord. **C.** A battery-powered light-emitting diode curing unit. **D.** A charging unit and rechargeable battery.

high-intensity commercial outdoor lighting. Light-emitting diodes are common in automobile dashboards and traffic signal lights. Features that aid the operator in controlling curing time include a timer, on/off switches, sound effects, and other "bells and whistles." Because the working time of light-cure materials is determined by the user, they are widely popular and have replaced chemically activated materials for most uses. Chemically activated composites are used when light cannot reach the composite material, such as when cementing a metal crown with a composite cement.

C. Types and Properties of Dental Composites

1. Macrofilled Composites

The first type of dental composite to be developed in the 1960s is now called a macrofilled composite. A **macrofilled composite** is illustrated in *Figure 5.8A*. The filler is a quartz material with particle sizes of 10 to 25 μm. Filler content is 70% to 80% by weight. There is a difference between filler content as measured by

weight and by volume. Because the filler phase is much denser than the resin phase, the volume percentage is typically 10% to 15% lower than the weight percentage. Manufacturers like to report the weight percentage because it is higher. Physical properties are determined by the volume percentage, so it is the favorite of scientists. Either percentage can be used to evaluate materials, but it is important to know which scale (weight percentage or volume percentage) is being used.

The large size of the filler particles in macrofilled composites results in a restoration that feels rough to the dental explorer and can appear rough to the eye. The likelihood of plaque accumulation and staining is greater with macrofilled than with other types of composites. The typical macrofilled composite will turn slightly gray when rubbed with an instrument. The hard filler abrades the metal instrument. This aids in the location of macrofilled composite restorations. Macrofills have little clinical importance at this time except that some orthodontists still use them. The rough feel and easy detection

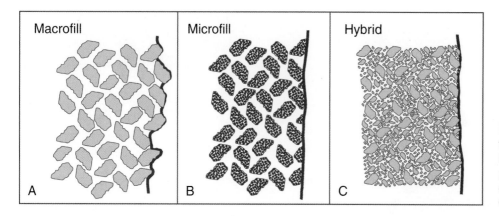

FIGURE 5.8. Schematic representation of different types of composites and their surface roughness after polishing or wear. **A.** Macrofilled composite. **B.** Microfilled composite. **C.** Hybrid composite.

give them an advantage during the removal of bonded orthodontic brackets or appliances and the accompanying bonding material.

Except for wear resistance and surface roughness, the strength and other physical properties of macrofilled composites are adequate for class III, IV, and V restorations. Excessive wear when used for class I and II restorations limited their posterior use. Macrofills were used before dentinal bonding systems were developed; placing them in posterior teeth resulted in postoperative sensitivity, leakage, and recurrent decay.

2. Microfilled Composites

In the late 1970s, microfilled composites were marketed. The particle size of **microfilled composites** is far smaller than in macrofill composites (0.03–0.5 μm). Microfill composites polish very smooth and lustrous (*Fig. 5.8B*), and the surface appearance is very similar to enamel. The very small filler particles are typically fused silica. The problem with microfilled composites is the low percentage filler (40–50%). The surface area of the very small filler particles requires much more resin to wet the surface of the filler particles. This high resin content results in an increased coefficient of thermal expansion and lower strength.

The polymerization shrinkage of microfilled composites is less than expected based on the total resin content. Some (or all) of the filler particles are actually "composite filler particles" (*Fig. 5.8B*). The resin of these "composite filler particles" has already been polymerized. Therefore, this resin cannot polymerize and does not increase polymerization shrinkage. It does increase the coefficient of thermal expansion. Additional uncured matrix components are combined with the "composite filler particle" to make the microfilled composite paste.

Microfill composites were enthusiastically received by the dental profession when introduced in the mid-1970s. Smooth, lustrous composite restorations were a significant improvement over the available macrofilled composites. Microfilled materials were tried in class I and II restorations, but the performance of most of the products was not much better than that achieved with macrofilled composites. Microfilled composites are used when esthetics are the dominant concern. Large composite restorations, such as an extensive class IV restoration, are built in layers of several different shades and translucencies. The first layers to be placed are a hybrid composite selected for strength. The final layer, a veneer of sorts, is a microfilled composite selected for surface luster.

Microfilled composites were also used in class V restorations at the cementoenamel junction. Microfills have a lower modulus of elasticity and flex with the tooth better than the strongest composite materials. Clinical research has shown class V microfill composite restorations are more likely to be retained than other composite materials.

3. Hybrid Composites

The next type of composite was developed in the late 1980s and is called a **hybrid composite**. These composites are strong and polish well. Their filler content is 75% to 80% by weight. The filler particles average 0.5 to 1 μm in size, but with a wider range of particle sizes (0.1–3 μm) (*Fig. 5.8C*). They are called hybrid (or blended) composites because they have a range of particle sizes. Hybrid composites are very popular; their strength and abrasion resistance are acceptable for small to medium class I and II restorations. Their surface finish is nearly as good as that of microfills; thus, they are also used for class III and IV restorations.

4. Improved Hybrid Composites

Hybrid composites currently on the market are a result of manufacturers' efforts to improve the clinical performance of composite materials. They continue to maximize the amount of filler present by controlling the particle size and distribution. The average particle size has decreased and nano-sized particles have been added. Nano-sized particles are approximately 100 times smaller than the thickness of a human hair. The results are slight improvements in strength and polymerization shrinkage. The most notable improvement is the smooth surface of modern well-polished composite materials. These materials have largely replaced microfilled compositions.

5. **Special Use Composite Materials**
Two special use composite materials are available. Most manufacturers market flowable composites, and some are marketing condensable composites. Because composite materials are more difficult to place in the cavity preparation than amalgam, both types are designed to make the placement of composite materials easier.

a. **Flowable composites** flow into the cavity preparation because of their lower viscosity. Manufacturers have decreased the filler content of the material to reduce the viscosity and increase the flow of these materials. A weaker, less abrasion-resistant material results. Flowable composites are typically used as the initial increment of a composite restoration and then covered with a hybrid material.

b. **Condensable composites** (or, more properly, composites that can be compacted) are another attempt to make placement of the material into the cavity preparation easier. In general, condensable composites have a filler particle feature that inhibits the filler particles from sliding by one another. A "thicker, stiffer feel" results, and the manufacturers call these products condensable. Clinical research has shown

these materials with a different "feel" are not an improvement over hybrid composite materials; most performed poorly and few are still on the market.

6. **Shades and Opacities of Dental Composites**
Dental composites, porcelains, and ceramic restorative materials are manufactured in several shades to match the color and translucency of teeth. By layering materials with different shades and translucencies, a more natural restoration can be placed. The most commonly used composite materials match the body of the tooth in translucency and have no specific designation. Opaque materials are designed to prevent the underlying color from showing through. Opaque composites are used to hide stained or discolored dentin. Over the opaque material, the typical dental composite is placed. The last layer may simulate the translucency of enamel; some products come with "incisal" or "translucent" shades. These shades may actually be more translucent to light, or they may just have a blue appearance that mimics the appearance of incisal enamel.

D. Use of Composites for Restorations

Composite restorations are the material of choice for directly placed esthetic restorations, as shown in *Figure 5.9* and summarized in Table 5.1. Composites are one of several materials called "tooth-colored" materials. Composites have the smoothest surface and best translucency of any direct esthetic restorative material, but they are still considered to be inadequate for the characteristic of life-like appearance when compared to all ceramic restorations. However, ceramic restorations, although superior in terms of esthetics, are more costly because they are indirect restorations that require a

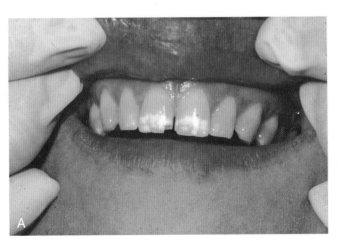
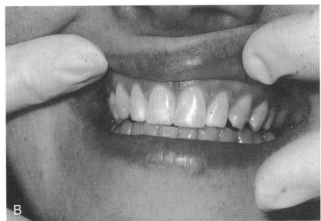

FIGURE 5.9. **A.** Patient with chipped mesial of a central incisor, small diastema, and enamel discoloration. **B.** Both central incisors were restored with a hybrid composite bonded to the mesial and facial surfaces, restoring the fracture, closing the diastema, and covering some of the discolored enamel.

TABLE 5.1. Types of Composites

Property	Microfill	Macrofill	Hybrid
Filler size (µm)	0.03–0.5	10–25	0.5–1
Filler (wt%)	40–50	70–75	75–80
Strength	Low	Fair	Good
Abrasion resistance	Good	Poor	Very good
Thermal expansion	Poor	Fair	Good
Current uses	Class III, IV, and V; veneers	Few	Class I, II, III, and IV
Polishability	Very good	Poor	Good
Examples	Helimolar	Adaptic	Tetric Ceram
	Renamel	Concise	Spectra
			Aelite
			Vitlescence
			Filtek Supreme

second appointment for cementation and involve a lab fee. Ceramic restorations are discussed in a later chapter.

Composite materials are also inadequate in the mechanical property of fracture toughness when compared to metallic restorative materials. The use of directly placed dental composites is often limited to restorations that are subjected to low to moderate stresses. The current practice of dentistry requires bonding the restoration to tooth structures.

Hybrid composites dominate composite materials currently in use. They function well in moderate stress restorations where esthetics are important. Their use has expanded to all surfaces of all teeth where isolation during placement is possible (see Figs. 1.15, 1.16, and 5.9). As the size of the restoration increases, the stress on the restorative material increases. Composites do not have the mechanical properties for long-term success in large high-stress restorations such as cusp replacement restorations. With proper treatment planning and placement, composite restorations will succeed for many years.

E. Factors Affecting the Placement of Composites

1. Depth of Cure

Typical use of dental composites involves etching of tooth structure, priming, and application of the adhesive and placement of the composite restorative material. Unfortunately, the curing light can only penetrate through several millimeters of composite to polymerize the underlying material. The thickness of composite that is cured by a light source is called the **depth of cure**. The depth of cure varies depending on the time of light exposure, the composite product, the shade of that product, and the curing light. If the composite material nearest the pulp is not fully cured, pulpal irritation and postoperative sensitivity are more likely to occur. To prevent this situation, the composite material is placed in a thin layer (>3 mm thick) at the bottom of the preparation and cured before the next layer or increment is placed.

2. Incremental Addition

Placing dental composites in layers, which is commonly called **incremental addition**, not only assures adequate polymerization but provides a secondary benefit as well. Composites shrink approximately 2% when they set. Polymerization shrinkage continues to be a problem with dental composites, just as it was (although to a much greater extent) with acrylic resin materials. Dentists learned to place acrylic resins in layers, allowing the first layer to set and shrink toward the tooth before adding additional layers. The same process is used with dental composites. The first layer is placed into the cavity preparation and is cured. If placed properly, the first layer shrinks toward the tooth. The second and any subsequent layers are then placed and cured until the tooth is adequately restored to form and function.

3. Air Inhibition

When composite materials are placed in increments, each increment chemically bonds to the previous one. Chemical bonding occurs because addition polymerization is inhibited by atmospheric oxygen. This inhibition of the reaction results in a thin layer of unreacted material on the surface of a newly set composite (if the surface was exposed to air when it set). The thin, air-inhibited layer does not cure, regardless of whether light activation or chemically activated material is involved. When a second layer is added, it excludes oxygen, and the air-inhibited layer and the new material are chemically bonded together when the second layer is cured. The air-inhibited layer on a dental composite has a tacky feel. Composite surfaces adjacent to the tooth structure or a matrix band are not exposed to atmospheric oxygen, and their setting reaction is not inhibited.

4. Unreacted C=C Bonds

Not only can composite materials be placed in layers and bonded together but also new composite will bond to old composite. Why? Not all C=C bonds react when a dental composite sets. Typically, only about 50% of the C=C bonds react. Therefore, it is possible to repair or add to a composite restoration by cleaning the surface and then properly adding new material. Some of the unreacted C=C bonds in the old material will react with the setting matrix of the new material. The strength of the bond is much lower than that of a newly placed, solid piece of material, but adding new composite material to an old composite is not uncommon.

F. Placement of a Composite Restoration

A brief summary of the placement of a composite restoration is provided:
1. Diagnose the lesion.
2. Determine the shade or shades that are needed.
3. Isolate the area to be treated, preferably with a rubber dam.
4. Cut the cavity preparation, including beveling enamel margins.
5. Determine the need for a cavity liner, and place if necessary. (The liner protects the pulp from the acid etchant when the cavity preparation is very deep.)
6. Etch, prime, place, and cure the adhesive.
7. Incrementally place and cure the composite material.
8. Finish (proper anatomical contours).
9. Check for proximal contacts.
10. Examine for voids and marginal defects with a mirror and explorer. Use dental floss to detect any overhangs.
11. Polish (lustrous surface).
12. Remove the rubber dam.
13. Check occlusion and adjust if needed.

G. Detecting Composite Restorations

Detecting a well-placed composite restoration can be difficult. A good shade match and excellent margins may make composite restorations nearly "invisible," but they do feel a bit softer than enamel to a sharp explorer. Composite restorations appear either radiopaque or radiolucent on radiographs, depending on the filler in the product. Composite materials have evolved from being very radiolucent to having a radiopacity somewhat like that of tooth structure. The radiopacity of composites aids in their detection and in the detection of recurrent caries. The radiopacity of composites is accomplished by making the fillers radiopaque. Barium and other heavier elements have been added to the engineered glass that is the starting material in the manufacture of fillers. Chapters 14 and 15 discuss the clinical detection and radiographic appearance of composite restorations, respectively.

H. Pit and Fissure Sealants

Pit and fissure sealants are preventive materials applied to the susceptible pits and fissures of teeth to prevent or reduce caries. Current recommendations for use of pit and fissure sealants are based on the clinical and radiographic assessment of the tooth and the caries risk of the patient. Caries risk factors include past history of caries, diet, salivary flow and buffering capacity, fluoride exposure, and oral hygiene.

1. Purpose

Fluoridation of water and toothpaste have greatly reduced smooth surface dental caries. However, pit and fissure caries continue to be common. If one examines a few patients older than 40 years of age, one commonly sees that the pits and fissures of their molars have been restored.

Pit and fissure sealants are effective in reducing caries and the need to restore teeth. The goal is to fill susceptible pits and fissures with a polymeric material, thus depriving cariogenic bacteria of a niche to colonize, as illustrated in Figure 1.11. Pit and fissure materials use the acid-etch technique to bond the material to enamel. It is an acceptable responsibility of the dental hygienist to place and maintain sealants.

2. Placement of Sealants

Placement of a sealant begins with isolation of the surface, usually using cotton rolls, a rubber dam, or other means. Next, the surface is typically cleaned with a slurry of pumice, rinsed, and dried. The tooth is then etched, rinsed with water, and aggressively dried (desiccated). The sealant is placed as a final step. The sealant is allowed to set if the material is chemically activated, but currently, light-activated sealants are more commonly used. This is the same acid-etching procedure that was used for composite restorations before the development of dentinal bonding agents. Isolation during the procedure is very important. Sealant products vary in filler composition and color. Some sealant materials have no filler; others have a small percentage of filler. Some products are clear; others are opaque white in appearance. The placement of pit and fissure sealants is presented in detail in Chapter 25.

3. Use of Primers with Sealants

If isolation is difficult, an alternative procedure is to etch, rinse, and dry, then use a primer from a dentinal bonding system or a one-step self-etching adhesive, and finally place the sealant. The primer is believed to help the sealant wet a slightly contaminated surface. Improved retention of the sealant occurs.

4. Maintenance of Sealants

Sealants commonly wear and chip during function as a result of occlusal forces. Periodic examination of sealants for loss, fractures, or caries is an important responsibility of the dental hygienist. Some sealants will need to be reapplied when they are lost. The clinical reduction of dental caries as a result of sealant use is well established.

I. Preventive Resin Restoration

Some research has shown sealed dental caries to remain inactive, but most clinicians are not ready to routinely leave decay in developmental pits by sealing over this potential problem. A conservative approach to pit and fissure decay, called **preventive resin restoration** (PRR), was developed in the 1980s.

1. Placement of PRR

The original description of a PRR is shown in *Figure 5.10*. It was a combination of a pit and fissure sealant and a composite restoration. In the first step, the suspicious pit is opened with a bur, and any existing caries are removed. If the preparation is solely in enamel, the restoration is classified as a PRR. If the caries extends into the dentin, the restoration is classified as a composite restoration. The tooth is then etched and primed, and the adhesive is placed. The prepared pit is filled with composite material. Any pits and fissures not filled by the composite or adhesive are filled with sealant. A great deal of tooth structure is preserved by placing a PRR compared to the traditional class I cavity

preparation developed by G.V. Black in the late 1800s.

2. Air Abrasion Systems

Some clinicians are using air abrasion systems to remove debris and decay from pits and fissures and then placing sealants, preventive resins, and composites. Air abrasion systems utilize high-velocity stream of air that carries very hard ceramic particles (aluminum oxide) and abrades the tooth, similar to industrial sandblasters. These systems are different from the "Prophy-Jet" that uses baking soda to remove stains from the surface of teeth. Air abrasion systems can effectively cut enamel and dentin, cut cavity preparations, and remove composite materials. Eliminating the use of pumice and prophy cup to prepare (clean) enamel surfaces is another advantage of air abrasion systems. However, a rubber dam is required to protect the patient's airway from the dust and debris that result from an air abrasion system.

3. Hard Tissue Lasers

Dental lasers that cut enamel, dentin, and composite materials are becoming common. Many patients do not require anesthesia for the use of such lasers. Hard tissue lasers are ideal for cleaning debris from pits and fissures when placing sealants, PRRs, and composites.

J. Composite Cements

1. Composition

Composite cements or luting materials have the same structure and composition as other dental composites. They are a resin matrix reinforced with filler. Composite cements have a greater percentage of resin to increase flow and smaller-sized particles for a lower film thickness. Composite cements are presented in greater detail in Chapter 7.

2. Use

One advantage of composite cements is their ability to bond restorations to the tooth structure. Composite cements are the luting material of choice for ceramic restorations. They are also used when retention of a preparation is less than desired. Examples include crown preparations that are short in height or of a shape with "little holding power" (excessive taper).

K. Other Uses of Composite Materials

1. Indirect Composite Restorations

Composite restorations can be made indirectly by a dental laboratory. To improve strength, indirect composite materials can be processed at higher temperatures and pressures than the oral cavity can tolerate. Laboratory-processed

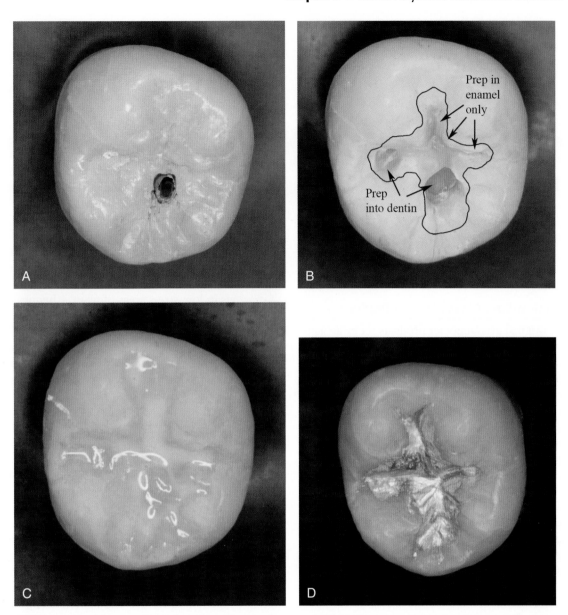

FIGURE 5.10. Photographs of **A.** molar with decay in several pits, **B.** the decay removed and the central groove opened, **C.** restored with a preventive resin restoration, and **D.** with the preventive resin restoration removed and restored with a conventional cavity preparation and amalgam. Note the amount of tooth structure conserved by the preventive resin restoration.

composite restorations require an impression of the prepared teeth and a cast. A second appointment is needed to cement the restoration. Recently, several innovative laboratory-processed composite materials have been introduced, including CAD/CAM techniques. Fiber reinforcement has been tried to increase strength to enable the construction of composite crowns and short-span bridges.

2. Composites as Alternatives to Acrylic Resins
Because composite materials are superior in strength and other properties to acrylic resin materials, they have begun to replace acrylic resin materials in a variety of uses. This replacement

has been slow to occur, however, because of the increased expense of composite materials. Some of these acrylic resin replacement composites are a polyester resin cross-linked with a bis-GMA–type monomer by addition polymerization monomer. (This is how fiberglass is made.) Composite materials are now used for temporary crowns, denture teeth, custom tray materials, and other laboratory uses. One example of a crown and bridge temporary material and mixing gun are shown in *Figure 5.11*. The construction of temporary crowns is presented in Chapter 35. Several products are laboratory light-cure materials, and again, additional details are presented in Chapter 11, Removable Prostheses.

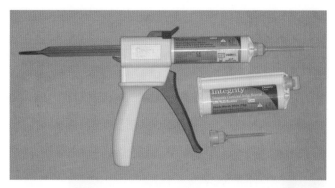

FIGURE 5.11. A crown and bridge temporary material. This paste/paste system is mixed in the baffle of the mixing tip, as is common with impression materials.

VI. Glass Ionomer Materials

A. Chemical-Cure Glass Ionomer Products

The original glass ionomer products set by an acid–base chemical reaction. These are sometimes called chemical-cure or conventional glass ionomers. Glass ionomer materials were the first truly adhesive restorative materials. They chemically bond to enamel and dentin as described in Chapter 4, Adhesive Materials. Glass ionomer materials release fluoride over time; it is commonly thought that this fluoride inhibits recurrent decay. The chemistry of glass ionomer and other dental cements is covered in Chapter 7. Glass ionomer restorations are "tooth colored" but opaque in appearance. Their esthetics are inferior to those of dental composites. In this chapter, the use and properties of glass ionomer restorative materials are presented.

Glass ionomer restorative materials (acid–base reaction only) are supplied as powder/liquid systems; a variety of shades are available for most products. Proper mixing and placement are critical. The proper powder/liquid ratio is mixed, and a viscous material (much like icing for a cake) results. Many products are available in preproportioned capsules that are mixed with an amalgamator (see Fig. 7.7B). The freshly mixed material is placed into the cavity preparation without delay and then contoured to the proper shape. Sometimes, plastic strips are used to hold the material in the proper shape while it sets.

Placement of chemical-cure (acid–base reaction only) glass ionomer restorations is technique sensitive. If mixing is too slow or placement is delayed, the adhesive property of the material is lost. In addition, these glass ionomer materials are susceptible to dehydration during the initial setting of the material and the finishing of the restoration. If not protected from dehydration, surface crazing occurs. **Crazing** is the formation of many shallow surface cracks. After the initial finishing, a protective sealant is painted on to cover the newly placed glass ionomer material. Enamel bonding resins, as described in Chapter 4, Adhesive Materials, or special varnishes are used as a protective sealant. The final polishing of these glass ionomer materials is typically delayed for 24 hours to allow the material to set completely. At a subsequent appointment, the final polish achieves optimum surface smoothness and esthetics. Chemical-cure glass ionomer materials have a high initial solubility in oral fluids, but their solubility is low after the setting reaction is complete.

The advantages of adhesion and fluoride release make chemical-cure glass ionomers useful materials, but their shortcomings have limited their clinical use. Glass ionomer products are very popular for use as luting cements and as restorative materials in low-stress areas of teeth. Chemical-cure glass ionomer restorative materials are brittle. Poor wear resistance and fracture toughness limit their use to class I and II restorations in deciduous teeth. The fluoride release makes glass ionomer restorative materials the material of choice for class V lesions in patients with a high risk of caries.

B. Resin-Modified Glass Ionomer Products

Resin-modified glass ionomer products were developed in the late 1980s (Table 5.2). They are also called resin-reinforced glass ionomers. They have the same acid–base setting reaction of conventional glass ionomer materials in addition to free radical polymerization, whether it is light or chemically activated. Light-activated polymerization products set when exposed to the same curing light that is used for composites. Light-activated products are popular because of their "cure on demand" setting reaction. They are still adhesive, and they release fluoride. Light-activated glass ionomer restorations are easier to place and finish, and they are not as sensitive to dehydration as their chemical-cure counterparts. At the time of placement, light-activated glass ionomers are finished and polished. They are a little stronger and tougher than chemically activated glass ionomers. Light-activated glass ionomers are currently quite popular for class III and V restorations; several class V restorations are shown in *Figure 5.12*. In addition, light-activated glass ionomer liners are popular products.

C. Acid–Base Chemically Activated Resin-Modified Glass Ionomer Products

The superiority of resin-modified glass ionomer restorative materials in terms of mechanical properties resulted in a market for similar luting materials. Because light is ineffective in curing material under a metal crown, chemically activated (addition

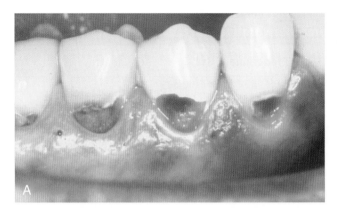
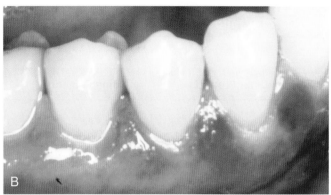

FIGURE 5.12. **A.** Several class V carious lesions and **B.** light-cure glass ionomer restorations. (Courtesy of GC America, Inc.)

polymerization) glass ionomer materials, which also incorporate the acid–base reaction, have been developed. They are considered by many to be the "state of the art" for luting metal and porcelain-fused-to-metal crowns.

D. Recharging Fluoride in Glass Ionomer Materials

Laboratory studies have shown that glass ionomer materials release fluoride. Dentists use glass ionomer materials in hopes of preventing decay by this fluoride release. This fluoride release decreases over time. Other laboratory studies have shown that glass ionomer materials can have their fluoride "recharged" with topical fluoride treatments. The result is a significant increase in the fluoride released by "old" glass ionomer material. Acid–base glass ionomer materials, both initially and after recharging, release more fluoride than resin-modified materials.

VII. Compomers

Because of the popularity of glass ionomer materials and composite/dentinal bonding systems, a combination of the two materials was developed and was once quite popular. The "**compomer**" label is used to describe materials that

bond and set like dentinal bonding/composite systems but that initially release some fluoride-like glass ionomers. Some of these products are a bit-like glass ionomers, but most are very much like composites. Compomers typically use the same dentinal bonding systems as composites do. Some initially release fluoride, but clinical data showing a reduction in recurrent caries are lacking. The promise of fluoride release and good handling characteristics resulted in the large number of compomer products, but few are currently available.

VIII. Selecting Restorative Materials

The current market in adhesive polymeric restorative materials is a continuum, ranging from chemical-cure glass ionomers at one end to composites at the other end, as illustrated in *Figure 5.13*. Many times, choosing a product for a particular restoration in an individual patient is a matter of the dentist's personal preference rather than a decision based on a material's physical properties or clinical data. The patient's desires for an esthetic material and the strength required by the location of a restoration are also significant factors in the selection of a product. Handling characteristics are an important consideration as well. Brand names of adhesive restorative materials are included in Tables 5.1 and 5.2.

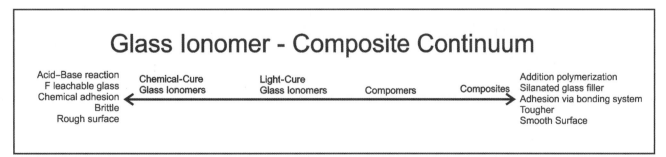

FIGURE 5.13. A continuum of direct esthetic restorative materials.

TABLE 5.2. Brand Names of Glass Ionomer and Compomer Restorative Materials

Glass Ionomer Products	Predominant Uses		
	Luting Cements	Liners	Restorative Material
Acid–base reaction only	Ketac-Cem	HI	Fuji II LC; Fuji IX; Fuji Triage
	Fuji I		Ketac-Silver; Ketac-Fil
			Fuji Miracle Mix
Acid–base reaction and chemically activated polymerization	GC Fuji Cem; GC Fuji Plus	N/A	N/A
	RelyX Luting Plus		
Acid–base reaction and light-activated polymerization[a]	HI	Vitrebond	Fuji II LC
		GC Fuji Lining LC	Ketac-Nano
		Vivaglass Liner	Vitremer
Compomers (light-activated polymerization)	N/A	N/A	F2000
			Dyract

[a]Some products also include chemically activated polymerization.
HI, mostly products of historical interest; N/A, not applicable.

Summary

The first acrylic resins used in dentistry were the "pink portion" of a denture base. Later, they were also used as a tooth-colored restorative material. Since then, materials scientists have developed composite materials with greatly improved properties. Filler particles made of ceramic materials were added to improve strength. Silane coupling agents, a coating over the filler particles, transfer the stress from the unfilled matrix portion of the composite to the filler particle.

Composite restorative material may be cured in two ways: chemical reaction (chemically activated) or light activation (photo cure). Chemically activated materials are two-paste systems that blend into one color. Working time to place and contour the material is limited because of the "auto" setting reaction. It is also easy to incorporate bubbles during mixing. Light-cure materials are more commonly used and are supplied as single-paste materials. No mixing is required; therefore, voids are minimized and result in a stronger restoration. With light-cure composites, working time is essentially unlimited because they will not set until the curing light is activated.

Dental composites fall into three categories: macrofilled, microfilled, and hybrid. The categories are named for their particle size. The current practice of dentistry is dominated by hybrid composite materials.

Hybrid composites are strong and result in a smooth surface. Microfills are indicated for class V lesions and times when surface luster is a major concern.

For the most part, pit and fissure sealants are unfilled (or slightly filled) resins that flow into the enamel pit and fissures areas of occlusal surfaces. They, too, are supplied as either light-activated or chemically activated products. The acid-etch process is used to bond sealants to enamel. It is the responsibility of the hygienist to periodically examine sealants for loss, fracture, or caries.

Preventive resin restorations are a combination of a pit and fissure sealant with a composite restoration. The suspicious pit is opened with a bur. Caries are removed, and the pit is then etched and primed. Finally, the adhesive is placed.

Another use of composite materials is for restorations made indirectly in a dental laboratory. This type of restoration requires an impression, and the patient must return for a second appointment for the cementation. Still other uses include temporary crowns, denture teeth, and custom tray materials.

Glass ionomers are another esthetic restorative material that chemically bond to enamel and dentin. They were the first truly adhesive restorative materials.

Glass ionomers have been improved by resin reinforcement and can be activated chemically or by light. All glass ionomer materials release fluoride into the adjacent tooth structure. Chemical-cure glass ionomers are supplied as powder/liquid systems. They may be used in low-stress areas of teeth; however, there are shortcomings. This type of glass ionomer is brittle, has poor fracture toughness, and has poor wear resistance.

Light-activated glass ionomers are also called resin-modified glass ionomers. They are easier to place and finish, less sensitive to dehydration, and a little stronger and tougher. They are used for class III and V restorations.

This chapter has presented many adhesive polymeric restorative materials from which a dentist may choose. The choice may be made based on the dentist's personal preference rather than on the material's physical properties or clinical data. The patient's desire for esthetics and the strength required of the restoration are other significant factors. Composites and glass ionomers are two of the many dental materials that the dental hygienist must be able to identify as well as assess and maintain during the patient's routine dental visits. The remaining chapters assist the clinician in accomplishing these goals.

Learning Activities

1. Cure a 1-mm-thick (5- by 5-mm) sample of composite with one side against a Mylar strip (bottom) and the other side exposed to air (top). Feel the sticky air-inhibited layer on the top, and compare this surface with the bottom.

2. Place additional composite material on the top surface of the above sample. Cure and attempt to push the second increment off the first. Describe the force required.

3. Make composite samples of several types of composites listed in Table 5.1. Feel the surface with an explorer. Compare the surfaces for roughness and surface luster.

4. Make Rice Krispies treats with different marshmallow/cereal ratios. How do the different mixtures feel when eaten? Crunchy? Chewy? What happens if too much cereal is added? Give the leftovers from the bad batches to your least favorite teacher. Send the good stuff to our troops overseas.

Review Questions

Question 1. One problem with polymers is their high coefficients of thermal expansion. These coefficients can be _____ to _____ times greater than that of tooth structure.

a. 1 to 3
b. 3 to 5
c. 2 to 5
d. 2 to 10

Question 2. Which of the following components of restorative resins acts as a "coating" and serves to transfer stress from a weak component to a stronger one?

a. Matrix
b. Filler particle
c. Silane coupling agent
d. Polymers
e. Adhesives

Question 3. What advantage do microfilled composites have compared to macrofilled composites?

a. Low coefficient of thermal expansion
b. Smooth and lustrous polished surface
c. Greater overall strength
d. Higher percentage of filler

Question 4. Which of the following characteristics best describes chemical-cure composite restorative materials?

a. Unlimited working time
b. Supplied as single-paste materials
c. May incorporate air bubbles during mixing
d. Contains less matrix and more filler particles

Question 5. A specific amount of composite (thickness) that is cured by a light source is termed:

a. Depth of cure
b. Incremental addition
c. Depth of addition
d. Incremental polymerization

Question 6. The size of the filler particles in a dental composite determines the:

a. Polymerization reaction
b. Technique for incremental additions
c. Etching time before the primer and adhesive are placed
d. Surface smoothness of the resulting restoration

Question 7. The _____ composite restorative materials are those with a lower viscosity (decreased filler) to aid in placement.

a. Preventive resin
b. Hybrid
c. Flowable
d. Condensable

Question 8. Hybrid composites are recommended for:

a. Surface luster
b. Areas needing strength
c. Low-stress areas
d. Class V restorations

Question 9. A combination of a pit and fissure sealant and a composite restoration is termed:

a. Flowable composite
b. Condensable composite
c. Compomer
d. Preventive resin restoration

Question 10. Abrasion resistance for hybrid composite restorative material is said to be:

a. Poor
b. Fair
c. Good
d. Very good

Question 11. Thermal expansion for microfill composite restorative material is considered to be:

a. Poor
b. Fair
c. Good
d. Very good

Question 12. Which composite material has the largest percentage of filler by weight?

a. Microfill
b. Hybrid
c. Macrofill
d. Flowable

Question 13. Composite materials that polymerize using light activation are:

a. Initiated by mixing
b. Not as popular as chemically activated resins
c. Supplied as a single paste
d. Lack the "set on demand" characteristic

Question 14. A restorative material that initially releases some fluoride (like glass ionomers) but bonds and sets like composites is called:

a. Flowable composites
b. Condensable composite
c. Compomer
d. Preventive resin restoration

Question 15. Which of the following best describes microfill composite materials?

a. Abrasion resistance is poor; filler size is 10 to 25 microns
b. Abrasion resistance is poor; strength is high
c. Polishability is poor; strength is high
d. Polishability is very good; strength is low

Amalgam

Objectives

After studying this chapter, the student will be able to do the following:

1. Differentiate between an amalgam alloy and a dental amalgam.
2. Compare the composition of conventional and high-copper dental amalgams.
3. Describe the function (effects) of the major elements of dental amalgams.
4. Discuss the self-sealing property of amalgam.
5. List and describe the three shapes of amalgam alloy particles.
6. Describe the effect of moisture contamination on amalgam.
7. Describe the use and advantages of direct gold restorations.

Optional

8. Discuss the trituration and setting processes.
9. Describe the reactions involved in both conventional and high-copper amalgams.
10. Recall the composition, relative strength, and relative corrosion resistance of the four most common amalgam phases.

Key Words/Phrases

admixed alloy
alloys
amalgam
amalgam alloy
amalgamation
amalgamator
blended alloys
cohesive gold
creep
delayed expansion
dental amalgam
direct gold
gold foil
lathe-cut alloys
precipitation
spherical alloys
trituration
triturator
working time

Introduction

Dental amalgam is a very old, but still widely used, restorative material. The present forms of amalgam evolved from the "silver paste" that was developed in the 1800s. The popularity of dental amalgam results from its cost-effectiveness and ease of use. During the 1970s and 1980s, more than a million amalgam restorations were placed each year. Dental amalgam is used in all surfaces of posterior teeth and, occasionally, in the lingual pits of anterior teeth. Use of dental amalgam is decreasing as caries prevention becomes more and more successful. Composites are also widely used as an alternative material.

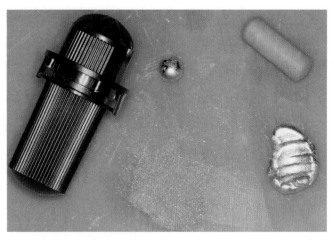

FIGURE 6.1. Starting at the *left* and moving *clockwise*: capsule, liquid mercury, pestle, freshly mixed amalgam, and powdered amalgam alloy.

I. What Is Dental Amalgam?

A. Amalgam is a metal alloy of which one of the elements is mercury (Hg). **Alloys** are metals that are a combination of several elements.

B. Dental amalgam is made by mixing approximately equal parts (by weight) of a powdered metal alloy with liquid mercury. These components are illustrated in *Figure 6.1*. The powdered metal is called an amalgam alloy and is predominantly silver (Ag) and tin (Sn). The mixing process of the alloy with the liquid mercury is called **amalgamation** or **trituration**.

A mechanical device called an **amalgamator** or **triturator**, as shown in *Figure 6.2*, "shakes" the capsule containing the alloy powder and mercury at high speed, mixing the two components into a plastic mass, as shown in *Figure 6.3*. The triturated material is reacting or setting while it is forced, or condensed, into the cavity preparation. The cavity preparation is always overfilled with amalgam. The excess is then removed (carved) to restore the original anatomy of the tooth. The condensation and carving procedures are illustrated in *Figure 6.4*.

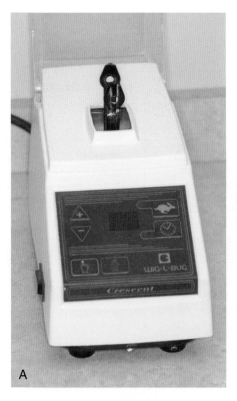

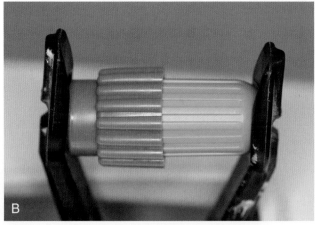

FIGURE 6.2. Photographs of **A.** a triturator and **B.** an amalgam capsule in place, ready to be triturated.

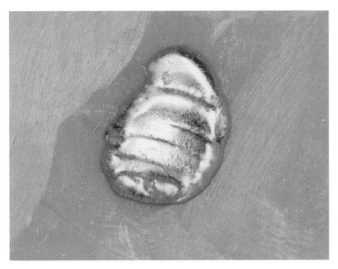

FIGURE 6.3. Photograph of properly triturated dental amalgam.

C. The setting reaction of amalgam starts during trituration and progresses while condensation and carving take place. The **working time** of amalgam (the time that is needed to condense and carve) is not directly controlled by the dentist, as it is with light-activated composites.

D. Amalgam is a direct restorative material that is held in place by mechanical retention. Examples of mechanical retention include undercuts and grooves that are placed by the dentist in the cavity preparation with a handpiece and bur. Examples of convergent undercuts and retentive grooves are shown in *Figure 6.5*.

E. The particles of the amalgam alloy may be formed by two methods.

   1. The first method used to produce dental amalgam particles is grinding an ingot of metal to produce filings. Such amalgam alloys are called

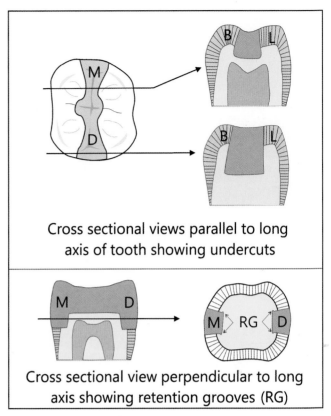

Cross sectional views parallel to long axis of tooth showing undercuts

Cross sectional view perpendicular to long axis showing retention grooves (RG)

FIGURE 6.5. Illustration of the retentive features of an amalgam restoration. Buccal (*B*), distal (*D*), lingual (*L*), and mesial (*M*) surfaces are labeled for orientation.

lathe-cut alloys, and an example is shown in *Figure 6.6A*.

   2. The second method used to produce dental amalgam particles is to spray molten metal into an inert atmosphere. The droplets cool as they fall, producing **spherical alloys**, as shown in *Figure 6.6B*.

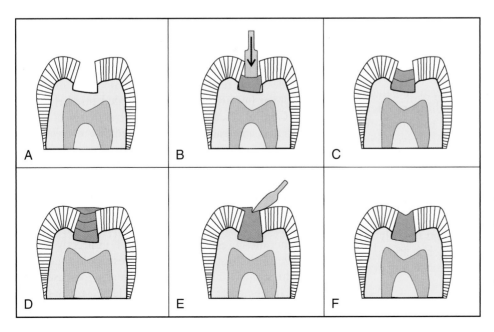

FIGURE 6.4. Illustration of condensing and carving procedures. **A.** The cavity is prepared. **B.** The first increment of amalgam is placed in the preparation and condensed to eliminate voids. **C** and **D.** The second and succeeding increments are placed until the preparation is overfilled. **E** and **F.** While still "soft," the material is carved to reproduce the proper anatomical contours.

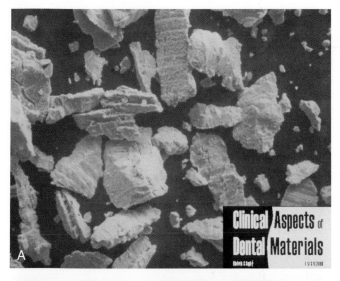

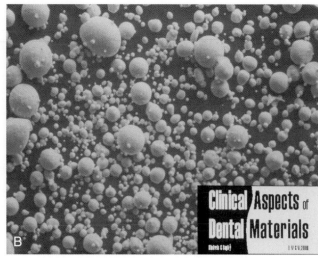

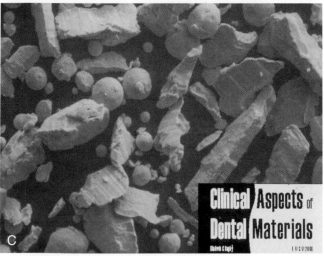

FIGURE 6.6. Scanning electron micrograph of amalgam particles. **A.** Lathe-cut amalgam alloy. **B.** Spherical amalgam alloy. **C.** Admixed amalgam alloy. (Courtesy of Special Metals Corporation, Ann Arbor, MI.)

3. Some products are a combination of both lathe-cut and spherical particles, as shown in *Figure 6.6C*. These products are called **admixed or blended alloys**.

4. Regardless of the production method used, the particles are mixed and react with liquid mercury. The result is dental amalgam.

F. It is important to note that the term "amalgam alloy" does not mean the same thing as "dental amalgam." **Amalgam alloy** is the silver–tin (Ag–Sn) powdered metal before it is mixed with mercury. Dental amalgam is the result of mixing the powdered metal with mercury and is used to restore teeth. Many times, including in this text, the terms "amalgam" and "amalgam alloy" are used. Most of the time little confusion results. Occasionally, however, it is important (usually for test questions) to understand which material is being discussed: amalgam alloy, the resulting dental amalgam, or both.

II. Advantages of Using Dental Amalgam

Because of its toughness and wear resistance, amalgam is a long-lasting, cost-effective restorative material. In addition, amalgam has the ability to seal its margins during service. As the margins corrode, the tooth/restoration interface fills with corrosion products so that microleakage is reduced. Often, margins of a dental amalgam may look broken down but are actually well sealed just below the surface. Clinical research has shown that marginal integrity of dental amalgams is a poor predictor of recurrent decay.

Amalgam is the least technique-sensitive permanent restorative material that is available to the dentist. In addition, it is the only material that might work when placed in a wet, contaminated environment.

The life expectancy of an amalgam restoration, like that of any other direct restorative material, is indirectly related to the size of the restoration. As the restoration increases in size, the stress within the restoration also increases, and the life expectancy of the restoration decreases. Based on clinical research, the life expectancy for a conservative class I amalgam is 15 to 18 years. A class II amalgam should last 12 to 15 years. It is important to remember that the patient has a great deal of influence on the longevity of restorations. The patient's diet and oral hygiene practices are very important and can contribute to a longer life expectancy of their restorations.

III. History of Dental Amalgam

A. Initial Development

Dental amalgam was developed in France in the 1800s and was introduced to the United States in 1833. At that time, the only alternatives for direct restorative materials were time consuming or ineffective. The clinical success of dental amalgam was improved greatly by the work of Flagg and Black.

B. Specification 1

In the 1920s, the National Bureau of Standards (now the National Institute of Standards and Technology) was asked by the US government to develop a set of standard tests for dental amalgam. The standard was enthusiastically received by the field of dentistry and became Specification #1 of the American Dental Association (ADA). Specifications are discussed in Chapter 1, Introduction. In the first half of the 20th century, most amalgam alloys followed the formula of G.V. Black because his composition was included in the specification.

C. Introduction of High-Copper Amalgam

Around 1960, an amalgam alloy with a higher copper (Cu) content was developed. Increasing the copper content reduced the percentage of the weakest phase of the resulting dental amalgam. Clinical performance improved markedly. Today, numerous high-copper dental amalgams are on the market, and a variety of particle shapes and compositions are available. The copper content ranges from 10% to 30%.

IV. Low-Copper Dental Amalgam

Low-copper amalgams are included in this text for historical perspective. In addition, they are a good starting point because of their simple composition and chemistry. Today, high-copper amalgams are the state of the art and dominate the market.

A. Composition

The composition of a low-copper, "traditional" or "conventional" amalgam alloy is based on Black's composition: approximately 65% silver, 25% tin, less than 6% copper, and, sometimes, 1% zinc.

B. Function of Components

1. Silver causes setting expansion and increases strength and corrosion resistance.
2. Tin causes setting contraction and decreases strength and corrosion resistance.
3. In low-copper amalgams, copper functions much the same as silver.
4. If the zinc content is greater than 0.01%, the amalgam is called a zinc-containing amalgam. If the content is less, the amalgam is called a non-zinc amalgam. During manufacture, zinc reduces oxidation of the other metals in the alloy. For many years, the clinical effect of zinc was debated. Recently, clinical research has shown that zinc-containing dental amalgams have a longer clinical life expectancy than do nonzinc amalgams.

C. Setting Reaction of Low-Copper Amalgam—Optional

$$\text{excess } Ag_3Sn\,(\gamma) + Hg \rightarrow$$
$$\text{unreacted } Ag_3Sn\,(\gamma) + Ag_2Hg_3\,(\gamma_1) + Sn_8Hg\,(\gamma_2)$$

Or, simply,

$$\gamma + Hg \rightarrow \gamma + \gamma_1 + \gamma_2$$

1. γ is the Greek letter gamma and is used to designate the Ag–Sn alloy, or gamma phase.
2. γ_1, or gamma-one, is used to designate the Ag–Hg phase.
3. γ_2, or gamma-two, is used to designate the Sn–Hg phase.
4. When the liquid mercury is mixed with the amalgam alloy, the mercury is bold absorbed by the alloy particles and dissolves the surface of the particles.
5. Silver and tin continue to dissolve in the liquid mercury, which then becomes saturated with silver and tin. New γ_1 and γ_2 phases begin to precipitate. These are new compounds, the result of the setting reaction. **Precipitation** is a process in which a solid is formed from material dissolved in a liquid. Examples of precipitation include freezing water (ice is the precipitate), sugar that forms in old honey, and the curdling of milk (milk protein is the precipitate).
6. Precipitation of the γ_1 and γ_2 phases continues until the mercury is consumed and a solid mass results. The reaction products bind the unreacted γ particles together resulting in a "cored" structure.

D. Mercury/Alloy Ratio

The composition of the set dental amalgam depends on several factors. The mercury/alloy ratio is the amount of mercury that is mixed with the amalgam alloy. Using more mercury increases the mercury-containing reaction products. Using less mercury decreases the mercury-containing reaction products. Proper trituration and condensation techniques can also reduce the mercury content of the set amalgam. Because the mercury-containing reaction products are weaker than the Ag–Sn starting material, minimizing mercury results in an improved restoration. The strength of the amalgam is increased, and marginal breakdown is reduced. Remember, as with other dental materials, the liquid mercury must wet all alloy particles and form a cohesive mass without voids. An inadequate mercury/alloy ratio results in voids and poor restorations.

E. Microstructure of Low-Copper Amalgams—Optional

Dental amalgams are a mixture of elements and phases.

1. The γ (Ag–Sn) phase is typically the strongest and most corrosion-resistant phase. It is approximately one-quarter of the volume of a dental amalgam.
2. The γ_1 (Ag–Hg) phase is somewhat strong and corrosion resistant, but it is also brittle. The γ_1 phase makes up approximately half of the amalgam and is the matrix phase that holds this multiphase material together.
3. The γ_2 (Sn–Hg) phase is the weakest and most corrosion prone. It makes up approximately one-tenth of the material, but is the "weak link" in the structure.
4. It is important to realize that the chemical formulas for amalgam phases do not include minor components, which affect the properties of each phase and of the resulting amalgam. The γ_1 (Ag–Hg) phase usually contains some copper, tin, zinc, and other amalgam alloying elements.

V. High-Copper Dental Amalgams

Starting in the 1960s, a variety of high-copper dental amalgams were developed. The clinical performance of many, but not all, of these amalgams is superior to that of the best low-copper amalgams. The significant factor that determined improved performance is elimination of the weak γ_2 phase. Strength is increased, and corrosion and marginal breakdown are reduced. Currently, high-copper amalgams dominate the dental market. These high-copper amalgams can be categorized into several groups.

A. Admix High-Copper Amalgam

"Blended," "admix," or "dispersion" alloys are a mixture of two kinds of particles, as shown in *Figure 6.6C.*

1. These high-copper amalgams contain lathe-cut particles with the same composition as those of the low-copper amalgam alloys, silver and tin. The other particles are spherical and contain 28% copper and 72% silver. This composition is called the Ag–Cu eutectic.
2. The first high-copper amalgam was "Dispersalloy," developed by Innes and Yondelis in Canada in 1963. It was originally sold to Johnson & Johnson, but the patent and trademark have since been sold several times to other dental materials companies. Several admix amalgams are available, but Dispersalloy maintains a significant market share.

B. Spherical High-Copper Amalgams

Single-composition, high-copper, spherical dental amalgams have only one shape of particle, as shown in *Figure 6.6B.* The particles are a combination of silver, tin, copper, and other elements.

The first single-composition spherical dental amalgam, "Tytin," was developed by Kamal Asgar. Again, the trademark has been sold. Many spherical single-composition alloys are available, but Tytin remains very popular and has a significant market share. Dispersalloy and Tytin are good examples of dentists' brand loyalty.

C. Setting Reactions of High-Copper Amalgams

The setting reaction of high-copper amalgams is a little more complex than in low-copper amalgams. The following is a simplified reaction; its notable feature is the lack of a γ_2 (Sn–Hg) product:

$$\text{excess AgSnCu (the alloy)} + \text{Hg} \rightarrow$$
$$\text{unreacted alloy} + \text{Ag}_2\text{Hg}_3\,(\gamma_1) + \text{Cu}_6\text{Sn}_5$$

1. The alloy contains 10% to 30% copper.
2. Silver reacts in the same manner as a low-copper amalgam, forming a γ_1 (Ag–Hg) reaction product.
3. Tin reacts with copper to form several Cu–Sn reaction products. No Sn–Hg reaction product is formed as occurs in the low-copper amalgam reaction. The microstructure of an admixed amalgam is shown in *Figure 6.7.*

D. Why So Many Different Amalgam Products?—Optional

Why do so many kinds of amalgam exist? The answer is that each has different handling characteristics.

1. Shape of the Alloy Particle
The shape of the alloy particle affects the handling characteristics of the material. Lathe-cut particles are rough and do not slide past each other easily. Therefore, the resulting freshly

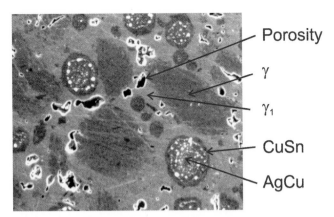

FIGURE 6.7. Scanning electron micrograph showing the microstructure of a high-copper admixed dental amalgam. (Courtesy of Drs. Bill and Sally Marshall, San Francisco, CA.)

triturated lathe-cut amalgam requires more force during condensation than is required with spherical particles. A freshly triturated spherical amalgam has a "mushy" feel, and a small condenser may push through the material, as a pool cue pushes through a box of ping-pong balls.

a. Particle shape greatly affects the amount of liquid mercury that is needed to wet the surface of the particle. Of all solids, a sphere has the lowest ratio of surface area to volume. Therefore, spherical particles need less mercury to wet the particles, and less mercury means that the reaction is finished sooner, with a faster-setting amalgam as the result.

b. With less mercury used or a lower mercury/alloy ratio, the relative percentage of mercury-containing reaction products is reduced. Because mercury-containing phases are the weaker phases, reducing the amount of mercury increases the strength and other properties of the dental amalgam.

c. Proper mixing and handling also affect the composition of the resulting dental amalgam. Proper mixing and condensation will keep porosity to a minimum. In addition, mercury can be "squeezed out" of the freshly triturated, nonspherical amalgams by using a proper condensation technique. The particles are forced together by condensation pressure, and the excess mercury is forced to the surface. Personal preference for the "feel" of amalgam when condensing and carving is a very important factor when selecting products for purchase.

2. **Silver Content of the Alloy**

The silver content of an amalgam alloy affects the cost. Several alloys have as much as 30% copper. As the copper content increases, the silver content decreases, and so does the cost of the product. The cost of amalgam itself is a minor factor in the overall cost of an amalgam restoration. On the other hand, recycling amalgam scrap is both environmentally and economically beneficial.

VI. Factors Affecting Handling and Performance

Both the manufacturer and the dentist control factors that affect the handling and performance of dental amalgam.

A. Manufacturer

The manufacturer controls
- Alloy composition
- Alloy particle shape
- Particle size
- Particle size distribution

The manufacturer also controls the rate of the setting reaction by heat treating the particles and by washing the surface of the particles with acid to remove surface oxides.

Manufacturers supply amalgam alloy in several forms, as shown in *Figure 6.8*. Amalgam alloy can be purchased as a powder, as a powder pressed into tablets (looking much like a silver aspirin), and as preproportioned disposable capsules containing both the alloy powder and mercury. With current concerns for mercury hygiene and clinical infection control, preproportioned disposable capsules are considered the standard form in most practice settings.

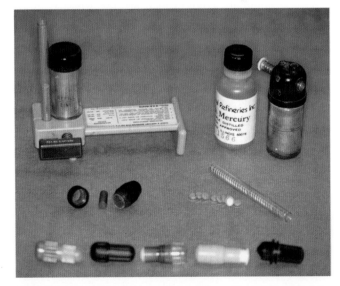

FIGURE 6.8. Several forms of amalgam alloy as supplied by their manufacturers. **Top row** (moving *left* to *right*): Alloy pellet and mercury dispenser, bulk mercury in a plastic bottle, mercury dispenser. **Center row:** Reusable capsule and amalgam alloy pellets. **Bottom row:** Several precapsulated amalgam products.

B. Dentist

Mixing and handling by the dentist and the auxiliary personnel also affect the properties of the set amalgam.

1. The manufacturer controls the mercury content when preproportioned capsules are used, but other forms of alloy require the assistant to precisely control the amount of mercury that is mixed with the alloy. Excess mercury increases the mercury-containing reaction products, which tend to be the weaker phases.

2. Proper trituration technique is required. Both the speed and time of trituration are set to obtain the proper consistency of the mix. Overtrituration and undertrituration also affect the working time and strength of the material.

   a. Overtriturated amalgam tends to crumble and is difficult to condense. It exhibits a shortened working time. In addition, voids will likely result in the restoration.

   b. Properly triturated amalgam is a cohesive mass that might be slightly warm to the touch. The surface is smooth, and the mass has a plastic feel. Such a mix is easily condensed and exhibits the proper working time.

   c. Undertriturated amalgam has a mushy-grainy feel because not all of the particles are broken up. The mass is difficult to properly condense.

   d. Examples of overtriturated, properly triturated, and undertriturated amalgam are shown in *Figure 6.9.*

3. Proper condensation techniques reduce or eliminate voids, which are the worst component of the amalgam. Although amalgam is probably the only material that might work in a wet environment, it should be condensed in a clean, dry cavity preparation. Contamination with saliva increases leakage of the restoration. If zinc-containing amalgams are contaminated by moisture when they are condensed, they will expand excessively.

4. The dentist controls the anatomical form and finishing techniques. Open interproximal contacts, overhanging margins, and other improper contours increase the likelihood of periodontal problems. Poor condensation with defects at the margins increases the likelihood of recurrent decay. Finally, undercarved occlusal surfaces cause trauma to the supporting tissues.

VII. Amalgam Properties

Several physical properties of amalgam hold particular interest for the clinician. Proper handling of the material is required for optimum results.

A. Dimensional Change

Minimal change in dimension after condensation is important. Excessive contraction leads to leakage and postoperative sensitivity. Excessive expansion can also cause postoperative sensitivity. Dimensional change is affected by many factors, such as the mercury/alloy ratio as well as trituration and condensation techniques. The best results are obtained by following the manufacturer's recommendations.

B. Strength

Amalgam restorations must resist the biting forces of occlusion. At one time, it was thought that the 1-hour compressive strength of amalgam was an important property, and this strength was incorporated into the specification. The 1-hour strength of spherical alloys is much greater than that of lathe-cut or admix amalgams. Strength at 24 hours is greater for all types of amalgams, and strength differences between the types of amalgams are much less after 24 hours. Again, the strength of the amalgam depends on the phases that are present. Having more of the stronger phases results in a stronger material.

Dental amalgam has a high compressive strength, but the tensile and shear strengths are comparatively low. Therefore, amalgam should be supported by tooth structure for clinical success in the long term, which is approximately 10 to 20 years. Also, amalgam needs sufficient bulk. A thickness of 1.5 mm or more is needed to withstand occlusal forces.

C. Creep

Creep was discussed previously in Chapter 3, Physical and Mechanical Properties of Dental Materials. **Creep** is a slow change in shape caused by compression. Creep of dental amalgam specimens is a common test and is included in the amalgam specification. It was once thought that creep provided a good indicator of clinical performance. However, when high-copper amalgams were

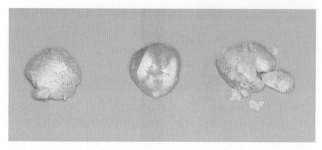

FIGURE 6.9. From *left* to *right*, undertriturated, properly triturated, and overtriturated amalgam.

developed, creep became less of a predictor of clinical success.

D. Corrosion of Dental Amalgam

Amalgam galvanically corrodes in much the same way that iron rusts. Galvanic corrosion occurs when two dissimilar metals exist in a wet environment. An electrical current flows between the two metals, and corrosion (oxidation) of one of the metals occurs. The likelihood of galvanic corrosion increases if two metallic phases are present in a metal. Dental amalgams always have more than two phases, and they also exist in a corrosive environment, the oral cavity. Therefore, amalgams corrode and, eventually, fail.

Corrosion occurs both on the surface and in the interior of the restoration. Surface corrosion discolors an amalgam restoration and may even lead to pitting. Surface corrosion also fills the tooth/amalgam interface with corrosion products, reducing microleakage. Internal corrosion (in the interior of the restoration) is hidden from the clinician. Such corrosion will lead to marginal breakdown and, occasionally, fracture. Assessing the status of an amalgam restoration for marginal breakdown and internal corrosion is beyond the current clinical diagnostic techniques. Instead, alleged recurrent decay is the dominant reason for replacing amalgam restorations. Although the restoration may look unesthetic and the margins may appear to be "ragged," the amalgam is still sealed at the interface and serves the patient well.

An acidic environment promotes galvanic corrosion. Poor oral hygiene and a cariogenic diet will expose both teeth and restorative materials to a destructive environment. The same factors that promote caries will accelerate corrosion. Therefore, patient behavior can affect the longevity of amalgam and other restorations.

E. Working and Setting Times

The working and setting times of dental amalgams are not well-standardized properties. Fast-set and slow-set versions of many brands are sold. The fast-set version of a given product will set faster than does the regular-set version of that product. However, that same fast-set version may not be faster than the regular-set version of a different product. Personal preference for working and setting times is a very important factor when selecting products for purchase.

VIII. Use of Dental Amalgam

Amalgam is used to restore many different types of carious lesions and tooth fractures, as shown in *Figure 6.10*.

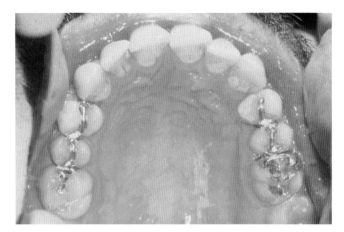

FIGURE 6.10. Photograph of a maxillary arch with several amalgam restorations. (Courtesy of Dr. Ted Stevens, Morgantown, WV.)

Again, amalgam is a very cost-effective restorative material and is used to restore class I, II, V, and VI carious lesions. At times, amalgam is used for small cingulum pits in the lingual of anterior teeth.

Amalgam is also used as a foundation for a future crown to restore a severely decayed tooth, as shown in *Figure 6.11*. The amalgam restoration is called an "amalgam buildup" or "amalgam core" when it is initially placed. An amalgam buildup that has been prepared with a dental handpiece for a crown is shown in Figure 8.1A. Such a large amalgam restoration may function adequately for 5 to 6 years, but not nearly as long as it would function when also restored with a crown (15–20 years) (see Fig. 1.4).

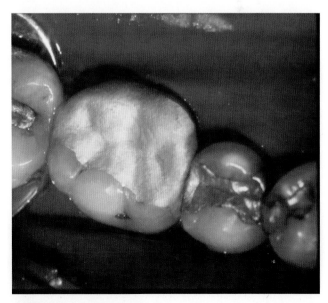

FIGURE 6.11. Photograph of a large amalgam restoring the mesial, distal, occlusal, and lingual surfaces of a mandibular first molar. This could function as a permanent restoration or be prepared and serve as a core for a crown, as shown in Figure 8.1A. (Courtesy of Dr. Ted Stevens, Morgantown, WV.)

A. Selection of the Amalgam Alloy

It is recommended that dentists use only ADA-accepted, high-copper alloys. Many outstanding products are on the market. These products have differences in particle shape, rate of set, and other factors that affect the "feel" of these materials. One must choose an alloy based on personal preference, but the product should have independent clinical research data available that detail its clinical life expectancy. Some products are definitely better than others.

B. Effect of Moisture

As with any dental material, the quality of an amalgam restoration is reduced if it is placed in a wet or contaminated preparation. Zinc-containing amalgams are more affected than nonzinc materials by moisture. Zinc reacts with water to produce hydrogen gas. The hydrogen gas causes the amalgam restoration to expand, seeming to push it out of the preparation. **Delayed expansion** is illustrated in *Figure 6.12*. Increased corrosion and reduced clinical longevity result. Amalgam should not be handled with bare hands because even the moisture from one's skin can cause problems. Current standard precautions, when mixing and placing amalgam make this a moot point.

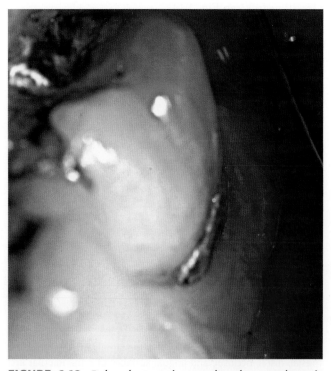

FIGURE 6.12. Delayed expansion results when amalgam is condensed in a contaminated cavity preparation.

C. Finishing and Polishing

The relative value of polishing amalgam restorations has been debated. It is not uncommon for the first few amalgams placed by a dental student or auxiliary to need finishing and polishing at a second appointment. In addition, an amalgam (placed by another dentist) may need to be recontoured or smoothed on occasion due to chipping or corrosion. It is important for the dentist to recontour any amalgam needing such care regardless of when or where it was placed. Providing such treatment is considered to be quality patient care.

The goal of finishing an amalgam restoration is to produce margins that are continuous with adjoining tooth structure and to produce proper contours. Polishing produces a smooth and lustrous surface that reduces both the likelihood of corrosion and the ability of plaque to adhere to the surface. Appropriate finishing and polishing of amalgam restorations improve their appearance, as illustrated in *Figure 6.10*. The finishing and polishing of amalgams are presented in Chapter 26 and are often the responsibility of the dental hygienist at recall appointments.

D. Mercury Toxicity

Mercury toxicity is a concern in dentistry because mercury and its chemical compounds are toxic to the kidneys and the central nervous system. Proper handling of mercury will prevent harm to office staff. The most significant danger is from mercury vapor. Mercury has a high vapor pressure and evaporates at room temperature. The lungs absorb most of the mercury vapor in air when inhaled. Poor mercury hygiene will subject office staff to unnecessary risk. It is important that the ADA recommendations for mercury hygiene are followed. These recommendations include proper handling and storage along with prompt cleaning of all mercury spills. Safety in the dental office is addressed in Chapter 20.

Mercury toxicity is not a problem for patients. Numerous government and nongovernment scientific panels have rebuffed claims of mercury toxicity in patients. The only exception is patients who are truly allergic to mercury. Very few cases (<0.1% of patients) of mercury allergy have been reported in the scientific literature. Dentists who urge patients to replace amalgam restorations to cure medical problems are not practicing ethical dentistry. Several such dentists have lost their licenses.

Mercury in the environment is an important problem. The role that dentistry plays in mercury contamination is under investigation. Significant mercury contamination problems are from industrial sources, however, and not from dentistry.

IX. Direct Gold Restorations

Another direct metallic restorative material is direct gold. Pure gold will cold-weld to itself at room temperature. In dentistry, pure or nearly pure gold was used to place small restorations, as shown in *Figure 6.13*. **Gold foil** is also called **direct gold** or **cohesive gold**. Gold foil restorations require extreme attention to detail and considerable skill.

Because chair time and labor costs (not the cost of the material) are high, other materials have significant economic and esthetic advantages. If properly placed, gold foil restorations are very long lasting. Use of gold foil is limited to small class I, II, III, and V restorations because it lacks strength compared to other metallic restorations. Direct gold is also used to repair defects in gold crowns. Due to cost and esthetics, direct gold is rarely used and would most likely be seen only in older patients.

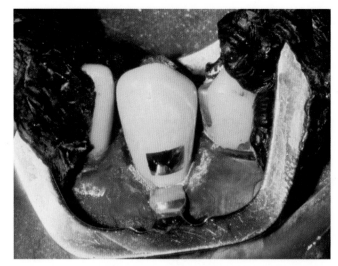

FIGURE 6.13. A gold foil restoration isolated with a #212 (butterfly) retainer and rubber dam. The retainer is stabilized with impression compound. (Courtesy of Dr. Birgitta Brown, Morgantown, WV.)

Summary

Dental amalgam is a direct restorative material that is used in all surfaces of the posterior teeth and, sometimes, in the lingual pits of anterior teeth. Dental amalgam is made by mixing approximately equal parts of a powdered metal alloy with mercury. It is held in the cavity preparation by mechanical retention. The particle shape of the alloy is manufactured in two forms: spherical and lathe-cut (filings). A combination of both comprises admixed (also called blended or dispersion) alloys. Use of dental amalgam has several advantages. It is long lasting, cost-effective, and able to seal its margins over time. The development of high-copper amalgams has significantly improved the clinical performance of amalgam as a restorative material. The restorations are stronger and have less marginal breakdown.

The manufacturer and the dentist both control the handling and performance characteristics of dental amalgam. The manufacturer controls the alloy composition, particle shape, particle size, and particle size distribution. The manufacturer also controls the rate of the setting reaction and the form in which it may be purchased. The dentist controls the trituration technique, the method of condensation, and the anatomical form and finishing techniques.

Dental amalgam reaches its maximum stress after 24 hours. The compressive strength is high, but the tensile and shear strengths are comparatively low. It is used for class I, II, V, and VI carious lesions. It can also be used as a foundation for a crown when the tooth is severely decayed. This is called an "amalgam buildup" or an "amalgam core."

Finishing and polishing of dental amalgam will extend the lifetime of the restoration. The goal of finishing is to produce a continuous margin with the adjoining tooth structure. Polishing produces a smooth and lustrous surface that reduces corrosion and plaque adherence. It is a well-accepted responsibility of the hygienist to finish and polish amalgams.

Mercury toxicity has been a concern in dentistry for decades. If not handled properly, mercury can be harmful to both patients and office staff. The recommendations by the ADA as well as mandates from Occupational Safety and Health Administration that address proper handling, storage, and cleaning greatly minimize the risk of using this material. As of this writing, no scientific evidence shows that dental amalgam is harmful to the patient or to dental personnel.

Learning Activities

1. Condense a spherical amalgam and an admix amalgam into a simple simulated cavity preparation, such as a washer from a hardware store. Note any difference in the handling or "feel" between the two materials.

2. Overtriturate (by increasing the speed and time settings on the triturator) an amalgam mix, and note the difference in handling characteristics compared to those mixed in learning activity 1.

3. Observe the amalgam restorations in the mouth of a classmate or the restorations charted for several patients. Which surfaces of their teeth are restored with amalgam?

Discuss the advantages of amalgam compared to alternative materials, such as a composite resin.

4. Working alone or in small groups, use a collection of extracted teeth to find amalgam restorations with the following conditions:
   - An amalgam overhang
   - A fracture
   - Pitting and/or corrosion
   - Submarginal area (see Chapter 26)
   - Overextensions or flash (see Chapter 26)
   - Delayed expansion

Review Questions

Question 1. Which of the following elements is used in the highest amount in an amalgam restoration?

a. Tin
b. Copper
c. Silver
d. Mercury
e. Aluminum

Question 2. Amalgam is strongest in _____ strength after it has set.

a. Shear
b. Tensile
c. Compressive
d. Bending

Question 3. The elements composing the gamma-two (γ_2) phase (the weakest and most corrosion-prone phase) of the amalgam reaction are:

a. Silver and tin
b. Silver and mercury
c. Tin and mercury
d. Tin and tin

Question 4. The function of silver in the amalgam reaction is to:

a. Reduce strength and corrosion resistance
b. Increase strength and corrosion resistance
c. Minimize oxidation
d. Maximize oxidation

Question 5. Control of the mercury content during mixing and condensing of amalgam must be carefully considered because:

a. The higher the mercury content, the higher the strength and the lower the marginal breakdown
b. The lower the mercury content, the higher the strength and the lower the marginal breakdown
c. The higher the mercury content, the higher the strength and the greater the marginal breakdown
d. The lower the mercury content, the higher the strength and the greater the marginal breakdown

Question 6. The single most important feature that accounts for the clinical success of amalgam restorations is:

a. Finish and polish
b. Marginal seal
c. Economy
d. Ease of manipulation

Question 7. The manufacturers of dental amalgam control all of the following except:

a. Alloy composition
b. Rate of setting reaction
c. Proper trituration technique
d. Particle size

Question 8. An amalgam restoration that has been finished and polished:

a. Reduces the ability of plaque to adhere

b. Resists tarnish and corrosion

c. Will not have any voids

d. Is more likely to have continuous margins with tooth structure

e. All of the above

f. a, b, and d

g. a, c, and d

Question 9. In the low-copper or traditional amalgam reaction, tin reacts with mercury. In the high-copper amalgam reaction, tin reacts with:

a. Silver

b. Copper

c. Zinc

d. Mercury

Question 10. The life expectancy of an amalgam restoration is indirectly related to the size of the restoration. As the restoration increases in size, internal stresses decrease, as does the life expectancy.

a. The first statement is true; the second statement is false.

b. The first statement is false; the second statement is true.

c. Both statements are true.

d. Both statements are false.

Question 11. Ashley was condensing an amalgam during lab, and she noticed that the triturated amalgam had a softer, "mushy" feel. What type of alloy did she most likely use in the mixed amalgam?

a. Spherical

b. Lathe-cut

c. Admixed

d. Blended

Question 12. Just after Jennifer triturated her amalgam, the appearance of it was "crumbly" and dry. It already looked set. The amalgam was most likely:

a. Mixed with an increased mercury/alloy ratio

b. Overtriturated

c. Properly triturated

d. Undertriturated

Question 13. Amalgam may be used for a variety of restorative procedures. ALL of the following pertain to the use of amalgam EXCEPT:

a. Good service to patients at a reasonable cost

b. For cingulum pit areas on the lingual of anterior teeth

c. Amalgam cores

d. Restoring class I, II, IV, and V caries

Question 14. It has been reported in the scientific literature that _____% of dental patients have a TRUE mercury allergy.

a. 0.01

b. 0.05

c. 0.1

d. 1.0

Question 15. The use of gold foil is limited to small restorations because of its:

a. Short-term longevity

b. Low strength compared to other restorative materials

c. High cost of gold foil compared to other materials

d. Unique handling characteristics

Dental Cements

Objectives

After studying this chapter, the student will be able to do the following:

1. Describe the use of dental cements as a:
   - Luting agent
   - Base/liner
   - Filling material
   - Temporary restoration
   - Intermediate restoration
   - Periodontal pack
   - Temporary cement
2. Explain the importance of adhesion and microleakage of dental cements.
3. Describe the use of a cavity varnish or cavity sealer.
4. Describe the differences between the two cement powders and three cement liquids.
5. Explain the setting reaction of a typical dental cement.
6. Based on the properties of the liquid and the powder, discuss the properties of:
   - Zinc oxide–eugenol (ZOE) cement
   - Zinc phosphate cement
   - Polycarboxylate cement
   - Glass ionomer cement
   - Composite cement
   - Calcium hydroxide base
7. Summarize the mixing process for the first four cements in objective #6 and how it relates to the setting reaction.
8. Describe the use and advantages of a (resin) composite cement.

Key Words/Phrases

base
composite cements
direct pulp cap
eugenol
glass ionomer cements
liner
luting agent
obtundent
polycarboxylate cement
resin cements
silicate cement
temporary cements
varnish
zinc oxide–eugenol (ZOE) cement
zinc phosphate cement

Introduction

Dental cements are used to lute (glue or cement) inlays, crowns, bridges, and other restorations in place, as shown in *Figure 7.1*. These are used similar to the cements and glues of everyday life. In addition, dental cements are used for a wide variety of other dental procedures depending on the material.

I. Use of Dental Cements

Each use of dental cement requires specific characteristics. Luting materials need to be very fluid when being used to cement a crown and should become very strong after they set. Other cements are mixed to a putty-like consistency to restore missing tooth structure or to help protect the pulp under a filling. Some cements are used for a variety of procedures; others have limited use. Chapter 23, Mixing Liners, Bases, and Cements, presents the laboratory and clinical application of five of the materials and may be used to supplement this chapter.

A. Luting Agent

The term "cement" implies that the material will be used to lute or glue things together. Although other uses are common, use as a **luting agent** has given this group of materials their name, cements. Dental cements hold appliances and restorations in place with micromechanical and macromechanical retention. Some dental cements are adhesive through chemical bonds, but most are not. Adhesion is discussed in Chapter 4.

When a crown is luted to the preparation, the cement is mixed and then painted inside the crown (or filled), as shown in *Figure 7.1A*. The crown is seated in place on the preparation, causing the excess cement to ooze out at the margins, as shown in *Figure 7.1B*. The cement is allowed to set either partially or completely, and the excess is removed, much like scaling calculus from teeth. It is critical that all the excess cement is removed because any excess cement left behind will become a plaque trap and cause gingival irritation.

Luting cements have the most demanding requirements of any dental material. They must set in the mouth, changing from a fluid liquid to a rock-hard solid in a matter of minutes. The resulting material must be biocompatible and insoluble in oral fluids. Because cements are much more soluble than the overlying restorative material, accurate fit of the restoration to be luted is critical. Crown margins should precisely fit the preparation to minimize the amount of cement that is exposed to the oral environment. Poorly fitting margins increase the solubility of the cement and the likelihood of recurrent decay.

A patient's oral hygiene and diet can also affect the longevity of a luted restoration. As bacteria ferment sugars, the pH in the mouth drops. Dental cements are much more soluble in an acidic environment. As the cement dissolves, a gap is created between the tooth and the restoration. The tooth structure at the gap will have a high risk for caries. Plaque control and proper diet will reduce the probability of recurrent decay and help maintain a less destructive environment for dental cements and other materials.

B. Pulp Protection

Dental cements are also used as an intermediate base or liner when the remaining dentin is believed to be less than 2 mm thick. A base or liner is placed on the dentin between the pulp and the restorative

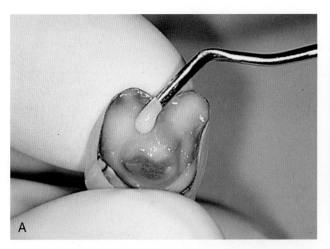
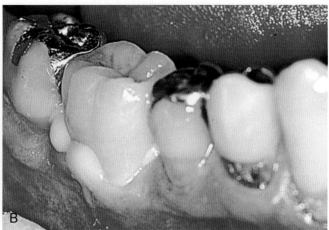

FIGURE 7.1. A. When luting a crown, the clinician paints the inside with cement. **B.** The crown is then seated on the prepared tooth, and the excess cement is forced out at the margins. (Courtesy of GC America, Inc., Alsip, IL.)

material. A base and a liner are illustrated in *Figure 7.2E and F*. Because the solubility of dental cements is much greater than is that of the overlying restorative material, bases and liners must not be placed on margins.

1. Liners

A **liner** is used to protect the pulp from chemical irritation, as illustrated in *Figure 7.2F*. A liner may stimulate secondary dentin formation (bioactive) or release fluoride. Liners are too thin (<0.5 mm) to provide thermal insulation, and they may be too weak to support the restorative material or to resist amalgam condensation forces.

2. Bases

A **base** is stronger and thicker than a liner, as illustrated in *Figure 7.2E*. A base provides thermal insulation. Some support the restorative material and may release fluoride, and some are irritating to the pulp before the setting reaction has completed. Such a base may be used in conjunction with a liner. Previously, the distinction between bases and liners was clear. Today, liner materials are much stronger, and the distinction between bases and liners is quite blurred.

C. Temporary Restoration

Some of the same dental cements that are used to lute crowns and that serve as a base may also be used as a temporary restorative material *(Fig. 7.2A–C)*. For some cements, the material is mixed to a thicker consistency than is used for luting. Other cements have formulations that are designed for use as temporary and permanent restorations.

1. Temporary Restorative Materials

Many dental cements are used as a temporary restorative material. The specific cement is chosen based on the particular clinical requirements of the situation. A temporary restoration (filling) may be placed as an emergency procedure when time restraints prevent a more complex treatment. Also, when pulpal pain and other symptoms do not result in a definitive diagnosis, such as reversible versus irreversible pulpitis, a temporary restoration might be placed.

2. Temporary Material as a Base

At times, a temporary filling is placed, and at a later appointment, part of the temporary filling material is removed. The remaining temporary material then becomes a base, which is covered with a permanent restoration. The advantage to such procedures is that the pulp is less irritated since the overlying dentin is not exposed a second time. These procedures are illustrated in *Figure 7.2A–E*.

3. Caries Control

When patients have a high number of carious lesions (>10), caries control procedures may be implemented. The goal of caries control is to change the oral environment from cariogenic to noncariogenic. It is hoped that caries control procedures change the oral flora from acid-producing and acid-loving bacteria to other nonpathogenic species. Caries control includes quick, efficient removal of as much decay as possible in the shortest time possible, placement of temporary restorations, improved oral hygiene, diet changes, and fluoride supplements. Two dental cements that are frequently used for caries control are zinc oxide–eugenol (ZOE) and glass ionomer cement. If all the decay is removed from a lesion, the temporary restoration can later function as a base, as previously described. Light-cure glass ionomer materials

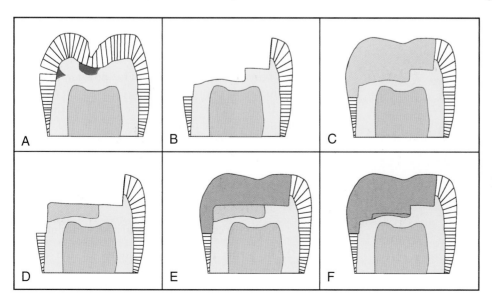

FIGURE 7.2. Several uses of dental cements for pulpal protection. **A.** Carious lesions are present. **B.** The tooth is prepared. **C.** A temporary filling is placed. **D.** At a later appointment, the temporary filling is cut back, leaving a cement base. **E.** The base is covered with a permanent restoration. **F.** A liner is much thinner than a base.

will bond to composite materials to a certain extent. Light-cure glass ionomers may be used for caries control and then veneered with composite material to improve esthetics and surface roughness. The ZOE materials are snow white in appearance and, for many patients, are not suitable for use in the anterior teeth.

D. Other Formulations of Dental Cements

Formulations of dental cements are also used as endodontic sealers and surgical/periodontal packs; these formulations are discussed later in this and in other chapters.

Still other cement formulations include impression materials and bite registration materials. These formulations are discussed in the following chapter.

E. Cavity Sealers

Cavity sealers are discussed in this chapter because both these and dental cements are used to protect the pulp.

1. Varnish

In dentistry, copal varnish and other varnish formulations are used much like varnishes are used to protect wood. **Varnish** is composed of resins dissolved in a solvent. *Figure 7.3* shows an example of a cavity varnish. The varnish is painted onto the entire cavity preparation, including the margins. The solvent then evaporates and leaves behind a very thin layer of resin. Varnish is frequently used to seal preparations for amalgam restorations. It can also function as a chemical barrier, protecting the pulp from an irritating base or a luting cement. It decreases the initial microleakage of the amalgam restoration until corrosion products form at the interface. Varnish is not thick enough to affect thermal sensitivity, and it is not used with composite materials because it would interfere with adhesion.

2. Dentinal Bonding Agents

Some dentists are substituting dentinal bonding agents for varnish. Several of these products will bond the amalgam to the tooth structure. Clinical studies of postoperative sensitivity, however, do not support the routine use of dentinal bonding systems to seal all amalgam restorations. Some dentists are using Gluma primer as a substitute for varnish. Gluma is a brand name for one of the original dentinal bonding systems. The original Gluma system has been completely reformulated, but the original primer is still available.

3. Order of Placement

If more than one base, liner, varnish, or dentinal bonding system is used, the properties of the materials determine their order of placement. Bioactive materials are placed first and then adhesive materials. Irritating materials are placed last.

II. Chemistry of Dental Cements

With the exception of composite cements, dental cements are brittle, ceramic materials. For many cements, the chemistry is a simple acid–base reaction. The resulting product is insoluble in water and oral fluids.

A. Formulation

1. Dental cements are often a powder/liquid system.
2. The liquid is an acid.
3. The powder is a base. The powder must be insoluble in oral fluids but reactive with the acid.
4. If one understands the properties of the components of a dental cement, then one will be able to predict the properties of the resulting set material.

B. The Reaction

1. The reaction is

   acid + excess base → residual base + insoluble salt

2. In terms of the components of the dental cement, the reaction is

   liquid + excess powder → residual powder + matrix

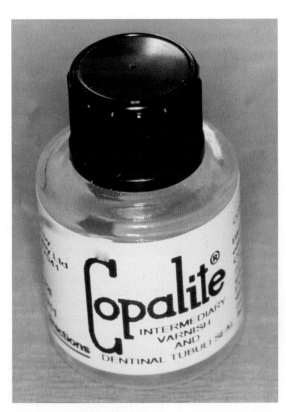

FIGURE 7.3. Cavity varnish.

3. The residual powder and the matrix must be insoluble in oral fluids.

4. The end result is a "cored structure," much like that of set amalgam.

C. Composite Cements

The chemistry of composite cements is the same as that of acrylics and composites. This chemistry was presented in Chapter 5, Direct Polymeric Restorative Materials.

III. Powders Used in Dental Cements

Two materials are used to make powders for dental cements: zinc oxide and glass. The manufacturing process grinds and sieves the powders to obtain the proper particle size. The size of the particles determines the film thickness of the resulting mixed cements. Film thickness determines how well a casting or other restoration can be seated on a preparation. Excessively large particles result in high film thickness, open margins, and recurrent decay.

A. Zinc Oxide

1. Zinc oxide is the only insoluble, nontoxic, reactive oxide or hydroxide that is available to react with an acid. Common additives to the zinc oxide powder are aluminum oxide (alumina) to strengthen and magnesium oxide to control the setting rate.

2. Zinc oxide has some antibacterial effects and is included in diaper rash, sunscreen, and foot powder products.

B. Powdered Glass

1. Silicon oxide, the chemical formula of glass, is very unreactive. However, if oxides of sodium, calcium, and potassium are added in sufficient quantity, the glass will react with a strong acid. As expected, the powder is white because it is made of small, translucent glass particles.

2. The glass formulation also contains fluoride. Fluoride is a common glass additive because it reduces the melting temperature and improves the flow of the molten glass. Fluoride in the glass powder gives the resulting dental cement the ability to release fluoride and inhibit recurrent caries.

C. Reactivity of Powders

The reactivity of the powder components is controlled by the manufacturer and is matched to the reactivity of the liquid component.

IV. Liquids Used in Dental Cements

The composition or strength of the acid determines the reactivity of the cement liquid. The manufacturer controls this.

A. Eugenol

Eugenol is an organic liquid that is also a weak acid. Eugenol is a major component of oil of cloves. As a result, eugenol has the distinctive smell and taste of cloves.

1. Eugenol is a phenol derivative that is antibacterial and also **obtundent** to the pulp. Obtundent means that it reduces irritation.

2. Eugenol inhibits free radical polymerization. This limits the use of eugenol-containing cements because they will inhibit the set of composite restorative materials.

3. Other organic liquids have been added to eugenol to formulate dental cements. The most notable of these added organic liquids is ethoxybenzoic acid.

B. Phosphoric Acid

The phosphoric acid used in dental cements is approximately two-thirds phosphoric acid and one-third water by weight. This formulation is very acidic and can be quite irritating to biologic tissues in or out of the oral cavity. The amount of water present affects the reactivity of the liquid by changing the ionization of phosphoric acid. Therefore, it is important to keep the cap on the bottle and not dispense the liquid until one is ready to mix the cement. High or low humidity will affect the water content and, therefore, the pH, reactivity, and properties of the resulting cement. If the liquid appears cloudy, it has outlived its shelf life and should be discarded.

C. Polyacrylic Acid

Several dental cements use an aqueous solution of polyacrylic acid. These solutions are 30% to 50% polyacrylic acid by weight and are very viscous liquids.

1. Dispensing

Dispensing these liquids requires more attention than does dispensing other cement liquids. If one is not careful, the viscous liquid does not form independent drops. Instead, the drops can "run together," and the amount of liquid dispensed will not be accurate and will vary greatly with each mix. Like phosphoric acid, the liquid should not be dispensed until one is ready to mix the cement because water can evaporate, changing the reactivity and the cement properties. These cement liquids should not be stored in the refrigerator because some will gel and become unusable.

2. Bonding

The carboxyl groups of polyacrylic acid bond to calcium in tooth structure. This bond is believed to be relatively stable in a wet environment. Adhesion of glass ionomer materials was presented in Chapter 4, Adhesive Materials.

3. Water-Hardening Cements

"Water-hardening" or "water-setting" cements use anhydrous, freeze-dried polyacrylic acid. The manufacturer mixes zinc oxide or glass powder with the powdered anhydrous polyacrylic acid. This combined powder is mixed with a companion liquid that is predominately water. When mixed, the polyacrylic acid first dissolves in the water and then reacts with the zinc oxide or powdered glass.

V. Powder/Liquid Ratios and Systems of Dental Cements

Dental cements combine these three liquids and two powders. Table 7.1 lists the resulting cements. The properties of the resulting cements are based on the properties of the components involved. The manufacturer adjusts the reactivity of both the liquid and powder components to obtain proper setting characteristics and other properties. Do not mix powders and liquids of different cements or different products of the same type.

A. Components Dictate Handling and Mixing

1. The ZOE cement and zinc phosphate cement are mixed with a powder/liquid ratio that depends on the intended use. A base or temporary restoration mix is thicker than a luting mix. The higher the powder/liquid ratio, the greater the strength, the lower the solubility, and, in general, the better the cement. On the other hand, working time decreases, and viscosity increases.

TABLE 7.1. Components and the Resulting Cements

Components	Zinc Oxide Powder	Glass Powder
Eugenol	Zinc oxide–eugenol (ZOE) cement	No reaction
Phosphoric acid	Zinc phosphate cement	Silicate cement
Polyacrylic acid	Polycarboxylate cement	Glass ionomer cement

If a luting mix becomes too thick, the restoration may not seat adequately. In this case, the marginal gap is increased, as is the likelihood of caries. In addition, micromechanical retention is reduced.

2. The powder/liquid ratio is limited in that the liquid must wet all the powder for the cement to function adequately.

3. Glass ionomer and polycarboxylate cements have powder/liquid ratios that are determined by the manufacturer; it is important to follow the manufacturer's directions. Mixing time is also important. If the mixing procedure is too slow, two problems can occur. The first involves the resulting mix becoming too thick. In this case, the restoration may not adequately seat when luted, which increases the marginal gap. The second involves adhesion. The mixed cement must be fluid enough to wet the tooth for both micromechanical and chemical adhesion. If the mixing process is too slow, the carboxylic acid groups react with the powder and are not available to react with the tooth structure. Chemical adhesion is then reduced or even eliminated.

4. Paper pads are available for mixing many dental cements and other dental materials. One must be careful, however, if a paper-mixing pad is used for mixing dental cement. Cement liquids may weaken the paper surface, causing it to become abraded. The abraded paper particles are then incorporated into and weaken the resulting cement. Some mixing pads use paper that has been coated with a thin layer of plastic. This type of pad is commonly used with glass ionomer and polycarboxylate cements. A thick glass slab is favored for mixing zinc phosphate cement; typically, the slab is cooled to improve the resulting mix.

B. Systems

Most cements come as powder/liquid systems, but some are paste/paste systems. Paste/paste systems are dispensed by equal lengths, as are other paste/paste dental materials.

Each dental cement has its own advantages and disadvantages. Use and mixing of dental cements are summarized in Table 7.2. The remainder of this chapter focuses on the following dental cements:

1. ZOE
2. Zinc phosphate
3. Glass ionomer
4. Polycarboxylate
5. Composite
6. Others

TABLE 7.2. Reference Guide for Liners, Bases, and Cements

Cement	Use	Mixing Technique	Mixing Time[a]	Characteristics of a Proper Mix	Setting Time[a]
Calcium hydroxide	Cavity liner	Mix quickly in a small area of paper pad	10 seconds	Uniform color	2–3 minutes
Zinc phosphate	Luting agent	Add divided increments in specified time, using large slab area	1–1.5 minutes	Mix will stretch 1 inch between slab and spatula	5.5 minutes
	Base	Same as luting agent (above)	1–1.5 minutes	Thick, putty-like (nonsticking) consistency	5.5 minutes
Glass ionomer	Luting agent	Add powder to liquid in one portion	30–45 seconds	Use while glossy	7 minutes
		Paste/paste; mix equal amounts	20–30 seconds	Uniform color	5 minutes
	Base	Same as luting agent (above)	30–45 seconds	Use while glossy	7 minutes
Zinc oxide–eugenol (ZOE)	Base and temporary restoration	Add half-scoop increments, using small mixing area	1.5 minutes	Thick, putty-like (almost crumbly) consistency	2.5–3.5 minutes
Polycarboxylate	Luting agent and intermediate base	Add powder to liquid in one portion	30 seconds	Use while glossy	10 minutes
Temporary	Temporary luting agent	Equal lengths; mix all at once	30 seconds	Uniform color	5 minutes
Composite	Luting agent	Mix equal amounts of pastes	30–45 seconds	Uniform color	5 minutes

[a]These are approximate time periods. Check the manufacturers' instructions for specific mixing times, measurements, and setting times.

VI. ZOE Cement

When zinc oxide is mixed with eugenol, **zinc oxide–eugenol (ZOE) cement** is the result.

A. Products

1. Unreinforced ZOE products are still on the market, but they should only be used when strength and solubility are not critical. Such ZOE formulations for temporary cements are popular and perform adequately.

2. Reinforced ZOE products are stronger and less soluble than unreinforced products. Reinforced ZOE products are used for temporary restorations and intermediate bases. Additives include alumina, rosin, and polymethyl methacrylate resin.

B. Properties

1. Formulations of ZOE have been developed for nearly every use of dental cements. This cement works very well for some uses, but not for all. Unfortunately, ZOE products including reinforced ZOE do not have adequate strength and are too soluble for use as permanent cement.

2. The ZOE cement is obtundent and, therefore, very useful when pulpal protection is desired or a sedative filling is needed.

C. Mixing

1. Paste/Paste Products
The two pastes are dispensed in equal lengths on a paper-mixing pad. The pastes have different colors. Mixing with a cement spatula swirls and strops the two pastes together. Stropping would be similar to a back-and-forth cake frosting motion. Mixing continues until a homogeneous color is obtained.

2. Powder/Liquid Products
The powder is measured and dispensed with a scoop, as shown in *Figure 7.4*. The liquid is dispensed as drops. A glass slab or coated paper pad is commonly used for mixing powder/liquid ZOE products. The powder is forced into the liquid with a cement spatula. The mixing process first incorporates large increments of powder, followed by smaller increments, as adding powder becomes more difficult. The mixing

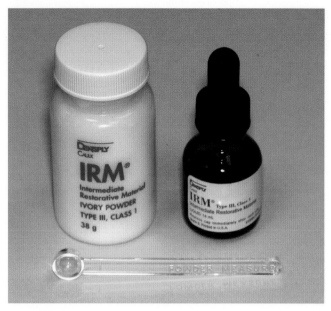

FIGURE 7.4. A zinc oxide and eugenol cement product.

process requires time to incorporate enough powder to obtain acceptable properties.

3. Cement Consistencies

When a luting mix is desired with a powder/liquid product, mixing is continued until a proper consistency is obtained. For example, a "1-inch string" of material occurs when the flat surface of the cement spatula is pulled from the mixed material (*Fig. 7.6E*). When a base consistency is desired, mixing is continued until the material has the consistency of pie dough (can be rolled into a ball with fingers covered with cement powder but has a bit of a crumbly nature). If too little powder is used, the mixed mass will be sticky and difficult to handle. A proper base mix will not stick to instruments and can be pushed or condensed into place and even carved.

4. Cleanup

As with all dental cements, the set material is nearly insoluble in water. Therefore, it is important that the cement spatula and glass slab are washed with water before the material sets. Soap assists with cleanup because eugenol is an organic liquid that is only slightly soluble in water. If one delays cleanup, the set material is difficult to remove from the instruments used. Set ZOE materials can be dissolved with a variety of organic solvents, such as alcohol, orange solvent, and others.

5. Setting Reaction

Water accelerates the ZOE setting reaction. Therefore, ZOE materials set faster in the mouth than they do when out of the mouth, making them quite useful and popular.

6. Removal of Excess ZOE

Removing excess ZOE luting material is very easy if the material is allowed to set and become a brittle mass, after which it cleanly breaks off at the margins. With an instrument such as a scaler or an explorer, it usually breaks off in large chunks. If one is impatient, the soft material breaks into little pieces, making removal more difficult.

D. Uses

1. ZOE cement is a very old and yet still useful material. Its obtundent property makes it very useful for sedative and temporary fillings. Its use as a base has declined greatly. Other cements that release fluoride have replaced ZOE.

2. A reinforced ZOE base can withstand amalgam condensation forces and support the overlying amalgam restoration.

3. Biocompatibility is very good because ZOE seals very well. However, eugenol causes hypersensitivity reactions in some patients. In addition, eugenol can irritate the skin of dental personnel.

VII. Zinc Phosphate Cement

Zinc phosphate cement is formed when zinc oxide powder is mixed with phosphoric acid. Zinc phosphate cement has been used in dentistry for centuries. At one time, it was the strongest and least soluble cement that was available. This is no longer true, but zinc phosphate cement remains an option for several uses.

A. Products

1. Zinc phosphate cement is supplied by manufacturers as a powder and liquid, as shown in *Figures 7.5 and 7.6A*. The powder and liquid are mixed to a thick or thin consistency depending on the clinical use.

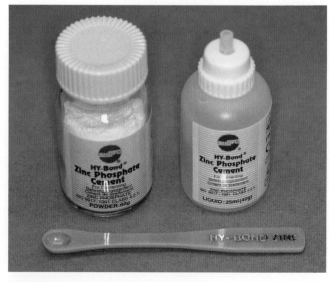

FIGURE 7.5. Zinc phosphate cement.

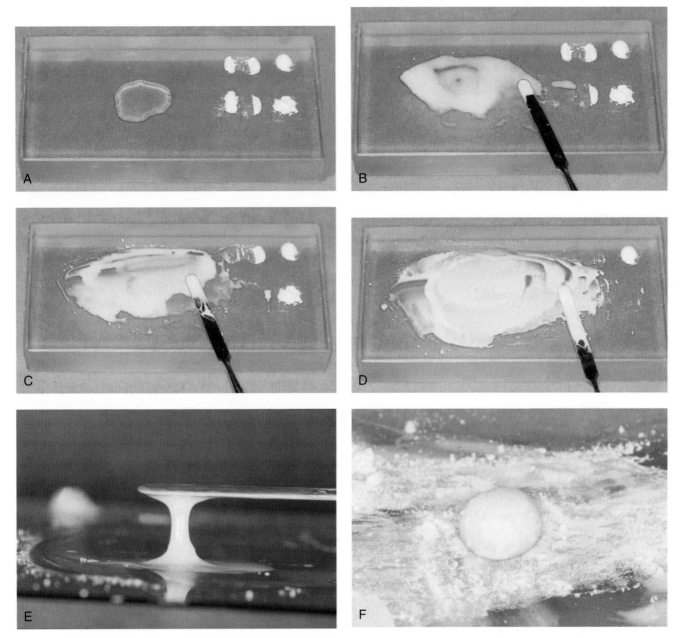

FIGURE 7.6. The mixing process for zinc phosphate cement. **A.** Powder and liquid are dispensed on a chilled glass slab. The powder is divided into increments. **B.** The first increment is mixed into the liquid. **C** and **D.** Increments are added to the mix, using the entire surface of the glass slab. **E.** When mixed for luting, the cement will "string" 1 inch. **F.** A mix for a base can be rolled into a ball.

2. Zinc phosphate cement powder comes in shades. The color of cement can affect the esthetics of a translucent restorative material. Zinc phosphate cement powder is mixed with water for trial cementing of the esthetic restoration.

B. Properties

1. As mentioned, zinc phosphate cement is strong and has a low solubility.
2. Because the mixed cement has a low pH until it has set, zinc phosphate cement is irritating to the pulp. When zinc phosphate cement is used as a base, often a liner is placed or a varnish is first applied to the preparation.
3. Zinc phosphate cement sets to a hard, brittle material. It can withstand amalgam condensation forces and support the overlying amalgam restoration. Removing excess luting material is very easy if the material is allowed to set and to become a brittle mass, after which it breaks off cleanly in large chunks. If one is impatient, the soft material breaks into little pieces, making removal more difficult.

C. Mixing

1. Zinc phosphate cement is dispensed as scoops of powder and drops of liquid. A cement spatula and glass slab are used to mix the material. The mixing process is shown in *Figure 7.6*.

2. Zinc phosphate cement is mixed to the proper consistency, which depends on the intended clinical use. The mix is thinner (lower powder/liquid ratio) when used as a luting agent and thicker (higher powder/liquid ratio) when used as a base. Proper mixing is critical. When improperly mixed, zinc phosphate cement is difficult to handle and has inferior properties.

3. The setting reaction is very exothermic. The heat of the reaction accelerates the setting rate. It is important to dissipate this heat. Zinc phosphate cement is mixed slowly and over a large area of a chilled glass slab to dissipate the heat of the setting reaction. Each increment of powder as shown in *Figure 7.6* is mixed for 10 to 15 seconds (for a total of 60–90 seconds) to facilitate the transfer of heat to the glass slab. The chilled glass slab absorbs the heat given off and slows the setting reaction, enabling more powder to be incorporated into the liquid. Using the entire surface of the slab facilitates heat removal, as shown in *Figure 7.6D*. The powder is incorporated into the liquid with force, as with ZOE cement. The significant difference is that the powder for zinc phosphate is added first in small increments and then in larger ones. The heat of the reaction of the initial small increments is dissipated into the glass slab if mixing is slow enough.

4. When a luting mix is desired, mixing is continued until a "1-inch string" occurs when tested with the cement spatula, as shown in *Figure 7.6E*. When a base consistency is desired, a higher powder/liquid ratio is used. In this case, mixing is continued until the material has the consistency of putty and can be rolled into a ball with fingers covered with cement powder, as shown in *Figure 7.6F*. If too little powder is used, the mixed mass will be sticky and difficult to handle. A proper base mix will not stick to powder-covered instruments and can be pushed or condensed into place.

5. As with all dental cements, the set material is nearly insoluble in water. Therefore, it is important that the cement spatula and glass slab are washed with tap water before the material sets. If one delays cleanup, the set material becomes very difficult to remove from the slab and the instruments. If the mix happens to set on the spatula or slab, cleanup is much easier if the instruments are soaked in a baking soda–water solution.

D. Uses

1. Zinc phosphate cement is used for luting inlays, crowns, bridges, orthodontic bands, and other appliances. Zinc phosphate cement has a long working time compared to other luting cements.

2. Zinc phosphate cement is also used as a base material. It is acidic, however, and the pulp may need to be protected with a liner or a varnish.

3. Years of clinical use have demonstrated the longevity of zinc phosphate cement.

VIII. Glass Ionomer Cements

Glass ionomer cements are formed when a glass powder is mixed with an aqueous solution of polyacrylic acid. Glass ionomer cements have become quite popular because of their physical and mechanical properties and their clinical performance. A multitude of products are on the market. The first glass ionomer cements set by an acid–base reaction, like most other dental cements. We will call them A/B (acid–base) cements. "Resin-modified" or "resin-reinforced" products have become more popular. They set via two reactions: acid–base and addition polymerization. Glass ionomer products are discussed in Chapter 5, Direct Polymeric Restorative Materials and are summarized in Table 5.2.

A. Products and Uses

1. Luting Materials
   Glass ionomer cement is one of the most popular luting materials. Both A/B and resin-reinforced products exist. Resin-modified glass ionomer cement has been called the material of choice for luting all-metal and ceramometal crowns. These glass ionomer products are stronger and tougher than those products that set solely by an acid–base reaction.

2. Restorative Materials
   Glass ionomer restorative materials were discussed in Chapter 5, Direct Polymeric Restorative Materials. The restorative materials have the same setting reactions as luting materials but are thicker, stronger materials with a much higher film thickness.

3. Base/Liner Materials
   A number of base and lining A/B materials have been developed. With the introduction of light-activated, resin-reinforced glass ionomer liners, however, use of A/B products has greatly diminished. Light-activated glass ionomer liners have adequate strength for use as a base and are quite popular. At times, dentists will use a glass ionomer restorative material for a temporary restoration or a large base.

4. Glass Ionomer Cements

Glass ionomer cements are available in three forms. One form is supplied as a powder and a liquid (*Fig. 7.7A*). The powder is measured with a scoop and is mixed with a specific number of liquid drops from a bottle. It is important that the cement is mixed quickly and the working time is not exceeded.

The second form is a premeasured, single-dose capsule (much like amalgam) (*Fig. 7.7B*). These unidose capsules are mixed with an amalgamator. The capsule has a "spout" where the mixed material is expressed from the capsule with a "gun or dispenser." Capsules are easy to use and very popular, but they are also more expensive.

The third system is a paste/paste system common for many dental materials (*Fig. 7.7C*). The pastes are dispensed and mixed until they become one homogenous color. Many resin-reinforced glass ionomer–luting materials are paste/paste products supplied in a double barrel dispensing device. These dispensing devices assure proper proportioning of the two pastes.

B. Properties

1. Glass ionomer materials are the strongest and least soluble dental luting cements (with the exception of composite cements). They are also adhesive, release fluoride, and have good biocompatibility. This combination of properties makes them quite popular.

2. Glass ionomer materials bond to tooth structure. In addition, they bond to stainless steel and alloys for ceramometal crowns.

C. Mixing

1. It is critical that glass ionomer cement is properly mixed and handled. If it is not, a nonadhesive material results. The powder is dispensed with a scoop, and the liquid is dispensed as drops. Cement spatula and paper pads are typically used. The cement manufacturer supplies special mixing pads that consist of sheets of plastic-coated paper. The plastic coating protects the paper from abrasion and prevents the liquid from being absorbed by the paper. It is

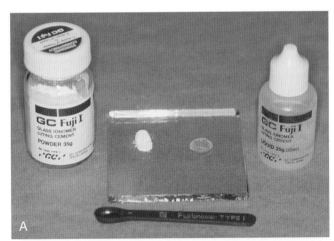
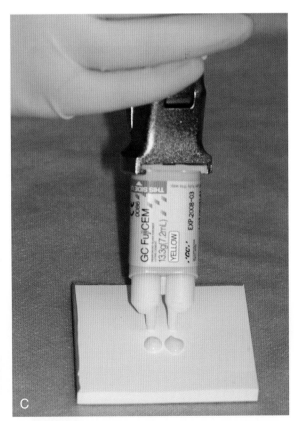
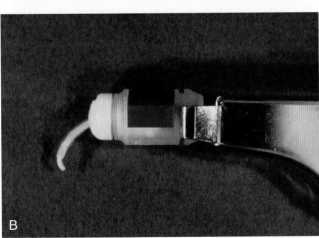

FIGURE 7.7. Glass ionomer products. **A.** Powder and liquid. **B.** Premeasured capsule. Note the cement being expressed from the capsule tip. **C.** Paste/paste dispenser.

important that the drops form and fall separately. Glass ionomer cement is not mixed to a specific consistency, as ZOE and zinc phosphate cements are. The manufacturer's recommended powder/liquid ratio should be followed.

2. The mixing process is much quicker than that for ZOE or zinc phosphate cement. Mixing should be completed in 30 seconds or less, and the restoration should be seated within 2 minutes from the start of mixing. Typically, the powder is mixed into the liquid in two increments. The mixed material must be placed while the cement surface appears glossy; beyond that time, adhesion is reduced or lost.

3. Cleanup with water is easy and should be done as soon as possible. Remember that the set material will bond chemically to the stainless steel cement spatula.

IX. Polycarboxylate Cement

A. Properties and Use

Polycarboxylate cement is formed when zinc oxide powder is mixed with an aqueous solution of polyacrylic acid (*Fig. 7.8*). Polycarboxylate cement was the first adhesive material developed for use in dentistry. Polycarboxylate cement bonds to tooth structure, and this results in very little leakage. It

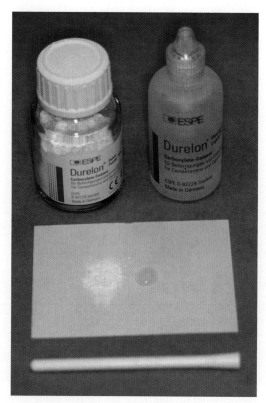

FIGURE 7.8. Polycarboxylate cement.

is not as acidic as zinc phosphate cement, is very biocompatible, and is used as a luting cement and an intermediate base. Unfortunately, polycarboxylate cement is not very strong and has a moderate solubility. Glass ionomer cements have the same adhesive properties along with better strength, solubility resistance, and fluoride release. Glass ionomer and zinc phosphate cements have a much greater market share than polycarboxylate cement.

B. Mixing

Polycarboxylate cement is mixed in the same manner as glass ionomer cements. The powder and liquid are dispensed and mixed on a paper pad with a cement spatula. The mixing time is similar to that of glass ionomer cements because adhesion depends on unreacted carboxylic acid groups. The mixed material must be placed inside the crown and the crown seated while the cement is still glossy.

X. Composite Cements

Composite cements are composite materials (see Chapter 5) with a higher percentage of resin and smaller particle sizes to reduce viscosity and film thickness. They are sometimes referred to as **resin cements**. Originally, they had a very high film thickness. Before the development of dentinal bonding systems, leakage of composite cements was common and caused postoperative sensitivity. Modern composite cements have an improved film thickness (thinner). With the use of a dentinal bonding system (*Fig. 7.9A*), composite cements are the favorite luting material of many clinicians. They are the material of choice for luting most ceramic restorations. If the ceramic material is properly etched and silanated, composite cement will bond the restoration to the underlying tooth structure. Composite cements are also useful for recementing poorly fitting crowns when the patient does not wish to have the inadequate crown remade. Composite cements also come in an automix format. The two pastes are mixed in a tip that includes a baffle that swirls and mixes the two pastes as they are expressed (*Fig 7.9B*).

Many types of composite cement systems are available. They come as chemically activated, light-activated, and dual-cure systems. The activation method of the cement should be the same as the activation method of the accompanying bonding system. This combination of cement and bonding system can be quite complex and requires attention to detail. Many times, an additional component is added to the dentinal bonding system to change a light-activated bonding system to a dual-cure bonding system. It is important to note self-etching one-step dentinal bonding systems are not compatible with chemically activated composite cements. Regardless of which product is used, the tooth must not be contaminated by oral fluids during the application of

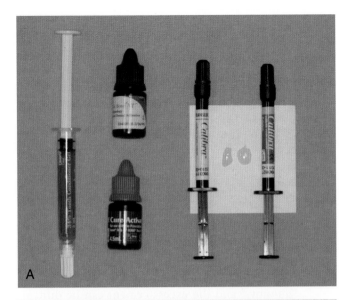

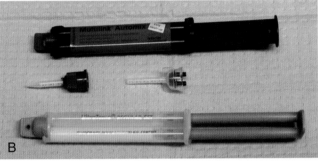

FIGURE 7.9. Paste cements. **A.** A composite cement kit containing etchant, dual-cure dentinal bonding agent, and the cement. **B.** Automix cements systems, a composite cement on the top and a temporary cement below. Note the mixing tips with baffles in the center.

the dentinal bonding agent and cement while the crown is being seated. Although one assistant may be adequate, for some products, use of a second assistant is wise.

Composite cements come as a single paste if light-activated. Single paste light-activated materials are used to bond veneers and orthodontic brackets. Dual-cure and chemically activated products are supplied as two pastes and are mixed on a paper pad with a plastic spatula. As composite cements are used with esthetic restorations such as veneers, composite cements come in a variety of shades. The color of the cement can change the appearance of an esthetic restoration. Some products include try-in pastes to allow evaluation of the restoration with a specific shade.

XI. Other Dental Cements and Cement Uses

A. Silicate Cement

Silicate cement is formed when a glass powder is mixed with phosphoric acid. Silicate cement was an old anterior restorative material and is not used today; however, a short discussion is included for historical perspective. Silicate cement is very acidic,

very irritating to the pulp, and highly soluble. It also leaks excessively. Silicate cement restorations needed to be replaced often; however, recurrent decay was rare. It was discovered that the infrequent occurrence of recurrent decay was caused by fluoride release. Fluoride was present in the glass powder. Thus, fluoride release became a desirable property for many dental materials.

B. Calcium Hydroxide Liners and Bases

At one time, calcium hydroxide liners and bases were very popular materials and were placed under most composite restorations. Calcium hydroxide products promote the formation of secondary dentin. They are still used when a cavity preparation leaves little dentin covering the pulp or when a "micro pulp exposure" is suspected. They were also used for direct pulp-capping procedures. A **direct pulp cap** is a material that is placed on vital pulp tissue when the overlying dentin is removed and the pulp is exposed. The tooth is then restored without root canal therapy. Success of a direct pulp cap is not guaranteed, and additional treatment may be required.

Calcium hydroxide materials are paste/paste systems, as shown in *Figure 7.10*. One paste contains calcium hydroxide; the other contains salicylate. Salicylate is a weak acid that is chemically similar to eugenol and reacts with the calcium hydroxide. Titanium oxide is added as a filler. With the development of dentinal bonding systems and our current understanding of the biocompatibility of composite materials, use of calcium hydroxide products has greatly diminished.

The setting reaction of calcium hydroxide materials is accelerated by water. The moisture

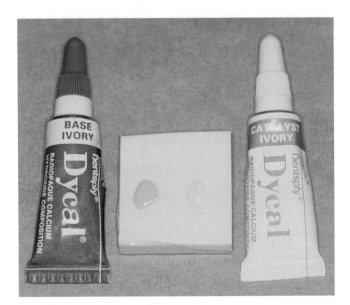

FIGURE 7.10. A calcium hydroxide product.

in dentin is sufficient to cause the material to set within seconds of its application onto the dentin surface. This feature makes calcium hydroxide very easy to use.

C. Calcium Silicate Materials

A new class of materials based on calcium silicate has become popular. They are very similar to Portland cement. These materials are very biocompatible and are often used as liners. However, they set very slowly and are difficult to handle. The oldest one is MTA or mineral trioxide. It was expensive, but the patent has expired and several similar products are now available.

D. Temporary Cements

Temporary cements are used to retain a temporary restoration while the permanent restoration is being fabricated. Temporary cements are typically paste/paste systems, as shown in *Figure 7.11*. They are a unique group of materials in that both a maximum and a minimum strength are required (remember Goldilocks?). If the temporary cement is too weak, the temporary restoration will be lost prematurely. If the temporary cement is too strong, the dentist may have trouble removing the temporary crown, and damage to tissues may occur.

Many temporary cements are paste/paste ZOE formulations. The composition of one paste is zinc oxide and vegetable oil. The other paste contains eugenol. The ZOE temporary cements mix easily and set quickly in the humidity of the mouth.

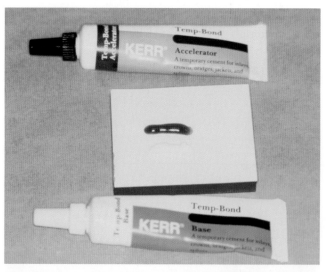

FIGURE 7.11. An example of a paste/paste temporary cement.

The set material is brittle, and the excess cement is easily removed. The obtundent property may even settle down an irritated pulp after it has been insulted by tooth preparation, impression procedures, and construction of a temporary crown. This describes a nearly ideal material—so what's the problem?

With the development and use of resin cements, many dentists believe that using ZOE temporary cement will inhibit the set of resin cement. Remember that eugenol inhibits free radical polymerization. As a result, temporary cements were developed that do not contain eugenol; instead, fatty acids and other chemicals are used to react with zinc oxide. These products have similar properties, but they do not handle as well. Many are not brittle. Rather, they are "gummy," and the excess cement can be difficult to remove.

At times, a temporary crown or bridge refuses to stay in place. It keeps coming off, frustrating both the dentist and the patient. When a stronger temporary cement is needed, a powder/liquid formulation of ZOE or even zinc phosphate cement can be used but should be mixed with a lower-than-recommended powder/liquid ratio to reduce the strength.

E. Surgical/Periodontal Packs

Surgical periodontal packs are paste/paste systems. They mix and handle much like ZOE impression materials, which are discussed in the next chapter. The composition is similar to ZOE temporary cements. These products are placed over surgical sites to protect the underlying tissues. They are temporarily held in place by using the undercuts and embrasures of teeth. Surgical packs are weak materials, so they are easily removed. Because ZOE products have an unpleasant taste and smell, noneugenol products have become popular. These products are formulated in the same manner as noneugenol temporary cements, and their use is presented with those of other specialty materials in Chapter 13. Mixing periodontal packs is presented in Chapter 33.

F. Endodontic Sealers

Many endodontic sealers are zinc oxide and eugenol preparations with added rosin and barium sulfate. Their use is presented with other endodontic materials in Chapter 13.

Summary

Dental cements are used to lute restorations and appliances into place. They are also used for a variety of other dental procedures. Luting cements have the most demanding requirements of any dental material. They must be insoluble, set in a wet environment, and be biocompatible.

Dental cements are also used as an intermediate base or liner when the thickness of dentin after cavity preparation is thin. The base or liner is placed between the pulp and the restorative material. In the past, liners were thin, soluble, and weak. Today, liners are stronger, and the distinction between liners and bases has become blurred. In the current practice of dentistry, use of liners has dramatically decreased. Bases are stronger and may release fluoride.

Temporary restorations are usually cements that have been mixed thicker than when used for luting. Sometimes, part of that temporary restoration is saved and then serves as a base material under the permanent restoration.

Many dental cements are a powder/liquid system, with the liquid being an acid and the powder constituting the base. The powder must be insoluble in the oral cavity yet must also react with the acid. The powders in dental cements are zinc oxide and powdered glass. The liquids are eugenol, polyacrylic acid, and phosphoric acid. Eugenol is a major component of oil of cloves and has an obtundent effect on the pulp.

Zinc oxide–eugenol (ZOE) cement is usually too weak and soluble to serve as permanent cement. Because of its sedative effect, however, it is useful for protecting pulp or for soothing an irritated pulp.

Zinc phosphate is a combination of zinc oxide powder and phosphoric acid. It is the oldest cement still in use today. This cement is strong, has low solubility, and involves a very exothermic setting reaction. The heat of the setting reaction accelerates the setting rate. Therefore, it is important to mix this cement over a large area of a chilled glass slab. This allows more powder to be added to the mix for the desired strength. This cement can be used as a base as well as permanent cement for crowns, bridges, orthodontic bands, and other appliances.

Glass ionomer cement is composed of glass powder and polyacrylic acid. It has been called the material of choice for luting metal and ceramometal crowns. Both chemically activated and light-activated materials exist. Glass ionomer materials are available in powder/liquid and paste/paste forms. Some products are supplied in premeasured single-dose capsules. Glass ionomer products are the strongest and least soluble dental cements, with the exception of composite cements. They also release fluoride, are biocompatible, and are truly adhesive to tooth structure.

Polycarboxylate cement consists of zinc oxide powder and polyacrylic acid. It, too, will bond directly to tooth structure. This cement is very biocompatible but not very strong. Its solubility resistance is rated as only moderate.

Composite cements are also called resin cements. They are used with dentinal bonding systems. They contain a higher percentage of the resin matrix material to reduce viscosity and are the materials of choice for luting all ceramic restorations.

Temporary cements are usually paste/paste systems and are used to retain a temporary restoration while the permanent restoration is being fabricated. They are unique in that both a minimum and a maximum strength are required. If the cement is too weak, the temporary restoration will be lost prematurely. If the cement is too strong, the dentist may have difficulty removing the temporary restoration and may damage tissue and tooth structure.

Dental cements are a broad category of materials with a broad range of uses. Proper mixing and handling typically have a greater effect on the resulting cements than on other categories of dental materials.

Learning Activities

1. Mix zinc phosphate cement on both chilled and room-temperature glass slabs. Note the amount of powder incorporated into each mix.

2. Mix ZOE cement with and without a drop of water. Use a consistent powder/liquid ratio. Note the setting time for each mix.

3. Mix glass ionomer cement. Apply it to a clean surface on an extracted tooth and to a surface contaminated with saliva. Allow the cement to set, and then scrape on the cement with an instrument. Keeping adhesion in mind, was there any difference between the two applications in the amount of adhesion?

Review Questions

Question 1. Which of the following cements is available in a single-dose capsule, much like that of silver amalgam filling material?

a. Polycarboxylate
b. Silicate
c. ZOE
d. Glass ionomer
e. Zinc phosphate

Question 2. Two dental cements that are used for caries control are:

a. ZOE and zinc phosphate
b. ZOE and polycarboxylate
c. Zinc phosphate and glass ionomer
d. Glass ionomer and polycarboxylate
e. Glass ionomer and ZOE

Question 3. All of the following are characteristics for ZOE EXCEPT:

a. Fluoride release
b. Lack of strength
c. An obtundent material
d. Pulp protection

Question 4. Which of the following cements is most soluble?

a. Glass ionomer
b. Zinc phosphate
c. ZOE
d. Polycarboxylate

Question 5. When glass ionomer is mixed too slowly, the resulting mix is:

a. Thin
b. Thick
c. Lumpy
d. Granular

Question 6. Cements are _____ soluble than the overlying restoration.

a. More
b. Less
c. Equally
d. None of the above

Question 7. During mixing, which of the following cements should use as much of the area on the slab as possible to reduce the exothermic reaction?

a. Polycarboxylate
b. Glass ionomer
c. ZOE
d. Zinc phosphate

Question 8. Which of the following dental materials promotes the formation of secondary dentin?

a. Composite cements
b. Silicate cement
c. Calcium hydroxide
d. Temporary cements

Question 9. Which of the following is a common additive to glass powder, reduces melting temperature, and improves the flow of molten glass?

a. Quartz
b. Fluoride
c. Silicate
d. Oxides

Question 10. The cement of choice for luting ceramic restorations to tooth structure is:

a. ZOE
b. Zinc phosphate
c. Polycarboxylate
d. Composite

Question 11. The disadvantage, or drawback, of using polycarboxylate cement is:

a. Lack of strength
b. Ability to bond to tooth structure
c. Biocompatibility
d. Lack of sufficient clinical data for long-term use

Question 12. ZOE may be used for the following:

a. Temporary restorations
b. Intermediate bases
c. Permanent restorations
d. Luting temporary crowns
e. Luting permanent crowns
f. a, b, and c
g. a, b, and d
h. a and d only

Impression Materials

Objectives

After studying this chapter, the student will be able to do the following:

1. Describe the use of impression materials during indirect restorative procedures.
2. List the oral structures from which impressions are made.
3. Differentiate between a model, a cast, and a die.
4. Describe the various types of impression trays.
5. List the desirable qualities of an impression material.
6. Differentiate between the following types of impression materials:
   - Elastic and inelastic
   - Reversible and irreversible
7. Describe the composition and setting mechanism of:
   - Wax and impression compound
   - Zinc oxide–eugenol (ZOE)
   - Agar or reversible hydrocolloid–optional
   - Alginate
   - Polysulfides
   - Condensation silicones
   - Polyethers
   - Addition silicones
8. Compare the properties, use, and cost of the above impression materials.
9. Describe the effect of water temperature on the setting rate of alginate.
10. Describe the effect of water and heat on the setting rate of polysulfides.

Key Words/Phrases

addition silicones
alginate
automix
bite registration tray
casts
condensation silicone
custom trays
die
gel
hydrocolloid conditioner
hysteresis
imbibition
impression compound
impression materials
impression tray
irreversible hydrocolloid
polyether
polysulfide
reversible hydrocolloid
retraction cord
sol
stock trays
study model
surfactants
syneresis
triple tray
viscosity
zinc oxide–eugenol (ZOE)

Introduction

Taking impressions may be one of the responsibilities of the dental hygienist in a busy practice. It is important to have an understanding of the various types of impression materials, their specific use, and their handling characteristics. Should you make athletic mouth guard or whitening trays, an impression will be a part of the appliance fabrication process. And it is not unlikely that you may be asked to assist with a "final impression" appointment should the dental assistant not be present that day. Taking impressions can be a welcome change from the typical daily routine of the hygienist.

I. Impression Materials

A. General Comments

Impression materials are used to make replicas (models or casts) of teeth and other oral tissues. In dentistry, we take impressions of teeth and their supporting structures. These supporting structures include gingiva, alveolar bone or residual ridge, hard and soft palate, and frenums, which are muscle attachments. The replicas are used to construct restorations and other appliances. The impression is a negative reproduction, whereas the replica (model or cast) is a positive reproduction, as illustrated in *Figure 8.1*. The impression must be an accurate duplication of the hard and soft tissues of interest and be stable enough to allow disinfection and production of an accurate model.

Not all impression materials are compatible with all model materials. Because impression materials are used for many purposes, a wide variety of products are available to make impressions of oral tissues. Some uses are simply to produce a physical model of the oral tissues for study, called a **study model**. Study models are used in diagnosis and treatment planning. Other uses require very exact (within 0.1%) replication of the size and shape of a preparation for the construction of a restoration or appliance. These replicas are called **casts**. A replica of a single tooth is called a **die**.

B. Impression Material Systems

Impression materials are supplied in a variety of forms. Some are powders that are mixed with water; others are paste–paste systems. Several materials are softened or melted by heating. Regardless of their form, impression materials are mixed (or heated) to make a thick paste or liquid. They are then loaded into an impression tray, placed in the mouth, and seated onto the tissues of interest. The tray functions as a carrier and can stabilize the set impression material. Several impression trays are shown in *Figure 8.2*. It is interesting to note that dental impression materials are also used to make impressions for medical prostheses (such as artificial eyes) and forensic investigations (bite marks).

Paste–paste impression materials (and many other dental materials) come in tubes, much like toothpaste tubes. The orifice of each tube is sized

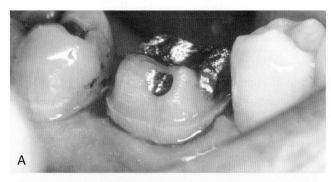

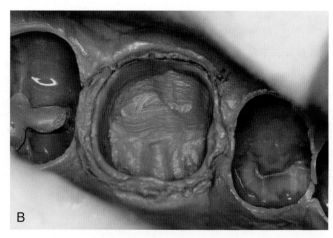

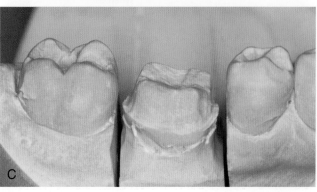

FIGURE 8.1. Photograph of **A.** a crown preparation, **B.** an impression, and **C.** a cast.

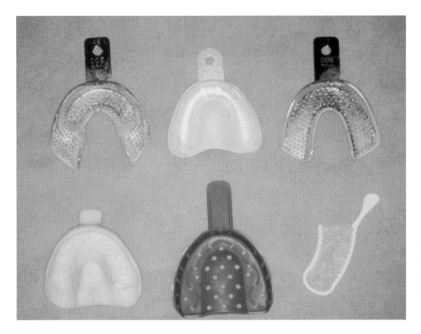

FIGURE 8.2. Several impression trays (from *upper left*, moving *clockwise*): a metal perforated tray for partially edentulous impressions, a solid metal tray for edentulous impressions, a metal tray for dentulous impressions, a bite registration tray, a plastic tray for dentulous impressions, and a custom tray.

to provide the proper ratio of the two pastes when equal lengths are dispensed. Thus, if the size of the two orifices is the same, one should dispense equal lengths. If the orifice of one tube is larger than that of the other tube, then again, one should dispense equal lengths. Examples are shown in *Figure 8.3*.

C. Cost

The cost of impression materials varies greatly, from pennies per impression to as much as several dollars. An accurate cost analysis needs to include the percentage of first impressions that are acceptable and the number of restorations that need to be remade. Unacceptable restorations made on casts from cheap impression materials can make dentistry a nonprofit enterprise.

D. Impression Trays

1. Use of Impression Trays

Impression trays are used to carry the impression material into the mouth, and the handle of the tray is used to remove the impression. The tray can also support the material impression and improve accuracy. Trays are supplied in a variety of shapes and sizes and are made from several materials. Plastic disposable trays are very popular and work well with current infection control practices. Plastic trays are inexpensive and convenient, but they do not support the impression as well as metal trays do. Metal trays are more expensive but reusable. In addition, metal trays are stiffer and, thus, are less likely to distort when

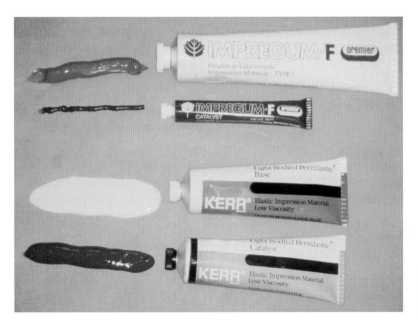

FIGURE 8.3. Polysulfide (*lower*) and polyether (*upper*) impression materials. Note that the lengths dispensed, but not the volumes, are equal.

removed from the mouth. Cleaning and sterilizing metal trays adds to the cost of their use.

2. Stock Trays

Stock trays are "off-the-shelf" items that come
in a variety of materials, shapes, and sizes. The
different-shaped trays are designed to take
impressions of different oral conditions: edentulous mouths, partially edentulous mouths, and
mouths with a full complement of teeth. Such
trays are illustrated in *Figure 8.2*. Stock trays also
come in a range of sizes, from very small trays
for pediatric patients to very large trays for large
adult mouths. Stock trays can be metal or plastic.

3. Custom Trays

The most accurate impressions are made with
custom trays. **Custom trays** are made on a
model of the patient's arch with acrylic or other
resin. Two impressions are necessary when a
custom tray is used. A preliminary impression
is taken with a stock tray and an inexpensive
material. A gypsum product is poured into the
impression, and the resulting model is used to
construct the custom tray. The custom tray is
then used to take a final impression.

Custom trays are used to take final impressions for full dentures, inlays, crowns, bridges,
and some removable partial dentures. Custom
trays use less impression material than do stock
trays because they fit around the teeth better
than a stock tray does. Some say that custom
trays are cost-effective because they use less
material. Others say that custom trays are cost-
effective because they make the impressions
easier to take and accurate impressions result
more frequently than with stock trays. Two
techniques for the fabrication of custom trays
for crown and bridge impressions are presented
in detail in Chapter 29, Fabrication of a Custom
Impression Trays. It is important to note that
proper mixing and handling of the impression
material are the factors most critical for success.

4. Special-Use Trays

A variety of special-use trays have been developed. **Bite registration trays**, as shown in *Figure
8.2*, record the occlusal surfaces of both arches.
Bite registrations are used to relate the upper and
lower casts in the dental laboratory in precisely
the same manner as they come together in the
patient's mouth. The use of a bite registration
without a tray is shown in *Figure 8.4*.

Another popular impression tray is the **triple
tray**, which is used with the dual-arch or closed-
mouth impression technique. The triple tray is a
quadrant tray with a "J" shape that curls around
the posterior of the most distal molars (*Fig.
8.5A*). With the dual-arch technique, the loaded

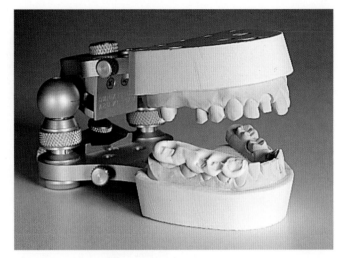

FIGURE 8.4. Models mounted on a simple articulator with
a bite registration on the mandibular right quadrant made of
impression material. (Courtesy of GC America, Inc., Alsip, IL.)

tray (on both sides) is seated on the arch with
the prepared tooth. The patient then closes the
mouth to his or her normal bite, and the tray
records an impression of the prepared tooth,
an impression of the opposing teeth, and a bite
registration, all at the same time (*Fig. 8.5B–D*).

E. Classification of Impression Materials

1. Chemical Reaction or Physical Change

Impression materials set either by a chemical
reaction or by a physical change. Impression
materials that set by chemical reactions to form
elastic rubber materials are called thermoset.
The chemical reaction involves chain lengthening, cross-linking, or both. Other impression
materials set by a physical change when they
cool, either by solidification or by gelation.
Solidification occurs when molten wax cools and
goes from a liquid state to a solid state. Gelation
is the process by which gelatin, such as Jell-O,
changes from a liquid state to a semisolid state
when it cools. Impression materials that undergo
a physical change when they cool are called thermoplastic. In general, thermoplastic materials are
not as stable as are thermoset materials.

2. Use

a. *Elastic/Inelastic*

Because impression materials are used for a
variety of purposes, the requirements of a
particular procedure determine which impression materials can be used. Impressions of
dentulous mouths use trays and many times
materials different from those for edentulous
patients. Teeth typically have undercuts
(nooks and crannies) that require an elastic material to be used. Edentulous impressions may use elastic or inelastic impression

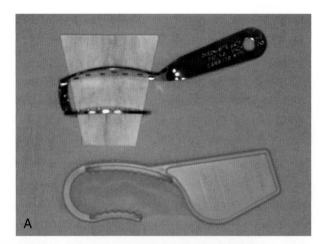

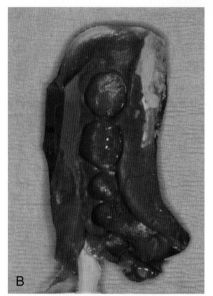
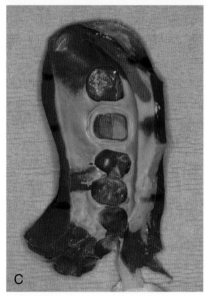
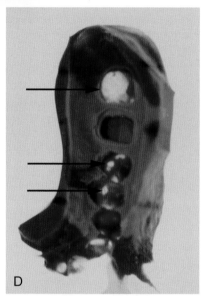

FIGURE 8.5. A. Reusable metal and disposable plastic triple trays. **B–D.** Three views of a triple-tray impression. **B.** Impression of the opposing arch. **C.** Impression of the preparation. **D.** Backlit view showing areas with teeth in contact during impression.

materials. Inelastic impression materials set hard and rigid compared with elastic impression materials and would "lock" around teeth if used on a dentulous patient.

b. *Accuracy*

The accuracy required by the restoration or prosthesis determines which impression materials can be used. Not all impression materials have sufficient accuracy for crown and bridge impressions. Study models are not considered to be highly accurate reproductions of oral tissues. Therefore, alginate is an acceptable impression material for study models, but it is an unacceptable impression material for the fabrication of bridges, crowns, and inlays. Nearly all impression materials are acceptable for full-denture impressions.

c. *Flow and Detail Reproduction*

Many kinds of impression materials come in a variety of viscosities. **Viscosity** is a measure of a liquid's ability to flow. There are (from thinnest to thickest consistency) light-body, medium-body, monophase, heavy-body, and putty materials. Light-body materials are typically used with an impression syringe and are injected around preparations. They are the most "runny" of the impression materials and best record the details of tooth preparations (small grooves, edges, and margins).

Many times, a **retraction cord** is placed in the gingival sulcus to facilitate crown and bridge impressions. In most instances, the patient will have had local anesthesia to ensure his or her comfort. The retraction cord pushes the gingiva away from the tooth, as shown in *Figure 8.6*. Frequently, the cord will contain a hemostatic or astringent medicament to control bleeding. After the cord has been in place for several minutes, it is usually removed, just before the impression is

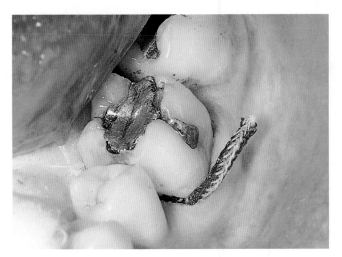

FIGURE 8.6. Retraction cord being placed in the sulcus during crown preparation. (Courtesy of Ultradent, Inc., South Jordan, UT.)

taken. There are exceptions, however, as the cord may be kept in place during the impression. The use of a retraction cord allows the low-viscosity material to flow to, and thus reproduce, areas of a preparation that are difficult to reach. The cord moves the gingival tissue slightly away from the tooth and also controls the moisture in the area.

Putty materials are the thickest impression materials, but they can still record the details of a fingerprint. Heavy-body and putty materials are placed in an impression tray, and

their high viscosity prevents running and dripping of the impression material out of the tray and onto the operator or patient. They are typically used with a light-body material. The light-body material records the preparation and its margins, while the thicker material becomes the bulk of the impression. The impression tray, which is filled with the high-viscosity material, is immediately seated over the light-body material. The materials then set together into one mass and are removed as one impression.

Medium-body impression materials may be injected or used in the tray depending on the dentist's preferences. Monophase materials are designed to be used for both injection and in the tray. Therefore, only one mix of monophase material is needed.

3. **Types of Impression Materials**
Each impression material has its own advantages and disadvantages for use in dentistry. The following sections will focus on each type of impression material and its use (Table 8.1).
   a. *Inelastic Impression Materials*
   1. Plaster
   2. Wax and impression compound
   3. Zinc oxide–eugenol (ZOE)
   b. *Aqueous Elastomeric Impression Materials*
   1. Alginate (irreversible hydrocolloid)
   2. Agar (reversible hydrocolloid)

TABLE 8.1. Classification and Use of Impression Materials

Type of Impression Material	Elastic versus Inelastic	Setting Process	Used for the Construction of:			
			Full Denture	Partial Denture[a]	Inlay, Crown, or Bridge	Study Models
Plaster	Inelastic	Chemical	Preliminary	No	No	No
Wax or impression compound	Inelastic	Physical	Preliminary	No	No	No
ZOE	Inelastic	Chemical	Final[b]	No	No	No
Reversible hydrocolloid (agar)	Elastic	Physical	Not used[c]	Yes	Yes	No
Irreversible hydrocolloid (alginate)	Elastic	Chemical	Preliminary	Yes	No	Yes
Polysulfide	Elastic	Chemical	Final[b]	Yes	Yes[b]	No[d]
Condensation silicone	Elastic	Chemical	Final[b]	Yes	Yes	No[d]
Addition silicone	Elastic	Chemical	Final[b]	Yes	Yes	No[d]
Polyether	Elastic	Chemical	Final[b]	Yes	Yes	No[d]

[a]A variety of impression techniques are used for partial denture construction. This table does not address all possible techniques.
[b]Use of a custom tray is recommended.
[c]Edentulous trays for hydrocolloid use are not common.
[d]These materials could be used, but their use is not economical.

c. *Nonaqueous Elastomeric Impression Materials*
1. Polysulfides
2. Condensation silicones
3. Polyethers
4. Addition silicones

II. Plaster

Plaster would seem to be an unlikely impression material. However, impression plaster is rarely used but still sold. It has the same setting reaction and properties as the gypsum products that are used for models and casts. Gypsum products will be discussed in Chapter 9.

III. Wax and Impression Compound

A. Wax

Wax was probably the first impression material used in dentistry. It is cheap, clean, and easy to use. A multitude of waxes are used in dentistry. Some are hard, much like paraffin wax that is used in canning jellies and jams. Others are soft and moldable at room temperature, similar to Play-doh. Wax used for taking impressions is solid at mouth temperature but is moldable at a temperature that is tolerated by oral tissues. Wax comes in many forms (sticks, strips,

tubes, etc.). Wax can be thought of as a low molecular weight polymer. It is a thermoplastic material. It is also very weak, and the technique must compensate for wax's poor mechanical properties. Wax is used by some dentists to take impressions for full dentures. Wax is often used to extend tray borders or adapt a stock tray when taking impressions.

More commonly, a variety of waxes are used as adjunctive materials in the dental laboratory for the fabrication of crowns, bridges, and other restorations. Wax is softened or melted and then formed into the desired shape of the restoration. Then, the wax piece is surrounded by a mold material. Later, the wax is melted away and the mold is filled with a restorative material, such as gold. These processes are described in more detail in subsequent chapters.

B. Impression Compound

Impression compound is wax with added filler to improve handling and stability. It is stronger and more brittle and, when softened, flows much less compared with wax. Impression compound is supplied as sticks or cakes of material, as shown in *Figure 8.7A*. It is softened in a warm water bath, as shown in *Figure 8.7B*. Because the thermal conductivity of impression compound is low, time and patience are required to soften the material

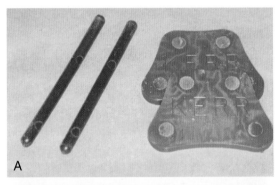

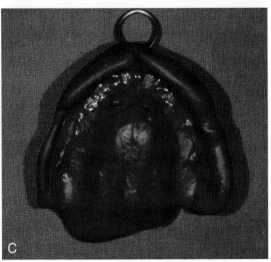

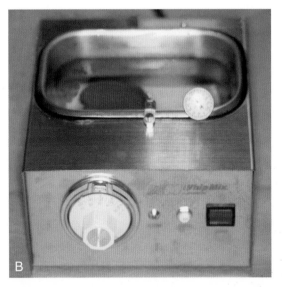

FIGURE 8.7. **A.** Impression compound sticks and cakes. **B.** Tray with impression compound in a water bath. **C.** Preliminary impression for a complete denture. (Courtesy of Dr. James Overberger, Morgantown, WV.)

properly. The heated, softened, and moldable material is placed in an impression tray, resoftened, and then seated in the mouth. When the material has cooled to mouth temperature, it returns to a rigid state and is removed. Impression compound is a stiff, thermoplastic material and is used by many dentists to make preliminary impressions for complete dentures, as shown in *Figure 8.7C*. Other impression materials that record fine details are better suited for final impressions.

IV. Zinc Oxide–Eugenol (ZOE)

Zinc oxide–eugenol (ZOE) has been formulated for a wide variety of uses in dentistry, including as an impression material. The chemistry of ZOE materials is covered in Chapter 7, Dental Cements.

A. Form of the Material

The ZOE materials come as two pastes. One paste contains eugenol and inert fillers; the other is formed by using zinc oxide powder mixed with vegetable oil. Eugenol is a major component in oil of cloves. Therefore, ZOE materials smell and taste like cloves. For some patients, this is unpleasant. The two pastes come in tubes, much like toothpaste, as shown in *Figure 8.8*. Equal lengths of material from each tube are dispensed. Typically, the two pastes of ZOE (and other materials that come in tubes) are of different colors.

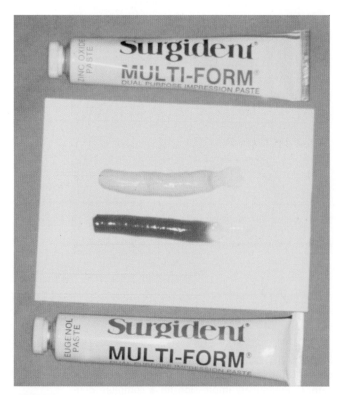

FIGURE 8.8. ZOE impression paste.

The pastes are swirled, stropped, and scraped together during mixing until one homogeneous color is obtained.

B. Use

The ZOE impression materials set to a hard and brittle mass, which limits their use to impressions of edentulous ridges for removable dentures. They are inexpensive and easy to use and were once very popular. They are commonly used in a custom tray for the final impression for a complete denture. Today, however, ZOE materials have been replaced by newer materials, such as addition silicones. Although the newer materials have little advantage in terms of performance and are much more expensive, the simple advantage of stocking one less impression material in the dental office is likely the reason for the declining use of ZOE impression materials.

V. General Aspects of Hydrocolloid Impression Materials

Two impression materials are considered to be hydrocolloid materials because their major component is water. Both materials change from a viscous liquid state, called the sol, to a semisolid, rubbery state, called the gel. The **sol** state is a solution of one material dissolved in another. In the **gel** state, two phases exist, much like a foam of soap bubbles. The first phase is a solid carbohydrate polymer network, like the soap used to create a foam. The second phase is water trapped in very small pockets of the material, like the air trapped in the foam formed by soap. Colloids are discussed in Chapter 2, Materials Science and Dentistry.

Hydrocolloid materials that set via a chemical reaction are called **irreversible hydrocolloids**, or, more commonly, **alginate**. Heating alginate that was set results in

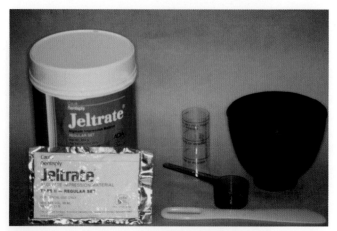

FIGURE 8.9. Alginate impression materials in a bulk container, premeasured envelope, scoop for bulk powder, water measure, mixing bowl, and spatula.

warm alginate; it does not reverse back to the sol (fluid) state. Hydrocolloid materials that gel by a physical change (cooling) are called **reversible hydrocolloids**. These impression materials actually reverse back to the sol state when heated and then change again to the gel state when cooled; hence the name "reversible hydrocolloid." Reversible hydrocolloid is also called agar or agar-agar (or sometimes simply hydrocolloid).

VI. Alginate (Irreversible Hydrocolloid) Impression Materials

A. Properties

Alginate materials are termed "irreversible impression materials" because they will not reverse to the sol state once they react and become a gel. They have advantages and disadvantages similar to those of reversible hydrocolloid materials because both types of materials are predominantly water. Alginate materials are not as accurate as reversible hydrocolloid materials, but they are much easier to use. Alginate materials are supplied as powders that are mixed with water as shown in *Figure 8.9*.

B. Composition

1. The powder contains potassium alginate. It is a carbohydrate polymer that dissolves in water, forming a sol. Carboxylate groups (–COOH) react with calcium ions and cross-link the material to form a gel. The reaction is similar to that of polycarboxylate and glass ionomer cements. Potassium alginate is derived from algae.

2. Another main component of the powder is an inert filler, such as diatomaceous earth (silica). The filler gives the mixed material "body," which allows acceptable handling. Without filler, the mixed material would be too runny for use.

3. Several other chemicals are present in the powder: the reactor for the cross-linking reaction (calcium sulfate), the retarder for working time (sodium phosphate), colorants, and flavor.

4. Some alginate products have antimicrobial agents added to the powder. The purpose is to reduce the microbial content of the powder as provided by the manufacturer more than to disinfect the impression after it has been taken.

5. Both reversible and irreversible hydrocolloid materials are predominantly water. Thus, several advantages and disadvantages result when their use is compared with that of other impression materials.

    a. Advantages
    Reversible and irreversible hydrocolloid will wet a tooth surface that is contaminated by oral fluids. Fewer air bubbles are trapped between the tooth and the impression material. Hydrocolloid materials will even absorb a limited amount of oral fluids. These two effects occur because water-based liquids mix together easily, like a mix of soda pop and fruit juice used to make punch.

    The second advantage of the material being composed predominantly of water is that pouring the impression with gypsum products is easier than with elastomeric impression materials. Again, the gypsum product, when mixed with water, easily wets the surface of the impression material, which is predominantly water. Hydrocolloid impression materials are quite hydrophilic, but the same cannot be said for all impression materials.

    b. Disadvantages
    The disadvantage of the material being predominantly water is that water evaporates from the surface of the impression if it is left exposed to air. When the water evaporates, the impression shrinks and is no longer accurate. To prevent evaporation of water from hydrocolloids (alginate and reversible hydrocolloid), impressions should be poured as soon as possible after disinfecting.

    Hydrocolloid materials contract slightly after setting and exude water. This process is called **synersis**. Synersis occurs very slowly, but it is a second reason to pour hydrocolloid impressions as soon as possible.

    When disinfecting a hydrocolloid impression, however, it is important to limit the time that the impression is exposed to an aqueous disinfecting solution. The hydrocolloid will absorb water, swell, and distort. This is called **imbibition**.

C. Setting Reaction—Optional

Alginate materials set by a chemical reaction that cross-links a carbohydrate polymer.

1. Working time is provided by a competing reaction that initially delays cross-linking. When the powder is mixed with water, the alginate powder dissolves, as does the calcium sulfate and sodium phosphate.

2. Initially, the calcium ions react with the phosphate ions and precipitate out of solution. The calcium ions do not react with the dissolved alginate until all the phosphate ions have reacted.

3. After the retarder (the phosphate ions) has reacted, the setting reaction becomes the dominant reaction. The calcium ions react with the alginate, cross-linking the polymer chains, and gelation occurs. The set material is a hydrogel that is composed mainly of water.

D. Use and Handling

1. Alginate is supplied in preweighed envelopes or bulk containers. With bulk containers, dispensing is achieved with a scoop that is supplied by the manufacturer. The alginate powder tends to settle in bulk containers during shipment and storage. Before opening a new bulk container, the material should be "fluffed" by shaking or turning the container upside down and right side up for about a minute. This will remix the heavier components with the lighter ones, resulting in the proper amount of material in each scoop.

2. The filler in most alginate materials is a silicate material. Silicate dust causes lung problems if inhaled. Additives have been included in some alginate products to reduce the dust that occurs when alginate is used; these products are called dustless alginates. Regardless, it is not healthy to breathe any dust. A mask, as commonly worn when treating patients, will reduce exposure to alginate dust.

3. Water is dispensed with a calibrated water measure that is also supplied by the manufacturer. If one is unhappy with the consistency of the mixed material, the solution is to change brands. Do not alter the water/powder ratio to make the mix thicker or thinner.

4. The temperature of the water controls the rate of the setting reaction. Warmer water increases the setting rate, and cooler water slows the setting reaction. Alginate is supplied by most manufacturers in regular-set and fast-set varieties. Regular-set materials gel in 3 to 4 minutes, whereas fast-set materials gel in 1 to 2 minutes.

5. Mixing the alginate material is an aggressive aerobic activity. First, the powder and water are gently stirred together. Once all the powder has been wetted by the water, the effort should be greatly increased. The paste is pushed against the side of the rubber mixing bowl to force the water and powder together. For better spatulation, the mixing spatula should have a curved side that follows the curve of the mixing bowl. Aggressive spatulation continues until a smooth creamy mix is obtained. The typical mixing time is 1 minute. The mixed alginate material is scooped from the mixing bowl with the spatula, placed in the tray, and seated in the patient's mouth. Procedures for making alginate impressions are presented in Chapter 27, Taking Alginate Impressions.

6. Regardless of the setting time of the alginate material, removal of the impression is delayed for 2 to 3 minutes after gelation. Strength and elasticity improve during this additional setting time. The impression is removed with a quick motion. Alginate tends to be stronger when it is stressed quickly. Removing impressions slowly can increase distortion and tearing, whether the material is a hydrocolloid or an elastomer.

7. As with irreversible hydrocolloid materials, alginate impressions must be disinfected and poured with care. Gain or loss of water (evaporation, syneresis, or imbibition) will affect the accuracy of the resulting cast. If an alginate impression cannot be poured immediately, it should be sprayed with disinfectant, sealed in a plastic bag, and poured as soon as possible. No satisfactory method exists to store hydrocolloid materials for more than 30 minutes.

8. Alginate impression material is used for a variety of purposes. It is inexpensive and easy to use but lacks the accuracy for precisely fitting restorations. Proper mixing and handling will result in acceptable study models and casts on which to fabricate mouthguards and whitening and fluoride trays.

VII. Agar (Reversible Hydrocolloid)—Optional

A. Form of the Material

Reversible hydrocolloid is premixed by the manufacturer and supplied as a semisolid material in tubes and sticks. The sticks look and feel like a long, thin pencil eraser, except they feel wet because of their high water content. Reversible hydrocolloid is predominantly water with added agar (a carbohydrate polymer). Agar is also the material used in microbiology as a growth medium. Other components of reversible hydrocolloid include colorants, flavors, mold inhibitors, and a sulfate compound. The sulfate compound improves the hardness of the gypsum material that is poured into the impression.

B. Use

1. Equipment
   Reversible hydrocolloid requires special equipment to heat, store, and temper the materials, as shown in *Figure 8.10*. In addition, special impression trays that circulate cooling water are needed. The special equipment that is required to use reversible hydrocolloid limits the popularity of this excellent material. Reversible hydrocolloid itself is very inexpensive and results in a very accurate impression.

2. Preparation of Material
   Reversible hydrocolloid must be prepared for use before taking the impression. This can be

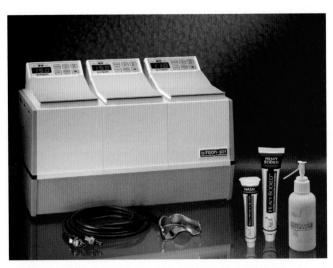

FIGURE 8.10. Hydrocolloid impression material (in tubes) and equipment for its use. The water bath (*top*) has three compartments with three different temperatures. (Courtesy of Dux Dental, Oxnard, CA.)

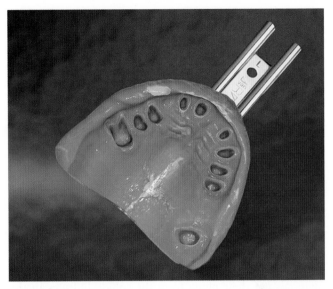

FIGURE 8.11. A hydrocolloid impression. (Courtesy of Dux Dental, Oxnard, CA.)

done at the beginning of the day or the week. Special equipment, called a **hydrocolloid conditioner**, is required (*Fig. 8.10*). This equipment has three compartments:

a. In the first compartment, the reversible hydrocolloid is boiled to change the rubbery material (the gel) into a viscous liquid (the sol).

b. In the second compartment, the material is stored in a 150°F (65°C) water bath until needed. Material can be stored for as long as several days.

c. Several minutes before it is to be used for an impression, the reversible hydrocolloid is placed in a 110°F (45°C) water bath. This step is called tempering. Tempering lowers the temperature to a point at which the oral tissues are able to tolerate the impression material. At mouth temperature, the material gels and returns to its elastic state. Circulating cold water through tubing and a special tray facilitates cooling. A hydrocolloid impression is shown in *Figure 8.11*.

3. Hysteresis

Hysteresis is unlike the common phase changes of water, which melts and freezes (or boils and condenses) at the same temperature. It is important to note that reversible hydrocolloid does not melt at the same temperature at which it gels. It melts at a much higher temperature than that of boiling water. On the other hand, it gels at a much cooler temperature, the mouth temperature. The characteristic of melting and gelling at different temperatures is called **hysteresis**.

4. Advantages and Disadvantages of Reversible Hydrocolloid

Reversible hydrocolloid works well in a wet environment. Therefore, reversible hydrocolloids are very useful for taking impressions when the margins of a crown preparation are subgingival or not easily kept dry. In fact, some dentists wet the teeth with water just before taking the impression. On the other hand, these materials require special equipment for heating, cooling, and use. Another shortcoming of these materials is their poor tear strength compared with nonaqueous elastomeric impression materials.

5. Popularity of Reversible Hydrocolloid

With the various advantages and disadvantages of reversible hydrocolloid material, one would expect dentistry to have a love–hate relationship with this material. Few dentists use reversible hydrocolloid, but those who do, love it. They work around the weaknesses of the material and are able to produce excellent results.

VIII. General Aspects of Nonaqueous Elastomeric (Rubber) Impression Materials

A number of rubber-like impression materials have been developed for dentistry. A variety of names are used to describe this group of materials: nonaqueous elastomeric impression materials, rubber base materials, elastomers, and others. These materials set via polymerization reactions and are more stable than hydrocolloid materials, but they are also more expensive. They are named based on their polymerization chemistry: polysulfide, condensation silicone, polyether, and addition silicone. Polysulfide, polyether, and silicone materials are also called nonaqueous elastomeric impression materials. They all undergo cross-linking and chain-lengthening polymerization reactions. They have similar, but not identical, mixing and handling properties. One very important difference between types of elastomeric impression materials is the adhesive that is used to bond the impression material to a nonperforated tray. Each impression material has its own adhesive, which will not work with other types of material.

IX. Polysulfides

Polysulfide impression material was the first nonaqueous elastomeric "rubber" impression material developed for dentistry. Often, polysulfide materials are called "rubber" or "rubber base" materials, even though polyether and silicone materials are also rubber materials. Polysulfide materials get their name from the sulfide linkages in the set material.

A. Condensation Polymerization

Polysulfide materials set via a condensation polymerization reaction. This is the same chemical reaction that joins together the building blocks of biologic polymers. Biologic polymers (proteins) are important components of the tissues in our body. In a typical condensation reaction, a hydrogen atom and a hydroxyl group (OH) are taken from monomers and are combined to form water (H_2O). The functional groups of the monomers can be carboxylic acid and amine groups that produce proteins (or nylon). The functional groups of polysulfide impression material are mercaptan groups (sulfur and hydrogen atoms) and oxygen from lead oxide, as shown in *Figure 8.12*. Reaction by-products other than water are produced by other condensation polymerization reactions, but water is the most common by-product. The name "condensation" polymerization is based on the production of water.

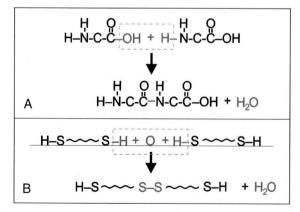

FIGURE 8.12. Condensation polymerization reactions that produce **A.** proteins and **B.** polysulfide impression material.

B. Composition of Polysulfide Impression Materials

Polysulfide impression materials are supplied as two pastes in tubes. Typically, one paste is dark brown, and the other paste is white. The white "base" paste contains a low molecular weight polysulfide polymer mixed with an inorganic filler, such as titanium oxide. The brown "accelerator" paste contains lead oxide and an "oily" organic chemical that does not react. A small percentage of sulfur is also included in the brown paste because it promotes the polymerization reaction.

C. Mixing Polysulfide Impression Materials

The two pastes are dispensed in equal lengths on a paper mixing pad. An impression material spatula is used to mix the two pastes. The impression material spatula has a long (~4 inches), straight-sided blade, as shown in *Figure 8.13A*. The pastes are swirled and stropped together until a homogeneous paste is obtained. Mixing may take from 30 to 90 seconds depending on the amount and viscosity of the material. The side of the spatula blade is used to scrape unmixed material off the paper pad and then to mix it into the rest of the material. The mixed material is loaded into the tray and placed in the mouth as a viscous paste. The same procedure is used to mix other nonaqueous elastomeric impression materials, such as polyether and silicones. The mixing process for polysulfide impression material is shown in *Figure 8.13*.

D. Polymerization Reaction of Polysulfide Impression Materials—Optional

The polymerization reaction starts when mixing begins and proceeds slowly. The low molecular weight polysulfide polymer has mercaptan groups (–SH) on the end of the short polymer chains and pendent groups hanging off the middle of the chains. Two hydrogen atoms from two different short polymer chains react with oxygen (from the lead oxide) to form water as shown in *Figure 8.12B*. The sulfur acts as a catalyst to link the two sulfur atoms and join the two polymer chains together. The same reaction lengthens and cross-links the polymer chains.

E. Properties of Polysulfide Impression Materials

Polysulfide impression materials are much more accurate than alginate. With proper handling, polysulfide impression materials can be used for inlays, crowns, and bridges. However, they are not as accurate as are other nonaqueous elastomeric materials. A polysulfide impression should be poured within several hours after mixing.

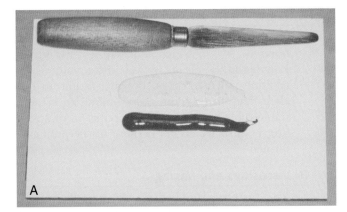
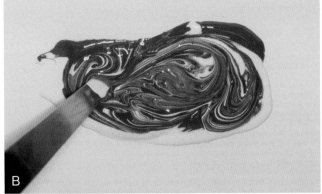
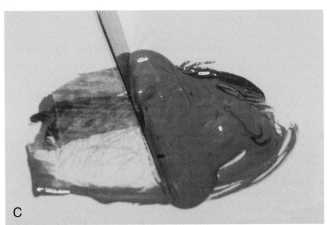
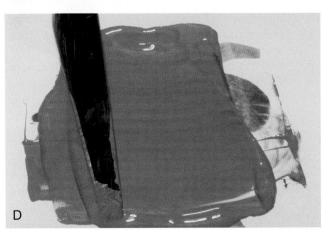

FIGURE 8.13. Mixing process for paste–paste impression materials as described in the text. The final mix should be of one homogenous color.

Custom trays are recommended for optimum results. Polysulfide impression materials have a disagreeable smell and taste. They stain clothing and are generally regarded as unpleasant materials. Polysulfide impression materials do have one advantage: they have the longest working time of any elastomeric material (4–6 minutes). As a result, they are useful for impressions of multiple preparations. Along with the long working time comes the longest setting time. Impressions need to be held in place in the mouth for as long as 15 minutes.

The water by-product of the setting reaction can be lost through evaporation, resulting in distortion. The working and setting times of polysulfide impression materials are significantly accelerated by heat and humidity. The setting time on hot, humid summer days will differ from that on cool, dry days. One technique using polysulfide impression material for a full-denture impression is to mix a drop of water with the material to accelerate the setting.

F. Use of Polysulfide Impression Materials

Polysulfide impression material is often used with custom trays to increase the accuracy of the impression. For impressions of crowns and bridges,

light-body material is injected around the preparation, and heavy-body material is used in the tray. Light- and medium-body materials are used for full-denture impressions.

Polysulfide impression materials are relatively inexpensive and easy to pour with gypsum materials. They are somewhat hydrophilic; however, so only a single pour (one model) is recommended. Subsequent pours using the same impression may not have the required accuracy.

X. Condensation Silicones

Condensation silicone impression materials were the next elastomeric impression material to be developed for dentistry. They are based on silicone rubber, which is commonly used in other industries. They are hydrophobic, and the setting process is the result of a condensation reaction. An alcohol by-product rather than water is formed. They are cleaner materials to use, but it is difficult to pour a model without voids and bubbles. As with polysulfide materials, loss of the reaction by-product through evaporation can result in distortion. Condensation silicone impressions must be poured without delay. These materials are not popular at present because newer materials provide better results.

XI. Polyethers

A. Development

Polyether impression material was developed in the late 1960s for use as a dental impression material. It was not borrowed from another industry. Polyether impression material was significantly different from the other materials available at that time.

B. Chemistry—Optional

These materials have an ether group in the molecular structure. An ether group is an oxygen atom that is bonded to two carbon atoms. Polyether impression materials set via a unique, ring-opening polymerization reaction that is thought to offset some polymerization shrinkage. The polymerization reaction is called cationic polymerization. Cationic polymerization is similar to addition polymerization except that instead of a free radical, a cation (positive ion) is the reactive molecule. No reaction by-product is produced.

C. Properties and Use

The working and setting times are shorter than those for polysulfide materials; they are more like those of addition silicone materials. Polyether impression materials are very stiff compared with other materials and set quickly. Polyether impression materials come in a single viscosity, much like the medium viscosity of other types of materials. They are clean materials to use but have an unpleasant taste. Polyether impression materials are very accurate and easy to pour with gypsum products. These properties and the ease of use make polyethers popular. The cost of polyether materials is similar to that of addition silicone materials. They are very stiff, which makes them well suited for use with a disposable triple tray, as shown in *Figure 8.5*.

Impregum is the most popular polyether product. The popularity of polyether impression materials has resulted in addition silicone "Impregum clones." The addition silicone clones have the same viscosity, stiffness, and even the purple color as Impregum. These clones are often called monophase impression materials. As with polyether materials, a single-viscosity addition silicone material is used in the syringe and the tray.

XII. Addition Silicones

Addition silicones are the most popular type of elastomeric impression material, especially for crown and bridge impressions. They are clean and do not have an unpleasant taste or smell. They are the most accurate, stable, and expensive impression materials. Addition silicone impression materials are also called vinyl polysiloxanes and polyvinylsiloxanes.

A. Polymerization Reaction

The reactive group is a carbon–carbon double bond (C = C), which is called a vinyl group. Polymerization occurs by way of free radicals and addition polymerization. Polymerization involves chain lengthening and cross-linking to create a stable rubber material. No evaporation of a reaction by-product occurs because no by-product is formed.

B. Viscosities and Mixing

The material supplied by the manufacturer is composed of short silicone rubber molecules with several reactive groups on each molecule. Fillers are added (to obtain the proper viscosity) along with a "catalyst," which functions as an activator. Manufacturers produce addition silicone materials in as many as five viscosities: light body, medium body, heavy body, monophase, and putty. Each viscosity comes in the form of two different-colored pastes. The pastes (except for putty) are mixed in the same manner as polysulfide materials. Addition silicones are also supplied in double-barreled cartridges for use in an "**automix** gun," as shown in *Figure 8.14*. The automix gun forces the two pastes through a tip, which contains a spiral-shaped "baffle." In the tip, the baffle causes the material to swirl around and flow in a turbulent manner that mixes the two pastes together. A second, smaller tip may be added to the main tip; this second tip is designed to dispense the impression material intraorally. The automix gun is very popular and has been adapted for other types of dental materials, such as cements and acrylic resins for temporary crowns and bridges.

C. Use of Putty

1. Purpose
   Putty is used in combination with a low-viscosity material. Putty fills the majority of the

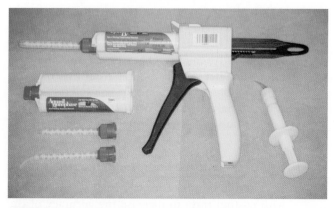

FIGURE 8.14. Automixing gun, cartridge of impression material, tips, and impression syringe.

tray. It is covered by a low-viscosity material in the tray, or the low-viscosity material is injected around the teeth of interest. The high viscosity of the putty forces the lower-viscosity materials around the teeth of interest.

2. Mixing, Working, and Setting Times

Kneading the two colored materials together with the fingers mixes impression putty. The palms of the hands should not be used because the material will be slightly heated by the clinician's body (hand) temperature. Polymerization is then accelerated, and working time is decreased. Also, latex gloves must not be worn when mixing addition silicone putties. Sulfur in the latex material inhibits the polymerization reaction; therefore, the material may not set. Instead, vinyl gloves should be worn over hands that have been washed with soap and water.

Impression putty typically sets faster than light-, medium-, and heavy-body materials. Working with two materials that set at different rates may be difficult. A variety of errors can occur when the two materials set at different times. It is very important to follow a standard impression procedure that uses a clock to time mixing, placement, and setting of materials; these are called the mixing, working, and setting times, respectively. Timing the mixing, placement, and setting of all chemically activated materials is recommended regardless of the material. Such procedures should follow the manufacturer's directions. Many manufacturers print the setting time on the tube to encourage proper use.

D. Additives to the Material

1. Surfactants

Current addition silicone impression materials have surfactants added to make pouring the model easier. **Surfactants** reduce the contact angle of the mixed gypsum product on the surface of the impression. Wetting is increased, and the likelihood of bubbles is decreased. Many manufacturers claim the surfactants also make taking an impression of wet teeth easier; however, such claims are without basis.

2. Hydrogen Absorbers

If the components of addition silicone materials are not formulated in the proper ratio or with the proper purity, hydrogen gas is produced by a secondary reaction. If such a material is poured too quickly, very tiny bubbles of hydrogen form at the interface of the impression material and the model material. Small bubbles on the gypsum cast are the result. Several products have hydrogen absorbers added to the formulation to prevent this problem.

Because disinfecting an impression takes from 10 to 30 minutes, hydrogen gas bubbles are less of a problem after such a delay. Also, addition silicone materials are very accurate and stable. Therefore, they are often sent to a commercial dental laboratory and poured there—even if the impression is shipped to a dental laboratory across the country. When the impression gets to the lab, sufficient time has passed for the hydrogen gas to have dissipated.

XIII. Miscellaneous Comments

A. Other Uses of Impression Materials

1. Bite Registration Materials

Most elastomeric impression materials can be used as a bite registration material. As shown in *Figure 8.4*, the mixed material is placed on the occlusal surfaces of the mandibular arch. The patient bites into the material. The impression material sets, recording the relationship of the maxillary arch to the mandibular arch. The bite registration is then removed and used in the dental laboratory to relate an upper cast to a lower cast in the same manner as the patient's natural bite.

2. Mold for Temporary Crowns

Putty can be used to make a "mold" for the fabrication of temporary crowns. Before the tooth is prepared for a crown, the mixed putty is placed over the tooth of interest. The putty sets and is removed, and the tooth is then prepared. The area of the prepared tooth of the putty impression is filled with a plastic temporary material. The most common temporary material is chemically activated acrylic resin. The putty impression is filled with the acrylic resin and is reseated in the patient's mouth. The prepared tooth forms the inside of the temporary crown, and the putty impression forms the outside of the mold of the temporary crown. After the acrylic resin sets, it is removed from the mouth and is trimmed, polished, and then temporarily cemented. Construction of temporary crowns is presented in greater detail in Chapter 35.

B. Compatibility of Impression Materials with Die Materials

Not all impression materials are compatible with all model materials. All impression materials can be poured with gypsum products. Hydrocolloid materials are not compatible with epoxy die materials. Impression material–model material compatibility is discussed in greater detail when model materials are presented in Chapter 9, Gypsum Materials.

C. Optical Impressions

Dentistry has embraced digital technology when it is economically advantageous. One example is digital radiography, which has been adopted by most practices. Several CAD/CAM systems have been developed for dentistry. CAD/CAM stands for computer-aided design/computer-aided manufacture. CAD/CAM requires a digital model of the tooth preparation. Several techniques are used to obtain this digital model. One involves the usual dental impression with an impression material. The resulting impression or cast is digitized in the dental office or at the dental laboratory. The restoration is then designed using interactive software and machined by milling (grinding) the restoration out of a piece of solid material. The dental laboratory assumes the financial burden of the cost of the equipment. The cost is spread among many dental practices.

The second technique uses an "optical" impression. The optical impression system may or may not be integrated with an in-office CAD/CAM milling machine. The optical impression is taken with an intraoral camera. The "optical" impression is stored digitally in a computer. The restoration could be designed and milled in the dental office if the equipment is present. A one visit crown is possible. The cost of the equipment is born by the individual dental office. In-office CAD/CAM systems are quite expensive but are increasing in popularity. Optical impressions are becoming more common when just the camera is purchased and the resulting data file is sent to a dental laboratory for construction of the restoration. The common crown and bridge impression may become a memory, as has the cassette audio tape.

D. Performance of Impression Materials

Impression materials are the best performing of all dental materials. The use of impression materials has fewer restrictions than are found with most other dental materials. Impression materials only need to function for a short time (several hours to a few days). In addition, simulating clinical use of impression materials is quite simple compared with restorative materials, such as amalgam and composite. Research, product development, and quality control are greatly facilitated when clinical use can be easily simulated in the laboratory.

E. Biocompatibility of Impression Materials

Some assistants have had a skin rash on their hands that has been attributed to the manipulation of impression material. With the current practice of wearing gloves when treating patients, skin problems are first blamed on latex gloves. However, one must not forget that other dental materials can cause skin irritation, even though this is rare. Polymeric dental materials are much more likely to be irritating before they are mixed; the cured or set polymer is typically much less of a problem.

Because impression materials are used in the mouth only for several minutes, biocompatibility is usually not a significant concern. However, if residual pieces of impression material remain subgingivally or between teeth, significant irritation will occur. The clinician should inspect the oral cavity for residual material after impression removal.

Summary

Impression materials are used to make replicas of teeth and other oral tissues. The replicas are then used to fabricate restorations and other appliances. Impression materials are supplied in a variety of forms. Some are powders mixed with water; others are paste–paste systems. They can be classified by use, type, or how they set.

The inelastic impression materials include plaster, ZOE, wax, and impression compound. Agar and alginate are aqueous elastomers. The nonaqueous elastomeric materials include polysulfide, addition silicones, condensation silicones, and polyethers.

Alginates are used frequently for diagnosis and treatment planning. They are also used to make fluoride and bleaching trays, mouthguards, and other appliances. The advantage of hydrocolloids is that while they are being poured, the gypsum easily wets the surface of the hydrocolloid because it is composed of water. The disadvantage of hydrocolloids is that they are susceptible to syneresis and imbibition, which can affect accuracy.

Addition silicones are the most popular impression materials used in the construction of bridges, crowns, and other precision restorations. They are easy to use, record detail well, and have excellent properties. Their advantages include cleanliness, ease of use, lack of odor, accuracy, and stability. Their disadvantage is cost.

Each kind of impression material varies in cost, ease of use, accuracy, purpose, and mixing and setting times. Overall, impression materials are the best performing of all dental materials. They have few restrictions and only need to function for a short time.

Learning Activities

1. Mix two different-colored toothpastes (or cake frostings). Dispense equal lengths and mix them with a cement spatula until a homogeneous color is obtained. Note the time that is required. The same can be done with two different-colored modeling clays to simulate the mixing of putty.

2. Obtain light-body, medium-body, and heavy-body impression material (of the same brand). Mix and place approximately equal volumes of each material in a mound on a mixing pad. Note the "slump" of each material and the area that each covers.

3. Mix the materials in learning activity #2 and make samples of equal thickness. Bend the samples and note the stiffness of each material.

4. With alginate and one nonaqueous elastomeric material, take an impression of a dentoform (or of several fingers) under water (in a bucket of water). Note the details recorded in the two materials.

5. Take three alginate impressions of a quarter. Store overnight—one in water, one in air, and one in a sealed plastic bag. Check each day-old impression for detail and elasticity. How well does the quarter fit into each impression?

6. Go to www. http://carestreamdental.com/. Click on Products, then Digital Imaging, and then Intraoral Scanners. Browse this Web site to see an overview of a digital impression and a CAD/CAM system.

Review Questions

Question 1. Alginate impression material is:

a. Expensive compared with other impression materials
b. Easy to use
c. Not affected by gain or loss of water
d. Well known for its long-term stability

Question 2. Impression materials that have mechanical properties permitting considerable elastic deformation but that return to their original form are classified as:

a. Thermoplastic
b. Elastomeric
c. Inelastic
d. Resins

Question 3. Dr. Jones requested that you mix alginate and take an impression. While measuring the water, you got involved in conversation and did not notice how warm it was. This oversight will:

a. Make the mix unusable
b. Lengthen the gelation time
c. Not affect the gelation time
d. Shorten the gelation time

Question 4. Which of the following dental materials is an example of an aqueous elastomeric?

a. Impression compound
b. ZOE impression paste
c. Polysulfide
d. Irreversible hydrocolloid
e. Addition silicone

Question 5. The brown paste used in rubber base is called the:

a. Polymer
b. Accelerator
c. Base
d. Filler

Question 6. Dental impression compound is known as a/an _____ material.

a. Chemoplastic
b. Irreversible
c. Hydroelastic
d. Thermoplastic

Question 7. Which of the following is an example of an inelastic impression material?

a. Polysulfide
b. ZOE impression paste
c. Alginate
d. Addition silicone

Question 8. The term used for the setting of hydrocolloid impression materials is:

a. Crystallization
b. Polymerization
c. Curing
d. Gelation

Question 9. The popularity of agar impression material is limited by the:

a. High cost
b. Need for special equipment
c. Poor reproduction of detail
d. Difficulty in pouring the impression

Question 10. When an alginate impression slightly contracts and exudes water, it is termed:

a. Imbibition
b. Gelation
c. Syneresis
d. Hysteresis

Question 11. Addition silicones are the most popular type of rubber impression materials. The reason for this is cost.

a. The first statement is true; the second statement is false.
b. The first statement is false; the second statement is true.
c. Both statements are true.
d. Both statements are false.

Question 12. Custom impression trays are made on a model of the patient's arch. Therefore, to make a custom tray, an alginate impression is also needed.

a. The first statement is true; the second statement is false.
b. The first statement is false; the second statement is true.
c. Both statements are true.
d. Both statements are false.

Question 13. Mrs. Smith had not been to the dentist for several years. She agreed to extensive restorative treatment that she needed. You were asked to take impressions as the first step of her care. The impression material of choice would be:

a. Agar
b. Alginate
c. Dental impression compound
d. Addition silicone

Question 14. The impression tray that is used to record the prepared tooth, a bite registration, and an impression of the opposing teeth is a:

a. Stock tray
b. Custom tray
c. Triple tray
d. Bite registration tray

Question 15. Which of the following impression materials sets by physical means?

a. Agar
b. ZOE
c. Alginate
d. Addition silicone

Gypsum Materials

Objectives

After studying this chapter, the student will be able to do the following:

1. Define the following terms: study model, cast, and die.
2. Discuss the major differences between dental plaster, stone, and improved stone.
3. Explain the meaning of initial and final setting times.
4. Give three examples of how to increase and decrease the setting times of gypsum products.
5. Discuss wet and dry strength as it relates to gypsum products.
6. Summarize the recommended technique for use of gypsum products for measuring, mixing, and filling the impression. Include hand and vacuum mixing.

Key Words/Phrases

accelerators
articulator
calcination
cast
die
dry strength
final setting time
gypsum products
high-strength stone
improved stone
initial setting time
plaster
retarders
stone
study model
water/powder ratio
wet strength
working time

Introduction

Gypsum materials are mixed with water to produce a replica from an impression. Gypsum materials are used in dental offices and laboratories by dentists, hygienists, assistants, and lab technicians. These materials are quite old but still popular due to their ease of use, their affordability, and the long-term stability of the resulting cast.

I. Gypsum Materials

A. Use of Gypsum Products in Dentistry

Gypsum products are supplied as fine powders that are mixed with water to form a fluid mass or slurry that can be poured and shaped and that later hardens into a rigid, stable mass. An example of this powder is illustrated in *Figure 9.1*. Gypsum products are used mainly for positive reproductions or replicas of oral structures. These replicas are called casts, dies, or models, and they are obtained from negative reproductions, such as alginate impressions. Each replica has a specific purpose.

1. A **study model** is used to plan treatment and to observe treatment progress (*Fig. 9.2A*).

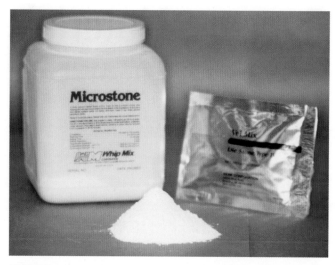

FIGURE 9.1. Gypsum powder (*front*): bulk package and pre-measured envelope.

2. A **cast** is a replica on which a restoration or appliance is fabricated. A cast is more accurate than a study model and is a replica of more than one tooth, such as a quadrant or a full arch. It may be partially or completely edentulous. Examples of dental casts are shown in *Figure 9.2B*.

3. A **die** is a working replica of a single tooth, as shown in *Figure 9.3*. Typically, it is a removable part of a cast.

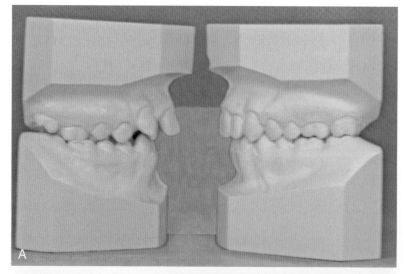

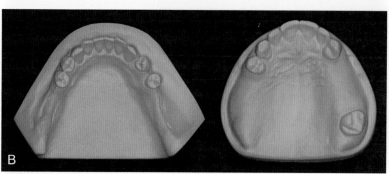

FIGURE 9.2. A. Preoperative and postoperative orthodontic study models. **B.** Dental casts made of stone for partial denture construction. (Part **B** reprinted from Richardson RE, Barton RE. *The Dental Assistant*. 5th ed. New York: McGraw-Hill; 1978, with permission.)

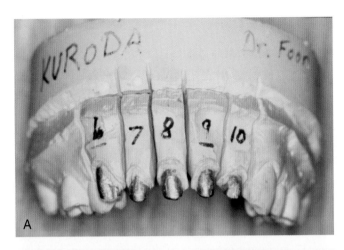

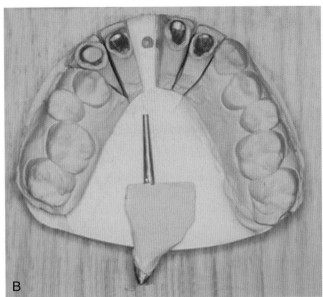

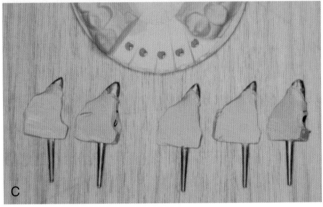

FIGURE 9.3. Cast with mounted dies. **A.** Five dies in cast. **B.** One die removed. **C.** All dies removed.

Because indirect dental restorations are fabricated on these cast or die replicas, it is essential that the particular gypsum product be carefully manipulated to ensure an accurate restoration.

B. Desirable Properties

Several properties are required of a material to be used for making casts, models, or dies. These properties are
1. Accuracy
2. Dimensional stability
3. Ability to reproduce fine detail
4. Strength and resistance to abrasion
5. Compatibility with the impression material
6. Color
7. Biological safety
8. Ease of use
9. Cost

Not all gypsum products display all of these desirable properties equally.

II. Types of Gypsum Products

Gypsum products are made from gypsum rock, which is a mineral found in various parts of the world. Gypsum rock is mined, ground into a fine powder, and then processed by heating to form a variety of products. Chemically, gypsum rock is calcium sulfate dihydrate ($CaSO_4 \cdot 2H_2O$). Pure gypsum is white, but in most deposits, it is discolored by impurities. Gypsum products are used in dentistry, medicine, homes, and industry. In homes, gypsum plaster is used to make walls; in industry, it is used to make molds.

In this chapter, three types of gypsum products are discussed: plaster, stone, and high-strength or improved stone. Chemically, all three are calcium sulfate hemihydrate. They are produced as a result of heating gypsum and driving off part of the water of crystallization. This process is called **calcination** and is shown in the following equation:

$$CaSO_4 \cdot 2H_2O + \text{heat} \rightarrow (CaSO_4)_2 \cdot H_2O$$
$$(\text{or } CaSO_4 \cdot \tfrac{1}{2}H_2O) + 1\tfrac{1}{2}H_2O$$

Plaster, stone, and improved stone differ in the physical characteristics of their powder particles as a result of differing calcination methods. These differences in powder particles are responsible for their different properties, which make them suitable for various uses. The manufacturers add other chemicals to improve handling and properties.

A. Plaster

Plaster was the first gypsum product available for dentistry. It is manufactured by grinding the gypsum rock into a fine powder and then heating that powder in an open container. This direct and rapid heating in open air drives part of the water of crystallization from the crystal and shatters the crystal. The resulting powder consists of porous, irregular particles (*Fig. 9.4A*). Plaster is the weakest and least expensive of the three gypsum products. It is used mainly when strength is not a critical requirement, such as preliminary casts for complete dentures and attaching casts to a mechanical device called an **articulator**. This device simulates the patient's occlusion and mastication process and is shown in Figures 1.8C and 11.6F; these photographs illustrate the use of plaster to secure the cast to the articulator.

Plaster is usually white in color and sometimes is referred to as beta-hemihydrate or Type II. In the past, plaster was modified for use as an impression material by the addition of chemicals and was called impression plaster (see Chapter 8, Impression Materials).

B. Stone

Stone is made from gypsum by carefully controlled calcination under steam pressure in a closed container. This method of calcination slowly releases the water of crystallization from the crystal so that the resultant powder particle (*Fig. 9.4B*) is more regular, more uniform in shape, and less porous compared to that of plaster. Stone is stronger and more expensive than plaster. It is used mainly in making casts for diagnostic purposes and casts for complete and partial denture construction, which require greater strength and surface hardness than that of plaster.

The stone is usually light tan in color, but it can be obtained in other colors. It is often referred to as alpha-hemihydrate, Type III stone, or Hydrocal.

C. High-Strength or Improved Stone

High-strength stone, or **improved stone**, is also made from gypsum by calcining the gypsum but in a calcium chloride solution. This method of calcination results in a powder particle that is very dense, is cuboidal in shape, and has a reduced surface area. High-strength stone is the strongest and most expensive of the three gypsum products, and it is used mainly for making casts or dies for crown, bridge, and inlay fabrication. *Figure 9.3* shows an example of an improved stone cast and several dies for the fabrication of crowns. This material is used because high strength and surface hardness are required during the fabrication process; the fabrication of crowns is described in the next chapter. High-strength stone is often referred to as Type IV stone, die stone, densite, or modified alpha-hemihydrate. A newly developed high-strength stone with a higher compressive strength than that of Type IV stone is also available. It displays higher setting expansion and is referred to as Type V stone.

D. Other Types of Gypsum

Other types of gypsum products are produced for special uses, such as fast set, mounting of casts on articulators, and impressions. Gypsum-based investments are presented in Chapter 10, Materials for Fixed Indirect Restorations and Prostheses.

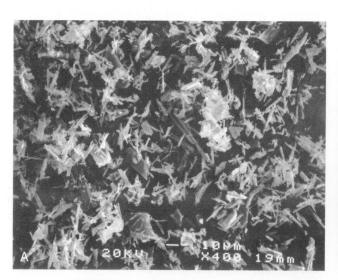
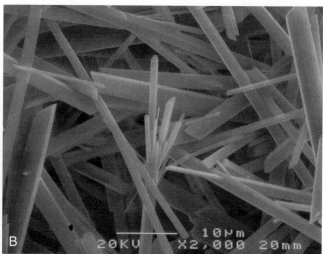

FIGURE 9.4. Scanning electron micrographs of **A.** dental plaster powder particles and **B.** dental stone powder particles. (Courtesy of Diane Schwegler-Berry, NIOSH, Morgantown, WV.)

III. Setting Reaction

When any of the various types of calcium sulfate hemihydrate are mixed with water, the hemihydrate is changed back to dihydrate by the process of hydration. Heat is liberated, as shown by the following reaction:

$$CaSO_4 \cdot \tfrac{1}{2}H_2O + 1 \cdot H_2O \rightarrow CaSO_4 \cdot 2H_2O + heat$$

The calcium sulfate hemihydrate dissolves in the mixing water. The dihydrate forms as it is less soluble than the hemihydrate. The calcium sulfate dihydrate precipitates out of solution as interlocking crystals forming a hard mass.

IV. Water/Powder Ratio

The proportion of water to powder used to make a workable mix of a particular gypsum product is called the **water/powder ratio.** For dental use, an excess amount of measured water above the theoretically correct amount required for hydration is always necessary. This excess amount is needed to make a workable mix or slurry that can be poured and shaped. The excess water is distributed as free water in the set mass without taking part in the chemical reaction, and it contributes to subsequent porosity or microscopic voids in the set product. The proper water/powder ratio for each product depends on the physical characteristics of the powder particles. Plaster requires more gauging water (measured water) to wet the powder surfaces, fill the pores, and float the irregular porous particles. The dense particles of stone require less gauging water to float them, and their regular shape allows them to roll over one another more easily. High-strength stone, because of its very dense and cuboidal type of particle as well as modifications made by the manufacturer, requires even less gauging water than does stone. For dental use, the proper water/powder ratios (fractions) are as follows:

- For the average mix of plaster, 45 to 50 mL/100 g (0.45–0.50)
- For the average mix of stone, 28 to 30 mL/100 g (0.28–0.30)
- For the average mix of improved stone, 19 to 24 mL/100 g (0.19–0.24)

This difference in the amount of measured water that is required to make a workable mix results in different consistencies for the products when first mixed at the proper water/powder ratio. Plaster is usually thin in consistency, like a "smoothie," whereas improved stone is like thick cake batter. Dental stone has an intermediate consistency. The water/powder ratio has a direct effect on the properties of each gypsum product and must be controlled for optimum results.

V. Setting Time

A. Definitions

Knowledge of the setting characteristics of a gypsum product is important for proper manipulation. The clinician should be aware of two time intervals in the setting process.

1. Working Time or Initial Setting Time
Working time or **initial setting time** is the length of time from the start of the mix until the setting mass reaches a semi-hard stage. It represents the available time for manipulating the product, and it indicates partial progress of the setting reaction.

2. Final Setting Time
Final setting time represents the length of time from the start of the mix until the setting mass becomes rigid and can be separated from the impression. The final setting time indicates the major completion of the hydration reaction.

B. Measurement

Setting times are usually measured with a surface penetration test. Gillmore needles are commonly used for this measurement and are shown in *Figure 9.5.* When the surface of the setting product

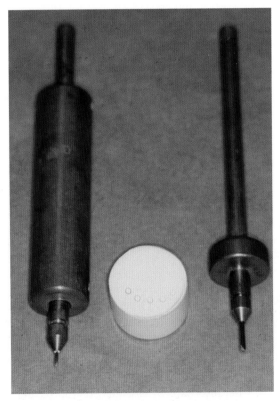

FIGURE 9.5. The 1-lb (*left*) and ¼-lb (*right*) Gillmore needles with a sample of a gypsum product.

has developed sufficient strength to support the weight of the ¼-lb needle and of the 1-lb needle, the initial setting time and the final setting time, respectively, have occurred. In other words, each designated setting time is reached when its respective needle no longer makes an indentation in the gypsum specimen. This method is somewhat arbitrary, and it is difficult to correlate directly with the setting reaction. In addition, the resulting values are mainly used for comparisons of different products. For practical purposes in a typical dental office, loss of surface gloss can be used as a determination of the working time; it is typically 5 to 7 minutes. The failure of penetration by a fingernail or dull knife would indicate relative rigidity and hardness and could be used as an indication of final set. Usually, a time of 30 to 45 minutes is used as a subjective criterion for the time of final set.

C. Variation in Setting Times

The setting time of a gypsum product is controlled by the manufacturer's particular formulation. Hence, several gypsum products are available with varying setting characteristics. Either a fast-setting or a slow-setting product can be purchased. Sometimes, it may be necessary to modify the setting time of a gypsum product in the dental office. Increased and decreased setting times may be obtained in the following ways:

1. Increased Setting Time (A Slower-Setting Product)
   a. Decreased mixing.
   b. Higher water/powder ratio (creates a thinner mix).
   c. Addition of certain chemicals called **retarders**. A commonly used retarder is borax.

2. Decreased Setting Time (A Faster-Setting Product)
   a. Increased mixing (the longer the mixing time, the shorter the setting time).
   b. Lower water/powder ratio (creates a thicker mix).
   c. Addition of certain chemicals called **accelerators**. A commonly used accelerator is potassium sulfate. Other chemicals can be used, but their effect on the setting time depends on concentration and other factors.

Improper storage and use of gypsum products can also change the setting characteristics. Because water is essential for the setting reaction, any moisture that inadvertently comes in contact with the product can change the setting time. Thus, gypsum products should be stored in airtight containers to prevent any uptake of water resulting from high relative humidity. As a result, preweighed packages have become popular for many gypsum products. The first indication of moisture contamination is faster setting of the product. If the contamination continues, slower setting occurs.

VI. Setting Expansion

All gypsum products expand externally on setting. Plaster expands the most, at 0.2% to 0.3%. Stone expands 0.08% to 0.10%. High-strength stone expands the least, at 0.05% to 0.07%. Theoretically, a contraction on setting can be calculated; however, the growing crystals of the gypsum push against each other and cause an outward crystal thrust. In turn, this thrust causes an external expansion with resulting internal porosity in the set mass. A minimal setting expansion is desirable to achieve accurate dimensional reproduction for most casts and dies. Manufacturers modify most gypsum products that are used for casts and dies to provide for minimal expansion. They do this by the addition of chemicals, which also control the setting characteristics. Thus, a particular gypsum product has both the setting time and expansion characteristics controlled by the manufacturer. The setting expansion can be controlled by manipulating variables. A thicker mix and increased spatulation will cause an increase in the amount of setting expansion; a thinner mix and decreased spatulation will cause a decrease in the amount of setting expansion. In most dental offices, however, there is little need to change the expansion characteristics of gypsum products.

If gypsum materials are immersed in or come in contact with water during the setting process, the setting expansion increases. This is called hygroscopic expansion, and it can be used to increase the setting expansion of casting investments. Casting investments are discussed in the next chapter. Although small, hygroscopic expansion is approximately twice as great as the normal setting expansion. Therefore, to prevent an inadvertent increase in size, routine casts should not be immersed in water during setting.

VII. Strength

The strength of the gypsum product is usually measured in terms of crushing or compressive strength. As expected from the setting reaction, strength develops rapidly during the first 30 to 45 minutes as hydration is completed. The strength depends on the porosity of the set material, and the porosity relates to the water/powder ratio necessary to make a workable mix. Plaster, which requires the most gauging water to make a fluid mix, is the weakest in strength, with improved stone being the strongest and stone being intermediate between the two. The 1-hour strengths of gypsum products are listed in Table 9.1.

TABLE 9.1. One-Hour Compressive Strengths and Water/Powder Ratios of Gypsum Products		
	Minimum 1-Hour Compressive	
Gypsum	**Strength in lb/in² (MPa)**[a]	**Water/Powder Ratio (fractions)**
Plaster (Type II)	1,300 (9)	45–50 mL/100 g (0.45–0.50)
Dental stone (Type III)	3,000 (21)	28–30 mL/100 g (0.28–0.30)
Dental stone, high-strength (Type IV)	5,000 (34)	19–24 mL/100 g (0.19–0.24)

[a]Adapted from Revised ANSI-ADA specification no. 25.

The presence or absence of excess free water also affects strength. Two types of strength are recognized: wet strength and dry strength.

A. Wet Strength

The **wet strength** is the strength that is measured when the sample contains some or all of the water in excess of the theoretical amount required for hydration. This is the typical condition after setting. The material feels wet to the touch for many hours.

B. Dry Strength

The **dry strength** is the strength that is measured when the excess water is not present in the sample. The dry strength may be two or more times the wet strength. Usually, the cast must sit in a dry environment overnight to approach these values.

C. Factors Affecting Strength

The strength of a particular product depends on the water/powder ratio; thicker mixes will increase the strength within limits, and thinner mixes will decrease the strength. However, extremely thick mixes, particularly those of stone and improved stone, are heavy in consistency and can cause distortion of the impression as well as entrapment of air voids. Extremely thin mixes will cause a decrease in strength. Therefore, it is a good practice to follow the manufacturer's recommended water/powder ratio for optimum strength and consistency properties.

VIII. Surface Hardness

The surface hardness is related to the compressive strength but reaches its maximum value more rapidly because the surface is the first to dry. The greatest surface hardness occurs when the product reaches its dry strength, which many times is not realized under practical conditions. Casts and dies should be allowed to set for 1 to 2 hours, or preferably overnight or longer, before beginning subsequent laboratory procedures. The surface hardness of set gypsum is not as high as desired. Use of a commercial hardening solution in place of water may increase the hardness and improve the abrasion resistance.

IX. Dimensional Stability

The dimensions of a hardened or set gypsum cast are relatively constant under ordinary conditions of room temperature and humidity; however, gypsum is slightly soluble in water. Occasionally, it is necessary to soak a cast in water for a laboratory procedure. If the cast is soaked in water for prolonged periods of time, the surface may be dissolved away. If the cast must be soaked in water, the water should be saturated with gypsum to prevent erosion of the surface. The safest way to soak a cast is to place it in a water bath containing particles of gypsum to provide a saturated solution of calcium sulfate at all times.

X. Technique of Use

The technical use of gypsum products is relatively simple, requiring only a mixing bowl, mixing spatula, room-temperature water, and the appropriate gypsum product. As mentioned earlier, the water and powder must be proportioned accurately for optimum properties to be obtained. The measuring and mixing technique can be summarized as follows.

A. Measuring the Water

The water is usually dispensed by volume in a graduated cylinder because 1 g of water has a volume of very close to 1 mL.

B. Measuring the Powder

The powder can be weighed in grams with a simple balance or scale. Volume dispensers may also be used, but are not as accurate because of the varying packing effect on the powder. First, the water is added to the mixing bowl and it is placed on the scale. Second, the scale is tared (reading is set to zero). Finally, the powder is added to the bowl with a suitable scoop until the desired weight of powder has been added.

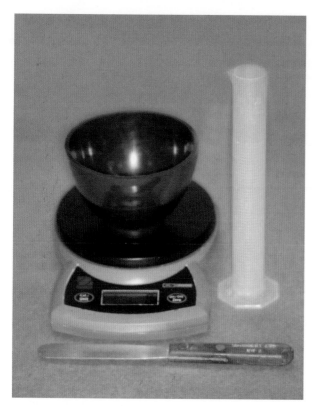

FIGURE 9.6. Equipment for mixing gypsum products: scale, rubber mixing bowl, graduated cylinder, and plaster spatula.

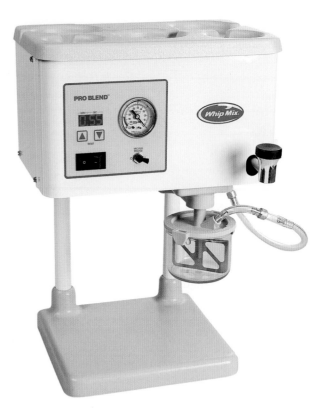

FIGURE 9.7. A vacuum mixing and investing machine. (Courtesy of Whip Mix Corp., Louisville, KY.)

A measuring scale, bowl, and graduated cylinder are shown in *Figure 9.6*. Weighing with the scale is a simple and convenient method to ensure accurate proportions. Preweighed packets are now available to ensure an accurate mix. They control the weight of the powder, reduce wasted powder, and require less time.

C. Adding Powder and Water

The preferred method of mixing is to add the measured water into the mixing bowl first, followed by gradual addition of the preweighed powder. The guesswork of repeatedly adding water and powder to achieve the proper consistency is to be avoided even though it is a common practice. It can result in low strength and inconsistent expansion.

D. Mixing

1. Hand Mixing

Hand mixing is usually done in a flexible plastic or rubber bowl with a stiff-bladed spatula to combine the powder and water. The mix should be smooth, homogeneous, workable, and free of air bubbles. A minimum of air inclusion in the mixed product is desirable to prevent surface bubbles and internal defects. Mixing is usually accomplished with a wiping motion against the sides of the bowl (to eliminate lumps and air bubbles). Use of a dental vibrator will reduce bubbles in the mix. A smooth, homogeneous

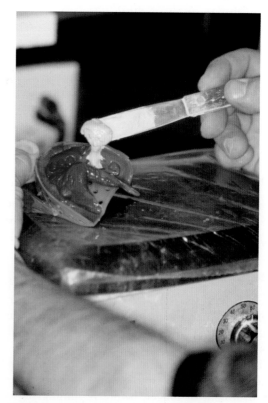

FIGURE 9.8. An impression sits on a dental vibrator as it is poured with stone.

mix should be obtained in approximately 1 minute. A whipping motion should be avoided.

2. Vacuum Mixing

Often, mixing is done mechanically with a vacuum mixing and investing machine. An example of this device is shown in *Figure 9.7.* This provides a gypsum mix that is free of air bubbles and is homogeneous in consistency. Many devices are available that will mix gypsum products mechanically with or without vacuum. They are used when the elimination of voids and surface bubbles is critical.

E. Filling the Impression

When filling the impression, the gypsum mixture needs to flow slowly "ahead of itself" to prevent the entrapment of air. This is usually accomplished with a dental vibrator, as shown in *Figure 9.8.* This is particularly important when filling elastomeric impressions, which in many instances are water repellent. Vibrating the mix after mixing can also be used to bring air bubbles to the surface. Although relatively simple, manipulation of gypsum products requires careful attention to detail for accurate results.

Summary

Gypsum products are used for making positive reproductions or replicas of oral structures. These replicas are called casts, dies, or models. Gypsum products are available in three basic types: plaster, stone, and improved stone.

The water/powder ratios vary for each type of gypsum. For plaster, the ratio is 45 to 50 mL/100 g. For stone, the ratio is 28 to 30 mL/100 g. For improved stone, the ratio is 19 to 24 mL/100 g. The plaster mix will be thin in consistency, whereas the improved stone mix will be like thick cake batter.

The working or initial setting time is the length of time from the start of the mix until the mass reaches a semi-hard stage. Practically speaking, the "loss of gloss" could be used as a determinant for the working or initial setting time. Final setting time is the length of time from the start of the mix until the mass becomes rigid and can be separated from the impression. Failure of a fingernail or a knife to penetrate the gypsum would indicate the final set.

Gypsum products expand externally on setting. Plaster expands the most, at 0.2% to 0.3%. Improved stone expands the least, at 0.05% to 0.07%. The strength of gypsum products is measured in terms of compressive strength. Strength develops within 30 to 45 minutes and depends on the porosity of the material. Plaster is the weakest of the three products, and improved stone is the strongest. Wet strength is the measured strength "just after it sets," and dry strength is the strength measured when excess water is not present. Casts should be protected from contact with water because gypsum is slightly soluble in water.

When mixing, the powder is added to the water. Gypsum may be mixed by hand or by vacuum. When filling the impression, the gypsum should "flow ahead of itself" so that air does not become entrapped. Use of gypsum products is relatively simple, but attention to detail ensures more accurate results.

Learning Activities

1. Place 40 g of plaster in a 50-mL graduated cylinder. Calculate the density. Now do the same for stone. Why is there a difference?

2. Mix plaster with several water/powder ratios in the range of 0.4 to 0.6. How is the setting time affected?

3. Mix plaster, using various spatulation times: 1, 2, and 3 minutes. How is the setting time affected?

4. Make one-quarter inch thick patties of plaster, dental stone, and improved stone. Let them set for at least 1 hour (a day is better). Compare the time and effort to trim one-half inch of the edge of the patty of each material using a model trimmer.

Review Questions

Question 1. The desirable strength of gypsum materials is _____ related to the amount of water used.

a. Directly

b. Indirectly

c. Not

d. Partially

Question 2. For gypsum products, a suitable accelerator and retarder, respectively, would be:

a. Ethyl alcohol and oleic acid

b. Oleic acid and glycerin

c. Borax and potassium sulfate

d. Potassium sulfate and borax

Question 3. The gypsum material known as "high-strength stone" may also be referred to as:

a. Plaster

b. Dental stone

c. Type III stone

d. Improved stone

Question 4. The final setting time in minutes for gypsum products typically is:

a. 15 to 30

b. 30 to 45

c. 45 to 90

d. 90 to 120

Question 5. To make a correct mix for dental stone when using 50 g of powder, the amount of water would be approximately:

a. 10 to 12 mL

b. 14 to 15 mL

c. 28 to 30 mL

d. 45 to 50 mL

Question 6. Cathy and her parents will meet with an orthodontist to discuss an orthodontic treatment plan. At a previous appointment, the orthodontist took impressions of Cathy's maxillary and mandibular arches. The replicas made from each impression to discuss the treatment plan are termed:

a. Casts

b. Dies

c. Study models

d. Molds

Question 7. Decreasing the setting time of a dental material results in a product that:

a. Will set faster

b. Will set slower

c. Does not affect the setting time

d. Enhances the properties

Question 8. The weakest gypsum product is:

a. Improved stone

b. Dental stone

c. Plaster

d. Die stone

Question 9. When excess water is not present in a gypsum product, it is known as the:

a. Wet strength

b. Dry strength

c. Initial setting time

d. Surface strength

Question 10. The best way to mix gypsum products is to:

a. "Eyeball" the amount of powder added to water

b. Add water to the powder

c. Add powder to the water

d. Add powder and water to bowl simultaneously

Question 11. Initial and final setting times of gypsum can be determined with the use of Gillmore needles. A practical, easy method to determine final setting time in a dental office would be to:

a. Set a timer for 20 minutes

b. Observe the change from wet to dry strength

c. Watch for the loss of gloss

d. Attempt to penetrate the material with the metal spatula

Question 12. When the setting time of a dental material is increased, which of the following is true?

a. The material sets slower

b. The material sets faster

c. The setting reaction does not change

d. The setting reaction is increased

Materials for Fixed Indirect Restorations and Prostheses

Objectives

After studying this chapter, the student will be able to do the following:

1. Discuss the factors that affect treatment planning for a fixed indirect restoration.
2. Explain the lost-wax casting process used in dentistry to make metal restorations.
3. Describe the types of alloys used to make all-metal crowns, ceramometal crowns, and partial denture frameworks.
4. Recall the types of porcelain used to simulate the color of teeth.
5. List the advantages and disadvantages of all-metal, ceramometal, and all-ceramic restorations.

Key Words/Phrases

abutments

alloys

bridge

buildups

burnishing

ceramometal restorations

coping

cores

crowns

crucible

divested

elongation

fixed restorations

glass–ceramic

gypsum-bonded investments

indirect restorations

ingate

inlays

onlays

pontics

provisional restoration

retainer

sintered

sprue

temporary restoration

veneer

wax pattern

Introduction

There are many types of fixed indirect restorations. **Indirect restorations** are those restorations that are constructed outside the mouth. **Fixed restorations** cannot be removed from the oral cavity; they are luted (cemented) in place. Fixed indirect restorations can be classified in two ways: by the amount of tooth structure they restore or by the material from which they are made.

I. Classification by Amount of Tooth Structure Restored

A. Inlays

Inlays are intracoronal (inside the crown) restorations that replace small to medium amounts of tooth structure, as shown in Figure 1.3. They are most commonly used to restore pits, fissures, and grooves (class I) as well as proximal surfaces (class II) of posterior teeth. They do not restore the cusps. They are retained by luting cements.

B. Onlays

Onlays (or overlays) involve replacing more tooth structure than inlays. In addition to the pits, fissures, and proximal surfaces of an inlay, onlays restore one or more cusps and, at times, the entire occlusal surface of a tooth. Onlays are used when the likelihood of cusp fracture is high. The onlay protects the cusps from occlusal forces. Onlays, like inlays, are retained with intracoronal retention and luting cements. An onlay is shown in *Figure 10.1.*

C. Veneers

A **veneer** is a thin layer of material that covers another material (like the shell of a hard-boiled egg). In dentistry, veneers are restorations that are

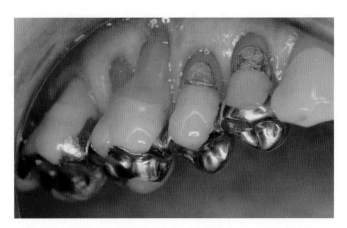

FIGURE 10.1. Photograph of several teeth restored with 30-year-old cast gold restorations. Tooth #3 is restored with an inlay. Tooth #4 is restored with an inlay/onlay combination. Tooth #5 is restored with an onlay.

placed on the facial surface of anterior teeth to treat an esthetic problem, such as discolorations, rotations, or spaces (diastemata) (*Fig. 10.2*). Veneers are often used in conjunction with orthodontic or periodontal treatment. Two types of veneers are used.

1. Direct veneers use bonded composites, as shown in Figure 5.9. Direct veneers may not involve the removal of significant tooth structure. If tooth structure is not removed, such veneers are considered to be a reversible treatment.
2. Indirect veneers use a ceramic material, such as porcelain. Usually, the facial surface is prepared to provide space for the veneering material. Therefore, indirect veneers are not a reversible procedure. Indirect veneers involve an impression, sometimes a temporary restoration, a second appointment, and a laboratory fee. Therefore, they cost more overall than direct veneers. At one time, composite materials were also used, but discoloration was a problem. Today, porcelain is popular because a single veneer can utilize a variety of porcelain

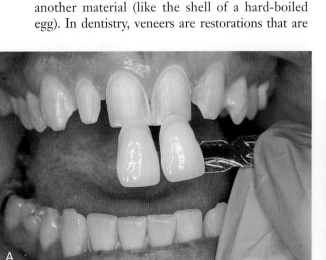
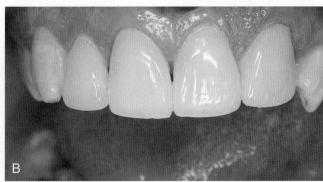

FIGURE 10.2. Photographs of teeth **A.** prepared for indirect veneers and **B.** the veneers cemented in place. (Courtesy of Ultradent Products, Inc.)

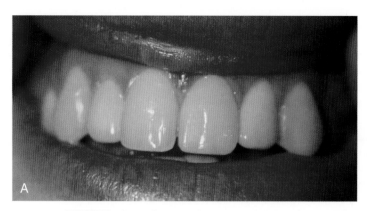
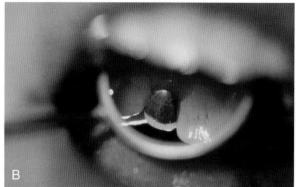

FIGURE 10.3. Photographs of porcelain-fused-to-metal crowns restoring teeth #7 and #10. **A.** Labial view of both teeth. **B.** Lingual view of tooth #10.

shades and translucencies. Indirect veneers are supported by, and are bonded to, the underlying tooth structure.

D. Crowns

Crowns are used to restore teeth that have lost a significant amount of tooth structure. They are used when intracoronal retention is unavailable or when the tooth needs to be surrounded and held together by the restoration. A full gold crown is shown in Figure 1.4. A porcelain crown is shown in Figure 1.10F. Ceramometal crowns are shown in *Figure 10.3*.

E. Complex Restorations

Complex restorations combine the features of inlay, onlay, and crown restorations, as shown in tooth #4 of *Figure 10.1*. A complex restoration is

designed by the dentist after caries, and the loss of tooth structure has been assessed.

F. Dental Bridge

A **bridge** replaces missing teeth. Typically, a bridge has a crown, called a **retainer**, at each end. The retainers are supported by teeth called **abutments**. The replacement teeth are called **pontics**. A bridge may replace one tooth or several teeth, as shown in Figure 1.5.

II. Classification by Material

A. Metals

A variety of metals are used to restore teeth, as shown in *Figures 10.1 and 10.4*. Most metallic

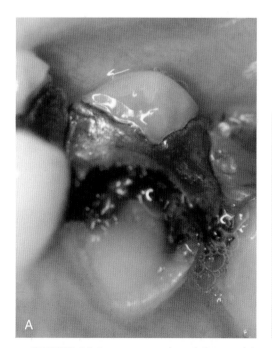
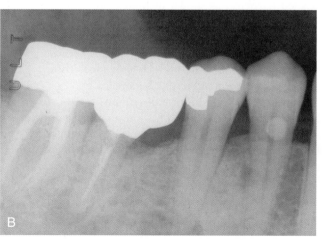

FIGURE 10.4. Two examples of the need for an indirect restoration. **A.** A fractured lingual cusp. **B.** A tooth #30 that has had a multitude of dental treatment, including root canal therapy, root amputation, and a crown. This tooth was deemed to be hopeless and extracted because of pain, mobility, and a periapical radiolucency.

indirect restorations are made by a casting procedure. Casting involves melting the metal and then pouring or forcing the liquid metal into a mold. The casting process allows custom, complex shapes to be easily produced. Metals are very tough and work well in high-stress situations, but their esthetics are poor.

B. Ceramic Materials

Ceramic materials are used when esthetics are important, as shown in Figure 1.10. Ceramic materials can simulate the natural colors and translucency of teeth. Porcelain is the ceramic material most commonly used in dentistry to obtain a variety of colors or shades for a single crown. A variety of materials and processing techniques are employed. Most ceramic materials lack the toughness and fracture resistance required by bridges, but their esthetics can be excellent.

C. Ceramometal

A metal–ceramic combination was developed for dentistry in the 1950s. This material is made by using the same process to bake enamel (porcelain) on metal as that was used to make old-fashioned pots and pans or sinks and bathtubs. The tough, strong metal supports the weak but esthetic ceramic material. The restorations are called **ceramometal restorations** (or porcelain-bonded-to-metal or porcelain-fused-to-metal crowns) and are considered to be an important "workhorse" in modern restorative dentistry. Ceramometal restorations are shown in *Figure 10.3*.

D. Composite Materials—Optional

Particle-reinforced composite materials (very similar to those discussed in Chapter 5, Direct Polymeric Restorative Materials) have been adapted for use as fixed indirect restorations. These materials are polymers reinforced by irregularly shaped particles, as shown in Figure 5.8C. They are cured at elevated temperatures, pressures, or both in the dental laboratory. Particle-reinforced composites have seen only limited success because their strength and toughness do not meet those required by crown and bridge materials.

Recently, fiber-reinforced composites have been developed for dentistry. These composites are similar to materials that have been developed for many other industries in which glass fibers are used to reinforce polymeric materials. Imagine a bowl of frozen, leftover spaghetti with sauce. The spaghetti represents the glass fibers; the frozen sauce represents the polymer matrix. The long fibers transfer stresses over a larger area than particles do. Automotive, aerospace, and sports equipment companies use fiber-reinforced composites to manufacture strong, lightweight products.

Fiber-reinforced composites are much tougher and stronger than particle-reinforced composites. Clinical results are promising, but these materials are not commonly used.

III. Procedures for Constructing an Indirect Restoration

A. Diagnosis, Treatment Planning, and Designing the Restoration

1. **Diagnosis**

   Lost tooth structure and missing teeth result from a variety of causes. Caries and periodontal disease are the most common. An extreme case involving caries and periodontal disease is shown in Figure 11.10. Trauma or fracture (*Fig. 10.4A*), esthetic concerns (Fig. 1.10), and congenital deficiencies (*Fig. 10.2A*) are other reasons to restore or replace teeth. Often, teeth are lost as the result of restoration and re-restoration and multiple dental treatments (*Fig. 10.4B*).

2. **Treatment Planning**

   A variety of factors affect the success of a restoration. These factors must be assessed during treatment planning.

   a. The periodontal status of the patient is critical. Without a stable foundation, the long-term success of any restoration is unlikely.

   b. The pulpal (endodontic) status of the tooth must be considered. A simple cold test for vitality is commonly used. A periapical radiograph is important to assess the periodontal and periapical condition of the tooth.

   c. Caries risk assessment and testing is becoming more common. If a crown or bridge will likely fail in several years because of recurrent caries, efforts to reduce the risk of caries should precede extensive and expensive restorations.

   d. Enough tooth structure must remain to retain the restoration. Badly broken-down teeth may require **buildups** (also called **cores**) to provide retention of the final restoration, as shown in Figures 6.11 and 8.1A.

3. **Restoration Design**

   Many factors influence the design of a restoration.

   a. The most common factor is the patient's desire for an esthetic restoration. Esthetic requirements include the shade and translucency of the restoration and influence the selection of the restorative material to be used.

   b. The attrition (wear) rate of the restoration should be considered.

   c. Biocompatibility of the material must be considered.

d. Location of the margins of a restoration may be placed above the gingiva or in the gingival sulcus. Margin location affects esthetics, retention, periodontal response to the restoration, and likelihood of recurrent caries.

B. Preparation

The tooth or teeth are prepared with specific restorative materials in mind. Different materials require different amounts of tooth reduction and shapes of the margins. Amalgam and inlay preparations are shown in Figure 1.3. Crown preparations are shown in Figures 1.10B and 8.1A.

C. Impressions

After the preparation is complete, an impression of the preparation, adjacent teeth, and opposing teeth is taken. Full-arch impressions result in more accurate articulation of models and less adjustment of a complex restoration before cementation. Several impressions were shown in Figure 1.8A and in Chapter 8.

D. Fabrication of a Temporary Restoration

The patient will not like the appearance and feel of the prepared tooth. In addition, exposed dentin can be very sensitive to heat, cold, and air. A **temporary restoration** (also called a **provisional restoration**) is constructed and cemented at the time of preparation, as shown in Figure 1.10C. The temporary restoration is left in place until the final restoration is received from the lab and permanently cemented. Chapter 35 presents techniques for the fabrication of a temporary crown.

E. Laboratory Procedures

The description and design of the restoration is written on a laboratory prescription (*Fig. 10.5*).

DiConcilis Dental Lab, LLC
Helping your practice build lasting smiles.

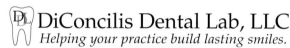

CHRIS DISCONCILIS
Owner/Operator ~25+ years experience
Specialty: Crowns and Bridges

DiConcilis Dental Lab, LLC
208 Willow Way
Uniontown, PA 15401

724-322-115

Call for pick up.

FROM _____   DATE _____

DR. _____   CASE # _____

ADDRESS _____   PHONE _____

_____

PATIENT _____   SEX ___ AGE ___

TYPE OF RESTORATION _____   TOOTH # _____

CUSTOM ABUTMENT _____ ATLANTIS _____ CMC _____

MANUFACTURER _____   SIZE _____

☐ TITANIUM _____   ☐ ZIRCONIUM _____

DATE WANTED _____ TIME _____   ☐ TRY-IN ☐ FINISH

SPECIAL INSTRUCTIONS:

_____
_____
_____
_____
_____
_____
_____

SHADES

1. _____

2. _____

DENTIST'S LICENSE # _____

DENTIST'S SIGNATURE _____

FIGURE 10.5. A laboratory prescription. (Courtesy of Christopher DiConcilis, Smithfield, PA.)

This prescription becomes a part of the patient record. Impressions are disinfected and then poured in the dental office or a commercial laboratory. The laboratory constructs the final restoration according to the dentist's instructions. A variety of restorations and prostheses are shown in Chapters 1, 10, and 11.

F. Cementation of the Restoration

At a second appointment, the temporary crown is removed, and the temporary cement is cleaned from the prepared tooth. Scaling instruments or pumice and a prophy cup are used. "Try-in" of the restoration is next. The restoration is seated on the preparation and carefully evaluated. The proximal contacts are checked with floss. The margins are examined with an explorer. The occlusion is evaluated with articulation paper, and the esthetics are examined with the patient's input. If all is acceptable, the restoration is cemented (see Fig. 7.1). Completed crowns are shown in Figures 1.4 and 1.10E.

G. Completion of the Treatment Plan

After the restoration is cemented, the remaining treatment plan is completed. The final step in the treatment plan should be to determine the recall status of the patient based on periodontal concerns, caries risk, chronic problems, and oral hygiene home care practices.

IV. Casting Process—Optional

Dentistry has used the "lost-wax casting technique" for a century to produce metal restorations. This process first constructs the restoration in wax. The wax is then replaced with metal in the same shape and size as the original wax pattern. The lost-wax casting technique is shown in *Figure 10.6*.

A. Wax and Waxing

1. Waxing

   Wax is easy to mold and shape. All that is required is a heat source and a few simple instruments. Creating the shape of the restoration in wax (**wax pattern**) requires skill and involves both the art and the science of dentistry, as shown in *Figure 10.6A*. The art is creating a reproduction of the shape of the lost tooth structure. The science is the requirement for the shape to function as the original tooth structure did (or should).

2. Dental Waxes

   Dentistry uses a variety of waxes with different melting, working, and handling properties.

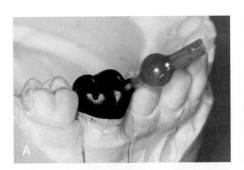
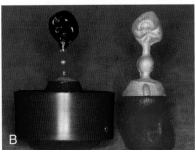
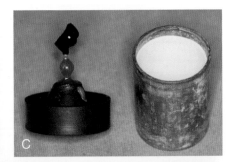
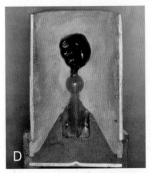
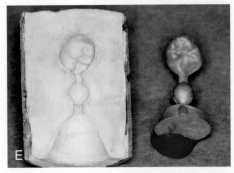
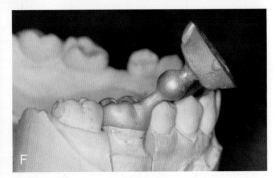

FIGURE 10.6. Photographs showing the fabrication of a full gold crown (the same crown as shown in Figs. 1.4 and 8.1). **A.** Wax pattern with the sprue attached. **B.** Wax pattern attached to the sprue base (also called crucible former) and the casting. Note the reproduction of shape and size. **C.** Wax pattern and casting ring with a paper liner. The casting ring slips over the wax pattern and fits into the sprue base. **D.** Sprued and invested wax pattern inside a sectioned casting ring. **E.** Cross section through a casting ring after burnout and a completed casting. **F.** Completed casting on the die.

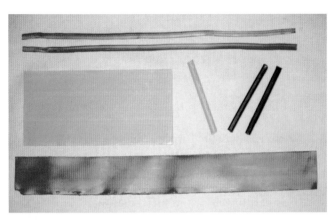

FIGURE 10.7. Photograph of several dental waxes: rope wax (*top*), baseplate wax (*middle left*), sticky wax (*middle center*), inlay wax (*middle right*), and boxing wax (*bottom*).

Several are shown in *Figure 10.7*. The composition of a wax product is usually proprietary and is typically a combination of natural and synthetic waxes. Wax is very soft compared to other dental materials. Distortion of wax is not typically visible to the unaided eye, but wax is unstable. A wax pattern can distort over time to a degree sufficient to affect the fit of restorations.

a. Inlay casting wax is used for casting inlays, crowns, and other restorations. Inlay casting wax is unique in that when it is heated to a sufficient temperature, it will burn away completely, leaving no residue. This feature is part of the specification for inlay casting wax. These waxes are hard and have higher melting temperatures compared to other waxes. Inlay waxes are not "sticky" to the touch. Other dental waxes have different handling characteristics.

b. Sticky wax is a hard wax that melts at a higher temperature. When sticky wax is applied to an object in the molten state and then allowed to cool to the solid state, it sticks well (for a wax).

c. Baseplate wax is a medium-hard wax that melts at an intermediate temperature and is not sticky. It is usually pink in color (to simulate the color of gingiva) and is used in the fabrication of dentures.

d. Other utility waxes, such as boxing wax (wide strips) and rope or beading wax (like a small rope or bead of caulk), are soft, flexible, and slightly sticky at room temperature. They are used to encircle an impression (also known as "boxing") before pouring with a gypsum material.

e. Dental waxes are quite costly when compared to paraffin wax used to preserve jelly and jam. The additional cost results from the purity of the components and the complexity of the formulation. Compared to other dental materials, dental waxes are very inexpensive. The different dental waxes work quite well and, surprisingly, have not been replaced by newer, "high-tech" materials.

B. Investing and Investments

1. Investing Procedures

The casting process forces molten metal into the empty space of the mold. The mold is made by investing a wax pattern. The wax pattern is surrounded by and embedded in a mold material, as shown in *Figure 10.6D*. When the wax is removed, the mold space is created. The wax pattern is the exact size and shape that the resulting casting will be. A **sprue** is a plastic or metal tube that will form an opening (or **ingate**) for the mold. It is attached to the wax pattern, as shown in *Figure 10.6A*. With the sprue used for support, the wax pattern is attached to the sprue base, as shown in *Figure 10.6B*. The casting ring, as shown in *Figure 10.6C*, is placed over the sprued wax pattern and then filled with mold material (investment). A casting ring is used to form the outside of the mold, as shown in *Figure 10.6D*. The sprue and sprue base are removed, and the mold space is actually formed by the investment material. The invested pattern is heated, and the wax is melted and flows out of the mold. As the temperature rises, any residual wax is burned away. This heating procedure is called "wax burnout." Burnout results in a mold space into which the metal is forced or "cast," as shown in *Figure 10.6E*.

2. Investment Materials

The most common investment materials are gypsum-based products. The same handling characteristics discussed in Chapter 9, Gypsum Materials, for gypsum products apply to gypsum-bonded investments. A silica material is added to dental stone to produce **gypsum-bonded investments**. The silica material improves the investment's resistance to heat and is called a refractory material. A second (and equally important) function is that the refractory material increases thermal expansion of the mold. The mold must be expanded to compensate exactly for the thermal shrinkage of the solid metal casting as it cools to room temperature. If mold expansion does not compensate for the thermal shrinkage, the casting will not fit. Metals typically shrink much more than ceramic materials. Luckily, the silica materials used in dental casting investments have unusual thermal properties. They exhibit a sudden increase in expansion at an elevated temperature. The amount of expansion and the temperature at which the expansion occurs depend on the silica material used in the investment. Different investment materials expand by different amounts at various temperatures.

C. Burnout

A temperature-controlled oven is used to burn out the wax pattern invested in the casting ring. The proper burnout temperature will result in proper mold expansion and a well-fitting casting. The casting ring is placed in the oven, and the mold is heated to 500°C to 600°C (900–1,100°F). The wax melts and is volatilized, leaving a clean mold space. The casting ring is left in the oven after reaching the desired temperature for approximately 30 minutes to 1 hour to "heat soak" the ring. Heat soaking the ring assures that the entire wax pattern has burned out and that the mold has reached the desired temperature.

D. Casting

Several types of equipment are used to make dental castings (*Fig. 10.8*). The casting process involves melting the casting alloy and then forcing it into the mold space. The technique used to melt the alloy depends on the melting temperature of the alloy. Gold casting alloys for all-metal crowns are easily melted with a "blow torch" using compressed air and natural gas (used to heat homes and offices). The alloy is melted while sitting in a refractory ceramic device, called a **crucible**, which is part of the casting machine. Alloys with higher melting temperatures require oxygen or acetylene gas. Other methods to melt casting alloys include electrical resistance heating (as in a toaster) and induction melting.

The most common casting machine used to force molten alloy into the mold is called a centrifugal casting machine. It rapidly spins the mold, crucible, and molten alloy in a circle. Casting occurs when spinning suddenly starts. While the crucible, molten alloy, and mold are rapidly accelerated, the

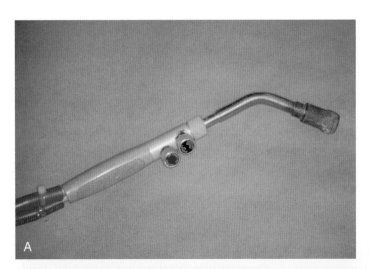
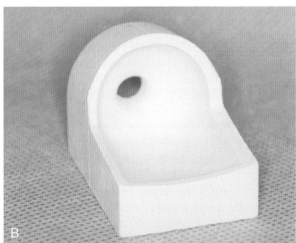
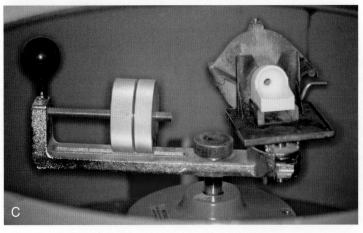
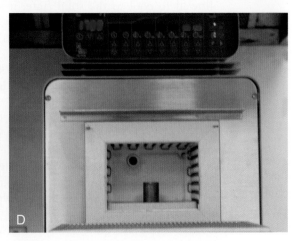

FIGURE 10.8. Equipment used to make dental castings. **A.** Torch. **B.** Crucible. **C.** Casting machine with crucible in place. **D.** Burnout oven with a casting ring inside.

inertia of the liquid metal causes the alloy to stay in place. The alloy seems to flow out of the spinning crucible and into the spinning mold. In reality, the molten metal stays in place; the casting ring spins and collides with the molten alloy. The liquid metal is forced to flow into the ingate of the ring previously occupied by the sprue. The molten alloy flows down the sprue space and into the mold, and it fills the space previously occupied by the wax pattern. When the metal cools, it solidifies, and the casting is complete.

The most common casting machine has a coiled spring that is wound up. The energy stored in the wound spring is used to rapidly spin (accelerate) the rotating arm of the casting machine. The mold is accelerated into the molten metal as the spring unwinds. The rotating arm is composed of two parts connected by a pivot point; thus, this device is called a "broken-arm" casting machine. The pivoting of the arm keeps it at the proper angle to allow the molten alloy to flow into the mold.

Other types of casting machines use a vacuum or compressed air to force the molten metal into the mold. The crucible and casting ring are stationary; only the molten metal moves. Details of spruing, investing, and casting are beyond the scope of this textbook; interested readers are referred to the excellent dental materials texts in the suggested readings section of the website.

E. Divesting, Finishing, and Polishing

After cooling, the casting is retrieved (or "**divested**") from the ring by carving away the investment and exposing the casting. The casting is cleaned, as shown in *Figure 10.6F*. The metal that represents the sprue and casting button (excess metal) is cut off and can be reused. The casting is finished and polished, as shown in Figure 1.4. This is done by using a variety of abrasives and is described in Chapter 16.

V. Alloys for All-Metal Cast Restorations

Cast metal restorations use alloys rather than pure metals. **Alloys** are metals that are a combination of several elements. Traditionally, casting alloys for all-metal restorations have been gold alloys, thus the name full gold crown or gold inlay. Pure gold is not used because it is too soft. Gold (~75% by weight) is combined with copper (~5%), silver (~10%), palladium (~2%), zinc (~1%), and other elements to form high-noble dental alloys. Percentages of elements vary depending on the type of casting alloy and the manufacturer. Gold alloys are easily cast with gypsum-bonded investments and relatively simple equipment.

The properties of dental casting alloys are described in the American Dental Association (ADA) specification. The specification has no composition requirements but does

have performance criteria for strength, elongation, tarnish resistance, and biocompatibility. **Elongation** is a measure of the ability of a material to be stretched before it breaks. Elongation is used to predict the ability of an alloy to be burnished. **Burnishing** margins of soft, malleable gold restorations pushes the metal against the tooth to close any gap between the tooth and the casting. Therefore, a margin or gap between the restoration and the tooth becomes smaller when it is burnished. Less cement is needed to fill in the space. Because dental cements are much more soluble than casting alloys, the likelihood of recurrent caries during clinical service is decreased when margins are burnished.

A. ADA Classification of Casting Alloys for All-Metal Restorations—Optional

Four types of casting alloys are described in the ADA specification: Types I, II, III, and IV. The differences between them are predominantly the strength and elongation of the casting alloy. Type I is the weakest, has the greatest elongation, and is used for inlays. Type IV is the strongest, has the least elongation, and is used for high-stress bridges and partial denture frameworks.

B. Terminology Used to Describe Metals

Many terms are used to describe metals. Some have precise meaning; others do not.
1. Metals are classified as noble elements based on their lack of chemical reactivity. The noble metals include gold, platinum, palladium, and other inert metals.
2. Precious metals are classified based on their cost. Precious metals are the noble metals and silver.

C. Classification by Gold Content

The gold content of alloys can be described several ways.
1. Percentage is parts per 100.
2. Carat is parts per 24.
3. Fineness is parts per 1,000. Therefore: 75% = 18 carat = 750 fine.

D. Classification by Composition—Optional

Dental alloys for all-metal restorations can be classified by their composition.
1. High-gold or high-noble alloys contain 60% or more gold and other noble elements. They are usually yellow metals.
2. Low-gold or low-noble alloys contain at least 25% noble metals, with gold typically being replaced by increased silver content. Low-gold alloys are yellow or white metals.
3. A third group is the silver–palladium alloys, with approximately 70% silver and 25% palladium. These alloys are white (silver) in color.

4. Alloys with less than 25% noble elements are called predominantly base metals.

5. The term "nonprecious" is used to describe alloys without any noble elements.

E. Alloys for Ceramometal Restorations

1. Requirements for Ceramometal Alloys
Casting alloys for ceramometal restorations have the same mechanical and biocompatibility requirements as alloys for all-metal restorations. One exception is elongation because it is not usually considered to be important when bonding porcelain to metal. The ceramometal alloy must withstand the very high porcelain firing temperatures. These temperatures are much higher than the melting temperatures of alloys for all-metal cast restorations. It is important that the metal not melt or distort because the ceramometal alloy supports the porcelain during firing and clinical use.

2. Bonding Porcelain to Metal—Optional
a. After the metal substructure (or **coping**) is waxed and cast, the metal surface is cleaned.
b. The next step is to oxide the surface of the metal by heating the casting in a porcelain oven. A porcelain oven reaches temperatures much higher than a typical burnout oven and has more precise temperature control. Adherent oxides form on the metal surface and function to chemically bond the porcelain to the metal. Small amounts (1–5%) of nonprecious elements are added to ceramometal alloys to form these adherent oxides on the surface. Common examples are tin, indium, and gallium.
c. Porcelain is supplied by manufacturers as powders, as shown in *Figure 10.9*. Each shade has its own powder. Porcelain powders are applied (or stacked) in layers. Each layer has esthetic properties to simulate the

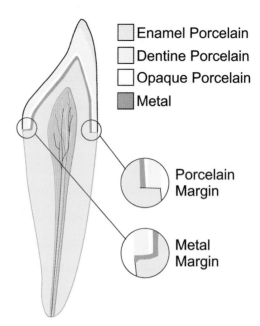

FIGURE 10.10. Illustration of porcelain layers used in construction of a ceramometal crown. A metal margin is shown on the lingual and a porcelain margin on the facial.

appearance of the layers of teeth, dentin, and enamel, as shown in *Figure 10.10*.
d. The first porcelain layer that is applied hides the color of the metal. It is called the opaque layer and covers the gray, oxidized surface of the metal. The opaque layer is fired before adding subsequent layers of porcelain.
e. The second porcelain layer is the dentin or body porcelain shade or shades. These porcelains make up the bulk of the restoration. More than one shade of body porcelain may be used because a single tooth may vary in shade between different locations on the same tooth.
f. After the body layer, the enamel or translucent layer is applied. This is the most translucent of the porcelain materials and gives the restoration a more natural appearance.
g. Each layer may be fired separately or in combination with another layer. Dental porcelains are fired at very high temperatures, such as 850°C to 1,100°C (1,550–2,000°F). Constructing a ceramometal restoration typically involves three to five firings.
h. The procedures for building porcelain to metal can be found on YouTube: opaque to a metal coping (https://youtu.be/w7hCB-FwOV8) and applying body and enamel porcelain (http://www.youtube.com/watch?v=kbP8eIxnBl4).

3. Sintering Porcelain
Firing porcelain causes the powders to become "**sintered**." Sintering changes the porcelain from a powder to a solid. The powder is not

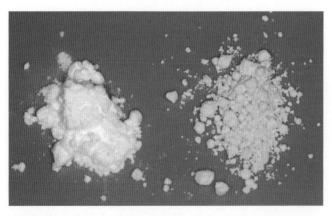

FIGURE 10.9. Two shades of opaque porcelain powder.

melted, so the general shape is maintained. The process of sintering is similar to that of making a snowball. The snow is not melted; instead, the snow is compacted together. Sintering porcelain is the same process that is used to fire clay pots, china, and ceramic tiles. Reducing the porosity of the resulting product is very important. The less porous (more dense) the product is, the greater the strength of the final product will be.

After sintering, the final shape of the restoration is refined by grinding. Stains and glazes can be applied and fired to produce the shade detailed in the laboratory prescription.

4. Types of Ceramometal Alloys
Ceramometal alloys can be classified in many ways. The following is one example.

a. *Noble Alloys*
The high-noble alloys for all-metal restorations were modified for porcelain bonding. Gold (~88%)–platinum (~4%)–palladium (~6%) alloys were developed first. No (or very little) silver and no copper are used. These alloys are yellow in color (like gold alloys for all-metal restorations) but have a higher melting temperature to withstand porcelain application firings.

Gold (~50%)–palladium (~40%) alloys are white in color. They possess better mechanical properties than gold-platinum–palladium alloys. Today, these are the noble alloys of choice for ceramometal restorations.

Palladium (~60%)–silver (~30%) alloys are less costly and are white metals.

High-palladium (~80%) alloys are also white in color. They are less costly than the gold-containing ceramometal alloys but more expensive than the palladium–silver alloys.

b. *Nonprecious Alloys*
Nickel (~80%)–chromium (~10%) alloys are white in color and have higher melting temperatures than the noble ceramometal alloys. They tend to be stronger and harder than the noble ceramometal alloys and are much less expensive.

Chromium (~65%)–cobalt (~25%) alloys are also white and inexpensive. They have the highest melting temperatures and are the most difficult to cast. Their mechanical properties are similar to those of the strongest nickel–chromium alloys.

VI. Titanium

Titanium is the most biocompatible metal. As a result, a great deal of effort has been devoted to developing

materials and methods that would allow crowns, bridges, and partial denture frameworks to be made from titanium. Current titanium use is limited. It will most likely increase in the future as titanium restorations become easier to produce. Titanium has been used as the material of choice for dental implants for decades. If handled properly, titanium can osseointegrate with bone. Osseointegration is a type of biologic bonding of bone to a material. Implants are discussed in Chapter 12.

VII. Partial Denture Frameworks

A. Alloys

At one time, the frameworks of partial dentures were made with gold alloys. The large amount of metal required to construct a framework makes using gold alloys quite expensive. As a result, less expensive alloys from the aerospace industries, such as nickel–chromium and cobalt–chromium alloys, were adapted for removable partial denture frameworks. When the price of gold increased greatly in the 1980s and in recent years, these nonprecious alloys were modified for use as crown and bridge alloys. The high-melting temperatures of these alloys require slightly different casting techniques and investment materials.

B. Silicate- and Phosphate-Bonded Investments

Silicate- and phosphate-bonded investments are used to cast high-melting partial denture framework alloys and ceramometal alloys. They can withstand much higher burnout temperatures and are more difficult to use than gypsum-bonded investments.

VIII. Ceramic Restorative Materials

Dentistry has been in love with porcelain ceramic materials for more than a century. The shades and translucency of porcelain materials are unmatched in their ability to simulate the appearance of teeth.

A. Porcelain

Porcelain jacket crowns were the first all-ceramic restoration used in dentistry. The entire crown is made of porcelain, as shown in Figure 1.10E and F. Unfortunately, the mechanical properties of this brittle material are inadequate for restoring most areas of the mouth. However, the outstanding esthetics of porcelain have maintained an interest in ceramic materials.

Porcelain jacket crowns are made by applying porcelain powders in layers onto a thin layer of platinum foil that is adapted to the die. Platinum is an element with a very high–melting temperature. The foil supports the porcelain powder during firing and is removed from the inside of the completed crown. No metal remains. A very translucent and natural appearing restoration results.

B. Techniques to Strengthen Porcelain Materials

1. Ceramometal

To strengthen the porcelain, it can be bonded to a metal substrate as with pots, pans, and bathtubs. The advantages of metal include tough mechanical properties and the ability to obtain a precise fit of the crown to the preparation. The disadvantage is that metals are opaque to light, even when used in very thin layers. Light is not transmitted through the restoration as it is through tooth structure. Therefore, a ceramometal restoration is not as natural or lifelike in appearance compared to an all-ceramic crown.

2. Aluminous Porcelain

Alumina (alumina oxide) was added to porcelain to increase strength much like the filler strengthens a dental composite. Alumina is a very strong ceramic material, and its addition slightly increases strength and clinical performance without affecting esthetics. Unfortunately, this marginal improvement was not sufficient to significantly improve clinical performance.

3. Improvements in All-Ceramic Restorations

The search for stronger ceramic materials resulted in significant improvements in materials and processing techniques for all-ceramic restorations.

a. Castable Glass. First, a castable glass–ceramic material was developed. The glass is cast much like metals are cast and is then given a strengthening heat treatment. The heat treatment precipitates a second strong ceramic phase resulting in what is called a **glass–ceramic** (again like a dental composite but two ceramic phases). This dental material was similar to the material used to make CorningWare baking dishes and was called Dicor. It was developed by Corning and was marketed by Dentsply. Only one white, translucent shade of castable glass–ceramic material was produced. The cast glass–ceramic core was veneered with a thin layer of porcelain to produce the desired shade. Dicor was an improvement over porcelain, but it was too weak for most clinical needs.

b. Pressed Ceramics. In the late 1980s and early 1990s, several new ceramic products were developed for dentistry. IPS Empress and In-Ceram are brand names. A strong, dense core of ceramic material is processed by melting an ingot of ceramic material and forcing or pressing the viscous ceramic material into a mold; think of injecting soft-serve ice cream into an ice-cream cone. The core may or may not be veneered with porcelain to obtain the desired esthetics. Because the core is a ceramic material, it is translucent to light. Esthetics similar to those of porcelain jacket crowns result. The improved strength of these materials and their excellent esthetics have made these ceramic products very popular, including the use for some bridges. Unfortunately, occasional fractures still occur even with this improved strength. Proper case selection is important.

c. CAD/CAM. Computer-aided design/computer-aided manufacture (CAD/CAM) continues to be developed for dentistry. An in-office computer-based system captures an "optical" impression, rather than a physical impression, of the preparation. The restoration is machined out of a solid piece of high-strength ceramic material through computer control in the dental office or dental laboratory. Porcelain and stains may be added to meet the patient's esthetic needs. This technology is an important technique for the manufacture of zirconium oxide high-strength ceramic restorations. Zirconium oxide (ZrO) high-strength ceramic materials require CAD/CAM techniques to produce dental restorations. ZrO has become an affordable alternative to ceramometal restorations. CAD/CAM technology has been adapted for use with other materials, such as metals, polymers, and composites. It is used in the production of crowns, bridges, veneers, and even dentures. 3D printing techniques continue to be developed for a variety of dental uses. It is very hard to keep up with the advances in dental technology.

IX. Advantages and Disadvantages of All-Metal/Ceramometal/Ceramic Restorations

A. Fracture

An all-metal restoration is least likely to fracture compared to ceramometal and ceramic restorations. Metals are tough, and fractures of metallic restorations are quite rare. On the other hand, all-ceramic restorations do fail and are only recommended for certain teeth. Restorations for teeth that do not experience high occlusal forces, such as a maxillary lateral incisor, have high success rates. Restorations for teeth that do experience high occlusal forces, such as first molars, have a lower success rate. Materials for all-ceramic restorations have improved greatly in recent years, and their use in moderate-stress areas of the mouth, such as anterior teeth and premolars, has been very successful. With proper case selection, molar crowns and short bridges are successful.

Ceramometal restorations are used in all areas of the mouth. Fracture of the porcelain is not common, but this is the most common mechanical failure. Mechanical failure of the metal substructure almost never occurs. Depending on the complexity of the restoration and the location of the porcelain fracture, this may be a nuisance or a disaster. The use of ceramometal restorations has significantly decreased with the improvements in all-ceramic restorations and the increase in the cost of gold.

B. Esthetics

All-metal restorations may have acceptable or unacceptable esthetics depending on the location of the restoration and the patient's preferences. Ceramometal restorations adequately simulate the natural dentition in most situations. All-ceramic restorations reproduce the translucency of the natural dentition better than ceramometal restorations.

All-ceramic restorations have the most life-like appearance of all restorative materials.

C. Wear

Unfortunately, the ceramic materials that are used for ceramometal and all-ceramic restorations are very hard. They wear the opposing enamel much more than natural tooth structure or gold alloys. Newer ceramic materials are a significant improvement but still may cause excessive wear in some patients. The softer gold alloys wear opposing enamel much like enamel does.

D. Margins

Casting techniques for metals result in more accurate margins than those for all-ceramic restorations. An excessive gap at the margin of an all-ceramic restoration increases the risk of recurrent caries. Luckily, modern dentistry has adhesive composite cements to fill the marginal gap of ceramic restorations.

E. Selecting Materials

Advantages and disadvantages exist for each restorative material and must be assessed on a case-by-case basis. The patient should be made aware of the "pros" and "cons" of each type of material and be included in the decision. It must be emphasized that proper handling of all dental materials by all dental personnel is important to the success of any procedure.

Summary

Fixed indirect restorations may be classified in two ways: by the amount of tooth structure restored or by the material from which they are made. Inlays, onlays, veneers, crowns, and dental bridges comprise the classifications based on the amount of tooth structure restored. Metals, ceramics, ceramometal, and composites comprise the classifications based on the material.

This chapter also discusses the procedures for constructing an indirect restoration, from diagnosis and treatment planning to casting and final cementation of the restoration. Classifications of alloys for all metal restorations include the ADA classification and others.

Ceramometal restorations involve many steps because the porcelain must be bonded to the metal. Ceramometal alloys include the noble and nonprecious alloys.

A porcelain crown is an all-ceramic restoration that is unmatched regarding ability to simulate the natural appearance of teeth. However, the mechanical properties of porcelain crowns limit their use mostly to anterior teeth. Other ceramic materials have been developed that have good esthetic properties and much better mechanical properties.

Composite indirect materials include particle-reinforced and fiber-reinforced composites. These materials are processed in dental laboratories by using pressure and heat to improve their polymerization and usefulness in dentistry.

Each of the all-metal, ceramometal, and ceramic restorations has both advantages and disadvantages. Areas of concern include fracture, esthetics, effects of wear, margins, and area of use.

Learning Activities

1. Assume that a member of the class needs to have a tooth restored with a crown. Discuss the advantages and disadvantages of the possible options for a maxillary lateral incisor, maxillary premolar, and mandibular molar.

2. Describe the clinical and laboratory procedures necessary to construct an all-metal or a ceramometal crown.

Review Questions

Question 1. If a mold that is created for investing and casting does not _____ to compensate for the action of the metal alloy, the casting will not fit.

a. Contract
b. Equate
c. Expand
d. None of the above

Question 2. The most obvious purpose of the investment is to:

a. Enlarge the mold by hygroscopic expansion
b. Enlarge the mold by thermal expansion
c. Form the mold for the casting
d. Provide compensation for contraction

Question 3. Porcelain is "best suited" for which of the following?

a. Full coverage posterior crowns
b. MODFL onlays
c. Veneers on anterior teeth
d. MOD inlays

Question 4. The crown(s) portion of a dental bridge is called the:

a. Pontic
b. Retainer
c. Abutment
d. Fixed partial denture

Question 5. Which of the following waxes is hard, leaves no burnout residue, and has a higher melting temperature?

a. Boxing
b. Rope
c. Sticky
d. Baseplate
e. Inlay

Question 6. During the casting procedure, a wax pattern is heated, the wax melts and then flows out of the mold. As the temperature continues to rise, any residual wax is burned away. This heating procedure is called:

a. Shrinkage compensation
b. Investing
c. Burnout
d. Crucible heating

Question 7. Identify the correct sequence in the centrifugal casting process.

a. Add sprue to pattern, place in crucible former, invest, and then cast.
b. Add sprue to pattern, invest, place in crucible former, and then cast.
c. Place sprue in crucible former, add pattern to sprue, invest, and then cast.
d. Place sprue in crucible former, invest, add pattern to sprue, and then cast.

Question 8. A 33% gold alloy may also be expressed as:

a. 10 Carat
b. 16 Carat
c. 333 Fine
d. 33 Fine

Question 9. The term used to define the process of firing porcelain powder to become a solid is:

a. Liquidating
b. Sintering
c. Burnishing
d. Investing

Question 10. One type of an all-ceramic restoration is castable glass. All-ceramic restorations are superior to ceramometal restorations in all respects.

a. The first statement is true; the second statement is false.

b. The first statement is false; the second statement is true.

c. Both statements are true.

d. Both statements are false.

Question 11. Which of the following is considered to be a fixed indirect restoration?

a. Amalgam

b. Direct gold (gold foil)

c. Onlay

d. Composite

Question 12. A restorative material that is placed on the facial surface of anterior teeth to "cover" or hide an esthetic problem is called a:

a. Coping

b. Veneer

c. Buildup (core)

d. Pontic

Question 13. Another name for a provisional restoration is a _____ restoration.

a. Conditional

b. Nonpermanent

c. Buildup

d. Temporary

Question 14. Silver is classified as a _____ metal.

a. Nonprecious

b. High-noble

c. Precious

d. Noble

Question 15. An advantage of bonding porcelain to metal is:

a. A precise fit of the metal

b. The resulting opacity

c. The resulting translucency

d. Ease in plaque removal

Removable Prostheses and Acrylic Resins

Objectives

After studying this chapter, the student will be able to do the following:

1. List the uses of acrylic resins in dentistry.
2. Explain the physical and chemical stages of polymerization of acrylic resins.
3. Describe the function of the components of heat activated and chemically activated acrylic resin systems.
4. Describe the steps involved in construction of a denture.
5. Summarize the procedures used to reline a denture.
6. Explain the dental hygienist's role in maintenance of an acrylic prosthesis.

Key Words/Phrases

acrylic resins

chemically activated

cold cure

complete denture

denture base

denture setup

flask

full denture

heat activated

immediate denture

monomer

relining

removable partial denture

vertical dimension

wax try-in

Introduction

As with a fixed bridge, a removable denture is a prosthesis; it replaces missing teeth. This chapter presents materials and procedures that are used to construct removable prostheses: partial and complete dentures. Alloys used for partial denture frameworks are very similar to those presented in Chapter 10, Materials for Fixed Indirect Restorations and Prostheses. This chapter focuses on acrylic materials and their use.

I. Acrylic Resins

A. What Is an Acrylic Resin?

Acrylic resins are hard, brittle, glassy polymers. The commercial plastic called Plexiglas is an acrylic resin product. Acrylic resin is clear and colorless, making it an excellent replacement material for glass in storm doors. Acrylic resins are easily colored. Technically, acrylic resins are classified as thermoplastic materials, and many commercial products are made by injection molding acrylic materials. In dentistry, however, acrylic resins are handled more like a thermoset material; after it sets, it is not heated and molded.

The most common acrylic monomer is methyl methacrylate. The chemical structure is shown in Figure 5.4A. Note the C=C bond in this illustration. Acrylic resins are long chains of such monomers. The chains have side groups that inhibit chain slippage and result in mechanical properties that provide more strength than polymer chains without side groups. Polyethylene (the same material used in "plastic" sandwich bags) is an example of a polymer without side groups.

B. Acrylic Resins as Biomaterials

Acrylic resins were developed in the 1930s and were first used in dentistry in the 1940s. They quickly replaced materials previously used in the construction of dentures. An acrylic resin denture is shown in Figure 1.6. They were also used (without success) as a direct restorative material. They have been adapted for many other uses in dentistry. Their handling characteristics and mechanical properties are quite satisfactory for a variety of applications. These uses include temporary crowns, as shown in Figure 1.10C, custom trays, as shown in Figure 8.2, and baseplates for denture construction, to be presented later in this chapter.

It is interesting to note that a dental biomaterials scientist (Dennis Smith) suggested to an orthopedic surgeon (John Charnley) that acrylic resin would be a good material to cement artificial joints in place. In the 1960s, acrylic resin was introduced as the first bone cement and was used in hip replacements. Today, acrylic resin is still commonly used to cement hip prostheses and other orthopedic devices in bone.

II. Acrylic Resin Systems Used in Dentistry

Acrylic resin systems set by addition polymerization in the same manner as dental composites, which were discussed in Chapter 5, Direct Polymeric Restorative Materials. The same terms and classifications are used. They are based on the method used to initiate polymerization.

A. Cold-Cure or Chemically Activated Acrylic Resins

Cold-cure or **chemically activated** acrylic resin systems are supplied as a powder and a liquid, as shown in *Figure 11.1*. These are the same materials used for the "brush-bead" buildup technique for artificial fingernails. The typical components are listed in Table 11.1.

1. Liquid

The liquid is mostly **monomer**, methyl methacrylate. A cross-linking agent, such as glycol dimethacrylate, is added. An inhibitor is always added to methyl methacrylate to prevent premature polymerization; hydroquinone is most

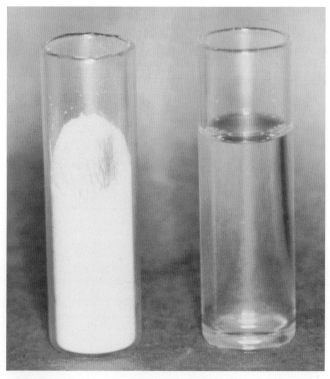

FIGURE 11.1. Photograph of an acrylic resin system, powder, and liquid.

TABLE 11.1. Components of an Acrylic Resin System

	Cold (Chemical) Cure	Heat Cure
Liquid	Methyl methacrylate	Methyl methacrylate
	Hydroquinone	Hydroquinone
	Ethylene glycol	Ethylene glycol
	Tertiary amine	
Powder	Acrylic resin powder	Acrylic resin powder
	Benzoyl peroxide	Benzoyl peroxide
	Fibers and colorants	Fibers and colorants

commonly used. Methyl methacrylate is a powerful solvent. It can dissolve permanent marker (used for labeling things) and even some polymers. The ability of methyl methacrylate to dissolve polymethyl methacrylate resin (acrylic resin) has a significant effect on the mixing and handling properties of acrylic resin systems. After mixing, the liquid dissolves some of the powder forming a workable dough.

2. Powder

   The powder is predominantly polymethyl methacrylate resin with added colorants and benzoyl peroxide. It is usually composed of very small beads of acrylic resin, as shown in *Figure 11.2.* When activated, benzoyl peroxide forms free radicals to initiate polymerization.

3. Physical Changes During Setting

   When the powder and liquid of an acrylic resin system are mixed, several stages in the setting process occur. These stages can be noticed when

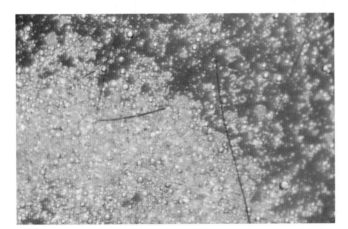

FIGURE 11.2. Low-power magnification photograph of acrylic resin powder. Note the fibers and the various sizes of beads. (Courtesy of E. M. Krouse, Department of Anatomy, West Virginia University, Morgantown, WV.)

a sufficient mass of material is mixed as in the construction of a custom tray. During the initial stages, the changes are physical. The mixed powder and liquid have a "grainy" or "sandy" feel. The powder and liquid are separate phases. As some powder dissolves, the mixed material becomes thicker and less "runny." As more powder is dissolved, the material reaches the "dough" stage. At this point, the material is easy to handle and mold, and up to this point, the changes are mainly physical.

4. Polymerization Reaction

   A cold-cure or chemically activated system has an activator, typically a tertiary amine, added to the liquid. When the powder and liquid are mixed, the benzoyl peroxide and the tertiary amine react to produce free radicals. The inhibitor in the liquid destroys the free radicals that are initially produced, and working time results. This occurs while the material goes from a grainy to a dough stage.

   When the inhibitor is used up, typically during the dough stage, chemical changes occur, and the polymerization reaction proceeds. The doughy material thickens and becomes stiffer. The reaction generates heat as well, and the material becomes warm. Many times when a mass of material is mixed as in the construction of a custom tray, the material becomes hot to the touch. The material becomes rigid and solid as polymerization reaches completion.

5. Residual Monomer

   Initially, the set material contains some residual monomer. Any monomer that does not polymerize soon evaporates, leaving little or no monomer or unreacted double bonds in the set material.

6. Cross-Linking

   Cross-linking the resin improves mechanical properties. A linear resin without any cross-linking agent is brittle. Addition of a cross-linking agent improves the toughness of the material.

B. Heat-Activated Acrylic Resins

1. Heat-activated acrylic resin systems are very similar to chemically activated systems. The major exception is that no chemical activator is present in the liquid. A minor difference is that less inhibitor is present in the liquid. The inhibitor is not needed to provide working time; it functions as a preservative, reacting with free radicals to prevent polymerization during storage.

2. Heat-activated systems are supplied as powder/liquid systems similar to those of cold-cure resins. When the powder and liquid are mixed, they go through the same initial stages of the setting process. Because no chemical activator is present, the mixed material stays in the dough stage for an extended period of time. Therefore, working time is much longer than it is for heat-cure acrylic resins. After the material is formed into the desired shape (to be explained later), the material is heated in a water bath. The heat breaks down the benzoyl peroxide, forming free radicals. Polymerization proceeds by changing the dough into a rigid material. Products that are properly heat cured are a bit stronger and tougher than cold-cure acrylic resins.

C. Light-Activated and Dual-Cure Acrylic Resins

Light-activated and dual-cure acrylic resin systems are available, but they are not as popular as light-activated and dual-cure composites. Recently, light-activated and dual-cure composite materials for temporary crowns, custom trays, and other acrylic resin uses have been introduced. Because these composite materials are stronger, they are gaining acceptance. As prices decrease, they may completely replace acrylic resins for some uses.

D. Acrylic Resin Systems and Porosity

Regardless of the type of activation of an acrylic resin system, porosity is a major concern. Methyl methacrylate and other monomers evaporate easily at room temperature. If monomer evaporates during handling or processing, the resulting material will be porous, as shown in *Figure 11.3*. Porosity weakens the material. Also, the denture is likely to collect debris in pores and develop an offensive odor and taste. A great deal of effort is made to prevent porosity when acrylic resins are processed. Pressure and temperature controls are used to minimize porosity.

III. Complete Dentures

A **complete denture** or **full denture** replaces an entire arch of missing teeth, as shown in Figure 1.6. A complete denture also replaces alveolar bone, which resorbs when teeth are missing. Dentures are made with acrylic materials that are colored to simulate the missing tissues.

Complete dentures are held in place by suction, which is the result of surface tension and atmospheric pressure. Therefore, a complete denture requires precise adaptation to the supporting tissues and a peripheral "seal" for adequate retention (like that of a suction cup). Saliva helps to achieve the seal and improves suction, just as water improves the effectiveness of a suction cup. An impression for a complete denture involves much effort to determine and record the supporting tissues and the proper extension of the denture borders. The borders of the denture that are recorded by the impression are reproduced in the denture. Proper extension of the borders of a denture determines the seal and much of the success of a denture. Most patients function reasonably well with an upper denture. The same cannot be said for lower complete dentures. The peripheral seal of a lower denture is much less effective than that of an upper denture. In addition, an upper denture has a larger surface-bearing area (the palate), and it usually has a better alveolar ridge to support the denture.

A. Components of a Denture

A complete denture has two major components: the white denture teeth and the pink denture base. Denture teeth, as shown in *Figure 11.4*, are purchased from a manufacturer. The denture base is made in the dental laboratory following the dentist's prescription; it is made on the master cast, which is a positive reproduction of the patient's alveolar ridge.

B. Denture Teeth

Denture teeth come in a variety of shapes, sizes, and shades. The shape is chosen to match that of the patient's natural teeth, usually as judged from an old photograph. Another technique is to use the shape of the face to select the tooth shape. The size

FIGURE 11.3. Closeup photograph showing porosity (*white spots*) in a poorly cured acrylic resin sample.

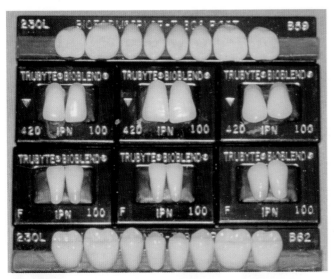

FIGURE 11.4. Photograph of acrylic teeth for maxillary and mandibular dentures (from *top* to *bottom*): maxillary posterior, maxillary anterior, mandibular anterior, and mandibular posterior denture teeth.

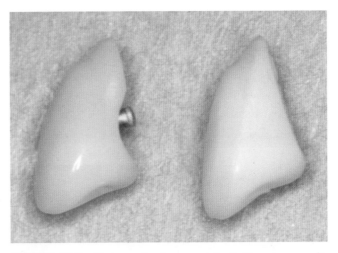

FIGURE 11.5. Photograph of a porcelain (*left*) and an acrylic (*right*) denture tooth. Note the pin protruding from the back of the porcelain tooth. The pin serves to anchor the tooth firmly in the denture base.

is determined by the size of the patient's arch. The shade of the teeth is chosen to match the patient's natural complexion. Often, the patient desires white teeth and must be counseled as to the true color of natural teeth, because bright white teeth will look artificial.

1. Acrylic Resin Teeth

Today, most denture teeth are made from acrylic resin much like that used to construct the denture base. Denture teeth have more cross-linking agents added. Because the teeth are constructed under tightly controlled conditions at a manufacturing plant, they are stronger than the acrylic material used for the denture base. Acrylic denture teeth are "chemically" bonded to the acrylic denture base during processing of the denture.

2. Porcelain Teeth

Porcelain teeth are made by manufacturers in much the same shapes, sizes, and shades as acrylic teeth. Porcelain teeth are much harder and more stain-resistant compared to acrylic teeth. Porcelain teeth are rarely used, however, both because they excessively wear the opposing teeth and because it is generally believed they cause trauma and bone loss in the supporting and opposing alveolar ridges. Porcelain teeth are held in the denture by the mechanical undercuts of pins that are embedded in the back of the denture tooth, as shown in *Figure 11.5*.

3. Composite Teeth

Composite denture teeth are made from materials similar to dental restorative composite

materials. The resin is slightly different, but fillers are added to improve strength and wear resistance.

C. Denture Base

The **denture base** is constructed on the master cast made from the final impression. The denture base is the pink part of the denture that sits on the alveolar ridge.

IV. Constructing a Complete Denture

A. Impressions and Casts

Typically, denture construction requires a number of dental appointments and laboratory procedures. Many dentists make a preliminary impression, preliminary cast, custom tray, final impression, and master cast (in that order). The denture is directly constructed on the master cast, such as that shown in *Figure 11.6A*.

B. Recording the Maxillary and Mandibular Relationship and Arranging Teeth

The relationship of the maxillary and mandibular ridges, or the "bite of the patient," is very important to the success of the prosthesis. An improper relationship can result in overworked muscles of mastication, poor phonetics, and unsatisfactory esthetics.

1. First, a "baseplate" and "wax rims" are constructed from chemically activated acrylic (or similar material) and baseplate wax, as pictured in *Figure 11.6B*. They are made to precisely rest on the patient's ridge, as shown in *Figure 11.6C*.

2. The wax rims on the baseplates are used to determine the patient's midline, "plane of

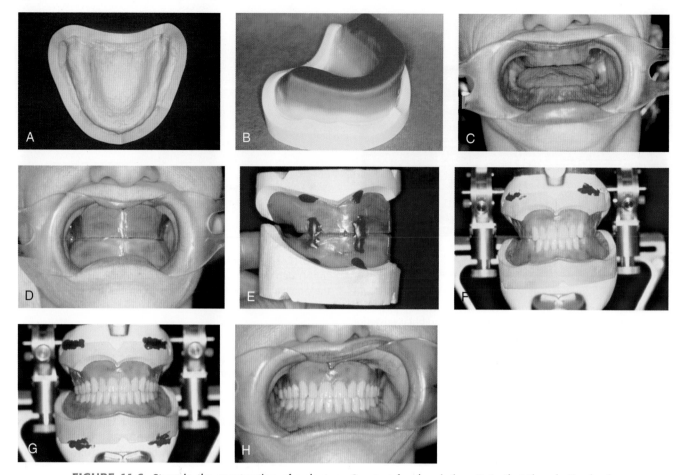

FIGURE 11.6. Steps in the construction of a denture. See text for description. Note that the plastic cheek retractors in **C**, **D**, and **H** are to aid photography and are not typically used during the dental procedure. (Courtesy of Dr. James Overberger, Morgantown, WV.)

occlusion," and size of the denture teeth. The plane of occlusion is the plane where the upper and lower teeth meet when a patient bites, as illustrated in *Figure 11.6D*.

3. At the same appointment, the patient's bite is recorded, as shown in *Figure 11.6D*. This bite is used to position the upper and lower casts in the same relationship as the supporting tissues in the mouth (*Fig. 11.6E*).

4. With the aid of baseplates and rims, the casts are mounted on an articulator using dental plaster, as pictured in *Figure 11.6F and G*.

5. The denture teeth are "set" in wax. Wax is easily softened with a hot instrument to allow the denture teeth to be partially set in wax and then easily moved into the proper position (*Fig. 11.6F*). When all the denture teeth are set in wax, it is called a **denture setup**. A setup simulates the proper bite (relationship of the two arches), the **vertical dimension** (distance between the two arches), and the esthetics of the final denture, as shown in *Figure 11.6G*.

6. Before processing, the setup (the baseplates with the teeth set in wax) is placed in the patient's

mouth. This procedure is called the "**wax try-in**" and is pictured in *Figure 11.6H*. The wax try-in allows patients to see the arrangement of teeth that their denture will have. It also allows the dentist to check function, occlusion (bite), and phonetics before the actual denture is processed.

C. Processing the Denture

1. Processing a denture involves embedding the master cast and the denture setup in a denture **flask** filled with gypsum materials. It is done in such a way as to create a split mold. The mold is opened, and the wax and the baseplate are removed while the denture teeth stay in position. Acrylic resin in the dough stage is placed in the mold space. The mold is then closed, and the acrylic resin replaces the wax and base plate, forming the denture base. This process is illustrated in *Figure 11.7*.

2. The closed mold is heated in a water bath to activate the heat-cure acrylic resin. The heating rate is controlled to reduce porosity. The application of pressure minimizes loss of the volatile

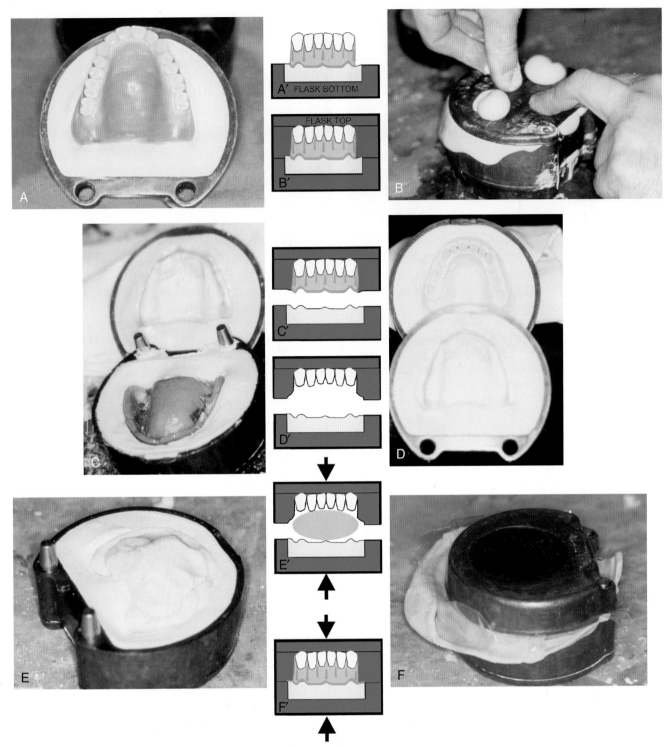

FIGURE 11.7. Processing a denture. First, **A** and **A′** the master cast and denture setup are embedded in plaster and stone in a denture flask (*dark outside line* in diagram). **B** and **B′** The first increment fills the lower component of the flask up to the level of the master cast. The rest of the setup is covered with dental stone and plaster until the flask is filled. **C** and **C′** Second, a mold space is made. After heating in hot water, the flask is opened, and the baseplate is separated from the cast. **D** and **D′** The baseplate is removed, and the wax is flushed out with hot water while the teeth stay embedded in dental stone. **E** and **E′** Mixed acrylic resin in the dough stage is then placed in the mold, and the mold is compressed. **F** and **F′** While under compression, the resin is adapted to the master cast and replaces the baseplate and wax. The teeth stay in proper relationship. Finally, the flask is heated, and the resin polymerizes.

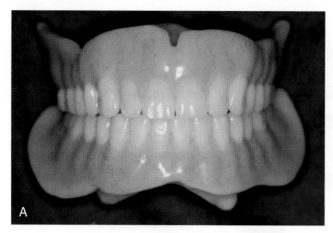
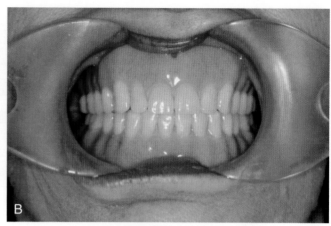

FIGURE 11.8. Photographs of completed dentures **A.** as received from the laboratory **B.** and in place. (Courtesy of Dr. James Overberger, Morgantown, WV.)

monomer. Loss of monomer results in porosity and weak spots.

3. After processing, the denture is removed from the mold by breaking the surrounding gypsum materials. It is then finished, polished, disinfected, and delivered to the patient. Completed dentures are shown in *Figure 11.8*.

V. Partial Dentures

Many patients are partially edentulous, and the remaining teeth are frequently used to support and retain a prosthesis. If the prosthesis can be removed by the patient, it is called a **removable partial denture** or simply a partial denture. Most partial dentures are supported by both natural teeth and the alveolar ridge, as shown in Figure 1.7. A lower partial denture with a few remaining natural teeth to hold it securely functions far better than a complete lower denture. The dental hygienist should stress to the patient the critical need to maintain the remaining natural teeth so that wearing a mandibular complete denture is avoided.

Patients with a mandibular complete denture often have problems chewing. The mandibular denture will lack suction or retention and will float and move around in the mouth. The lack of stability of a mandibular denture may cause "sore spots" (ulcerations of the oral mucosa) and make speech difficult. Helping the patient to retain several mandibular teeth will allow a patient to wear and use a mandibular partial denture. This is an important preventive responsibility of the dental hygienist.

A. Frameworks

A partial denture uses a cast metal "framework" for retention, as shown in *Figure 11.9A*. The framework is composed of clasps, connectors, and mesh.

1. The framework has clasps that rest on and go around the abutment teeth. A clasp is shown in *Figure 11.9B*. Because the clasps are metal,

they can be bent to adjust their fit, as pictured in *Figure 11.9C*.

2. Connectors are the thicker parts of the framework that connect the mesh and clasps together.

3. The framework also has an area of mesh that the acrylic resin flows into and around when the partial denture is processed. This results in the mechanical attachment of the teeth and the denture base to the framework.

B. Denture Base

The denture base is constructed and used in much the same way as a complete denture. However, the mesh areas of the partial denture framework are embedded in acrylic resin.

C. Teeth

The same teeth used to construct complete dentures are used to construct partial dentures. Teeth are chosen with the proper shape, size, and shade to replace the missing natural teeth.

D. Processing a Partial Denture

A partial denture is processed much like a complete denture. However, the acrylic resin must flow through and around the mesh of the framework.

VI. Relining a Denture

Dentures lose their "fit" after a period of time, because the alveolar ridge atrophies and resorbs when teeth are not present. Most resorption occurs when the teeth are first extracted, but resorption continues slowly throughout a patient's life. Therefore, as the alveolar ridge changes, the fit of the denture changes as well.

Indications that a denture is not fitting as well as it should include frequent use of denture adhesives or over-the-counter denture "cushion" materials or liners. Use of

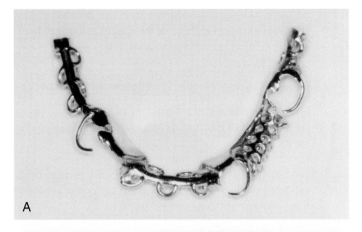

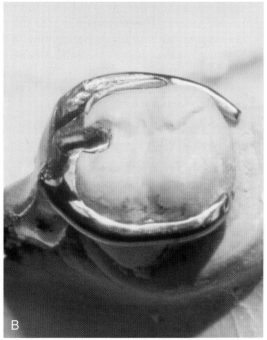

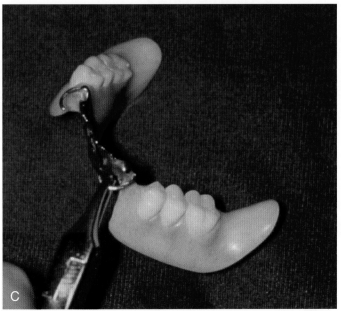

FIGURE 11.9. Components of a partial denture. **A.** Framework. **B.** Clasp. **C.** Denture base. Note the clasp being adjusted or bent.

these materials makes cleaning the denture difficult and can result in a foul smell. Long-term use of adhesives may cause tissue inflammation. Liners may change the bite or occlusion of a denture, causing trauma to the supporting tissues. The dental hygienist must be aware of these problems and educate patients about the proper use of over-the-counter products and treatment options.

An "old" denture can have its fit improved by a process called relining. **Relining** adds a small amount of new material to the inside tissue area of the denture base to replace the additional alveolar ridge that has been lost since the denture was made. Relining a denture can be done either in a dental laboratory or at chairside.

A. Laboratory-Processed Reline

A laboratory-processed reline involves making an impression, much like the final impression that is made when a denture is constructed. The existing denture functions as the impression tray. A variety of impression materials are used depending on the clinician's personal preference. The denture containing

the impression is sent to a dental laboratory. A cast is poured. The impression and cast are separated, and the impression material is removed from the denture. New acrylic material is added to fill the space between the denture and the cast (the space previously occupied by the impression material). The acrylic material is cured, finished, and polished in the same manner as during the construction of a new denture. The denture is returned to the dentist and given to the patient. A laboratory reline is generally superior to a chairside reline; however, patients must go without their denture for a day or more when the reline is processed at a dental laboratory.

B. Chairside Reline

A chairside reline uses a different material. The same material that functions as the impression material also becomes the added material. The material is mixed, placed in the denture, and then placed in the patient's mouth. The material sets in the mouth and becomes rigid. The excess is trimmed, and the denture is polished and returned to the patient. The advantage is that the patient does not go without his or her denture. The disadvantage is that the new material is more porous and, typically, not as smooth as that of a laboratory reline. This will make it more difficult for the patient to keep clean.

VII. Immediate Dentures

Most dentures are made for patients who have had their teeth previously extracted. An **immediate denture** is a denture that is placed at the same appointment during which the remaining teeth are extracted. Typically, when an immediate denture is constructed, many of the teeth in the arch to receive the denture are already missing, and most of the remaining teeth are hopeless. An impression is made by the dentist, and the denture is constructed in the laboratory, similar to a complete denture. At the delivery appointment, the remaining teeth are extracted, the denture is placed, and postoperative instructions are given to the patient (*Fig. 11.10*). An immediate denture not only restores function and esthetics, it can protect the extraction sites during healing. In most cases, an immediate denture is relined several months after it is placed.

VIII. Repairing Acrylic Prostheses or Appliances

It is not unusual for a denture or other acrylic prosthesis or appliance to fracture. It seems that dogs love to chew on them. Repairs are made by using new, chemically activated acrylic material as a glue to repair the fracture. In many offices, the dental hygienist may be the professional who repairs simple fractures of partial or complete dentures. The process involves several steps.

A. Clean the Surface

First, clean the surfaces being repaired. Often, this involves grinding the surface to remove a thin layer of the surface and any contaminants.

B. Apply Monomer

Next, monomer is applied to the clean surfaces to dissolve some of the set material. One end of

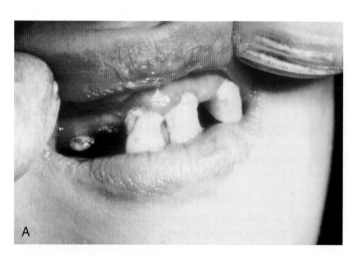
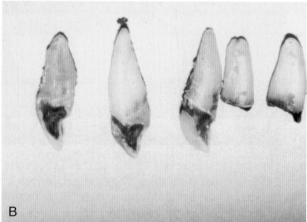
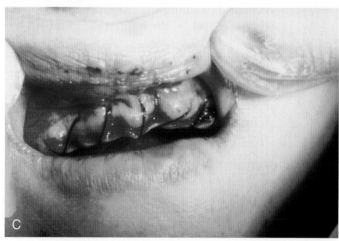
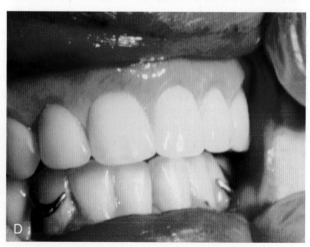

FIGURE 11.10. Photographs of **A.** teeth destroyed by caries and periodontal disease, **B.** the extracted teeth, **C.** the alveolar ridge after the extraction, and **D.** the immediate denture in place.

some of the polymer chains dissolves in the monomer; the other end remains embedded in the solid acrylic resin.

C. Apply New Material

New material is then mixed, applied to the surface, and allowed to set. The polymer chains of the old material become entangled in the new material. Because no residual double bonds are available for a chemical reaction, the bond is quasi-chemical.

The same process is used to "chemically" bond acrylic denture teeth to the denture base during denture processing.

D. Finish and Polish

Finally, the repaired prosthesis is finished and polished by using acrylic burs, pumice, and other materials as for a complete denture. This too can be done by the dental hygienist.

IX. Handling Acrylic Devices

It is important that patients regularly clean their dentures. Patients should be instructed to brush their prostheses with a denture cleaner and a denture brush or to use other denture cleaning procedures. Calculus may form on the denture in similar areas as in natural teeth. It is the dental hygienist's responsibility during the recall appointment to remove the calculus in a manner that is not harmful to the acrylic.

Most dentists prefer that their patients do not sleep with dentures in the mouth. Therefore, patients should store their dentures in water at night.

During dental appointments, it is important to store acrylic appliances in water. Do not let them dry out, because they may warp. This applies not only to dentures but also to acrylic orthodontic retainers. The dental hygienist should play an active role during recall visits and educate patients who wear complete and partial dentures.

Summary

This chapter presents the materials and procedures that are used to construct both complete dentures and removable partial dentures. These oral appliances involve the use of acrylic resin. In dentistry, acrylic resins are used for temporary crowns and custom trays in addition to the bases for complete and partial dentures.

Two forms of acrylic resins are used for the fabrication of dentures: chemically activated (cold-cure) and heat-activated (heat-cure) resin systems. The chemically activated resin is supplied as a powder and a liquid, the liquid being mostly methyl methacrylate with added cross-linking agent. The powder is polymethyl methacrylate resin with added colorants and benzoyl peroxide. The powder is in the form of very small beads.

Heat-activated resin systems are very similar to chemically activated systems. The major difference is that no chemical activator is present in the liquid. The mixed material also stays in the dough stage for a longer period of time. Heat-activated products are usually stronger than chemically activated resins.

Dentures are composed of two components: the denture base and the denture teeth. Denture teeth may be made of porcelain or acrylic resin. Acrylic teeth are used most often, are bonded to the denture base, and do not excessively wear the opposing natural teeth.

Constructing a denture involves several steps. A resin baseplate is made on a master cast, wax rims are added, and both are mounted on an articulator. Teeth are then embedded in the wax, and the patient and dentist approve the wax try-in. Next, the denture is flasked, heat cured, finished, and polished.

Partial dentures are supported by both natural teeth and the alveolar ridge. A partial denture is composed of a metal framework, the denture base, and denture teeth. The framework includes the clasps, connectors, and mesh. A partial denture is processed much like a complete denture.

Dentures will lose their "fit" as the alveolar ridge continues to resorb; however, an "old" denture can be relined to restore the fit. Resin material is added to the tissue side of the denture either at chairside or using a dental laboratory.

Immediate dentures are dentures placed during the same appointment in which teeth are extracted. The denture serves to restore function as well as to protect the extraction sites during healing. The denture is usually relined several months after it is placed.

Repairing acrylic prostheses or appliances involves grinding a thin layer off the surface, adding monomer, and then applying new mixed material. Once this is set, it is finished and polished.

The role of the dental hygienist in treating patients with complete and partial dentures includes simple repairs and significant patient education on preventing the need for dentures, home care for these oral removable prostheses, and overuse of adhesives.

Learning Activities

1. Discuss the periodic dental and dental hygiene care that a patient with complete maxillary and partial mandibular dentures should have.

2. Wet a paper towel, and stick it to a smooth wall or blackboard. What holds it in place?

3. With a dissecting microscope, observe acrylic powders. Note the color of the beads and fibers.

4. Collect several plastic objects of no value. Place a few drops of methyl methacrylate (the liquid from an acrylic system) onto the different plastic materials. What happens to the surface? Can you use the same liquid to remove "permanent marker"?

5. Observe patients in the clinic who have complete and partial dentures. Notice the different shades and shapes of denture teeth. How do these relate to the patient's complexion or the shape of his or her face?

6. Go to YouTube and view the video at https://youtu.be/KV_tCpfnh5w

Review Questions

Question 1. The term used when the denture teeth are set in wax is:

a. Denture arrangement

b. Denture setup

c. Articulated setup

d. Articulated arrangement

Question 2. To repair a broken denture, a thin layer is ground off. Next, monomer is applied to the surfaces so that:

a. Some of the set material is dissolved

b. The setting reaction of the repair is accelerated

c. The finishing and polishing of the repair is made easier

d. The color of resin powder does not change

Question 3. Heat activated acrylic resin systems are very similar to chemically activated systems. The major difference (or exception) is:

a. Heat-activated systems have much less strength than chemically activated systems

b. More inhibitor is present in the liquid of heat-activated systems

c. Chemical activator is present in the liquid of heat-activated systems

d. No chemical activator is present in the liquid of heat-activated systems

Question 4. Most denture teeth used today are acrylic rather than porcelain. Porcelain teeth are softer than acrylic teeth and do not cause excessive wear on natural opposing teeth.

a. The first statement is true; the second statement is false.

b. The first statement is false; the second statement is true.

c. Both statements are true.

d. Both statements are false.

Question 5. Partial denture frameworks usually include:

a. Clasps, denture base, and connectors

b. Teeth, clasps, and connectors

c. Clasps, connectors, and mesh

d. Teeth, denture base, connectors, and clasps

Question 6. Cross-linking of acrylic resins will improve the mechanical properties. The most important or beneficial property it would improve would be:

a. Resilience

b. Toughness

c. Fatigue

d. Creep

Question 7. Mandibular dentures are easier to wear than maxillary. Saliva helps to improve the suction needed to hold a denture in place.

a. The first statement is true; the second statement is false.

b. The first statement is false; the second statement is true.

c. Both statements are true.

d. Both statements are false.

Question 8. The wax rims used for denture construction serve to determine the patient's:

a. Midline
b. Plane of occlusion
c. Size of denture teeth
d. All of the above

Question 9. The acrylic resin of a partial denture is processed the same way as a complete denture EXCEPT:

a. It takes less time because fewer teeth are involved
b. The finishing and polishing technique is much different
c. The acrylic resin must flow through and around the mesh of the framework
d. It takes longer because of the design of the framework

Question 10. Listed below are the steps of constructing a denture. Numbering from 1 to 10, place the steps in sequential order.

_____ Casts and rims are mounted on an articulator.

_____ The master cast and denture setup are embedded in stone within the denture flask.

_____ Acrylic resin is mixed and placed in the mold, and the mold is then compressed.

_____ The patient has the wax try-in.

_____ The mold is created by heating in hot water, the baseplate is removed, the wax is flushed out, and the teeth remain in stone.

_____ The baseplate and wax rims are constructed on the master cast.

_____ The denture is removed from the mold, finished, polished, and disinfected.

_____ The baseplate and rims are fitted on patient; midline, plane of occlusion, and bite determined.

_____ The flask is heated and the resin polymerizes.

_____ Denture teeth are set in wax.

Dental Implants

Objectives

After studying this chapter, the student will be able to do the following:

1. List the indications and contraindications for dental implants.
2. Describe the materials used for dental implants.
3. Recall the types and uses of dental implants.
4. Describe osseointegration.
5. Discuss the dental hygienist's role in the maintenance of dental implants.

Key Words/Phrases

abutment

atrophic edentulous mandible

dental implant

endosseous implants

hydroxyapatite

osseointegration

perimucosal seal

titanium

tooth form implants

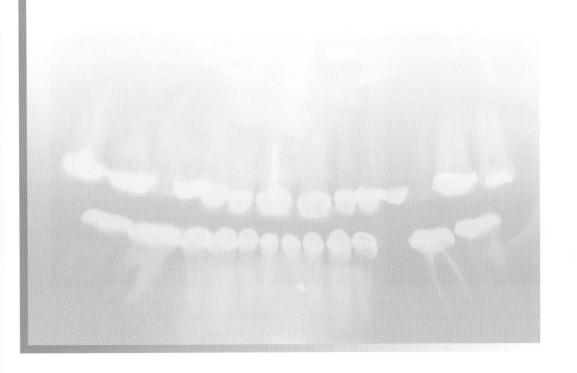

I. Medical versus Dental Implants

The typical medical implant is a device that is placed entirely inside the body. The typical **dental implant** exists both inside and outside the body. A dental implant projects through the oral mucosa and, thus, is not completely surrounded by tissues, as with most medical implants (e.g., silicone breast, artificial hip, knee, and lens implants). An implant existing both inside and outside the body is susceptible to infection. The interface of the surface of the implant and the surrounding tissues is a potential entry site for bacteria and other microorganisms.

II. Indications and Contraindications for Dental Implants

A. Indications

1. Restoring an Edentulous Atrophic Mandible
   Originally, dental implants were used predominantly for prosthodontic patients for whom no other treatment options were satisfactory.

The most common prosthodontic problem has been making dentures for a patient with little or no mandibular ridge. When the teeth are lost, the alveolar bone (bone that supports the teeth) is no longer stimulated and will resorb. As the alveolar bone reduces in size or atrophies, the ridge available to support a denture shrinks. This is called an **atrophic edentulous mandible**. Dental implants have greatly improved the treatment of this condition, as shown in *Figure 12.1*. With the development and success of osseointegrated implants, dental implants are now used as an alternative or adjunct to other conventional prosthodontic treatments.

2. Restoring a Single Missing Tooth
   For patients with a single missing tooth, a crown supported by a single endosseous implant is becoming a popular treatment option, as shown in *Figure 12.2*. The conventional option of a three-unit bridge requires that the two

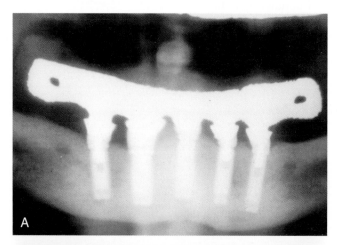
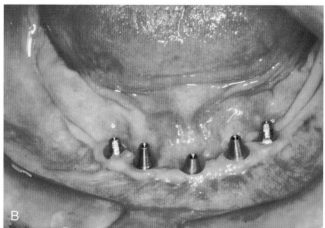
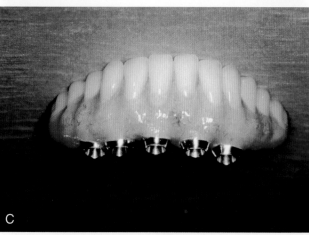
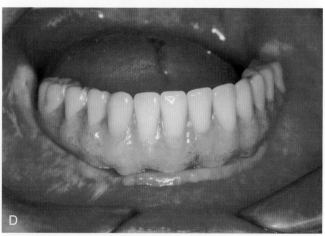

FIGURE 12.1. A mandibular fixed prosthesis supported by implants. Shown are **A.** a panorex of an implant-supported fixed prosthesis as well as **B.** photographs of the atrophic mandible with five implants, **C.** the prosthesis, and **D.** the implant-supported prosthesis in place. (Courtesy of Dr. Paul A. Schnitman, Wellesley Hills, MA, and Noble Biocare, Yorba Linda, CA.)

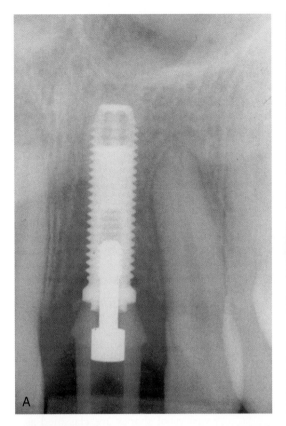

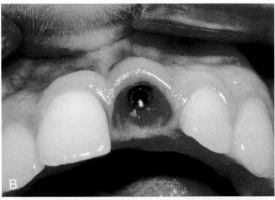

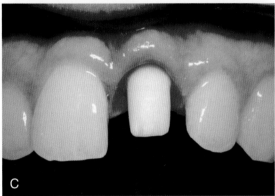

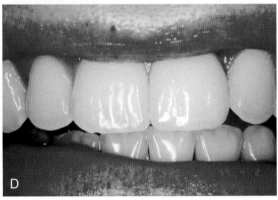

FIGURE 12.2. An endosseous single-tooth implant restored with a crown. Shown are **A.** a radiograph of the implant, abutment, and abutment screw as well as **B.** clinical photographs of the implant, **C.** esthetic abutment and cylinder, and **D.** the crown supported by the implant. (See color images.) (Courtesy of Dr. Roger A. Lawton, Olympia, WA, and Noble Biocare, Yorba Linda, CA.)

abutment teeth be prepared for crowns, as discussed in Chapter 1 and shown in Figure 1.5. Using an implant and a crown to replace a missing tooth may save previously unrestored (no fillings) abutment teeth from crown preparations. Often, the cost of one implant and a crown is comparable to the cost of a three-unit bridge. The specific cost will depend on the implant chosen, the placement procedures, and the final restoration.

B. Contraindications

Patients with systemic diseases that affect connective tissues may not be good candidates for dental implants. The most common of these diseases is diabetes. Smoking is the other major, common contraindication. Another factor to consider is the patient's ability to maintain the implants. Effective plaque control, regular dental prophylaxis, and recall examination are critical to the long-term success of implants. It is also important for the patient to have realistic expectations about the resulting prosthesis. Considering the large amount of time, effort, and expense involved, some patients may expect more than can be delivered. With patients having expectations that cannot be met, it is best they avoid any extensive expensive dental treatment.

III. Materials Used for Dental Implants

It is important to realize that although the implant material is a significant factor, how the material is placed and used is more critical to the success of dental implants.

A. Titanium

Titanium was briefly discussed in Chapter 10. Titanium and titanium alloys are very common implant materials in dentistry and medicine. Unfortunately, titanium is very difficult to cast; it is commonly manufactured for implants by machining into preformed shapes. The major advantage of titanium is that it will osseointegrate with bone if handled properly. Osseointegration is a kind of biologic bonding of bone to a material. Titanium is used for endosseous and most other types of implants. Numerous early researchers had worked with titanium implants but had limited success. Dr. P.I. Brånemark (an orthopedic surgeon) concurrently developed surgical procedures and implant materials; the results were the first reliable dental implants.

1. "cp Ti," or "commercially pure" titanium, is used for many types of medical and dental implants. As with other pure metals, cp Ti is not very strong, but it is strong enough for some dental implant uses.
2. "Ti-6 Al-4 V," or titanium with 6% aluminum and 4% vanadium, is a common aerospace alloy that has been used for dental implants. It is much stronger and stiffer than cp Ti. Dental and medical versions of this alloy have more restrictive composition requirements compared with other industries.

B. Apatite-Coated Titanium

Another popular implant material is **hydroxyapatite** (HA) bonded to titanium metal. Apatites are a broad class of calcium phosphate materials. The hydroxyapatite of hard tissues, such as teeth and bone, is one example. Hydroxyapatite materials also osseointegrate. Titanium coated with HA is commonly used successfully for many different types of implants. HA-coated implants have had increased clinical success when compared to Ti in certain clinical situations.

C. Other Materials

Dental implants have been made from many other materials. The results were not good; therefore, the search continued until titanium was tried with the proper techniques. These materials included metals, ceramics, and polymers.

1. Metals
   Gold, stainless steel, and cobalt–chromium alloys were used with little success.

2. Ceramics
   Hydroxyapatite and other calcium phosphate materials are currently used as implant materials. Vitreous (glassy) carbon, pyrolytic carbon, and aluminum oxide (sapphire) have also been tried with little success.

3. Polymers
   A variety of polymers, including acrylic resin, have been used. Polymers have had little success as prosthodontic implants, but other uses have been developed. Gore-Tex is a polymer material that is implanted as a "barrier" to tissue growth in periodontics. Gore-Tex is expanded polytetrafluoroethylene, the same polymer as Teflon.

IV. Various Types of Dental Implants

A. Endosseous or Tooth Form Implants

Endosseous implants or **tooth form implants** are screwed or pressed into a hole that is cut into the mandible or maxilla. All the implants shown in the illustrations of this chapter are endosseous implants. They reside inside the bone, thus the name "endosseous."

A variety of shapes are classified as endosseous implants. Some are cylinders, with threads on the surface like a bolt or a screw; others have straight sides. Still others, called blade implants, are shaped somewhat like a blade, with notches cut into it. Current use of implants is dominated by cylindrical endosseous shapes. Endosseous implants are used to support a single crown, multiple crowns, a bridge, or a denture.

B. Transosseous or Staple Implants—Optional

A transosseous implant was used to stabilize a mandibular denture. It consists of a plate and several bolts that transverse the mandible in the anterior region. The plate is placed on the underside of the mandible, and the bolts extend through the bone and gingiva into the oral cavity. The bolts have nuts screwed onto the intraoral side of the mandible to keep the implant in place. An extraoral incision under the chin is required to place a transosseous implant.

C. Subperiosteal Implants—Optional

Subperiosteal implants were also used to stabilize a mandibular denture. Subperiosteal implants are placed on the mandibular bone below the periosteum and involve two surgical procedures.

1. The first surgical procedure reflects or "flaps" (peels back) the mucosa and periosteum of the mandible, exposing the denture-bearing alveolar bone. An impression is made of this denture-bearing bone. The soft tissue is then sutured back over the bone.

2. Next, a cast is poured, and framework that supports the eventual denture is cast by a dental laboratory. The framework sits directly on the bone and has several posts that extend through the mucosa and support the denture. Chromium–cobalt is the most common alloy used to cast the framework. Chromium–cobalt is not as biocompatible as titanium; therefore, titanium is also used.

3. The second surgical procedure again reflects the soft tissues covering the alveolar bone, and the framework is put into place. The soft tissue is then put back into place and holds the framework in position. At times, surgical bone screws are used to stabilize the implant.

4. Clinical examples of subperiosteal implants can be found with a web search.

V. Osseointegration of Dental Implants

Osseointegration is attachment of molecules, fibers, cells, and tissues to the implant. The outcome is the result of biocompatible materials, kind surgical techniques, and proper healing conditions. Osseointegration is dependent on material biocompatibility, implant surface, status of bone, surgical technique, healing conditions, and biting forces. Successful osseointegration transfers bite forces to bone and stimulates the growth of bone.

A. Tissue Compatibility

The implant must be compatible with bone and must integrate for mechanical stability. The implant must also be compatible with epithelial cells to seal out the oral environment. The implant must be placed so that these two criteria are met.

B. The Interface with Bone

The interface of an implant that is osseointegrated with bone is depicted in *Figure 12.3*. It includes the following:
1. Titanium metal
2. Metal surface coated with either of the following:
   a. Titanium oxides, 50 to 100 Å (10^{-10} m) thick (the outer layer is actually TiOH)
   b. A ceramic coating, usually hydroxyapatite
3. Proteins, 100 Å thick
4. Healthy bone composed of fibers, cells, and hydroxyapatite

VI. Soft Tissue Attachment to Implants

The attachment of epithelial cells to the implant is called the biological or **perimucosal seal**. This seal forms a barrier, which inhibits the microorganisms' entrance into the tissues supporting the implant. Just as teeth may be lost due to periodontal problems, implants may fail if the supporting tissues are not healthy.

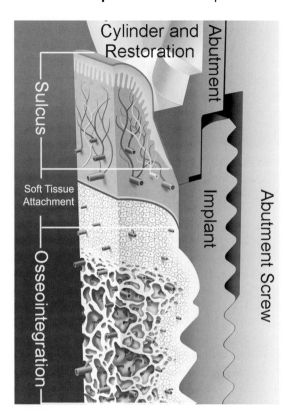

FIGURE 12.3. An artist's rendition of an osseointegrated dental implant. (Courtesy of Nobel Biocare, Yorba Linda, CA. Labels of the implant parts and the tissue/implant interface have been added.)

VII. Placement of Endosseous Dental Implants

When placing endosseous dental implants, the surgical technique must not injure the bone. Bone-cutting procedures must not heat the bone to greater than 47°C (117°F). Overheating or excessive trauma to the bone prevents osseointegration of the implant; the implant becomes surrounded by poorly organized connective tissue (scar tissue). For a dental implant to succeed, adequate healthy bone is needed to support the implant under an occlusal load. Implants may be placed by using one or two surgical procedures, depending on the location of the implant, the esthetic concerns, and the preference of the surgeon. Either way, the placement techniques described below are nearly identical.

A. Two-Stage Implant Placement Procedures

1. The first surgical procedure cuts the hole into the bone and places the implant. First, a soft tissue flap is laid, exposing the bone of the implant site. Next, a hole or channel is cut by using a surgical handpiece with special speed and temperature controls. The size and shape of the hole in the bone is matched to that of the implant. The body of the implant is then placed and covered by the soft tissue flap. The implant is left covered for weeks to several months to allow healing and osseointegration to occur without exposure to oral contamination and mechanical loading, as shown in *Figure 12.4A*.

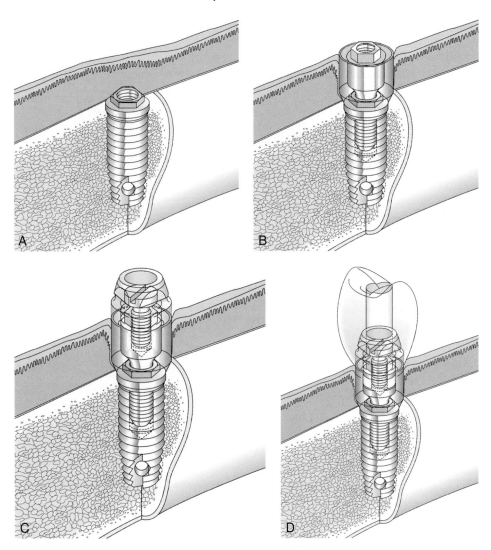

FIGURE 12.4. Placement and restoration of an endosseous implant. **A.** Implant. **B.** Implant with abutment. **C.** Cylinder added. **D.** Implant with restoration. See text (Section VII. *Placement of Endosseous Dental Implants*) for description. (Original artwork, part **D**, is provided courtesy of Noble Biocare, Yorba Linda, CA.)

2. The second stage attaches a healing cap to the body of the implant. The soft tissue covering the implant is removed, and the healing cap is held in place with a screw. The healing cap extends out of the mucosa and is exposed to the oral cavity. This allows epithelial tissue to form around a fixed (nonmovable) object. After the soft tissue has healed for several weeks, the prosthodontic phase begins.

B. Single-Stage Implant Placement Procedures

A soft tissue flap and hole in the bone are created as in the two-stage procedure. The implant is placed with the body extending above the tissue. The soft tissue is repositioned and sutured around the implant. The healing cap is placed. After healing, the prosthodontic phase begins.

C. The Prosthodontic Phase

1. The healing cap is removed, and an **abutment**, as shown in *Figure 12.4B*, is placed on the implant. The abutment functions as an abutment of a bridge; it is attached to and supports the prosthesis. A precision-fitting cylinder, typically made of gold, is placed on the abutment, as illustrated in *Figure 12.4C*. An impression of the cylinder is used to construct models for crown fabrication. Some systems combine the abutment and the cylinder.

2. The crown is fabricated on top of the cylinder, as depicted in *Figure 12.4D*. The crown and cylinder become one piece. The fabrication technique for the crown is determined by the restorative material prescribed. The crown may be made of gold, porcelain fused to metal, composite, or ceramic materials.

3. The restoration (crown and cylinder) may be retained on the implant by several means. It may be cemented in the same manner as a tooth-supported crown. Alternatively, it may be retained with a screw that threads into the abutment, as shown in *Figure 12.4D*.

4. Occlusion is a critical factor if an implant is to be successful. Proper loading of the implant stimulates bone growth and continued

osseointegration. Many implants use polymeric restorative materials to cushion biting forces. Overloading the implant will interfere with osseointegration, and mobility will develop. Excessive mobility may interfere with the epithelial attachment. Occlusion and other forces are very important!

VIII. Maintenance of Implants

Maintenance of dental implants is critical so that the epithelial attachment and the biologic seal remain in a state of health and continue to support the prosthesis.

A. By the Patient

Effective plaque control must be maintained by the patient along with regular prophylaxis at recall appointments. For single-tooth implants, the usual toothbrush and floss may be adequate for plaque removal and health of the surrounding tissue. For a complex prosthesis, the use of interdental brushes, flossing aids, and other auxiliary devices may be necessary as part of the homecare regimen.

B. By the Hygienist

The role of the hygienist in the care and maintenance of dental implants includes patient education, oral hygiene instruction, prophylaxis, and recall appointments. These topics are covered in depth in other texts, such as that of E. M. Wilkins, and in courses on periodontics. Without proper maintenance, the risk of implant failure greatly increases.

From a dental materials perspective, care must be taken not to damage the surface of the implant. Scaling and root planing with conventional instruments will damage the titanium or HA surface. There are now a variety of hand scaling instruments on the market that have tips that are "surface friendly" to the titanium and HA. Power instrumentation, both magnetostrictive and piezoelectric, as well as reciprocating handpieces, are also indicated provided a low setting is used with the correct tip (or tip covering).

Air-powder polishing with sodium bicarbonate–water slurry does not disrupt the surface characterization or the biologic seal around the implant. The typical rubber cup with a very mild abrasive is commonly used to clean the implant prostheses.

IX. Uses of Implants

A. Restorative Dentistry

The most common use of dental implants was to stabilize a prosthesis for an atrophic edentulous mandible. A variety of restorative options are used. Five or six implants can totally support a fixed prosthesis that restores an entire arch. At times, two implants are used with precision attachments to stabilize a complete denture. Precision attachments are clip-like devices that snap together and retain a complete or partial denture. The implants and attachments keep the denture in place (down), but the alveolar ridge supports the denture against biting forces.

With the long-term success of implants to stabilize dentures and other prostheses, dental implants are now frequently used to support single crowns. At times, several implants are placed to support a bridge replacing several teeth.

B. Maxillofacial Prostheses

Many maxillofacial prostheses are retained by osseointegrated implants. The most common are prostheses replacing ears, noses, and other facial structures. Osseointegrated implants eliminate the use of sticky adhesive materials to retain these prostheses. Both function and patient acceptance have greatly improved since the incorporation of osseointegrated implants.

C. Orthodontic Uses

Implants are now being used in orthodontics to provide anchorage for tooth movement.

D. Orthopedic Devices

Rather than being retained with bone cements, titanium orthopedic devices (e.g., hips, knees) use osseointegration for fixation.

Summary

Dental implants are indicated for restoring an atrophic edentulous mandible and single missing teeth. Implants may be contraindicated for patients who smoke, have diabetes, or exhibit poor oral hygiene.

Titanium is the metal of choice for implants because it will osseointegrate with bone. Osseointegration is a type of biological bonding to a material.

The three types of implants include endosseous, transosseous, and subperiosteal. Endosseous implants are quite common and are placed by pressing or screwing them into a hole that is cut into the alveolar bone. Transosseous and subperiosteal implants are used to stabilize dentures.

Endosseous implants may involve a one- or two-stage placement procedure. During the first surgery, a hole is cut into the bone, and the implant is placed. It is then covered by the soft tissue flap that was cut to expose the bone for implant placement and is left covered for several weeks. The second surgical procedure removes the soft tissue covering so that a healing cap can be placed. This extends out into the mucosa, and the epithelial tissue heals and forms around it. It is then replaced with an abutment. The one-stage procedure reduces the two-stage procedure into a single surgery. The abutment supports the prosthesis, such as a crown.

Maintenance of implants is critical so that the epithelial attachment and seal are maintained. The dental hygienist will perform the prophylaxis, select the necessary auxiliary aides, provide chairside education, establish a home care regimen, and schedule an appropriate recall date.

Learning Activities

1. Review patient charts, and discuss the possible use of dental implants to aid in the restoration of missing teeth.

2. Assume that a student has a congenitally missing maxillary lateral incisor. Discuss the various treatment options.

3. Assume that one of your clinical patients has implants and a prosthesis such as that pictured in *Figure 12.1*. Discuss your treatment plan for this patient. Include your dental hygiene care, recommended auxiliary aids, home care instructions, and recall schedule.

4. Go online and search the catalogs of dental instrument companies. Find implant scaling instruments. Compare the following to typical scaling instruments:
   • Cost
   • Design
   • Material

Review Questions

Question 1. The type of implant that involves cutting a hole into the alveolar bone and then pressing or screwing in the implant is called:

a. Subperiosteal

b. Staple

c. Transosseous

d. Endosseous

Question 2. Which of the following takes place during the second endosseous implant surgery?

a. An impression is taken for crown fabrication

b. An abutment is attached to the body of the implant

c. A healing cap is attached to the body of the implant

d. The amount of osseointegration is measured

Question 3. To ensure longevity and function of the implant, the patient is responsible for:

a. Eventual payment in full of all implant procedures

b. Plaque control

c. Application of tray-delivered fluoride

d. Proper occlusion

Question 4. The surgical procedure for placing implants must not injure the bone. Overheating the bone prevents osseointegration of the implant. Recommended temperatures are not to exceed:

a. 98.6°F

b. 47°F

c. 117°C

d. 117°F

Question 5. **All of the following conditions are contraindications for implant placement except:**

a. Recurrent caries
b. Poor oral hygiene
c. Diabetes
d. Smoking

Question 6. **Titanium is very difficult to cast. It is not very strong but is acceptable for implant uses.**

a. The first statement is true; the second statement is false.
b. The first statement is false; the second statement is true.
c. Both statements are true.
d. Both statements are false.

Question 7. **A patient who has a very small, or essentially no mandibular ridge, is said to have a (an):**

a. Atrophic dentulous mandible
b. Atrophic edentulous mandible
c. Iatrogenic edentulous mandible
d. Dysfunctional edentulous mandible

Question 8. **The patient's home care regimen of implant maintenance may consist only of a toothbrush and floss. Without proper maintenance, the possibility of implant failure greatly increases.**

a. The first statement is true; the second statement is false.
b. The first statement is false; the second statement is true.
c. Both statements are true.
d. Both statements are false.

Question 9. **The prosthodontic phase of implant treatment involves the placement of several "parts" or attachments. A patient who has completed the surgeries and restorative care would receive, in order:**

a. Cylinder, implant, abutment, crown
b. Implant, cylinder, abutment, crown
c. Cylinder, implant, crown, abutment
d. Implant, abutment, cylinder, crown

Question 10. **All of the following should be included in the postcare maintenance of a patient with an implant except one. Which one is the EXCEPTION?**

a. Necessary chairside, home care instruction
b. Recommended auxiliary aids
c. Selecting the restorative material for an adjacent restoration
d. Specific length of time between recall visits

Specialty Materials

Objectives

After studying this chapter, the student will be able to do the following:

1. Describe the components of a fixed orthodontic appliance.
2. Discuss the caries risk of orthodontic patients and the dental hygienist's role in preventing caries and periodontal disease in these patients.
3. Summarize the procedures involved in root canal therapy.
4. Explain the use of periodontal packs and sutures.
5. Discuss the rationale for the following procedures:
   * Pulpotomy
   * Stainless steel crown
   * Space maintainer

Key Words/Phrases

apicoectomy
appliances
band
bracket
debonding
elastic
elastic ligatures
endodontic files
endodontic sealers
fluoride varnish
gutta-percha
irrigants
lateral condensation
lingual arch
obturation
periodontal packs
pulpotomy
retainers
retrofill
root canal therapy
space maintainers
stainless steel crown
sutures
tube
wires

Introduction

Dental specialties use many of the same materials common in general practice of dentistry. Other materials are unique to one or several specialties. This chapter presents some of the more common materials used by orthodontists, endodontists, periodontists, oral surgeons, and pediatric dentists that the dental hygienist will encounter in a general practice setting.

I. Orthodontic Materials

The specialty of orthodontics seeks to align teeth in their most esthetic and functional position. Orthodontists use a variety of materials and devices. Some are the same materials used in other areas of dentistry; others are unique to orthodontics. Orthodontists use devices called **appliances** to move teeth and to affect growth of the maxilla and mandible. Orthodontists use both fixed and removable appliances. The most common fixed orthodontic appliance consists of brackets, wires, and bands, as shown in *Figures 13.1 and 13.2*. An orthodontic retainer is a removable appliance and is shown in *Figure 13.3*.

A. Materials Similar to Those Commonly Used in General Dentistry

1. Impression Materials and Gypsum Products

Impression materials used in orthodontics are the same as those discussed in Chapter 8, Impression Materials. Alginate is the most commonly used impression material because orthodontic appliances do not require the precision of a cast restoration. Orthodontists use dental stone to pour casts for the construction of appliances. Orthodontic stone is used for study models. It is not as strong as dental stone because this facilitates model trimming. Whiteners are added to orthodontic stone to improve the appearance of study models. Opital (digital) impressions are becoming common in orthodontics. This digital information is interfaced with digital radiographs and treatment planning software.

2. Bonding Materials and Composites

The same bonding materials used in restorative dentistry are used by orthodontists to bond appliances to teeth. Both light-cure and chemical-cure composites are used. Generally, orthodontists use only acid-etched enamel for bonding because no dentin is available. Use of dental bonding primers improves bonding if contamination of the etched surface is a problem.

Nearly all composite products are strong enough for use in orthodontics when bonding to anterior and premolar teeth. Strength of the bonding material is not a problem, but adhesion is. A macrofilled composite has the advantage in that when fixed appliances are removed at the end of treatment (**debonding**), it is much easier to locate residual composite bonding material. Macrofilled composites are rough and turn gray when the composite material is abraded with a metal instrument. The filler particles in macrofilled composites are harder than the metal of

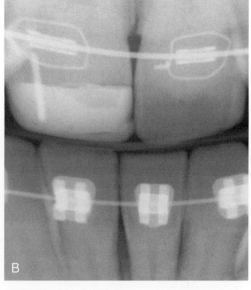
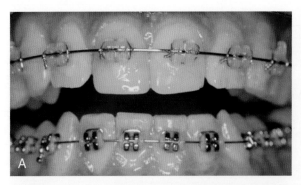

FIGURE 13.1. A. Orthodontic fixed appliance consisting of polycarbonate brackets with metal ligatures and rectangular wire on the upper arch and stainless steel brackets with elastic ties and a round wire on the lower arch. **B.** Radiograph showing the appliance. Note the composite restoration retained by a pin.

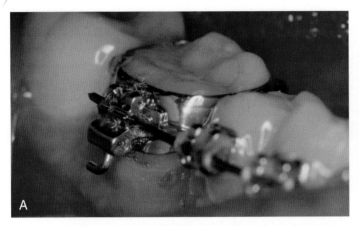

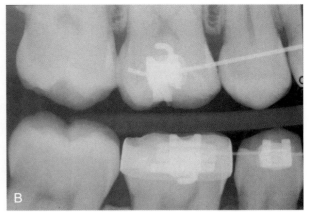

FIGURE 13.2. A. Photograph of a buccal tube that is part of the appliance shown in Figure 13.1. Note the hook for attaching elastics. **B.** A posterior bitewing of the same area. Note that the mandibular tube uses a band, whereas the maxillary tube is directly bonded to the molar.

the instrument; hence, they abrade the instrument and turn gray. General dentists and dental hygienists have spent significant time and effort removing orthodontic bonding material left on teeth after orthodontic treatment. Debonding of orthodontic brackets is presented in Chapter 32.

3. Acrylic Resins

The acrylic resins used to construct orthodontic appliances are the same chemically activated materials discussed in Chapter 11, Removable Prostheses and Acrylic Resins. The adolescent patients seen by orthodontists have encouraged the use of colors that stand out rather than match oral tissues. At times, acrylic orthodontic appliances do not blend in with the oral environment but are a fashion statement. Red, green, orange, and even sparkle colors are common.

B. Wires

Wires are used in orthodontics as springs and stabilizers. Many wires are bought preformed to match an ideal arch form from the manufacturer.

Others are bent by the orthodontist to the desired arch form. Wires are attached to the patient's teeth with brackets, ligatures, tubes, and bands. Elastic deformation of the wire (bending) is used to apply force to the teeth, much like with a spring. The force applied by wires pushes, pulls, or rotates teeth into the proper position, as shown in *Figure 13.4*.

Many metals have been used for orthodontic wires. Stainless steel is the most common. Nickel–titanium wires are also popular because they can store more energy for tooth movement than can other wires. Wires are manufactured in a variety of shapes and cross-section sizes. As the size of the wire increases, so does the stiffness of the wire and the force it can apply. Some wires are round; others are rectangular, square, or even several wires braided together.

C. Brackets, Bands, and Tubes

1. Brackets

A **bracket** is a device that is attached to teeth, holds the archwire in place, and is used to trans-

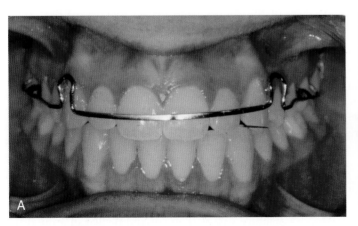

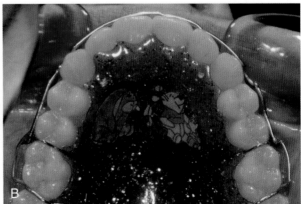

FIGURE 13.3. Photographs of an orthodontic maxillary retainer. **A.** Facial view. **B.** Occlusal view. (Courtesy of Dr. Daniel Foley, Beckley, WV.)

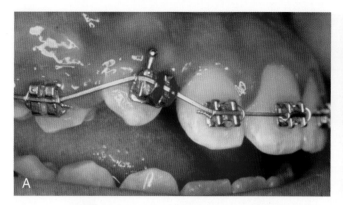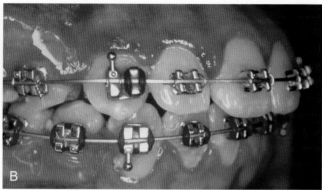

FIGURE 13.4. A. Initially a wire is ligated to a maxillary arch with a malposed canine. **B.** After the force of the wire has moved the canine into a more ideal position. (Courtesy of Dr. Daniel Foley, Beckley, WV.)

fer the forces of wires, springs, and elastics (rubber bands) to the teeth. A variety of materials is used to make orthodontic brackets, as shown in *Figures 13.1, 13.2, and 13.4.* Historically, stainless steel has been the most widely used material. A metal mesh is attached to the back of metal brackets. The undercuts of the mesh lock in the bonding material and attach the bracket to acid-etched enamel with composite resin material. Metal brackets have excellent mechanical properties, but they suffer from poor esthetics. They are relatively easy to bond to and remove from teeth.

Other materials used to make brackets are polymers, such as polycarbonate resin, and ceramic materials, such as aluminum oxide. Polymers tend to be too weak for this use, as they are subject to creep over time. Some manufacturers have added a metal reinforcement to the bracket slot to improve the strength and stiffness of polycarbonate brackets. Ceramic brackets have had mechanical problems as well. Although strong in compression, ceramic brackets are quite brittle. Bracket fracture during treatment has been a problem. On the other hand, the high compressive strength of ceramic brackets has made them difficult to remove from teeth. Many innovations and improvements have been made to both polymeric and ceramic brackets because the esthetic appearance of these brackets is commonly demanded by patients. Bonding polymeric and ceramic brackets to teeth is more technique sensitive than is bonding metal brackets. If directions are followed, success is common.

2. Bands and Tubes

An orthodontic **band** encircles the crown of the tooth. Bands were used to attach brackets to teeth before acid etching became available. Brackets were welded to the bands, and the bands were cemented around each tooth.

Current orthodontic practice uses bands only on molar teeth because molars require more force to move compared to other teeth.

Orthodontic bands and tubes are made from stainless steel. An orthodontic **tube** is just that, a tube that allows a wire to slide through it, as shown in *Figure 13.2A.* Most orthodontic tubes are actually a combination of several tubes, both round and square. An orthodontist may use more than one wire at a time. One wire is used to apply force to one or more teeth, and a second wire is used to stabilize the "anchor" teeth. Orthodontic tubes are welded to bands, and the bands are cemented on molars. The cement of choice is glass ionomer cement (because of fluoride release). At times, tubes are bonded to molars by using acid-etched composites.

D. Elastics and Ligatures

The term **elastic** is used in orthodontics for several types of products and thus can be confusing. The "rubber bands" worn by orthodontic patients are used to apply force to teeth. They are called elastics. These rubber bands are changed by the patient several times each day as the force (pull) of the rubber band decays (decreases) over time. They are made from latex rubber and come in a variety of sizes, force levels, and colors.

Other "elastics" are used to secure the archwire into the bracket. These are called **elastic ligatures**. They look like little rubber donuts and are stretched around the "wings" of the bracket, forcing the wire into the bracket slot. These elastic ligatures are typically made from thermoplastic rubber, such as polyurethane. Other commonly used ligatures are thin, stainless steel wires that are wrapped around the archwire and bracket wings and twisted to secure the archwire in the bracket. The end of the ligature wire is then cut and tucked in around the bracket, tying the wire into the bracket. Both types of ligatures are shown in *Figure 13.1.*

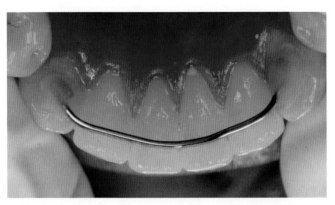

FIGURE 13.5. Photograph of a bonded lingual retainer.

E. Retainers

After the teeth are moved into the proper position, the orthodontist removes the bands and brackets. The patient is typically very happy that day. If left alone, however, the teeth would tend to "relapse" or partially return to their original position. To prevent relapse, orthodontists use **retainers** to keep the teeth in the desired position. There are many kinds of retainers, and many are similar to functional removable orthodontic appliances.

The common retainer for the maxillary arch consists of an acrylic palate with several wire clasps (much like a partial denture framework) and a wire that sits on the labial surface of the teeth. A retainer is shown in *Figure 13.3*. Sandwiched between the acrylic and the wire, the teeth are held in place.

A common mandibular retainer is a **lingual arch**. With this type of retainer, a heavy wire sits on the lingual surface of the lower anterior teeth and is bonded to the canines with a mesh pad using composite. A lingual arch retainer is shown in *Figure 13.5*.

F. Stainless Steel

Stainless steel devices are common in orthodontics. Stainless steel typically has a significant nickel content (~8%). Many patients are sensitive to nickel, and orthodontists find themselves in a dilemma with these patients. Until recently, many products were only available as nickel-containing, stainless steel products. More and more, however, manufacturers are using stainless steel with little or no nickel or other metals. Titanium is a popular alternative to stainless steel.

G. Oral Hygiene and the Orthodontic Patient

All orthodontic patients are considered to be at high risk for caries. Oral hygiene is difficult with orthodontic appliances because food debris is retained after every meal. Many orthodontic patients have "white spots" on their teeth when their brackets are removed. These white spots are the visible sign of initial decalcification (caries). Some orthodontic patients develop cavitated lesions. It is critical that the dental hygienist stress the importance of oral hygiene and proper diet to the orthodontic patient. Poor plaque control frequently results in gingival inflammation. Food debris stuck on the wires and brackets is a continuous source of carbohydrate for acidogenic bacteria. The orthodontic patient's swollen gums quickly heal after the "hardware" is removed, but carious lesions must be restored. It is very frustrating to the general dentist to restore the facial surfaces of anterior teeth in young patients when they know that these carious lesions could have been—and should have been—prevented. Many orthodontists will recommend fluoride rinses and auxiliary oral hygiene aids to their patients in an effort to prevent decay. In addition, orthodontists are using fluoride-releasing bonding materials and fluoride varnish to reduce the patient's risk of caries.

II. Endodontic Materials

A. Endodontics in General

Endodontics is the specialty of dentistry that treats pathology of the pulp and periapical tissues of teeth. Typically, endodontic treatment involves root canal therapy.

1. Diagnosis

Diagnosis involves determining which tooth, if any, requires root canal therapy. The status of the dental pulp and periapical tissues is important to determine the diagnosis. Occasionally, a patient is certain which tooth is causing the pain; other times, the involved tooth is difficult to identify. The clinician must use diagnostic tests to make a definitive diagnosis. Diagnostic tests include percussion tests (tapping the tooth with the handle of a dental mirror), mobility, reaction to hot and cold stimuli, periodontal probing, electric pulp tests, and radiography. A radiograph of tooth #7 with a periapical radiolucency is shown in *Figure 13.6A*. Before root canal therapy is performed, the clinician must determine if the tooth can be restored to adequate form and function. This involves examining the tooth's periodontal health and extent of caries.

2. Root Canal Therapy

Root canal therapy involves removing the contents of the dental pulp space: the pulp chamber and the canal system. Depending on the status of the pulp, local anesthesia is the first step. The pulp may be vital connective tissue, necrotic debris, or a combination of both. Pulp removal

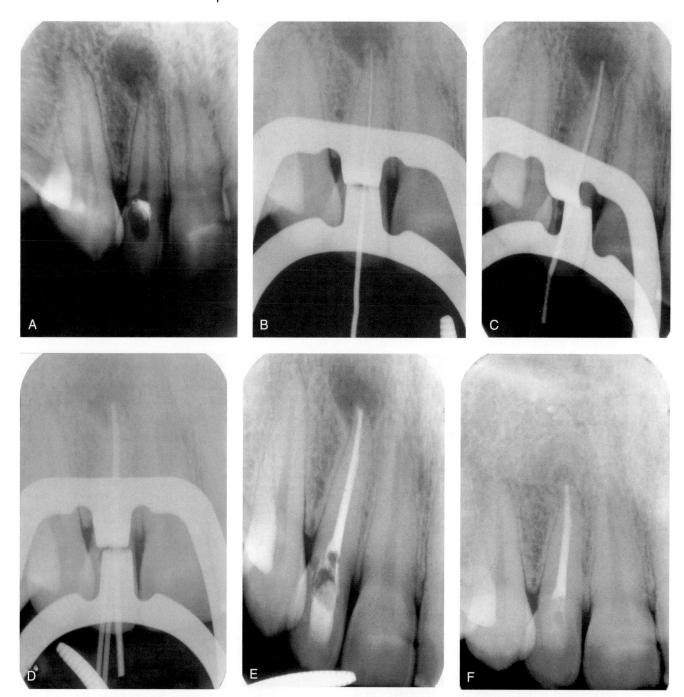

FIGURE 13.6. Radiographs of root canal therapy. **A.** Initial condition with a periapical radiolucency. **B.** Initial working file. **C.** Master apical file. **D.** Master cone and several accessory gutta-percha points. **E.** Completed root canal therapy. **F.** One-year recall. Note the decrease in the size of the periapical radiolucency. **B, C,** and **D** radiographs exposed with rubber dam and retainer in place.

is accomplished with files and irrigants, which will be described later in this section. The canal space is prepared to a shape that is designed to receive the filling material. The filling material is gutta-percha (a rubber-like material) in combination with an endodontic sealer. The filling material should fill the canal space in three dimensions and prevent leakage of oral fluids and contaminants into the periapical tissues.

3. Restoration

Restoration of an endodontically treated tooth may be as simple as a filling (amalgam or composite) or as complex as a post/core and crown. The complexity of the restoration depends on the location of the tooth and the amount of tooth structure that is missing. The restoration must fill the pulp chamber and protect the root canal–filling material from oral fluids.

Current adhesive restorative materials should be employed when restoring endodontically treated teeth to reduce the amount of coronal leakage. Inadequate coronal restoration has caused many well-performed root canal therapies to fail. Many clinicians believe that posterior teeth should receive full coronal coverage to prevent fracture of the tooth. Anterior teeth can be restored with a simple filling if the remaining tooth structure is adequate. Many teeth requiring root canal therapy have lost a large amount of tooth structure. These teeth may require a post, made of stainless steel or dental casting alloy, that is cemented into a canal and supports the core buildup. Core buildups are made of amalgam or composite. They replace the missing tooth structure and retain the crown, as shown in Figure 15.2.

B. Cleaning the Canal Space

1. Preparation of the Access Cavity

   After diagnosis, treatment options are discussed with the patient. Local anesthetic is administered, and a rubber dam is placed for isolation. A rubber dam is mandatory when performing root canal therapy to protect the patient from swallowing or aspirating small endodontic instruments or irrigating solutions. Access to the canal space is gained by use of a high-speed handpiece. Each canal is located with an endodontic explorer and endodontic files. Many times a microscope is used to locate small canals.

2. Endodontic Files

   Endodontic files and other instruments are used to remove the contents of the canal system. Files enlarge and shape the canal to receive the filling material. Files can be divided into two groups: hand files and rotary (handpiece-driven) files. Traditionally, endodontic files were made from stainless steel, but recently, files made of nickel–titanium have become popular. Files are moved in an up and down motion with a slight rotation at times to mechanically clean and shape the canal system. An international standardization for endodontic file sizes has been established (American Dental Association and International Standards Organization). Corresponding gutta-percha and paper points also exist. Files and gutta-percha points are shown in *Figure 13.7*. Files are placed in the canals, and the length of the canal is determined with the use of radiographs, as shown in *Figure 13.6B and C*. As the canal is enlarged, several radiographs are used to determine the exact working length of the canal. The file used to shape the most apical

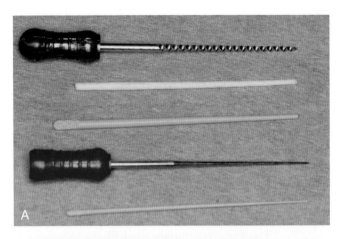
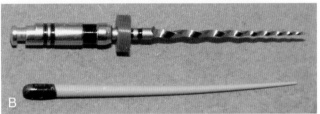

FIGURE 13.7. A. Photograph of (from *top* to *bottom*) an endodontic file, paper point, gutta-percha point, spreader, and accessory gutta-percha point. Note that the file, paper point, and gutta-percha are all of the same shape and diameter. **B.** Rotary file and corresponding gutta-percha point of the same size/taper.

portion of the canal is called the master apical file and is shown in *Figure 13.6C*.

3. Irrigants

   Irrigants are aqueous solutions that are used to disinfect the canal system by killing bacteria and dissolving pulpal tissue. Irrigants also flush out debris and lubricate the canal during instrumentation. Common irrigants include sodium hypochlorite (5.25%, or diluted to 2.5%), chlorhexidine gluconate (0.2%), or sterile saline. They are placed in the canal with a syringe and needle. As they flow out of the canal and crown of the tooth, they are removed with suction.

4. Paper Points

   A paper point is shown in *Figure 13.7*. Paper points are used primarily to dry the canal before it is filled with gutta-percha and sealer.

C. Filling the Canal (Obturation)

1. Gutta-Percha

   Various materials can be used to fill or obturate the root canal. The most common **obturation** material used is gutta-percha in combination with an endodontic sealer. **Gutta-percha** is a polymeric material that has been used for a variety of purposes for centuries. Dental gutta-percha is composed of zinc oxide (~66%), gutta-percha (~20%), heavy metal sulfates such as barium sulfate (~11%), and waxes/resins (~3%). Barium sulfate is added to make it radiopaque, as seen in *Figure 13.6D–F.* Two gutta-percha cones are shown in *Figure 13.7.* Gutta-percha is a flexible material at both room and body temperature; it softens when heated above 65°C (150°F). Gutta-percha is used with a variety of filling techniques. It can be softened with heat or a solvent and then placed into the canal space.

2. Lateral Condensation
The most commonly used filling technique is cold **lateral condensation**. In this technique, a master gutta-percha cone is selected that matches the size and length of the master apical file. The master cone is coated with an endodontic sealer and placed in the canal so that it reaches the entire length of the prepared canal. An endodontic spreader, as shown in *Figure 13.7,* is then placed beside the master gutta-percha cone and pushed into the canal to create a space beside the master cone. The spreader is rotated and removed from the canal, and an accessory gutta-percha cone is placed into the space that was created. A radiograph of a master cone with several accessory cones is shown in *Figure 13.6D.* The process of cold lateral condensation is continued until a dense, three-dimensional fill is achieved, as shown in *Figure 13.6E.*

3. Endodontic Sealers
Endodontic sealers are a type of dental cement. Sealers coat the canal space and fill any voids between the canal wall and the gutta-percha. Endodontic sealers are predominantly zinc oxide–eugenol (ZOE) products with additives. The most common additives are other essential oils and chemicals, such as barium sulfate or silver, that make the material radiopaque. Calcium hydroxide sealers are also available. Sealers are purchased as either a paste/paste or a powder/liquid system.

D. Restoration and Recall

After root canal therapy is completed, the tooth needs to be restored in a timely manner. Restoration may begin immediately or be delayed until certain symptoms resolve. The patient needs to be informed that placement of a permanent restoration is critical to the success of the root canal therapy. The patient should be informed to return to the office if the temporary filling is lost. Most dentists will take periapical radiographs of teeth with root canals at recall appointments, such as

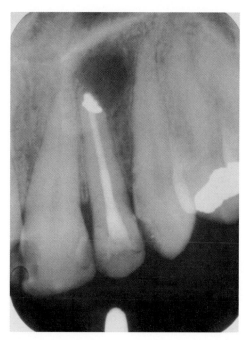

FIGURE 13.8. Radiograph of an apicoectomy and amalgam retrofill. (Courtesy of Dr. C. Russell Jackson, Morgantown, WV.)

that shown in *Figure 13.6F,* to assess the success of the treatment.

E. Apicoectomy and Retrofills

Root canal therapy is successful in approximately 95% of cases. If failure occurs, treatment options include conservative retreatment, extraction, or an apicoectomy. An **apicoectomy** is a surgical procedure that removes from 1 to 3 mm of the root apex. In addition, the apical portion of the canal is prepared, and a filling is placed to seal the end of the root (**retrofill**). *Figure 13.8* shows a radiograph of this treatment. In the past, retrofill materials included amalgam or cements. Now MTA (mineral trioxide aggregate) is the material of choice, see Chapter 7, Dental Cements.

III. Periodontal and Other Surgical Materials

Because periodontics and oral surgery involve the manipulation of soft tissue, both groups of materials will be discussed in this section. Because dental hygiene programs have significant course work in their curriculums covering periodontics, these materials will not be covered in detail.

A. Periodontal/Surgical Packs

Periodontal packs are used to protect surgical sites and promote healing. Periodontal packs are mixed to a putty-like consistency and then placed over the surgical site. The pack is retained in place by forcing the material into the embrasures of the teeth, as shown in *Figure 13.9.* The placement

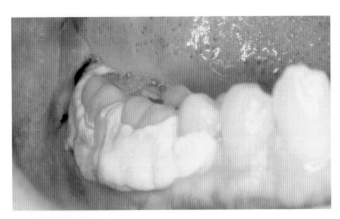

FIGURE 13.9. Photograph of a periodontal pack in place. (Courtesy of Dr. Louise Veselicky, Morgantown, WV.)

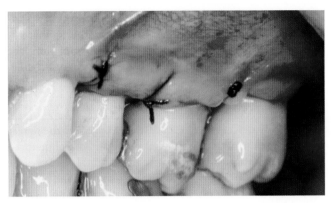

FIGURE 13.10. Photograph of sutures in place. (Courtesy of Dr. Louise Veselicky, Morgantown, WV.)

and removal of periodontal packs are presented in Chapters 33 and 34.

1. Chemistry

Many periodontal packs are based on the typical ZOE formulation described in Chapter 7, Dental Cements. When noneugenol temporary cements were developed, noneugenol periodontal packs soon followed. The set material is not as strong as cements and makes them easy to remove when desired.

Light-cure periodontal packs have also been marketed. The setting reaction is the same addition polymerization reaction as previously described in Chapter 5, Direct Polymeric Restorative Materials. The monomer and resulting polymer are a little different from the usual dental composite. The set material is much weaker than a composite, making it easier to remove.

2. Systems

Most systems are powder/liquid or paste/paste, similar to those of temporary cements. Light-cure materials come as a putty and do not need to be mixed.

B. Sutures

Sutures are threads or filaments that are used to reposition tissues that have been displaced by surgical procedures or trauma. Examples are shown in Figures 11.10C and *13.10*. A variety of sutures and suture materials are available. They are made from naturally occurring as well as man-made materials. Both absorbable and nonabsorbable sutures are available.

1. Absorbable Sutures

Absorbable sutures are resorbed by the body and, therefore, do not need to be removed at a second appointment. Absorbable sutures include surgical gut, both plain and "chrome,"

and synthetic polyglycolic acid. Glycolic acid is polymerized via addition polymerization and is formed into fibers.

2. Nonabsorbable Sutures

Nonabsorbable sutures include surgical silk and other threads, of either natural or synthetic materials. It is important that these sutures be removed at a later appointment. The sutures carry a risk of infection because they exist both inside and outside the body while in place. Suture removal is presented in Chapter 34.

3. Physical Characteristics of Sutures

Sutures may be single filaments or twisted or braided, multifilament materials. The size of sutures (diameter) is designated by a number of zeros. The smallest is 0 and is called "ought," 00 is called "double ought," and 3-0 is called "triple ought." The largest size is 8-0, or "eight ought."

4. Needles

Placing sutures requires pulling the filament through the tissue with a needle, similar to sewing with a needle and thread. Most needles are stainless steel, and they come in a variety of shapes. Most surgeons use swaged needles (needles that do not have an eye). Swaged needles do not use a knot to tie the suture to the needle. Instead, the end opposite the tip is a tube. The suture material is inserted into the tube, and the sides of the tube are crushed or swaged onto the suture, binding it to the needle. Swaged needles pass through the tissues much more easily and cause less tissue damage than do needles with an eye and a knot.

C. Bone Replacement Materials

Many materials have been developed to replace bone that has been lost to periodontal disease. Some are natural materials; others are synthetic. Various forms of human and animal bone are available.

They are treated with chemicals to prevent transmission of pathogens. Other synthetic materials, typically a calcium phosphate formulation, are used to replace bone. Some of these are resorbable, whereas others are not.

D. Membranes

Polymer membranes are used to prevent the apical downgrowth of epithelial tissue and attachment to cementum at the base of a periodontal pocket after periodontal surgery. Both absorbable and nonabsorbable membranes are available. Placement of a nonabsorbable membrane requires a second surgery to remove it.

E. Antibiotic Devices

Researchers have experimented for more than 20 years with materials that release antibiotics into the gingival crevice and periodontal pockets. New absorbable and nonabsorbable products have received U.S. Food and Drug Administration approval. Examples are Atridox and Arestin. Their use in the treatment of periodontal disease is common and widely accepted.

F. Bone Plates and Screws

Oral surgery is the field of dentistry that treats fractures of the maxilla and mandible as well as other facial structures. At times, a fixation device is used to stabilize sections of bone. Plates and screws or heavy-gauge wires are used. These materials may be left in place or removed after sufficient healing has occurred. They are made of titanium or a resorbable material.

IV. Pediatric Dentistry

Although pediatric dentistry is a recognized specialty, most children are treated in a general dentistry office. A dental hygienist working in such an office will see many young patients. Most of pediatric dentistry can be described as general dentistry for younger patients. A few cases, however, do not quite fit into the typical adult patient restorative procedures. Several are described here.

A. Pulpotomy

A **pulpotomy** is the removal of a portion of the pulp. Usually, this involves removal of only the coronal portion of the pulp of a primary or permanent molar; the pulp tissue in the canals is left in place. After the coronal pulp tissue is removed, various medicaments are placed in the chamber to sterilize or mummify the accessible remaining pulp tissue. The pulp chamber is filled with a dental cement, typically a reinforced ZOE product.

For primary molars (*Fig. 13.11A and B*), a pulpotomy is a permanent procedure. On the other hand, a pulpotomy is a temporary (frequently emergency) procedure on permanent molars that is followed by root canal therapy (as described earlier). A primary molar with a pulpotomy is typically restored with a stainless steel crown (*Fig. 13.11C–E*).

B. Stainless Steel Crown

In young patients, molars that are badly broken down can be restored with a preformed **stainless steel crown** (*Fig. 13.11C–E*). The crown is a metal shell (thin layer) with preformed anatomy. Stainless steel crowns come in a variety of sizes for each molar. This includes primary and permanent, maxillary and mandibular, and first and second molars. The tooth is prepared in a manner similar to that for a cast crown. The preformed crown with the proper mesial–distal dimension is chosen. The crown is adapted and then cemented by filling the crown with cement and seating it on the prepared tooth. The excess cement is removed after setting. A stainless steel crown on a primary tooth is designed to restore the tooth until it is exfoliated. A stainless steel crown on a permanent tooth is designed to restore the tooth until the patient is older, the tooth is completely erupted, and the risk of caries is more normal.

C. Esthetic Crowns

A variety of preformed anterior crowns are available for deciduous teeth. The esthetics of many are not suitable for many parents' perceptions. Recently preformed yttria-stabilized zirconia crowns have become available for pediatric patients. Similar to stainless steel crowns, they come in a variety of sizes for specific teeth. The shade selection is very limited but adequate for most patient needs (*see Fig. 13.11H and I*).

D. Space Maintainer

Some patients lose primary molars before the permanent tooth is ready to erupt. Teeth adjacent to that space may drift into the space formerly occupied by the lost tooth. Loss of this space for the permanent tooth often results in crowding when the permanent tooth erupts. Orthodontics may be necessary to correct the crowding problem.

Space maintainers are appliances that prevent the drifting of adjacent teeth in such cases. They keep the space open for the permanent tooth to erupt. This reduces the likelihood of orthodontics. When the permanent tooth begins to erupt, the space maintainer is removed. A unilateral band-loop and a bilateral lower lingual holding arch space maintainer are shown in *Figure 13.11F and G*, respectively.

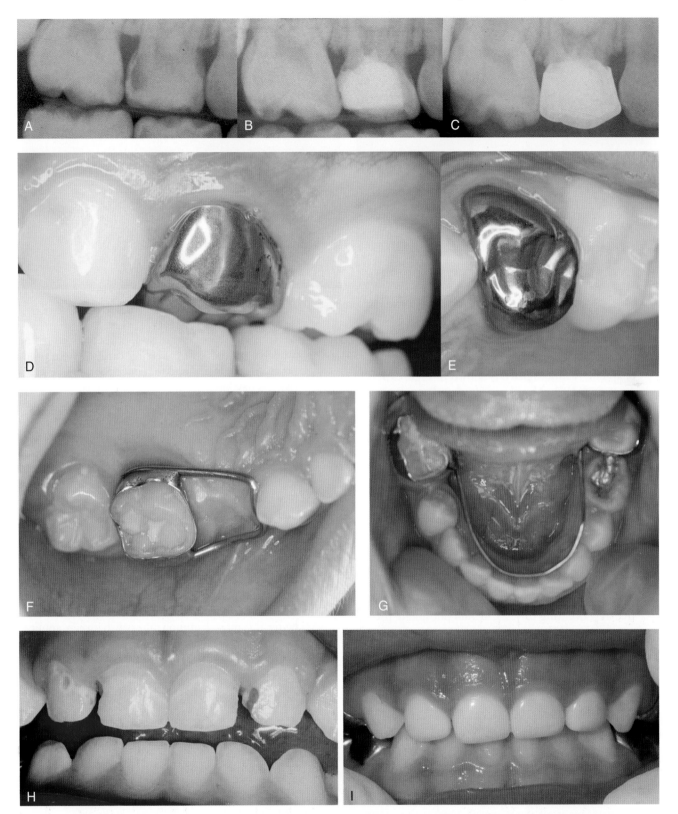

FIGURE 13.11. Radiographs of a deciduous tooth with **A.** deep carious lesion, **B.** pulpotomy, and **C.** stainless steel crown. Photographs of crown from the **D.** buccal and **E.** occlusal perspectives. **F.** Photograph of band-loop space maintainer. **G.** Photograph of a lower lingual holding arch. **H.** Preoperative photograph showing carious lesions. **I.** Post-op view on zirconium oxide crowns on deciduous anterior teeth, #**D**, #**E**, #**F**, and #**G**. (Courtesy of NuSmile Dr. William Waggoner, Las Vegas, NV.)

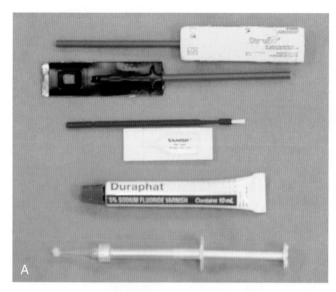
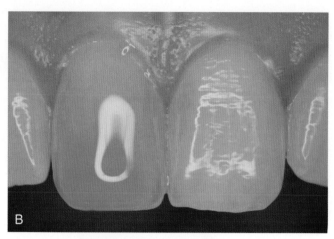

FIGURE 13.12. **A.** Several fluoride varnish products. **B.** Fluoride varnish applied to tooth #8.

E. Preventive Materials

A variety of preventive materials is covered in other chapters. A mouthguard is shown in Figures 1.12, 18.1, and 18.3. Mouthguards absorb energy and prevent trauma. A sealant is shown in Figure 1.11. Sealants prevent caries by filling caries-susceptible pits and fissures with a polymeric material. Pits and fissures are caries-susceptible ecological niches of teeth where bacteria colonize and toothbrush bristles cannot clean. The application of dental sealants is presented in Chapter 25. Some may consider glass ionomer materials to prevent recurrent caries. However, definitive supportive research is not available. Several categories of dental products prevent oral diseases. Mouthwashes are available that reduce gingivitis. Fluoridated toothpastes, gels, and rinses have long been known to be effective in preventing caries. Calcium phosphate products, such as MI paste, aid in caries prevention and recalcification.

Recently, fluoride varnish has been added to the available products for reducing caries. These products were originally used to reduce root surface sensitivity. They have become a quite popular preventive adjunct for high-caries-risk patients. They reduce caries by approximately 40% depending on the clinical study. A typical **fluoride varnish** contains 5% (22,600 ppm) NaF, a carrier resin, and a volatile solvent. The teeth need not be dried. Teeth are painted with the varnish. The patient is instructed to not brush or floss for 2 hours after placement. A soft diet is recommended for at least 2 hours. Some of the fluoride in the varnish is absorbed by the enamel, changing hydroxyapatite to fluoroapatite and reducing the solubility of the enamel in an acid environment. Fluoride varnishes are recommended for all ages assuming no medical contraindication is present. A variety of schedules have been used, 6 months being the most common interval between applications. Several products are shown in *Figure 13.12A*. A number of products result in a temporary yellow tint of the teeth (*see Fig. 13.12B*).

Summary

The dental materials discussed in this chapter include those from the specialties of orthodontics, endodontics, periodontics, oral surgery, and pediatric dentistry. In orthodontics, many of the materials used are the same as those used in general dentistry. These would include impression materials, gypsum products, bonding agents, composites, and acrylic resins. Wires are used in orthodontics to apply force to the teeth. Brackets are bonded to the teeth surfaces and provide a "slot" to hold the archwire. The archwire then extends through many brackets and "connects" all the teeth together. Brackets are made of metal, polymer, or ceramic. Orthodontic bands, which are made of stainless steel, encircle the crown of the tooth. Elastics and ligatures are also orthodontic materials. These materials apply force to the teeth or secure the archwire into the bracket depending on the type of "elastic" used. Retainers are used to prevent relapse of treated teeth.

Root canal therapy uses endodontic files to remove the pulp contents. Some files are used by hand; others are handpiece driven. Gutta-percha is a polymeric material that is used to fill the canal space. Barium sulfate is added to gutta-percha to make it radiopaque. Endodontic sealers are a type of dental cement that coats the canal space and fills in voids between the canal wall and the gutta-percha.

After periodontal surgery, periodontal packs are used to protect surgical sites and promote healing. They are usually supplied in powder/liquid or paste/paste form and are mixed to a putty-like consistency. Sutures are used in many types of surgical procedures to reposition tissues that have been displaced by surgery or trauma. Sutures may be absorbable (do not need to be removed) or non-absorbable (must be removed). Sutures may be single filaments or twisted/braided multifilament materials. To place a suture, a needle is required. Needles are made

of stainless steel and are usually swaged onto the suture material. Other surgical and periodontal materials include membranes, antibiotic devices, bone plates and screws, and those materials used for actual bone replacement.

Dental materials and procedures used in the treatment of pediatric dental patients include pulpotomies, stainless steel crowns, and space maintainers. Pulpotomies involve the removal of a portion of the pulp. It can be a permanent or a temporary procedure depending on the tooth that is involved. Stainless steel crowns can serve as a functioning restoration until the primary tooth is exfoliated. For permanent teeth, a stainless steel temporary restoration is replaced when the patient is older. Space maintainers are appliances that prevent the drifting of adjacent teeth until a permanent tooth erupts.

Learning Activities

1. Examine students in the class undergoing orthodontic treatment. Determine what types of materials are being used. Discuss the possible oral hygiene aids these students could use.

2. Examine radiographs of patients who have had endodontic therapy. Discuss the benefits of root canal therapy and the materials used to restore these teeth.

3. Place and remove a periodontal pack on a dentoform.

4. Place and remove sutures in a piece of fabric, an orange, or a piece of chicken.

5. Ask classmates if anyone has ever had a stainless steel crown or space maintainer. Discuss the treatment that the student experienced.

6. With a small group of students and several radiographs, look for the following films:
   • Any orthodontic appliance
   • Any root canal materials
   • Any surgical fixation devices

Review Questions

Question 1. The word "obturation," when used in discussion of root canal therapy, means:

a. Accessing the canal
b. Filling and sealing the canal
c. Placing the final restoration
d. Removing the contents of the pulp

Question 2. Which type of composite gives the clinician an advantage when removing orthodontic resins during bonding?

a. Microfilled
b. Macrofilled
c. Hybrid
d. None of the above

Question 3. The endodontic surgical procedure that removes 1 to 3 mm of the root apex is called a/an:

a. Endodontic retreatment
b. Retrofill
c. Root resection
d. Apicoectomy

Question 4. What is used to disinfect the canal system by killing bacteria and dissolving pulpal tissue?

a. Endodontic sealers
b. Paper points
c. Irrigants
d. Gutta-percha

Question 5.
Which orthodontic device prevents "relapse" of the teeth?

a. Archwire

b. Ligature

c. Bracket

d. Retainer

Question 6.
The debonding procedure is done after orthodontic treatment is completed. The dental material removed from tooth surfaces is:

a. Composite resin

b. Cold-cure resin

c. Dental cement

d. Ligature material

Question 7.
The most commonly used technique to fill a root canal with gutta-percha is termed:

a. Direct compression

b. Lateral compression

c. Direct condensation

d. Lateral condensation

Question 8.
A pulpotomy usually serves as a/an _____ procedure on permanent molars.

a. Temporary

b. Permanent

c. Either temporary or permanent

d. Neither temporary nor permanent

Question 9.
Which of the following materials used in orthodontic treatment serves to secure the arch wire on the facial surfaces of a tooth?

a. Band

b. Bracket

c. Composite resin

d. Retainer

Question 10.
Surgical silk suture is:

a. Another name for surgical gut suture

b. Absorbable and removed at a later appointment

c. Nonabsorbable and removed at a later appointment

d. Absorbable and exists both inside and outside the body while in place

Clinical Detection and Management of Dental Restorative Materials during Scaling and Polishing

14

Objectives

After studying this chapter, the student will be able to do the following:

1. Using the criteria listed in Table 14.1, differentiate between ceramic materials and composite materials.
2. Discuss how the following criteria may help a clinician to distinguish between tooth tissues and restorative materials or between two types of restorative materials:
   - Radiographic characteristics
   - Surface smoothness
   - Tactile and auditory sensations
   - Location
3. Describe some common procedures routinely performed by a dental hygienist that could be detrimental to teeth and restorative materials.
4. Verbally compare the expected differences in the surfaces of enamel and a gold crown after polishing with an abrasive agent.
5. Recall the recommended instrumentation technique around the margins of cast restorations.
6. Explain the causes of possible damage to restorations from the use of high-speed instrumentation.
7. Propose a possible scaling-and-polishing protocol for a patient with the following oral findings:
   - 4 mm of recessed gingiva
   - Class V glass ionomer restorations in the maxillary left quadrant
   - Two gold crowns in the mandibular right quadrant
   - Three composite restorations in the maxillary anterior segment

Key Words/Phrases

beveled margin

cavosurface margin

margination

tine

Introduction

Much has been written about the various techniques, instruments, and materials that are used during scaling and polishing. It is difficult, however, to find adequate references to document potential damage to the surfaces of teeth, restorations, and fixed prosthetic appliances.

In this chapter, the characteristics of restorative materials and tooth structure are described to aid the dental hygienist in providing the appropriate treatment during scaling and polishing. Criteria will be presented to help identify the various restorative materials that are used most frequently today.

After identifying the patient's restorative materials, the effects of instrumentation and the use of fluorides and polishing agents must be considered. Suggestions will be made as to which cleaning devices, instruments, and agents are acceptable for use on the given dental restorative materials.

I. Clinical Detection of Tooth Structure and Dental Restorative Materials

A. Identification of Tooth Structure and Restorative Materials

Many areas of tooth structure and types of restorative materials are easily identified. At times during an examination or scaling, however, it will be difficult to distinguish between exposed dentin and a recent, well-placed composite resin restoration. In such instances, the restorations can be overlooked, and an inappropriate polishing procedure may result.

Table 14.1 was developed as a guide for the hygienist to differentiate between tooth structure and restorative materials and between the different types of restorative materials.

1. An Example

Using Table 14.1 to distinguish between dentin and a glass ionomer restoration, several statements may be made: both may appear radiopaque. In addition, dentin feels smooth to the explorer, whereas glass ionomer feels rough.

A detectable margin also differentiates these two materials. If a sharp explorer were to pass over these two surfaces, a variance in sound would be noted, with the dull sound being peculiar to the glass ionomer. The sound referred to as sharp or dull is slight and, in all probability, is a combination of auditory and tactile sensations perceived by the operator. Another way to explain this concept is that most clinicians would agree that enamel has a certain hardness

and smoothness to it, whereas restorations may have a different texture and feel.

Using only the criteria listed in Table 14.1, rapid identification can be made. If the hygienist is unaware of the presence of the restoration and scales from the dentin surface of the tooth (in an area of gingival recession) onto the composite with heavy pressure, damage could be done to the restoration. A careful analysis of the restorative materials used on the patient must be carried out before initiating any form of treatment.

2. Other Criteria to Aid in Identification
   a. *Radiographic Characteristics*
   The shades of gray between the extremes of radiolucency and radiopacity aid the trained clinician in identifying tooth structures and materials. This information is discussed in Chapter 15, Radiographic Appearance of Dental Tissues and Materials.

   b. *Visual Appearance*
   Tooth enamel is the only natural material in the oral cavity that is translucent to visible light. Dentin has more color (yellow) and is much more opaque. In recent years, considerable efforts have been made to develop tooth-colored restorative materials that transfer light in a manner similar to that of tooth structure. This was discussed in detail in Chapter 5, Direct Polymeric Restorative Materials. These characteristics are evident in both ceramic materials and resin; the restorations made from these materials are difficult to be detected by casual observation. At times, an experienced clinician will detect a restorative material because it looks very homogenous in appearance rather than the slight variations present in enamel and dentin.

   c. *Surface Smoothness*
   In respect to surface smoothness, it could be stated that all exposed tooth surfaces in the oral cavity should be smooth. When a surface is smooth, it is free of irregularities. An explorer passed over this type of surface will glide freely with the change in contour and will not meet resistance.

   One of the goals of the hygienist is to produce smooth surfaces on both natural tooth structure and restorative materials. Less plaque and debris accumulate on smooth surfaces.

   d. *Sound and Touch*
   A sharp explorer can be one of the most helpful diagnostic tools available to the astute hygienist. Passage of the tip of the explorer

TABLE 14.1. Characteristics of Tooth Structure and Restorative Materials

CRITERIA:	TOOTH			POLISHED METAL RESTORATIONS				TOOTH-COLORED RESTORATIONS			OTHER	
	Enamel	Cementum	Dentin	Amalgam	Cast Gold	Gold Foil	Base Metal Alloys	Composite	Glass Ionomer	Ceramic Material	Pit and Fissure Sealant	Cements
Opaque		X	X	X	X	X	X	1	X	1		X
Translucent	X							X		X	X	
Smooth to Explorer	X		X	X	X	X	X	X		X	X	
Rough to Explorer		X							X			X
Tooth-Colored	X	X	X					X	X	X	2	
Glossy Surface	X		X	X	X	X	X	X		X	X	
Dull Surface		X						X	X			X
Detectable Margin[a]					X		X	X	X		X	X
Dull Sound		X						X	X		X	X
Sharp Sound	X		X	X	X	X	X			X		

1. The degree of opacity and translucency for resins and ceramic materials depends on the thickness of the material and the shade.
2. In many cases, pit and fissure sealants are clear, unfilled resins and are difficult to detect. Tints or coloring agents have been added to make them easier to detect; also, it is easier to determine if they need replacement.

[a]It has been assumed that all restorations are correctly finished and polished.
Modified from Krouse MA, Gladwin SC. Identification and management of restorative dental materials during patient prophylaxis. Dent Hyg. 1984;58:456–461, with permission.
Graphic by C. A. Hoffman.

at right angles to the surface with minimal pressure and force will transmit two distinct sensations to the hygienist.

1. The tactile sensation refers to the character of the surface: it could be smooth, as in tooth enamel, or it could be rough, as in a worn composite restoration.
2. Sound also plays a part in the diagnosis. The **tine** (sharp point) of the explorer is silent on smooth enamel but scratchy or noisy on rough tooth surfaces, worn composite restorations, and residual orthodontic bonding resin. When the tine passes over faulty or worn margins of a restoration, it produces a "ping" sound.
3. Some restorations could be so well matched to tooth structure that, without the "sound-feel" difference, they may go undetected. The ideal margin of all restorative materials is undetectable by passage of the explorer from tooth to restoration or from restoration to tooth. The tine of the explorer serves as an aid not in identification of the material but in determination of the condition of the restoration at the cavosurface margin. The **cavosurface margin** is the junction of the restoration with the external tooth surface.

e. *Location*
The location of the restoration can make the identification of tooth-colored restorations difficult. Depending on the material used, the age and marginal integrity of the restoration, the junction of the enamel, and the restorative

material are often visually indiscernible. For this reason, the clinician should make the most of radiographs and proper transillumination with the mouth mirror to identify the exact location of the restoration before using any instrument.

B. Management of Restorative Dental Materials during Scaling and Polishing

After the dental hygienist has identified the patient's various restorative materials, the selection of cleaning agents, instruments, and specific techniques is made. Polishing agents, instruments, and procedures are designed to aid the clinician in producing highly polished surfaces on the teeth, restorations, and appliances.

Smooth surfaces on tooth structure and restorative materials are less receptive to bacterial colonization and dental plaque formation. Coronal polishing, which may take place after scaling and root planing, must be accomplished in a way that is not damaging to the tooth and restorative materials. Fairly common examples of detrimental procedures include production of excessive heat during polishing, excessive use of abrasives, damage to the margins of cast restorations, and the use of high-speed instrumentation.

1. Production of Excessive Heat during Polishing

Heat is generated when an abrasive rubber cup and handpiece is used against a natural tooth surface. Rotating a bristle brush, rubber cup, or rubber wheel on a thumbnail readily demonstrates how quickly excessive heat can be generated by speed or pressure. Adding mouthwash, water, or glycerin to make a slurry when abrasives such as silex or tin oxide are being used will reduce the amount of heat that is produced.

Prophylaxis pastes supplied in unit doses are moist so that less heat is produced. It only takes once or twice for a patient to jump during polishing for the clinician to learn that excessive heat has been generated. The cause could be the cup is left on the tooth too long, too much pressure is applied, or too much speed is used by the clinician.

Temperatures of 140°F or greater will alter the surface characteristics of an amalgam restoration because of a release of mercury. This will result in accelerated corrosion and marginal breakdown.

2. Excessive Use of Abrasives

Excessive use of abrasives can be injurious to patients in several respects. Improper use of an abrasive agent and a rubber cup at the gingival margin can cause trauma to or removal of the surface epithelium in that area.

As is discussed in Chapter 16, Polishing Materials and Abrasion, abrasive agents can be harmful because of the following factors:

- Particle size of the polishing agent
- Number of particles applied per unit of time
- Speed of the application
- Amount of pressure applied

It is for these reasons that selective polishing has become an accepted alternative treatment to polishing with abrasives.

A study of the surface roughness of restorative materials after polishing with polishing pastes showed that many restorative materials were rougher after polishing. Gold, amalgam, and microfilled composites were used in this study. It must be remembered that for cast gold restorations, such as inlays, onlays, or crowns, the final polish applied in the dental lab provides the smoothest surface these restorations will have during patient service. Many polishing agents can create fine scratches in several restorative materials because of speed, pressure, and particle size. The hygienist should make a dedicated effort to use a polishing agent containing the smallest abrasive particle that will remove surface stain and attached plaque.

3. Damage to Margins of a Cast Restoration

A third way in which damage could be incurred on a restored surface during scaling is by opening a margin of a cemented casting. This particular type of restoration is likely to have a detectable margin. More so than gold foil or amalgam restorations, cemented castings (inlays, onlays, and crowns) will have a "cement line" margin. A properly mixed cement should have a film thickness of less than 40 microns. The margins of cast restorations are delicate, and they have been adapted to the preparation by the dentist. **Margination** is the process of using hand instruments from cast metal to tooth, to adapt the margins of the gold casting to the tooth preparation. Because the longevity of the cast restoration depends, in part, on the condition of the margin, it is critical that the margin be identified. When scaling in the area of a cast restoration, the dental hygienist should alter his or her scaling technique so as not to jeopardize the margin of any cemented casting.

Figure 14.1A illustrates the casting in place and a thin, fragile gold edge over the **beveled margin** (the sloping or angled edge of the preparation) of the tooth. A potential position of a curette scaler is shown in *Figure 14.1B*, and *Figure 14.1C* depicts the results of an applied working stroke. The scaler has engaged the gold edge and lifted the gold up and away from the tooth. The margin of the restoration is now "open." Note that destruction of the marginal integrity can lead to recurrent decay, which can be seen in *Figure 14.1D*.

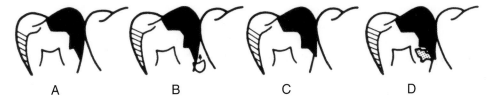

FIGURE 14.1. The cemented casting. **A.** Casting cemented into place. **B.** Curette blade improperly positioned. **C.** Results of an applied working stroke. The margin is now open (lifted). **D.** Recurrent decay resulting from an opened margin. (Reproduced from Krouse MA, Gladwin SC. Identification and management of restorative dental materials during patient prophylaxis. *Dent Hyg.* 1984;58:456–461, with permission.)

To prevent this damage, the use of an explorer and/or a scaling instrument is necessary to first locate the margin of the casting. Once the margin is identified, the working stroke must be kept within an area below the margin. On the facial or lingual surface, a more oblique or horizontal stroke (rather than a vertical stroke) should be used, always keeping in mind the location of the margin of the casting. If a student is in doubt of whether he/she is feeling a cast margin or subgingival deposit when exploring, it is recommended to get the assistance of a clinical instructor to help with this determination.

4. Power Instrumentation

Use of high-speed instrumentation, such as sonic or ultrasonic scalers or air polishers, may cause damage to or removal of several types of restorative materials.

a. *Ultrasonic Scalers*

The vibrating tips of ultrasonic scalers may harm composite resin restorations, laminate veneers, crowns, and titanium implant abutments. Amalgam margins may be altered, and restorations fabricated from ceramic materials may be fractured. *Figure 14.2* illustrates damage to a gold crown.

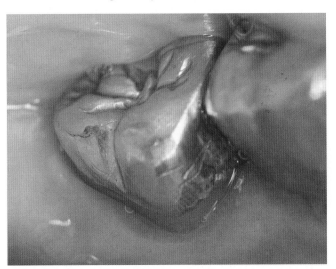

FIGURE 14.2. Note the scratches on the mesial of #18 from the inappropriate use of an ultrasonic scaler.

b. *Air Polishers*

Dental restorative materials, such as cements, composite resins, and other nonmetallic materials, may be removed or pitted by use of the air abrasive technique. Margins of cast restorations may be significantly damaged with the use of this instrument.

5. Application of Fluoride

Some restorative materials may be altered or damaged by the application of topical fluorides.

a. *Stannous Fluoride*

Tooth-colored restorations and the enamel margins adjacent to the restoration may discolor with the application of stannous fluoride.

b. *Acidulated Phosphate Fluoride*

The dental hygienist must be aware of the possible deleterious effects of applying acidulated phosphate fluoride to porcelain, composite, and glass ionomer restorations. A 4-minute application may create a loss of reflection or dull the appearance of these restorations. The fluoride will microscopically "etch" the outer surface of these materials.

It is recommended that the hygienist place petroleum jelly over the restoration before application of the acidulated phosphate fluoride. Another option is to apply a 2.0% sodium fluoride (NaF) gel or foam instead of acidulated phosphate fluoride.

II. Suggestions for Polishing Specific Restorative Materials

There are many acceptable methods to finish and polish typical restorative materials. This section will include standard protocols for amalgam, composite, gold, and ceramic materials.

A. Amalgam

For new or recently placed amalgams, the finishing and polishing consists of using finishing burs with a low-speed handpiece, followed by the use of silex and then whiting mixed in a slurry consistency. Rubber cups or prophy brushes may be used and should be changed when changing to the next abrasive agent.

Another polishing regimen consists of using finishing burs and then brown and green rubber polishing points. These points are impregnated with polishing agents and eliminate the use of liquids and powders. However, it is important to keep the point wet (with saliva). Excessive heat created when these polishing points are being used will cause discomfort for the patient and may injure the pulp. In addition, excessive heat may accelerate marginal breakdown and corrosion of the amalgam restoration. Both methods of finishing and polishing amalgams are described in detail in Chapter 26, Amalgam Placement, Carving, Finishing, and Polishing.

For older amalgams, finishing burs are usually used for a longer period of time to produce a smooth surface. Brown and green polishing points are then used.

B. Composites

As mentioned previously, there are many methods to finish and polish composite restorations. Interproximal areas may be finished by contouring the surface with a scalpel blade. It can be used to remove overhangs of composite and shape the line angles. Next, finishing strips may be used from most abrasive to least abrasive grit.

A sequence of aluminum oxide–coated discs may be used for the facial surfaces. For lingual surfaces, an egg-shaped finishing bur is used for finishing. Abrasive points and cups are then used to polish. Finally all surfaces may be polished with a composite polishing paste. A technique for finishing and polishing composites is described in detail in Chapter 36, Composite Finishing and Polishing.

In recent years, one-step diamond micropolishers have become available in cup and point shapes (PoGo by Dentsply/Caulk) and are recommended for composite, glass ionomer, and compomer restorations.

C. Cast Gold and Gold Foil

To polish gold restorations, either regimen mentioned for amalgam restorations may be used: the brown and green polishing points or a sequence of polishing powders, such as silex, and whiting or tin oxide. Tin oxide produces an excellent result when used as a final polishing agent for gold.

D. Ceramic Materials

For ceramic veneers and crowns, a variety of prophylaxis pastes may be used to clean and polish. Remember that ceramic materials are fired at very high temperatures, which result in a very hard material. For this reason, most prophylaxis pastes may be employed to polish the surfaces of ceramic veneers and crowns. As presented in Chapter 10, Materials for Fixed Indirect Restorations and Prostheses, all ceramic materials are not porcelain; differentiating nonporcelain ceramic materials from porcelain is clinically very difficult. Remember it is not unusual to veneer nonporcelain ceramic materials with porcelain to develop acceptable esthetics. As a result of this, all ceramic crowns, veneers, etc. should be treated as if they are porcelain to prevent damage to the restoration.

Summary

It is the professional responsibility of the dental hygienist to determine the composition of the surface being scaled and/or polished. Several criteria aid in the identification of tooth structure or restorative materials. Once identified, restorations should be managed as follows:

- *Temperatures of 140°F or greater should not be created when polishing amalgam restorations. Such temperatures accelerate corrosion and marginal breakdown.*
- *Abrasive agents are not to be used in excess. Remember that the particle size of the abrasive, the amount of abrasive applied, and the speed and pressure of the rubber cup or brush all play a role in potential trauma to the tissue or creation of a rough surface on tooth structure or restoration.*
- *Well-adapted margins of the castings should not be opened from the blades of curettes and scalers. An oblique or horizontal stroke (rather than traditional vertical stroke) should be employed.*
- *Ultraspeed cleaning devices should be used with caution and only after identifying existing restorative materials.*
- *Acidulated phosphate fluoride is not used on ceramic materials, composite, or glass ionomer restorations. This fluoride may etch the outer surface of these materials and create a dull appearance.*
- *The least abrasive polishing paste is selected to remove stains and plaque.*

There are many ways to finish and polish restorations. The last section of this chapter provides suggestions for finishing and polishing specific restorative materials, such as amalgam, composite, cast gold, gold foils, and ceramic materials.

Learning Activities

1. In a clinical setting, make an attempt to identify restorative materials in the mouths of classmates.

2. List any precautions for managing the materials found in learning activity #1 when scaling or polishing.

3. An elderly female patient presents with the following dental and periodontal findings:
   - Older, tarnished amalgams on #30 and #31
   - 3- to 4-mm facial recession on #3, #4, and #5

- Two class V glass ionomer restorations on #12 and #13
- Two gold inlays on #18 and #19
- Coffee stain on the linguals of #22 to #27

4. Ideally, what would your scaling and polishing protocol be for each of the situations listed above? What would you include in your home care instructions to the patient?

Review Questions

Question 1. Which of the following restorative materials may be affected by numerous applications of acidulated phosphate fluoride?

a. Cast gold

b. Zinc oxide–eugenol (ZOE) temporary restorations

c. Glass ionomers

d. Amalgam

Question 2. Margins of cast restorations can be altered by instrumentation with curettes and explorers. A suggested technique for deposit removal in these areas is to employ:

a. A vertical stroke, as used on natural tooth structure

b. A vertical stroke, but with anterior instruments only

c. An oblique or horizontal stroke, with appropriate instruments

d. Any stroke, but with ultrasonic scalers

Question 3. A dull sound when an instrument is being used on these surfaces should be evident with which of the following materials?

a. Gold foil and base metal alloys

b. Enamel and dentin

c. Amalgam and cast gold

d. Composite and glass ionomer

Question 4. Tactile sensitivity and a sharp explorer will aid the clinician in identifying:

a. Opacities from translucencies

b. Glossy surfaces from dull surfaces

c. Dull sounds from sharp sounds

d. Rough surfaces from smooth surfaces

Question 5. Creating temperatures of 140°F or greater when amalgam restorations are being finished and polished will:

a. Arrest corrosion and marginal breakdown

b. Accelerate corrosion and marginal breakdown

c. Create a roughened surface

d. Change a sharp sound to a dull sound when using an explorer

Question 6. What are the agents of choice for polishing a gold crown intraorally?

a. Silex and tin oxide

b. Brown and green polishing points

c. A correct sequence of prophylaxis pastes

d. A sequence of aluminum oxide–coated discs

Question 7. One benefit of a moist polishing agent is:

a. Heat reduction

b. Aid in swallowing

c. Faster stain removal

d. Ease in rinsing

Question 8. When a cast gold crown has been marginated, it means that the:

a. Casting fits precisely in the preparation

b. Margins have been closely adapted to the crown preparation

c. Casting fits within the gingival margin

d. Casting is in relation to the adjacent marginal ridge

Question 9. When clinically polishing gold and gold foil, the regimen is similar to that of:

a. Composite
b. Amalgam
c. Glass ionomer
d. Porcelain fused to metal crown

Question 10. Acidulated phosphate fluoride is not recommended for the following materials:

a. Composite and porcelain only
b. Composite and glass ionomer only
c. Gold, composite, and porcelain
d. Glass ionomer, composites, and porcelain

Radiographic Appearance of Dental Tissues and Materials

15

Objectives

After studying this chapter, the student will be able to do the following:

1. Identify various dental tissues and restorative materials on a radiograph.
2. Explain, radiographically, why dental tissues and materials appear radiopaque or radiolucent.
3. Integrate the radiographic appearance of dental tissues and materials with clinical information to assess the patient's status of health or disease.

Key Words/Phrases

attenuation
electromagnetic radiation
radiographic contrast
radiolucent
radiopaque
retrofill

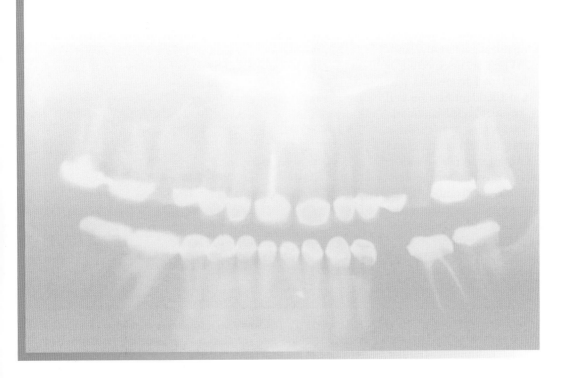

Introduction

Oral radiographs are useful supplements for use in assessing the patient's present oral and dental status. Although many adjunct assessment tools can assist in determining the diagnosis and prognosis of a specific dental disease or condition, the dental radiograph remains an important component of total patient care. The radiograph provides the diagnostician/practitioner with critical information that cannot be collected by any other method. Dental radiographs are also used to compare and identify patients after death, especially victims of disasters. The unique characteristics of a person's dentition reveal reliable and accurate information.

I. Essentials for Radiographic Interpretation

It is essential that the dental hygienist be competent in radiographic techniques, patient safety regarding radiation, and proper handling and processing of radiographs. It is also imperative that the dental hygienist has a basic knowledge in both general and dental anatomy, periodontics, pathology, and dental materials so that he or she can interpret the radiographs.

II. Rationale for Integrating Dental Radiology in a Dental Materials Text

To distinguish dental tissues from dental materials, health from disease, and normal aspects from abnormal aspects, it is essential that dental hygienists competently recognize what is "within normal limits" both clinically and radiographically. When viewing radiographs, the "mind's eye" scans each radiograph looking for normal anatomy, landmarks, and typical restorations. When an unexpected or uncommon area is identified, the dental hygienist's past knowledge and experience assist in the identification and naming of the material, object, or anatomical landmark. The ability to analyze critically what is seen or not seen in regard to oral anatomical structures, dental materials, and objects is essential for an accurate interpretation and/or diagnosis. While it is not legally permissible for the dental hygienist to prescribe radiographs or diagnose dental disease, this information is used not only to educate the patient but also to provide the dentist with accurate data for diagnosis, treatment planning, and treatment.

III. Producing the Radiographic Image

X-rays are a form of electromagnetic radiation. **Electromagnetic radiation** occurs as waves of photons that vary in wavelength, frequency, and energy. Because electromagnetic radiation may have biologic cellular effects, it is important that the dental hygienist understand the correct use and consequences of radiation.

The primary beam of radiation encounters and passes through hard and soft tissue before it reaches the X-ray sensor. Hard tissues include tooth tissues (enamel, dentin, and cementum) and bone. Soft tissues such as epithelium, muscles, nerves, glands, pulp, and blood vessels also occur in the oral cavity. Tissues and dental materials absorb the X-ray beam according to their thickness and density. As a result, the radiograph consists of "darks," "lights," and varying shades of gray (**radiographic contrast**).

This process of reducing the energy of the primary beam as it passes through the differing objects/materials is called **attenuation**. Attenuation results in the respective levels of blacks, whites, and grays on the processed radiograph that assist in distinguishing normal radiographic findings. The thickness and composition (object density) of the tissues and materials contribute to determining the overall appearance of the radiograph. These subtle variations of light (radiopacities) and dark (radiolucencies) can aid in the diagnosis and interpretation of patient information.

IV. Restorative Materials Categorized by Radiographic Appearance

A. Radiopaque Restorative Materials

Restorative materials that are clearly radiopaque include amalgam, cast gold, cohesive gold, nonprecious alloys, and the metal portion of a porcelain-fused-to-metal crown. Two large amalgam restorations including metallic retentive pins are shown in *Figure 15.1*. Retentive pins are used in several ways and with various materials to increase retention where natural tooth structure is not available. The metal of the ceramometal restorations, as seen in *Figure 15.2*, is depicted by the white areas. The darker shadows on the incisal

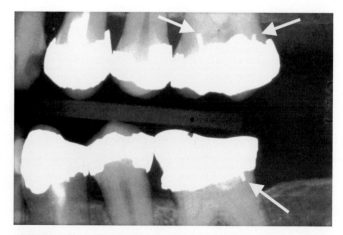

FIGURE 15.1. The amalgam restorations on teeth #14 and #19 include retentive pins (*arrows*) that enhance the resistance and retention of the restorative material.

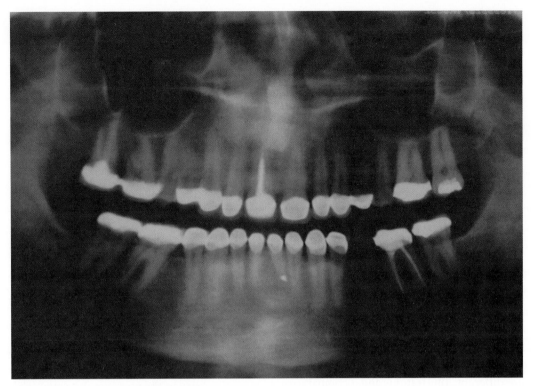

FIGURE 15.2. Numerous porcelain-fused-to-metal crowns are visible on the maxillary and mandibular arches on this panoramic radiograph. The radiolucent shadow at the incisal (#6–#11) and occlusal (#2, #3, #14) surfaces is the radiolucent porcelain.

surface of these teeth depict the porcelain portion of the crowns. Stainless steel and aluminum temporary crowns may be radiopaque depending on the thickness of the material.

B. Radiolucent/Radiopaque Restorative Materials

Other restorative materials may also appear as varying degrees of gray (dark and light or radiographic contrast). These materials include composite resins, sealants, cements, bases, and porcelain. Depending on the material, some of these products may appear more radiolucent than opaque, and vice versa. Look at the anterior porcelain and metal restorations shown in *Figure 15.2*. Depending on the type and amount of the material, varying degrees of radiolucencies and radiopacities are present. Refer to Table 15.1 to recognize the comparative radiographic characteristics of dental materials. Because of varying compositions, cements used for luting and bases may appear darker (radiolucent) or lighter (radiopaque) than the overlying restorations. Radiolucent bases under a metal restoration, particularly amalgam, and excessive adhesive materials under composites may imitate a carious lesion on the radiograph. For example, see Figure 1.9D, which shows a base under an existing amalgam restoration (tooth #3).

A dental sealant may be visualized on a radiograph depending on the type and amount of filler in its composition. A posterior composite restoration may also be visualized on a radiograph depending on the type of restorative material and the amount of filler in its composition. In both cases, the radiographic appearance would be radiopaque. *Figure 15.3* demonstrates a composite restoration on the occlusal of tooth #28. Although the restoration is opaque, it is less opaque than a metal restoration would appear.

C. Radiolucent Restorative Materials

Some restorative materials may appear more radiolucent because of the lack of fillers or density. These materials include temporary crowns and/or bridges made of acrylic or plastic tooth-colored materials, such as resins and porcelain. Again, refer to Table 15.1 for the radiographic characteristics of the various dental materials. *Figure 15.4* demonstrates an older composite resin that is radiolucent. The mesial of tooth #6 shown in *Figure 15.4* is not a carious lesion; it is a resin that does not contain radiopaque fillers and therefore appears lucent. The distal of tooth #7 in *Figure 15.4* has a radiopaque composite restoration compared to a more radiolucent composite in the mesial of tooth #6.

TABLE 15.1. Radiographic Appearance of Dental Materials[a]

Tissues and Materials		Enamel	Dentin	Cementum	Pulp	Amalgam	Cast Gold	Implants	Composite	Glass Ionomer	Cements	Bands	Gutta-Percha	Sealants	Porcelain	Other Ceramics
Radiographic Appearance	Radiopaque	X	X			X	X	X	X	X	X	X	X	X	X	X
	Radiolucent		X		X				X		X			X	X	X

[a]Certain categories have some products that are radiolucent and other products that are radiopaque.
Modified from Krouse M, Gladwin SG. Identification and management of restorative dental materials during patient prophylaxis. Dent Hyg. 1984;58:456, with permission.

V. Radiographic Descriptions of Dental Tissues, Disease, and Materials

A. Radiographic Description of Tissues and Disease

Radiographically, a variety of dental materials are similar to the natural tooth structure, and others are quite different. Illustrations and a comparative table in this chapter assist you in distinguishing the radiographic "looks" that are associated with tooth tissue and dental materials.

1. Soft Tissues

Soft tissues are not dense (compact and hard) and do not greatly attenuate the X-ray beam (the beam passes through nearly undiminished). Soft tissues appear black or dark on the processed radiograph and are called **radiolucent**.

Therefore, soft tissue is not generally visible on a radiograph.

Figure 15.5 illustrates soft tissue radiolucency. The interdental papilla and pulp canal are both radiolucent. The less dense the tissue or material, the less radiation it absorbs. Therefore, when the primary beam of radiation strikes the receptor, it is translated into a dark or radiolucent area on the radiograph.

Some dental materials are radiolucent and are not visible on the radiograph. Such materials transmit the primary beam of radiation so that they are not clearly distinguishable on

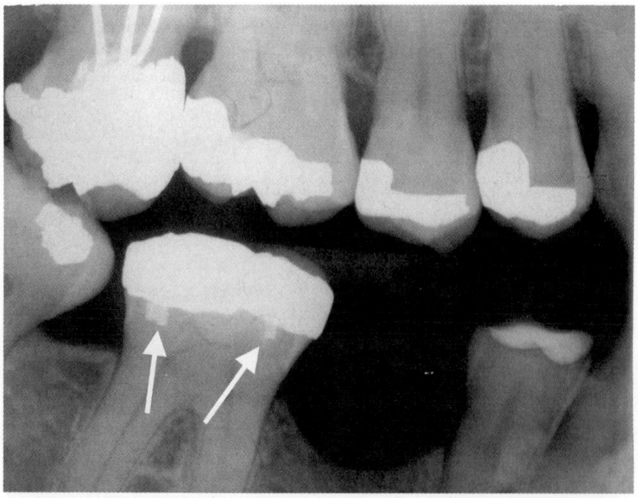

FIGURE 15.3. Note the composite resin restoration on the occlusal surface of tooth #28. Although it is radiopaque, its radiographic appearance is not as opaque as a metal restoration. Also note the retentive pins in tooth #31 (*arrows*) and the root canal therapy in tooth #2.

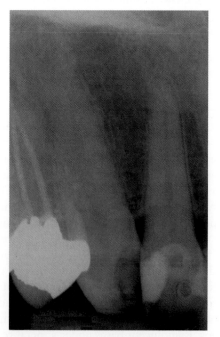

FIGURE 15.4. A radiolucent area is present on the mesial surface of tooth #6. This is not dental decay; it is a composite that appears radiolucent. The distinct outline differentiates it from caries, which would have a more diffuse outline. Root canal therapy is evident in tooth #5. The root canal filling material is gutta-percha.

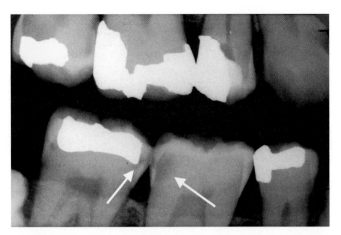

FIGURE 15.5. The radiolucent interdental papillary areas are located between adjacent teeth on this bitewing radiograph. Note the pulp chambers in the crown and root areas. Soft tissue is not visible radiographically and appears radiolucent. Caries are present in the distal of tooth #30 and the mesial of tooth #31 (*arrows*).

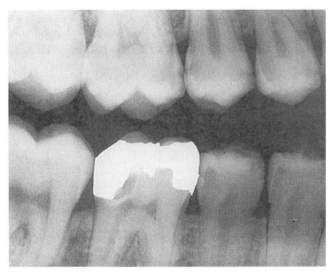

FIGURE 15.6. Radiographically, carious lesions appear radiolucent. The proximal carious lesions on this radiograph are noticeable (mesial of tooth #3, mesial and distal of tooth #4, mesial and distal of tooth #5, distal of tooth #29, and possibly under the large amalgam restoration on tooth #30). The enamel outline is radiopaque because of its density, and the dentin is comparably less opaque than the enamel (more *gray*). (Courtesy of Dr. Thomas F. Razmus, Department of Diagnostic Sciences, West Virginia University School of Dentistry.)

the radiograph. Examples are acrylic resin, porcelain, and most impression materials.

Figure 15.2 illustrates maxillary and mandibular porcelain-fused-to-metal crowns. On this radiograph, the porcelain is a shadow at the incisal and occlusal surfaces of the teeth. Also, note the numerous areas of radiopacities, which denote the metal of the crowns.

2. Hard Tissues

The enamel of the tooth is a very compact tissue. In fact, it is the densest tissue of the body, and it significantly attenuates the X-ray beam. In comparison, bone is slightly less dense than enamel and similarly absorbs the X-ray beam. On the other hand, dentin and cementum are considerably less dense than enamel or bone, and the X-ray beam can penetrate these tissues much more readily. The more dense the tissue or material, the more radiation is absorbed and fewer photons reach the X-ray sensor. This translates into light or **radiopaque** areas on the radiograph. As a result, the radiographic appearance of tooth enamel is light. The dentin is less dense and less radiopaque than the enamel. The dental pulp appears dark or radiolucent.

Figure 15.6 illustrates varying hard tissue radiopacities. *Figure 15.2* also depicts numerous areas of radiopacities denoting the metal of porcelain-fused-to-metal crowns.

The alveolar bone is a combination of trabecular bone and compact bone. The trabecular bone consists of shades of gray and a combination of opacities and lucencies. Compact bone is typically more radiopaque than is trabecular

bone. Some dental materials (metals) are very opaque; others have opacities similar to dentin and enamel. Differentiating a radiopaque dental material from enamel or dentin is accomplished by comparing the shape of the radiopacity with the expected anatomical features of a tooth. *Figure 15.7* illustrates the differences between tooth tissues and dental materials. The expected shape of class II restorations is evident. The same can be said for radiolucencies, but the possibility of caries complicates the identification. Observations from the clinical examination

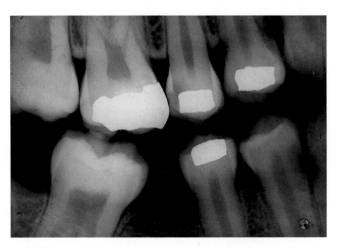

FIGURE 15.7. The carious lesion on the distal of tooth #4 is radiolucent. The amalgam restorations are radiopaque.

must also be considered when differentiating radiopacities and radiolucencies from normal anatomy. Note the trabecular pattern of alveolar bone of the radiograph in *Figure 15.6* and the radiopaque crestal bone in proximal areas.

3. Caries

Destruction of the calcified tissues of the tooth (enamel, dentin, cementum) results in dental caries. Radiographically, the carious area is radiolucent when compared to enamel or dentin. It is important that the diagnostician view the radiographs in an appropriate viewing situation and with a critical eye to differentiate between normal tooth anatomy, restorations, and carious lesions. *Figure 15.6* illustrates proximal carious lesions (radiolucencies) on the bitewing radiograph. For example, carious lesions can be seen on the mesial of tooth #3, the mesial and distal of tooth #4, and the mesial and distal of tooth #5. In addition, a radiolucency appears on the distal of tooth #28, the mesial and distal of tooth #29, under the MOD amalgam restoration of tooth #30, and on the mesial of tooth #31. *Figure 15.7* illustrates a distal radiolucency on tooth #4.

B. Radiographic Description of Dental Materials

1. Dental Amalgam Restorations

As previously described in Chapter 6, Amalgam, dental amalgam is a commonly used direct restorative material. Because of its color, it is used primarily in the posterior teeth and in the pits of lingual surfaces of the anterior teeth. Dental amalgam is an alloy of several dense metals, so it absorbs the primary beam of radiation. The corresponding area of the processed radiograph is radiopaque. *Figures 15.1 to 15.3 and 15.5 to 15.8* demonstrate amalgam restorations.

2. Resin Composite Restorations

Resin composite materials are commonly used as direct restorations. As with other dental materials, both advantages and disadvantages are found when resin composite restorations are used in posterior teeth. For more discussion on this topic, see Chapter 5, Direct Polymeric Restorative Materials. Many older resin restorative materials appear radiolucent on radiographs. *Figure 15.4* demonstrates a radiolucent resin in anterior teeth. Technology in biomaterials has advanced whereby fillers included in composite resins are now radiopaque to the degree that much less confusion occurs regarding the existence of recurrent caries.

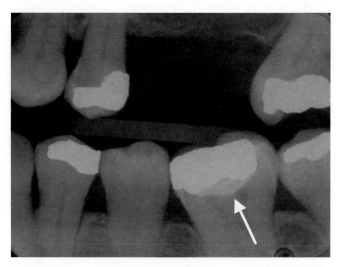

FIGURE 15.8. Amalgam restorations are present on teeth #13, #15, #18, #19, and #21. A base (*arrow*) is under the amalgam on tooth #19. A mesial radiolucency (carious lesion) is present on tooth #13. The radiopaque crestal bone is clearly depicted on this bitewing radiograph.

3. Crown and Bridge (Prosthodontic) Materials

Some materials for crown and bridge are radiopaque, whereas others are radiolucent. Metals are radiopaque, as shown in Figures 1.3B and 1.5. Porcelain can be either radiolucent or radiopaque. Porcelain fused to metal restorations have both areas (see *Fig. 15.2*). Temporary crowns can be either, depending on the material used. Acrylic resins are radiolucent. Bis-acryl temporary materials can be either radiolucent or radiopaque.

4. Dental Bases

During removal of dental decay and preparation of the tooth for a restoration, the pulp may be traumatized or irritated by the procedure. To reduce pulpal irritation, a dental material called a "base" may be placed in the floor of the cavity preparation to insulate the pulp from thermal stimuli. For the base to be effective as a thermal insulator, it must have sufficient thickness and low thermal conductivity. Thus, the base may be more radiolucent than the overlying amalgam or composite restoration and may imitate a carious lesion. For example, tooth #3 in Figure 1.9A, tooth #30 in *Figure 15.3*, and tooth #19 in *Figure 15.8* show a base under an existing amalgam restoration. Refer to Table 15.1 for the radiographic characteristics of the various dental materials.

5. Dental Temporary (Provisional Restorations) Fillings

Some dental procedures cannot be completed in one appointment due to various reasons, that is, diseased pulp. Between appointments, the

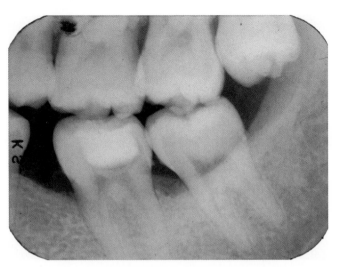

FIGURE 15.9. A temporary restoration exists in the occlusal of tooth #19. It is considered radiopaque, yet more radiolucent than metal. Note the irregular borders. Possible decay (radiolucency) remains between the tooth and restoration. Note the bone loss between #18 and #19.

tooth preparation must be temporarily sealed to prevent further irritation. Zinc oxide–eugenol (ZOE) cement, composite, or glass ionomer materials are commonly used. Tooth #19 in *Figure 15.9* demonstrates a temporary restoration in the occlusal surface.

6. Endodontic, Orthodontic, Periodontal, and Surgical Materials

Materials used in, on, and around teeth to treat, repair, or restore them are often metallic. Because most metals are dense, they appear on radiographs as radiopaque. *Figures 15.10 to 15.15* demonstrate the various metals used in dental specialties.

a. *Endodontic Materials*

Endodontic therapy is often a portion of the restorative treatment plan. Radiopaque endodontic instruments used during therapy include files, rubber dam clamps, and frame. The radiograph in *Figure 15.10* illustrates endodontic files used to clean and shape the pulp canals of the teeth during root canal therapy. Endodontic filling materials include gutta-percha, a thermoplastic polymer, or silver points along with an endodontic sealer. Tooth #7 in *Figure 15.11* contains a gutta-percha root canal filling. Gutta-percha is an inert polymer to which barium sulfate is also added for opacity. Tooth #28 in *Figure 15.12* shows a silver point. Sealers commonly used are zinc oxide–eugenol materials with barium sulfate added. Other sealers are based on other dental cements. In certain cases, a retrofill of amalgam or MTA (mineral trioxide aggregate) may

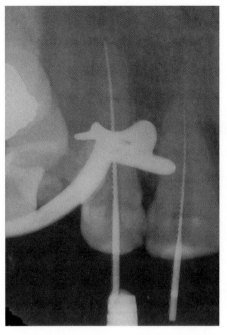

FIGURE 15.10. Teeth #7 and #8. Files are present in the pulp canals to locate the apices during the root canal therapy. Also note the radiopaque rubber dam clamp. (Courtesy of Dr. A.L.C. Kayafas, Akron, OH.)

also be used. A **retrofill** is a surgically placed restoration at the root apex. *Figure 15.11* illustrates root canal therapy with an amalgam retrofill. In some instances, a retentive post or dowel pin may be used to strengthen or enhance retention of the tooth's foundation, (see tooth #8 in *Fig. 15.2*) especially when used for a fixed or removable prosthesis.

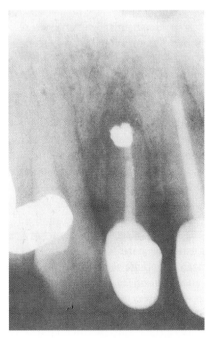

FIGURE 15.11. Tooth #7 exhibits a retrofill amalgam restoration.

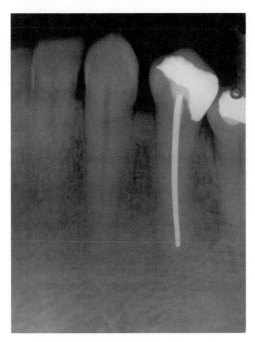

FIGURE 15.12. Tooth #28 has been endodontically treated. A silver point fills the root canal space.

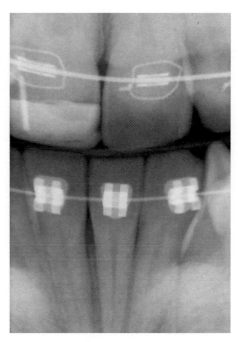

FIGURE 15.13. Anterior vertical bitewing radiograph with brackets, wires, and stainless steel ligatures. Also note the threaded pin and composite restoring the fractured incisal edge. Bilateral mandibular tori are present and appear radiopaque.

The endodontic files, silver points, retrofill amalgams, rubber dam clamps and frame, metal post materials, and some film/sensor holding devices are metal. These materials appear radiopaque on a radiograph. Although gutta-percha is not metal, it contains barium sulfate, which appears radiopaque or as a varying shade of opacity on a radiograph, as illustrated in *Figure 15.4* for tooth #5.

b. *Orthodontic Materials*
Metal orthodontic materials used in dentistry are primarily stainless steel orthodontic bands, brackets, and wires. Bands interfere with radiographic detection of dental caries. Brackets directly bonded to the tooth are now commonly used and may not interfere. Other frequently used radiopaque orthodontic materials include springs, fixed and removable retainers, space maintainers, appliances that discourage oral habits, and bite planes. Cements and bonding materials may be radiopaque or radiolucent. Refer to Table 15.1 for a comparison of dental materials. Figures 13.2, 15.13, and 15.14 illustrate a buccal tube, bands, brackets, and stainless steel ligatures.

c. *Oral and Maxillofacial Surgical Materials/ Objects of Trauma*
The majority of oral and maxillofacial surgical materials are radiopaque. Radiopaque materials can be located on radiographs, whereas radiolucent materials cannot.

Surgical items include implants or the implant fixtures, healing caps, and other tissue replacement materials. Radiographs assist in the continuing assessment of implant healing and stability (see Chapter 12, Dental Implants, for radiographs of dental implants). Other surgical items that may be used are wires, plates, or screws for stabilization of bone segments after trauma as shown in *Figure 15.15.*

d. *Periodontics*
The dentist and the dental hygienist view radiographs for changes in the periodontium. Radiographs are an adjunct to the clinical examination as they often illustrate

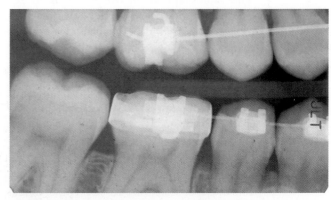

FIGURE 15.14. Posterior bitewing radiograph with orthodontic brackets, bands, wire, and buccal tube.

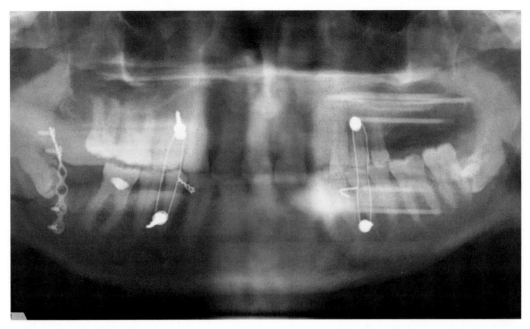

FIGURE 15.15. Panoramic radiograph of bone plate, screws, and wires for stabilization of bone segments after trauma.

periodontal destruction that has occurred in the past. However, they do not demonstrate whether the areas of destruction are currently undergoing periodontal disease activity. Bone loss from periodontal disease is evident on the mesial of tooth #19 in *Figure 15.1*, the distal of #3 in *Figure 15.3*, the mesial of tooth #30 in *Figure 15.5*, and interproximal of #18 and #19 in *Figure 15.9*.

To provide corrective therapy for periodontal disease, periodontists use resorbable and nonresorbable materials to assist in repairing and/or regenerating the periodontium. Periodontists determine which materials to use based on their knowledge, experience, philosophy, location of the therapy, type of defect, and specific therapy to be performed. Nonresorbable materials (e.g., ridge augmentation materials) are visible on a radiograph as shown in *Figure 15.16*. Resorbable materials generally are not visible on a radiograph, yet the healing response to these materials may be visible.

Overhanging restorations, poorly contoured margins, and open contact areas are plaque retentive and contribute to gingivitis and periodontitis. Overhanging restorations in the posterior region of the mouth are usually composed of composite resin or amalgam. The overhanging restoration on tooth #19 in *Figure 15.1* appears as a radiopacity and has contributed to alveolar bone loss.

VI. Dental Materials and Other Imaging Techniques

Several other imaging techniques are used in medicine and dentistry. The CAT (computer-aided tomography) scan that is common in medicine has been developed for dentistry. CBCT, or cone beam computed tomography, similarly creates a three-dimensional image of a portion of the head

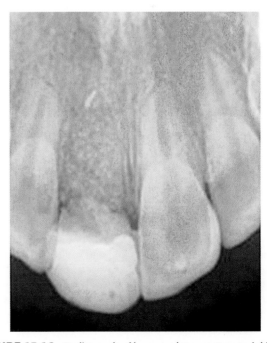

FIGURE 15.16. Radiograph of bone replacement material in the socket of #8 used for ridge augmentation of a future implant site. The crown of #8 is temporarily bonded to #7 and #9. (Courtesy of Dr. Eros Chaves, Morgantown, WV.)

and neck. CBCT is being used for orthodontic treatment planning, implant placement, endodontic retreatment, and other invasive oral maxillofacial surgeries. Biologic and dental materials interact with these X-ray photons in the same manner as previously described for dental radiographs.

Magnetic resonance imaging, MRI, is very useful for imaging soft tissues of the body. Although not commonly used in dentistry, some knowledge of the interaction of the very high magnetic field utilized by the MRI device is valuable. The very high magnetic field creates a hazard if a magnetic metal object is in the room. Luckily, few dental materials are magnetic. The exceptions are magnets used to move teeth in orthodontics or retain a denture. Some orthodontic stainless steel brackets, wires, and so on are slightly magnetic. Occasionally, the patient will have the orthodontic appliance removed prior to an MRI procedure for safety purposes. Currently, ultrasound is not used for dental imaging. Researchers are developing ultrasound techniques to image the bony defects of periodontal patients. Such equipment would be very beneficial to image bone loss at each recall appointment without the risk of ionizing radiation.

Summary

A patient's dental radiographs are critical components in the decision-making process of a dental hygiene diagnosis or a definitive dental diagnosis. The dental hygienist/practitioner must be competent in accurately identifying and interpreting dental materials used in dental treatment.

Products used in dental treatment/procedures appear as varying degrees of radiolucent or radiopaque images on dental radiographs. This variation depends on the density or compactness of the materials that attenuate or absorb the primary beam of radiation. For example, an amalgam restoration is dense and appears on the radiograph as radiopaque. Resin or porcelain is less dense than amalgam and appears on the radiograph as a gradient of radiolucent.

The dental hygienist must not only be able to consistently produce high-quality radiographs but also recognize and bring to the dentist's attention various and sometimes subtle gradations of opacities and lucencies that correspond with the clinical examination. With knowledge, a "keen eye," skills, and experience, the dental hygienist serves as an important partner in the oral health team and as the primary patient educator at chairside.

 ## Learning Activities

1. Participate in pairs or groups of three students to explore a full-mouth series of radiographs that include a variety of dental materials. Locate radiolucencies and opacities that correspond with tooth anatomy (i.e., enamel, dentin, pulp) and periodontal structures. Identify and discuss various other types of dental materials in the radiographs. Speculate as to the composition of any restorative material or other dental material that is present.

2. Perform a clinical oral examination on one of your classmates in clinic. Chart the findings: amalgams, composites, gold restorations, prostheses, and so on. After the charting, view the radiographs of your partner to correlate the radiographic appearance of oral findings with the clinical examination findings. Discuss your findings with an instructor.

3. Work in pairs to develop a case-based scenario using various periapical and/or bitewing radiographs with dental materials. Use these cases for discussion in lab sessions or class as a learning activity. Develop a mock clinical exam.

4. Using full-mouth radiographic series and sets of intraoral photographs from several patients with various types of restorative dental treatment, match the intraoral photographs with the radiographs.

5. Match the same radiographs to the dental charts included in the patient's record.

Review Questions

Question 1. To competently integrate dental radiographs into patient treatment, the dental hygienist must:

a. Diagnose dental disease from the dental radiographs

b. Recognize normal anatomy, landmarks, and restorations from abnormalities, pathologies, and artifacts

c. Prescribe radiographs and determine a dental hygiene diagnosis

d. Collect data and determine the definitive diagnosis

Question 2. Oral tissues and dental materials in the oral cavity result in radiographic contrast on a processed radiograph. These structures attenuate the primary beam of the X-rays.

a. The first statement is true; the second statement is false.

b. The first statement is false; the second statement is true.

c. Both statements are true.

d. Both statements are false.

Question 3. The more dense the object/material in the oral cavity, the more radiolucent the area will appear on a dental radiograph. The less dense the object/material in the oral cavity, the more radiopaque the area will appear on a dental radiograph.

a. The first statement is true; the second statement is false.

b. The first statement is false; the second statement is true.

c. Both statements are true.

d. Both statements are false.

Question 4. An endodontically treated tooth may be sealed with gutta-percha. The gutta-percha appears radiolucent on the radiograph.

a. The first statement is true; the second statement is false.

b. The first statement is false; the second statement is true.

c. Both statements are true.

d. Both statements are false.

Question 5. A porcelain-fused-to-metal crown appears both radiolucent and radiopaque on the radiograph. This radiographic appearance is caused by the various types of electromagnetic radiation.

a. The first statement is true; the second statement is false.

b. The first statement is false; the second statement is true.

c. Both statements are true.

d. Both statements are false.

Question 6. The presence of an orthodontic band interferes with the detection of a carious lesion because:

a. The band encircles the tooth, and its radiolucent appearance prevents the identification of proximal or occlusal decay

b. The band encircles the tooth, and its radiopaque appearance prevents the identification of proximal or occlusal decay

c. The band is cemented with zinc phosphate cement and fogs the detection of proximal or occlusal decay

d. The band is bonded with composite resin and fogs the detection of proximal or occlusal decay

Question 7. Resorbable materials used to repair or regenerate the periodontium are not generally visible on radiographs. The resultant healing of the resorbable material may be identified on the radiograph.

a. The first statement is true; the second statement is false.

b. The first statement is false; the second statement is true.

c. Both statements are true.

d. Both statements are false.

Question 8. A base may be placed under a new restoration and act as a thermal insulator to the pulp. Compared to a metal restoration, the radiographically visible base material is:

a. Opaque

b. Radiopaque

c. Radiolucent

d. Translucent

Question 9. To differentiate a radiopaque dental material from enamel or dentin, one should compare the:

a. Composition of the material with the anatomical parts of the tooth

b. Size of the material with the anatomical layers of the tooth

c. Shape of the radiopacity with the expected anatomical features of the tooth

d. Amount of the material with the anatomical parts of the tooth

Question 10. In recent years, it has become less confusing to radiographically distinguish composite resin restorations from carious lesions. The reason is that composite restorative material:

a. Has improved compressive strength

b. Has coefficients of thermal expansion closer to that of enamel

c. Contains radiopaque filler particles

d. Has improved elastic properties

Polishing Materials and Abrasion

Caren M. Barnes, R.D.H., M.S.

16

Objectives

After studying this chapter, the student will be able to do the following:

1. Briefly define the following terms:
   - Cutting
   - Abrasion
   - Finishing
   - Polishing
   - Abrasive
   - Cleaning Agent
2. Recall six common abrasives that may be used for clinical or laboratory procedures.
3. Explain the difference between two-body and three-body abrasion. Provide an example of a polishing procedure that exemplifies each type of abrasion.
4. Summarize factors that may influence the rate of abrasion, and explain why the dental hygienist must have a clear understanding of these factors when providing patient care.
5. Discuss the reasons why tooth structure and restorations are polished.
6. Recall the details of the polishing process. Include the series of steps, scratches produced, and wavelength of visible light.
7. Describe the difference between selective polishing and essential selective polishing.
8. Describe the characteristics of an acceptable prophylaxis paste.
9. Describe the difference between a cleaning agent and a polishing agent.
10. Identify the types of restorations that cannot be polished with an air powder polisher.
11. Identify the restorative materials, dental tissues, and periodontal tissues that are compatible with the following air polishing powders: sodium bicarbonate, aluminum trihydroxide, calcium sodium phosphosilicate, calcium carbonate, and glycine.

Key Words/Phrases

abrasion
abrasive
air abrasion
aluminum oxide
chalk
cleaning agent
cutting
cuttle
emery
essential selective polishing
facial emphysema
finishing
garnet
grit
polishing
pumice
sand
selective polishing
Silex
slurry
three-body abrasion
tin oxide
traditional air powder polishing
tribology
tungsten carbide burs
two-body abrasion

Introduction

One of the major responsibilities of the dental hygienist is the cleaning and polishing of teeth and restorations. This responsibility also includes any removable appliances, such as complete and partial dentures.

Before discussing polishing materials and abrasion, it is important to distinguish between the terms "cleaning" and "polishing." Polishing, by definition, involves the abrasion of a surface by an abrasive agent that is harder than the surface to be abraded, or polished. When a dental hygienist is truly polishing, the paste or slurry containing an abrasive agent will microscopically alter the tooth or restorative surface. Section V of this chapter, "The Polishing Process," addresses this topic in greater detail. Cleaning, sometimes referred to as plaque removal, is done with agents that do not contain abrasive particles. A **cleaning agent** is not abrasive and will not alter the surface characterization of enamel or esthetic restorative materials. The surface being cleaned is not altered or abraded as it would be in polishing.

I. Definitions

The topic of polishing materials and abrasion will be easier to discuss if we first define the basic terms that are involved in these procedures.

A. Cutting

Cutting refers to removing material by a shearing-off process. Examples of cutting would be milling, machining, or drilling. The process results in a somewhat smooth surface. In dentistry, cutting is done with metal burs and hand instruments to create cavity and crown preparations, which receive permanent restorations. An assortment of hand-cutting dental instruments is shown in *Figure 16.1*. When dental burs are used, the cutting process is affected by:

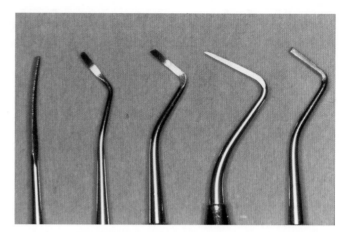

FIGURE 16.1. Examples of hand-cutting dental instruments (from *left* to *right*): Wedelstaedt chisel, spoon excavator, gingival margin trimmer, hoe, and hatchet.

1. Design of the Bur
   Dental burs are available in many shapes that aid the dentist in creating the correct design of the cavity or crown preparation. Examples of typical burs are illustrated in *Figure 16.2*.

2. Sharpness of the Bur
   The "lifetime" (or longevity) of a dental bur depends on the material from which it is made. Usually, cutting burs are made of carbon steel or tungsten carbide. **Tungsten carbide burs** are made by packing powdered metal constituents into a mold and then sintering (see Chapter 10, Materials for Fixed Indirect Restorations and Prostheses) at high temperatures. These burs are harder and maintain a sharper cutting edge than do carbon steel burs. Therefore, they last longer; however, they are more expensive.

B. Abrasion

Abrasion is the wearing away of a surface. It may also be referred to as grinding. Irregular grooves or scratches are produced on a surface as the result of abrasion.

C. Finishing

The process of producing the final shape and contour of a restoration is termed **finishing**. After

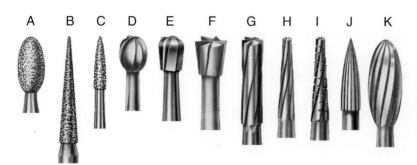

FIGURE 16.2. Names and shapes of dental burs. **A.** Egg or football diamond. **B.** Needle diamond. **C.** Flame diamond. **D.** Round. **E.** Pear. **F.** Inverted cone. **G.** Straight-fissure plain. **H.** Tapered-fissure plain. **I.** Tapered-fissure crosscut. **J.** Needle finishing. **K.** Egg or football finishing. (Courtesy of Brasseler USA.)

an amalgam restoration is placed, it may need to be finished and polished at a later appointment. Most other restorations are finished and polished when they are first placed. The instruments and armamentarium for finishing differ from those that are used for polishing. Examples used in finishing would be burs and stones.

D. Polishing

Polishing is the process of abrading a surface to eventually reduce the size of the scratches until the surface appears shiny. This concept not only applies to dentistry in regard to tooth structure and restorative materials but also extends into everyday life as well. We know that jewelry is polished, and we "polish" our sinks and bathtubs with certain kinds of cleansers that are recommended for those surfaces. This kind of polishing is different from polishing shoes or furniture. The shoe and furniture polish acts as a surface coat, similar to that of car wax.

E. Abrasive

The material doing the "wearing" (abrading) is the **abrasive**. In nature, wind and water carry abrasive particles and can wear away the surface of rocks.

In dentistry, abrasive particles may be bound together onto burs, disks, stones, wheels, or strips or they may be used with liquids to form a paste or slurry. These are discussed later in this chapter.

F. Tribology

Tribology is the science of interacting surfaces in motion; it incorporates the study and application of the principles of friction, lubrication, and wear. In dental polishing procedures, an abrasive agent creates friction and wear when it comes in contact with the surface being polished. The abrasive agent can be found embedded either in a surface such as a polishing wheel or in a moist paste; the moist ingredients in the paste serve as the lubricant. Within the science of tribology, polishing can be considered as two-body abrasion or three-body abrasion.
1. With **two-body abrasion** polishing, the abrasive agent particles are solidly fixed to a substrate, such as a dental bur, disk, wheel, strips, or in rubber cups impregnated with abrasive agents that do not require polishing paste.
2. **Three-body abrasion** occurs when abrasive particles move in a space between the surface being polished and the application device. The best example of three-body abrasion is polishing with a rubber cup and prophylaxis paste. The abrasive particles are mixed in the prophylaxis paste. The abrasive particles move in the space

between the tooth surface being polished and the surface of the rubber cup. Dental hygienists primarily use three-body abrasion.

II. Types of Abrasives

Many types of abrasives and polishing agents are used in dentistry, and to mention all of them would go beyond the scope of this text. Listed below are some of the more common ones that may be used when performing typical clinical or laboratory procedures:

A. Chalk

A mineral form of calcite is called **chalk**. It is also called whiting or calcium carbonate. Chalk is a mild abrasive and is used to polish teeth, gold and amalgam restorations, and plastic materials.

B. Pumice

Pumice is a silica-like, volcanic glass that is used as a polishing agent on enamel, gold foil, and dental amalgam and for finishing acrylic denture bases in the laboratory. It is the abrasive agent in "Lava" hand cleaner and is used to remove dried or callused skin in the form of a "pumice stone." Pumice, also found in clay, is the most common abrasive used in commercially prepared prophylaxis polishing pastes. Both chalk and pumice are illustrated in *Figure 16.3*.

C. Sand

Sand is a form of quartz and may be seen in various colors. Sand particles are rounded or angular in shape. They are typically bonded to paper disks for grinding metals and plastics.

D. Cuttle

As we know it today, **cuttle** is a fine grade of quartz. These particles are also bonded to paper disks and are beige in color. They are available in coarse, medium,

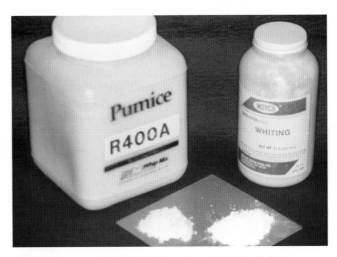

FIGURE 16.3. Chalk (whiting) and pumice in bulk form.

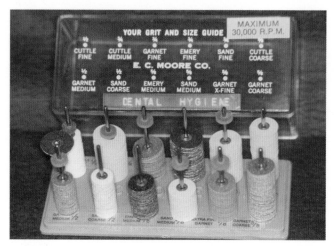

FIGURE 16.4. Kit of assorted disks coated with sand, cuttle, garnet, and emery.

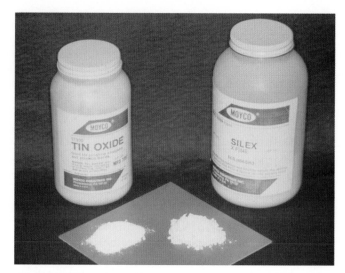

FIGURE 16.5. Silex and tin oxide in bulk form.

and fine grits. In the past, it was manufactured from the inside shell of a Mediterranean marine mollusk. A "cuttle bone" mounted in a parakeet's cage is made of the same material.

E. Garnet

Garnet is usually dark red in color. Because it is very hard, garnet is a highly effective abrasive. It is found on coated disks and is used for grinding plastics and metal alloys. The term **garnet** refers to several different minerals that have similar properties. These minerals are the silicates of manganese, magnesium, iron, cobalt, and aluminum.

F. Emery

Emery is sometimes also called "corundum." We are familiar with this abrasive because of "emery boards," which are used to file our fingernails. **Emery** is a natural form of aluminum oxide, and it looks like grayish-black sand. It is commonly found on arbor bands that attach to a dental lathe for grinding custom trays and acrylic appliances. Sand, cuttle, garnet, and emery disks can be seen in *Figure 16.4*.

G. Silex

Silex, a commercial product, is a silica-like material such as quartz and is used as an abrasive agent in the mouth. It is supplied as a powder and is mixed with various liquids to form a paste or slurry.

H. Tin Oxide

An extremely fine abrasive, **tin oxide** is supplied as a white powder and is used as a final polishing agent for teeth and metallic restorations. It is used as a paste or slurry in the same manner as Silex. Both Silex and tin oxide are illustrated in *Figure 16.5*.

I. Aluminum Oxide

Aluminum oxide is a common abrasive used in dentistry, and it has essentially replaced emery for several uses. This abrasive, shown in *Figure 16.6*, is widely used in the form of disks and strips. It is also impregnated into rubber wheels and points. It is the abrasive used in the popular "white stones" to adjust enamel or to finish metal alloys and ceramic materials.

III. Bonded and Coated Abrasives

To use the abrasives previously discussed, they must be attached to devices that permit an abrasive action. This action is usually rotary-powered, but in the case of finishing strips, it is accomplished by hand. Examples of these items include the following.

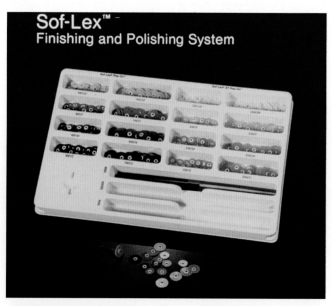

FIGURE 16.6. Aluminum oxide–coated disks and strips. (Courtesy of 3M/ESPE Dental Products.)

A. Diamond Burs

Diamond burs are actually very small diamond chips that are bonded to a shaft. Diamonds are very hard materials and make very good abrasives. Depending on the size of the chips, diamond burs can be used in many dental procedures.

B. Stones

Stones are available in various shapes, sizes, and grits, and they are made from a variety of materials. A "heatless stone" is illustrated on the right in *Figure 16.7*. Stones are used in clinical and laboratory procedures.

C. Rubber Wheels or Points

Molded rubber is impregnated with an abrasive into a wheel or point shape. The rubber acts as the matrix (or binder) of the abrasive agent. Examples are shown in *Figure 16.7*. Rubber wheels and points are designed for both clinical and laboratory procedures.

D. Rubber Cups

Abrasive agents are embedded in rubber cups intended for polishing. These rubber cups are available on disposable prophylaxis angles for use in polishing procedures during an oral prophylaxis, as shown in *Figure 16.8*. Rubber cups with embedded abrasives are not intended to be used with prophylaxis polishing pastes.

E. Disks and Strips

Abrasive particles are bonded to a paper, metal, or plastic backing to form disks or strips. Examples of coated disks and strips can be seen in *Figure 16.9*. They are used for intraoral and laboratory procedures.

F. Polishing Powders

Polishing powders, such as those illustrated in *Figures 16.3* and *16.5*, are used in conjunction with

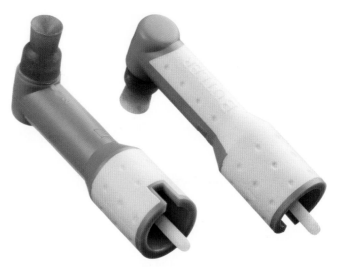

FIGURE 16.8. Disposable prophylaxis angle with abrasive particles embedded in the rubber cup. (Courtesy of Sunstar Americas, Inc.)

other agents and devices. These agents and devices include the following:
1. "Vehicles," such as water, alcohol, glycerin, fluoride, or mouthwash, are used to make pastes or slurries for polishing.
2. Brushes, rubber cups, felt cones and wheels, and cloth wheels are used to move an abrasive or polishing agent over the surface to be polished. *Figure 16.10* shows an assortment of cloth wheels, felt cones, bristle brushes, and rubber cups.

Some powders are used for laboratory and clinical procedures, whereas others are used only in the laboratory.

IV. Factors Affecting the Rate of Abrasion

Chances are, even though a class of dental hygiene students is taught to polish the same way, each student probably polishes differently. Depending on how much paste is

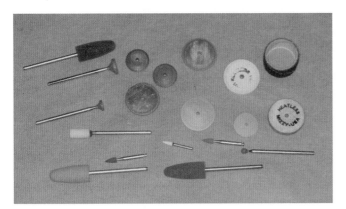

FIGURE 16.7. An assortment of bonded abrasive instruments (stones, rubber wheels, and rubber points) used in dentistry.

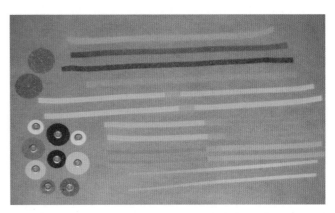

FIGURE 16.9. An assortment of coated disks and strips used in dentistry.

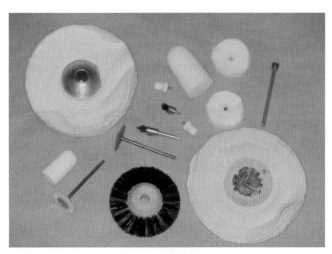

FIGURE 16.10. An assortment of cloth wheels, felt cones and wheels, brushes, and rubber cups used in dentistry.

put into the cup, the size and type of cup, the amount of pressure used against the tooth, how fast the cup is rotating, and what type of abrasive is in the cup, the surface being polished (technically abraded) will be significantly affected. The following factors affect the rate of abrasion.

A. Hardness

The abrasive particle must be harder than the surface being abraded if an acceptable rate of abrasion is to occur. Otherwise, the abrasive will be worn, and the surface will not be greatly affected. The abrasion rate can be "temperature dependent" (the abrasive heats up during use). The object being abraded could become heated, which may make it softer and affect the rate of abrasion.

Abrasives are usually made of very hard, ceramic materials. Table 16.1 lists Knoop and Mohs hardness of several restorative materials, abrasives, and tooth tissues.

B. Size

Common sense tells us that larger abrasive particles will produce deeper scratches than will smaller particles. Deeper scratches result in a greater amount of surface material removed. **Grit** is a term that is used to describe the size of the abrasive particle. Finer abrasives such as powders or flours are graded F, FF, and FFF as the fineness increases. When the particles are bonded to paper, the grit is designated as O, OO, and OOO in the order of increasing fineness. When a prophy paste is labeled "coarse" or "fine," the label is referring to the grit (or particle size) of the abrasive. It is important to note that there is no standardization in the definition of fine, medium, and coarse grit in prophy pastes among the manufacturers. The "fine" grit paste of one manufacturer may be nearly equal to the "coarse" grit paste of another manufacturer.

TABLE 16.1. Mohs and Knoop Hardness Values of Restorative Materials, Abrasives, and Tooth Tissues

Material	Mohs Hardness	Knoop Hardness
Composite (microfill)	2	30
Cementum	2	40
Composite (hybrid)	2–3	55
Dentin	3–4	70
Amalgam	3	90
Gold alloy (inlay)	3	100
Calcite (chalk, whiting)	3	135
Enamel	5	340
Pumice	6–7	560
Porcelain	6–7	590
Sand, quartz, cuttle	7	800
Garnet	8–9	1,400
Tungsten carbide (dental bur)	9	1,900
Aluminum oxide, emery	7–9	2,100
Diamond	10	7,000

Adapted from Weast R., ed. Handbook of Chemistry and Physics. 64th ed. Boca Raton, FL: CRC Press; 1983; Anusavice KJ. Phillips' Science of Dental Materials. 11th ed. Philadelphia, PA: Saunders; 2003:362; Callister WD. Fundamentals of Materials Science and Engineering. 2nd ed. Hoboken, NJ: Wiley; 2005:217.

C. Shape

Most individuals would agree that spherically shaped particles would be less abrasive than irregularly shaped particles. The sharp edges on irregularly shaped particles tend to dig into the surface rather than roll across it as rounded abrasive particles would, thus increasing the rate of abrasion. Cleaning agents have very soft or flat particles and do not abrade.

D. Pressure

Using excess pressure during finishing and polishing causes a higher abrasion rate because the abrasive particle cuts deeper into the surface. Increased pressure may also result in an increased temperature of the material being polished. An example of this would be using heavy pressure on an amalgam restoration. Raising the temperature of the amalgam could release mercury to the surface, which may increase corrosion and contribute to a marginal breakdown.

E. Speed

The term "speed" refers to the rate at which the polishing device is rotating. Like pressure, the speed at which the abrasive is applied will increase the rate of abrasion. Higher speed also results in a temperature increase. It is important to control the speed of the polishing cup or brush during polishing so that the abrasion rate and increase in temperature are kept to a minimum.

F. Lubrication

The most frequently used lubricant in dentistry is water. It is used with handpieces and burs to cool the tooth when cavity preparations are being made. During finishing and polishing, lubrication is also recommended to diminish the heat that is created by the abrasive action. This is accomplished by mixing lubricating agents, such as water, mouthwash, fluoride solutions (usually neutral sodium fluoride), glycerin, or alcohol, with the abrasive agent, which is usually in powder form. We refer to the resulting mixture as a "paste" or **slurry** depending on the liquid content.

V. The Polishing Process

A. Why We Polish

Tooth structure and restorative materials are polished for several reasons.

1. To Reduce Adhesion

    As discussed in Chapter 6, Amalgam, a smooth surface inhibits adhesion. Plaque, stain, and calculus are less likely to adhere to a smooth surface. Polishing removes the acquired pellicle. When the acquired pellicle reforms, it provides a medium for the adherence for dental plaque. This applies to tooth surfaces and restorative materials.

2. To Make the Surface Feel Smooth

    Patients expect a smooth surface on any permanent restoration that is placed in their mouths. In addition, they may comment on how they look forward to and value the smoothness that is produced after scaling and polishing during a routine dental hygiene recall appointment.

3. To Increase Esthetics

    An unpolished amalgam or gold crown is not as attractive as the one that appears smooth and shiny. This also holds true for the tooth surfaces of a heavy cigarette smoker before and after polishing. Esthetics play a very important role in dentistry, and polishing helps to create an attractive dentition for the patient. For the smoker, the subject of stain removal becomes an opportunity for the dental hygienist to discuss the subject of smoking cessation with the patient.

4. To Reduce Corrosion

    When metallic restorations are polished, it reduces the formation of tarnish and corrosion. In turn, this may extend the lifetime of the restoration.

B. Preparation for Polishing

Three steps should be taken prior to polishing.

1. First, the health history should be completed. No dental treatment procedures should ever be initiated without completion of the patient's health history to confirm there are no contraindications for polishing.

2. The second preparatory step prior to polishing procedures is the completion and/or review of the patient's chart of existing oral conditions and restorations. Some esthetic restorations are so artfully created and the colors so perfectly matched that detection of the restoration with the naked eye is almost impossible.

3. Finally, current radiographs should be reviewed and matched with the patient's intraoral chart to confirm the presence or absence of esthetic restorations or any restorations or conditions not previously charted.

C. What Happens During Polishing

Polishing procedures requires a series of steps. Each step removes a layer of material by abrasion. Because we use a series of finer and finer abrasives, the scratches become smaller and smaller, until they are smaller than the wavelength of visible light (<0.5 μm). With scratches of this size, the surface appears shiny. In short, the smaller the size of the scratches, the shinier the surface.

The same approach should be used when polishing teeth during routine oral prophylaxis. If heavy stains are present, a coarse abrasive, which could be a commercial paste or a powder and liquid mixed at chairside, should always be followed by a different abrasive with a finer grit and a different rubber cup.

Another approach to polishing is to use the same abrasive material in a progression of larger to smaller grits to produce increasingly smaller scratches. This technique is used more commonly in finishing and polishing restorations than it is during prophylaxis.

D. A Polishing Dilemma Resolved

In recent years, it was theorized that it was not necessary to polish all surfaces during every dental hygiene recall appointment. The only teeth that required polishing were the ones that were stained. The theory was based on the fact that stain removal is not a therapeutic procedure and plaque removal can be performed by the patient. This theory is known as **selective polishing**. When the selective polishing theory was met with reality, it placed dental hygienists in an ethical dilemma. Patients expect to have all of their teeth polished during an oral prophylaxis; want that "smooth clean, polished feeling"; and feel they are not receiving their money's worth if their teeth are not polished. In fact, some patients accused dental hygienists of being lazy! Further, dental hygienists who had been taught the selective polishing method learned they were removing the fluoride-rich outer layers of enamel during polishing and to only polish teeth that were heavily stained. The complexity of the dilemma was made even more confusing by the fact that even the definition of "oral prophylaxis" by the American Dental Hygienists' Association and the American Academy of Periodontology includes the polishing of teeth.

It is now recognized that there is no scientific proof of how much enamel is removed during polishing procedures, if at all. And with the use of cleaning agents, such as ProCare (Young Dental Mfg., Earth City, MO), all teeth can be polished without abrading teeth or restorative materials. Selective polishing takes on a new meaning and has been termed **essential selective polishing** by Barnes: it is essential that cleaning and polishing agents be selected according to the patient's needs. If a patient has stains, the polishing agent that will remove that amount of stain should be selected for use. For example, heavy stain should be removed with coarse prophylaxis paste, followed by the use of medium and fine prophylaxis pastes. If a patient with heavy stain has esthetic restorative materials present, those restorations should not be polished with any prophylaxis paste. Esthetic restorations should be polished with a polishing paste recommended by the manufacturer that is intended for use on esthetic restorative materials. Or a cleaning agent that will not compromise the surface or integrity of the esthetic restoration should be used. For teeth with no stain present, a cleaning agent that contains no abrasives should be utilized. The essential selective polishing approach solves all dilemmas related to polishing. Additionally, the essential selective polishing method eliminates the "one polishing paste for all polishing procedures" approach. Dental hygienists who have adopted this method will use either the "whatever grit is available" approach (fine–medium–coarse or extra-coarse) or the "coarse polishing paste on everything" approach. The use of this latter approach is based on the theory that if a coarse polishing paste can remove heavy stains, then of course, it can remove any stain less than heavy. These two approaches are unethical for two reasons: (1) they do not account for the patient's individual needs and (2) restorative materials can be severely compromised to the point of having to be replaced.

It is important to emphasize that enamel is in a constant state of "mineralization flux," demineralizing at times and also remineralizing. If a microscopic layer of enamel is removed from polishing with abrasive agents, it will remineralize in time with salivary minerals and exposure to fluorides, especially if the patient receives a fluoride treatment or fluoride varnish after polishing procedures.

The goal of polishing should be to create a smooth surface on teeth and restorations with the least abrasive agent to prevent adhesion of deposits. A summary of "Dos and Don'ts" when polishing teeth and restorative materials is provided in Table 16.2.

TABLE 16.2 General Summary of "Do and Do not" When Polishing

Do	Do not
• Recognize that polishing materials and devices are potentially harmful to soft tissue. • Avoid pulpal trauma and amalgam deterioration by using slow-speed, moderate to light pressure and adequate coolant when necessary. • Remember cementum and dentin abrade much easier than enamel. • Most polishing abrasive agents are harder than restorative materials and should be polished with an agent recommended by the material's manufacturer or use a cleaning agent that will not abrade. • Use high-polish, low-abrasion prophylaxis pastes. • Employ selective polishing procedures where indicated; select the appropriate cleaning or polishing agent to meet the patient's individual needs.	• Traumatize gingival tissue. • Generate excessive heat. • Overlook potential damage to root surfaces, especially on tooth-colored restorations. • Polish restorative materials with prophylaxis paste. • Use excessively abrasive prophylaxis pastes. • Polish every patient's teeth with the same polishing agents.

E. The Polishing Technique

When a polishing sequence is employed, it is important to remember that to prevent abrasive contamination, prophy cups and/or brushes must be changed before the next, less abrasive agent is used. The surfaces being polished should be thoroughly rinsed before the next agent is applied. In addition, if the clinician wants to use a fine abrasive on tooth-colored or cast restorations, and a coarse abrasive on the tooth structure, the coarse one should be used first. The clinician should avoid the restorative materials with the coarse abrasive, have the patient rinse, change the prophy cup, and polish with the finer agent.

The recommended polishing technique is the one of slow speed with light, intermittent pressure. Prophy brushes are usually limited to areas such as occlusal surfaces. Brushes get into the irregularities of occlusal surfaces better than does a cup but are more likely to abrade and cause trauma to gingiva.

Demineralized tooth surfaces can be considered as weak tooth structure. Rubber cup polishing may cause a significant amount of surface structure to be removed on demineralized teeth compared to intact enamel.

Polishing restorations may create a roughened surface. Restorative materials such as gold, composite, amalgam, and glass ionomer could be affected by the abrasive agents in prophy pastes. The surfaces could be roughened, and in some cases, the margins of the restoration could be damaged. For implants, there are nonabrasive pastes available for polishing the abutments and pontics.

We must remember that the purpose of polishing is to produce the smoothest possible surface. Whether we are polishing tooth structure or restorative material, we defeat this purpose when we use coarse abrasive agents. Grooves and scratches are created on the surface that may not have previously been there. This uneven surface is now more conducive for the formation and adhesion of plaque, stain, and calculus. These accumulations now occur more rapidly than they did before the surface was improperly polished.

VI. Prophylaxis Pastes

A vast assortment of prophy pastes are available from which the hygienist may choose. In recent years, they have been marketed not only by companies that make toothbrushes but also by those that manufacture disposable and autoclavable prophy angles. There are a few on the market that are supplied in bulk form, such as a jar shown in *Figure 16.11*. However, most are supplied in unit-dose cups as

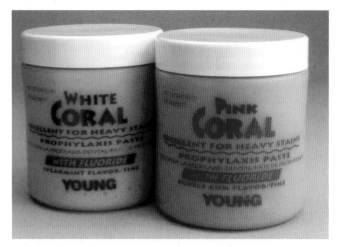

FIGURE 16.11. Prophylaxis pastes supplied in bulk form. (Courtesy of Young Dental Mfg.)

shown in *Figure 16.12*. Prophy paste is manufactured in a variety of colors, textures, flavors, grits, and formulations. Prices also vary depending on the brand and the quantity purchased.

In 1982, a journal article published by research associates Putt, Kleber, and Muhler from Indiana University addressed enamel polish and abrasion by prophylaxis pastes. This article became a "keystone" publication for this topic because it provided the hygienist with important information about polishing. It also rated 10 commercial prophy pastes for their enamel polish and abrasion properties. Unfortunately, this was more than 30 years ago. Most of the pastes rated in this article are no longer on the market. A few of the major points follow.

A. Polishing Ability

A polishing agent should not create deep scratches and grooves, as discussed earlier. Instead, it should produce very fine, shallow scratches and grooves so that light may be reflected and, therefore, "shine."

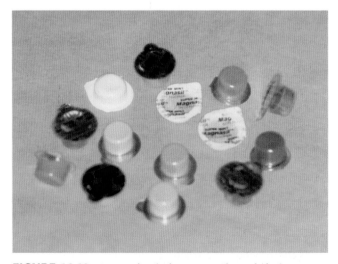

FIGURE 16.12. Assorted unit-dose cups of prophylaxis paste.

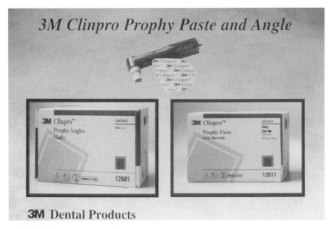

FIGURE 16.13. "Clinpro" prophylaxis paste. (Courtesy of 3M/ESPE Dental Products.)

In recent years, a prophylaxis paste has been developed that has both cleaning (abrasive) and polishing abilities in one paste. This product is illustrated in *Figure 16.13*. Sheet-shaped particles, known as "perlite," convert from coarse to fine with 15 seconds of use. *Figure 16.14* presents the particle shape and conversion after 15 seconds of polishing. However, it must be pointed out that all abrasives used in prophylaxis pastes break down into smaller and smaller particles during polishing procedures.

B. Abrasive Properties

The abrasive particle used in the paste should not produce a detrimental effect on the surface. It must, however, remove the stain.

An acceptable prophy paste will possess properties of both a high-polish rate and a low-abrasion rate. The Putt, Kleber, and Muhler publication identified a few pastes that exhibit these qualities, as well as some that produced a low-polish and a high-abrasion rate.

The Putt, Kleber, and Muhler research also commented on the use of polishing agents in areas of gingival recession. It must be remembered that dentin will abrade 25 times faster than enamel. Cementum, which is only temporarily present in areas of gingival recession, will abrade 35 times faster than enamel because of its thin layer and "softness." Common practice would dictate that abrasive polishing agents be contraindicated in gingivally recessed areas.

C. "Specialty" Prophylaxis Pastes

Manufacturers have developed prophy pastes that do more than clean and polish. The dental hygienist may typically have an assortment of products on hand that contains a prophy paste as well as a therapeutic agent. Some pastes, such as Clinpro (3M/ESPE) will transition from coarse to fine product. This was discussed in Section VI A: Polishing Ability and is shown in *Figures 16.13* and *16.14*. (However, all abrasive agents in prophylaxis paste break down to smaller and smaller particles as each tooth is polished.) Others may contain various amounts and types of fluoride such as "D-Lish" (Young Dental), "Topex" (Sultan Healthcare, Inc.), and "Enamel Pro" (Premier), to name a few. Yet others, such as "NuCare" (Sunstar Americas, Inc.), and "ProClude" (Ortek Therapeutics), have been reported to reduce sensitivity. It is important to point out that there is a void of research regarding the efficacy of some of the prophylaxis polishing pastes that contain additives, such as amorphous calcium phosphate or bioglass that claim to strengthen enamel or reduce hypersensitivity. Clinpro, NuCare, and Enamel Pro are pictured in *Figure 16.15*.

D. Prophy Pastes for Esthetic Restorations

In recent years, there has been a great demand by patients for esthetic restorations. The typical ones include microfills, hybrids, and compomers. Due to their "softer composition," many traditional prophy pastes should not be used on these restorations since they may create a very rough surface and/or remove the resin coating and expose the filler particles in the esthetic restorative materials. Instead, prophylaxis pastes specially formulated for esthetic restorations are recommended. These contain abrasives such as perlite, aluminum oxide, or diamond powder to name a few. When in doubt, a cleaning agent that will not abrade esthetic restorative materials should be used.

If the hygienist knows the brand name of the restorative material, it is important to follow the

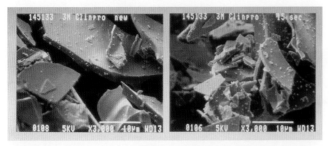

FIGURE 16.14. "Perlite" abrasive particle (in Clinpro): coarse **(left)** and resulting fine **(right)**. (Courtesy of 3M/ESPE Dental Products.)

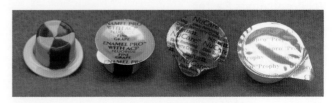

FIGURE 16.15. Assorted "specialty" prophylaxis pastes in unit-dose packaging.

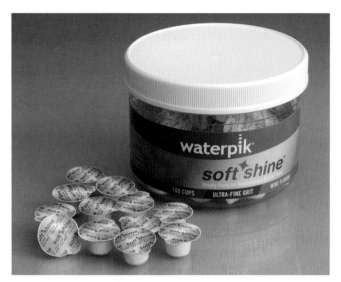

FIGURE 16.16. "Soft Shine" cosmetic restorative paste for restored and natural teeth. (Courtesy of Water Pik, Inc.)

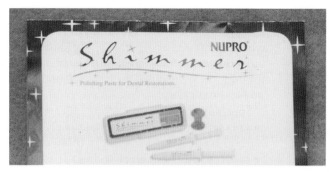

FIGURE 16.18. A polishing agent specifically developed for hygienists to polish restorations.

manufacturer's recommendations for polishing. In many cases, one of their own products will be recommended for polishing. These polishing agents contain very fine abrasives and are available in the form of pastes in unit doses and dispensing syringes, cups, points, and disks. Examples of these products are shown in *Figures 16.16 to 16.18*.

Identifying the types of materials used for these restorations (Clinical Detection and Management of Dental Restorative Materials during Scaling and Polishing: Table 14.1) and using the correct agents to polish them will indeed require some planning and time. But it is our responsibility as a professional to use the appropriate agents on teeth and restorations. The end result is a smoother, longer-lasting restoration, and your extra care and effort will be greatly appreciated by your patient.

VII. Air Powder Polishing

A. Traditional Air Powder Polishing

Traditional air powder polishing utilizes air, water, and a specially formulated polishing powder. The original air polishing powder and now "gold standard of the air polishing powders" is specially

processed sodium bicarbonate. The air powder polishing combines the compressed air, water, and sodium bicarbonate into a spray that uses kinetic energy to propel the powder polishing particles to the tooth surface.

B. Air Polishing Powders

Prior to using any air polishing powder in an air powder polishing unit, refer to the warranty for the unit. Using an air powder polishing agent not approved by the unit manufacturer may void the warranty on the unit. Specifically selected powders (glycine and erythritol) can be used subgingivally and have been reported to improve inflammatory responses in peri-implantitis and periodontally involved teeth.

1. **Sodium Bicarbonate**
Sodium bicarbonate is the original powder used in air powder polishing and is specially formulated with scant amounts of calcium phosphate and silica to keep it free flowing. This sodium bicarbonate formulation is not the same as over-the-counter sodium bicarbonate. Over-the-counter sodium bicarbonate will clog air powder polishing units. The only sodium bicarbonate that can be used is that which is specially formulated for air powder polishing units. Sodium bicarbonate particles for air powder polishing average 60 to 74 μm in size. It should be noted that various brands of sodium bicarbonate powder differ in the size of the particle and some brands are more abrasive than

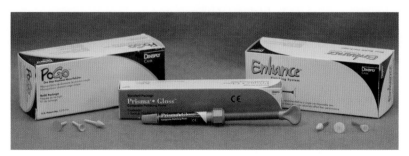

FIGURE 16.17. Products containing an assortment of pastes, cups, points, and disks for polishing esthetic restorations.

others. The Mohs hardness number for sodium bicarbonate is 2.5 and ranks in hardness with hybrid composite restorative material. Sodium bicarbonate powders are available in flavors; however, the patient will taste the salt and smell the flavoring.

Specially processed sodium bicarbonate can be safely used on enamel, especially for removal of heavy stains such as those created by tobacco use and chlorhexidine. It is especially useful for stain removal in hard-to-reach areas. Additionally, sodium bicarbonate is safe for use on amalgam, gold, porcelain, implants, orthodontic brackets and bands, and preparing occlusal surfaces for dental sealants. The use of sodium bicarbonate is contraindicated for use on sealants and tooth-colored restorative materials that include composites and glass ionomers.

2. **Aluminum Trihydroxide**
Aluminum trihydroxide was the first alternative air polishing powder developed for patients who cannot tolerate sodium bicarbonate. There are health conditions that would preclude the use of any sodium product. Those conditions would include patients on a physician-directed sodium-restricted diet or patients with high blood pressure or renal disease (see Section VII C: Contraindications for Air Powder Polishing). The Mohs hardness number for aluminum trihydroxide is 4 and the particles range in mesh size from 80 to 325 µm.

Aluminum trihydroxide is indicated for patients who have heavily stained enamel. Contraindications for aluminum trihydroxide include use on dentin, cementum, amalgam, gold, all composite types, glass ionomers, and implants. Aluminum trihydroxide does not cause surface disruption to porcelain. However, the luting agents used for placement of porcelain restorations are removed by aluminum trihydroxide, causing a compromise in the margin integrity that could quickly lead to development of dental caries.

3. **Glycine Powder**
Glycine is an amino acid. For use in powders, glycine crystals are grown using a solvent of water and sodium salt. Glycine particles for use in air polishing are 18 to 22 µm in size and have a Mohs hardness number of 2. Glycine is the least abrasive air polishing powder available for use in the United States as of this writing.

4. **Calcium Carbonate**
Calcium carbonate is a naturally occurring substance that can be found in rocks. The size of the calcium carbonate particle is 60 to 70 µm. It is a main ingredient in antacids and is also used as filler for pharmaceutical drugs. Calcium carbonate has a Mohs number of 3 and is also called chalk or whiting and is discussed in Section II: Types of Abrasives.

5. **Calcium Sodium Phosphosilicate (Novamin)**
Calcium sodium phosphosilicate (Novamin) is a bioactive glass and has a Mohs hardness number of 6, and particle sizes range from 20 to 120 µm making it the hardest air polishing particle used in air powder polishing powders. Research has confirmed that calcium sodium phosphosilicate is currently one of the most abrasive and possibly the most abrasive air polishing powder and is contraindicated for use with air polishing. Calcium sodium phosphosilicate will cause excessive abrasion to enamel, composite materials, and glass ionomers. It is important to note that air powder polishing should not be confused with air abrasion systems. **Air abrasion** involves removing some tooth structure with a high-velocity stream of air that carries a very hard abrasive particle (aluminum oxide) as part of a restorative procedure. Air abrasion systems were discussed in more detail in Chapter 5, Direct Polymeric Restorative Materials.

6. **Erythritol**
Erythritol is a sugar alcohol that occurs naturally in plants. As of this writing, erythritol is not available in the United States for air polishing but likely will be in 2017. Erythritol has shown promise, when used subgingivally, in reducing inflammation both in periodontal pockets and when used in cases of peri-implantitis. Erythritol is the softest of all air polishing powders and has been shown to be compatible with composite, enamel, and periodontal soft tissues. There is a growing body of research on erythritol and dental hygienists who use air polishing are advised to follow the research on erythritol.

C. Contraindications for Air Powder Polishing

Air powder polishing should not be used on:
1. A physician-directed sodium-restricted diet
2. Patients with respiratory disease
3. Conditions that limit swallowing or breathing (chronic obstructive pulmonary disease)
4. Patients with communicable infections
5. Immunocompromised patients
6. Patients taking
   a. Potassium
   b. Antidiuretics
   c. Steroid therapy

D. Air Powder Polishing Technique

Most dental hygiene clinical textbooks present the technique for air polishing in detail. A review of the procedure follows:

1. The handpiece should be angled:
   a. 60 degrees to the anterior teeth
   b. 90 degrees to the posterior teeth
   c. 90 degrees to the occlusal surfaces

2. High-speed evacuation should be used at all times and patients should wear eye protection.

3. The handpiece nozzle should be kept moving in a constant circular motion and 4 to 5 mm from the tooth surface.

4. Correct angulation is the single best method of controlling excess aerosol production.

5. Facial emphysema
   a. Occurs when the handpiece is angled incorrectly; the handpiece nozzle should never be directed subgingivally into pockets where there is little or no bony support, into extraction sites, or near or into traumatic lacerations or surgical wounds.
   b. Definition—**Facial emphysema** occurs when air is entrapped in the soft tissues of the head and neck.
   c. Normally treated with antibiotics.

   d. Symptoms: area feels "hard to the touch" or patients experience a "crackling" noise in the affected area.
   e. These can develop into more serious conditions such as thrombosis and embolism, among others.

VIII. Implants

As mentioned previously, dental implants may be cleaned with air powder polishing units using sodium bicarbonate powder or with a rubber cup and an appropriate *cleaning* agent. When polishing, the incompatibility of titanium with other metals and some chemicals must be taken into consideration during the prophylaxis appointment. True polishing agents are contraindicated for dental implants because the goal is not to alter (abrade) the surface integrity of the titanium.

An ideal agent for removing soft debris is the cleaning agent called ProCare (Young Dental Mfg.). The round, "softer," flat particles in this powder are not described as a grit. This product is one of the prophylaxis pastes that researchers Putt, Kleber, and Muhler (described previously in this chapter) had found to possess low abrasion and high polishing properties. The powder and liquid that are combined for this prophylaxis paste are pictured in *Figure 16.19.* Needless to say, to remove hard deposits

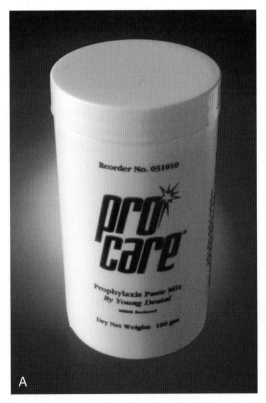

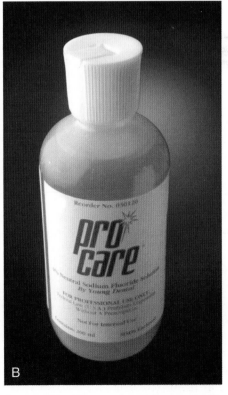

FIGURE 16.19. ProCare is a cleaning agent that comes in **A.** a powdered form and must be mixed with water or **B.** a neutral sodium fluoride that is provided. (Courtesy of Young Dental.)

from implants, special plastic hand instruments have been developed in addition to plastic sheaths for ultrasonic scaling instruments.

IX. Denture Cleansers

Full and partial dentures will accumulate plaque, stain, and calculus in the same manner as natural teeth. It is the dental hygienist's responsibility not only to examine the condition of removable appliances but also to return them to the patient in a deposit-free condition at the end of the appointment.

Denture base materials and denture teeth are, indeed, dental materials for which the hygienist provides professional services. Dentures may be cleaned and polished in several ways, and textbooks devoted to the clinical practice of dental hygiene discuss these in detail.

The goal in cleaning and polishing dentures, as when cleaning and polishing natural teeth and other restorative surfaces, is to remove deposits in a manner that is not detrimental to the surface. Care must be taken so that abrasives, rotary devices, or caustic ultrasonic solutions do not damage the surface of the removable denture appliance.

X. Dentifrices

As with denture cleansers, dentifrices are discussed in detail in clinical practice textbooks. From a dental materials standpoint, the most important constituent in a dentifrice is the abrasive agent.

A. Abrasive Content and American Dental Association Acceptance

One of several types of abrasives may be added to the dentifrice formulation. Several years ago, dentifrices were on the market that were considered to be very abrasive, such as those recommended for smokers. To reassure the consumer today, the American Dental Association (ADA) evaluates dentifrices in their Acceptance Program. This was discussed in more detail in Chapter 1, Introduction. A dentifrice is "ADA accepted" if it meets the specific requirements set forth by the ADA. In summary, these requirements are as follows:

1. Safety and Efficacy

The dentifrice must be safe and effective. Currently, the U.S. Food and Drug Administration (FDA) regulates dentifrices and their abrasivity. The American Dental Association (ADA) and the International Standards Organization (ISO) also have standards for dentifrices that are discussed later in this chapter.

2. Scientific Data

The manufacturer of the dentifrice must provide scientific data to the ADA to support any claims made in advertisements and on the packaging of the product. These data are usually the result of extensive clinical trials.

B. Abrasives Used in Dentifrices

There are three major categories of dentifrice abrasives:

1. Phosphates

These contribute to a whiter look and cleaner "feel" to the teeth. Two phosphates used in dentifrices are dicalcium phosphate dihydrate and calcium pyrophosphate.

2. Carbonates

Carbonates have been used for almost 100 years to make products and environments smell better, in addition to their abrasive properties.

a. *Sodium Bicarbonate*

This is also known as baking soda. In the 1920s, it was used to clean silver; in the 1940s, it was the deodorizer for refrigerators. The 1970s saw baking soda used as a laundry detergent and carpet deodorizer. In the past 20 years, it has been used as a dentifrice abrasive. In addition, research studies have shown that "sodium bicarbonate is compatible with fluoride, bactericidal against most periodontal pathogens, safe, as well as low in abrasivity and cost. It may be said that sodium bicarbonate is the consummate dentifrice ingredient."

b. *Calcium Carbonate*

As discussed previously, this abrasive is also known as chalk. It is one of the most economical mechanical abrasives available. Sodium monofluorophosphate is used with calcium carbonate.

3. Silica

Silica provides abrasion or cleaning when used in proprietary prophylaxis pastes and dentifrices and is available in various particle sizes. Additionally, silica can be formulated to take on certain characteristics. For example, silica particles can be manufactured to be opaque or translucent. Translucent silica particles are typically found in gel-type dentifrices or nonopaque prophylaxis pastes. Silica is largely nonreactive with prophylaxis paste and toothpaste ingredients. Silica has become the most frequently used abrasive in recent years and is compatible with soluble fluorides. Silica is often found in dentifrices that claim to whiten teeth.

C. Factors Affecting Abrasion Rate by Dentifrices

Intraoral and extraoral factors will influence the rate of abrasion from a dentifrice:

1. Intraoral factors include xerostomia, saliva consistency and quantity, exposed root surfaces, quality and quantity of deposits, and presence of certain restorative materials.
2. Extraoral factors include the type, size, and amount of abrasive in the dentifrice as well as the quantity of dentifrice used. The type of toothbrush, method of use, amount of force delivered, and frequency of brushing are other extraoral factors.

As mentioned earlier in this chapter, there is an abrasive index for toothpastes called the Relative Dentin Abrasivity Index (RDA Index) or Radioactive Dentin Abrasivity Index (RDA), which was initially developed by the American Dental Association. The ADA utilizes the RDA Index for comparing the abrasivity of dentifrices, as shown in Table 16.3. The RDA Index is based on a standardized method for determining abrasivity of dentifrices called Radioactive Dentin Abrasion (RDA). The RDA is determined by making extracted human teeth radioactive using mild neutron irradiation, as a first step. Second, the irradiated teeth are stripped of enamel. Third, the dentin samples are placed in a brushing machine under standardized conditions of pressure and brushing speed using the dentifrice of interest. The rinse water from the brushing machine is measured for radioactivity (abraded dentin). Finally, a score is calculated by comparing results of the test dentifrice to those of a standard abrasive reference material. Any value over 100 is considered to be abrasive. A dentifrice must obtain an abrasivity score of 200 to 250 or less to satisfy the abrasivity test requirements proposed by the ADA and the International Standard Organization (ISO). The FDA limit is 200. This means that a test dentifrice must abrade dentin 20% to 25% of the rate of the reference standard to be considered safe for normal usage. The shortcoming of this method is that it is performed in a laboratory and does not represent in vivo conditions.

Acknowledgment

This chapter is dedicated to the memory of Dr. Esther Wilkins (1916–2016), a dear and beloved friend, Caren M. Barnes.

TABLE 16.3. Relative Dentin Abrasivity Index for Some Commonly Recognized Brands of Dentifrices[a]

Toothpastes	RDA Value
Straight Baking Soda	7
Arm & Hammer Tooth Powder	8
Arm & Hammer Dental Care	35
Oxyfresh	45
Tom's of Maine Sensitive	49
Arm & Hammer PeroxiCare	49
Rembrandt Original	53
CloSYS	53
Tom's of Maine Children's	57
Colgate Regular	68
Colgate Total	70
Sensodyne	79
Aim	80
Colgate Sensitive Max Strength	83
Aquafresh Sensitive	91
Tom's of Maine Regular	93
Crest Regular	95
Mentadent	103
Sensodyne Extra Whitening	104
Colgate Platinum	106
Crest Sensitivity	107
Colgate Herbal	110
Aquafresh Whitening	113
Arm & Hammer Tarter Control	117
Arm & Hammer Advance White Gel	117
Close-up with Baking Soda	120
Colgate Whitening	124
Crest Extra Whitening	130
Ultra Brite	133
Crest MultiCare Whitening	144
Colgate Baking Soda Whitening	145
Pepsodent	150
Colgate Tarter Control	165
Colgate 2-in-1 Tarter Control/White	200
FDA Recommended Limit	200
ADA Recommended Limit	250

[a]0 to 70 = low abrasive; 70 to 100 = medium abrasive; 100 to 150 = highly abrasive; 150 to 250 = regarded as harmful limit.
Adapted from http://dukeslc.wordpress.com/2008/11/20/toothpaste-abrasion-ratings/. Accessed February 1, 2011.

Summary

The dental hygienist should have a fundamental understanding of the terms associated with the cleaning and polishing of teeth and restorations. Cutting is removing material by a shearing-off process. Abrasion is the wearing away of a surface. Finishing is the process of producing the final shape and contour of a restoration, whereas polishing is the abrasion of a surface to eventually reduce the size of the scratches until the surface appears shiny. The material doing the wearing or abrading is the abrasive.

The chapter includes descriptions of several abrasives commonly used in the practice of dental hygiene. To use these abrasives, they must be attached to devices that permit abrasive action. These devices include diamond burs, stones, rubber wheels or points, disks, strips, and powders.

The factors of hardness, size and shape, pressure, speed, and lubrication may affect the rate of abrasion. Polishing with a very dry abrasive and a hard-bristle prophy brush with significant pressure and speed is likely to produce an excessively abraded surface on tooth structure and restorative materials. In contrast, when the hygienist uses a wet, fine-grit paste or powder and a rubber prophy cup with gentle pressure and slow speed, a surface of high polish and low abrasion is more likely to be produced.

Reasons for polishing include reducing adhesion to discourage deposits, creating a smooth surface, increasing esthetics, and reducing corrosion of metallic restorations. During the polishing procedure, progressively finer scratches are produced as abrasives are used in a sequence from coarse to fine. However, a decision must be made regarding whether to polish at all. Many dental hygiene programs have instituted "selective polishing" as a recommended protocol.

Prophylaxis pastes are supplied in a variety of colors, textures, flavors, grits, and formulations. Recommended pastes are those with high polish and low abrasion levels. There are prophy pastes that now contain fluoride and desensitizing agents as well as one that transitions from a coarse to a fine abrasive agent. Yet others are formulated to contain a very mild abrasive or no abrasives to essentially be cleaning agents.

Denture base materials and denture teeth are dental materials that deserve attention during the dental hygiene recall/maintenance appointment. Plaque and calculus must be removed in a manner that is not detrimental to the prosthesis.

An important constituent in dentifrices, from a dental materials standpoint, is the abrasive agent. A U.S. FDA-approved and "ADA-accepted" dentifrice must meet requirements concerning level of abrasion and have scientific data to support any claims regarding effectiveness.

Air powder polishing uses air, water, and an abrasive to remove stain and biofilm on teeth, orthodontic bands and brackets, and implants. Selective powders can be used subgingivally and have been reported to improve inflammatory responses in peri-implantitis and periodontally involved teeth. Because the surface of titanium implants must not be altered, only cleaning agents, not abrasive agents, should be used for traditional polishing on implant surfaces.

There are three major categories of dentifrice abrasives: phosphates, carbonates, and silica. The carbonates include sodium bicarbonate, which is compatible with fluoride, bactericidal, safe, and low in abrasivity and cost. Silica has become the most frequently used abrasive in dentifrices in recent years.

Learning Activities

1. Take a small piece of brass or Plexiglas, a slow-speed handpiece, and a few prophy cups or brushes. Use three different grits of abrasive agents to polish as follows:
   a. Using the abrasive with the largest grit, finish the entire surface of the brass plate with scratches going in one direction only (see **A** at right).
   b. Change the cup or brush, use the second most abrasive agent, and rotate the surface 90 degrees so that the new scratches are perpendicular to the previous scratches. Polish approximately two-thirds of the surface (see **B** at right).
   c. Change the cup or brush again, use the finest-grit agent, rotate surface 90 degrees back to the original position, and polish one-third of the surface (see **C** at right).
   d. With the same cup and agent, polish the entire bottom half of the surface going across all the previously polished areas (see **D** at right).

   Evaluate your specimen, and describe the results. Note the appearance of scratches in the various areas. What does this tell you about polishing in proper sequence? Now, compare the bottom and top halves. What is the result of polishing with the finest abrasive directly over the rougher sections?

2. Squeeze a long sample of composite restorative material onto a resin strip. Fold the strip over, and flatten the sample. Light cure until set. Divide the strip into three sections, and polish in the same manner as described in learning activity #1, using Sof-Lex aluminum oxide disks in sequence from coarse to fine. Evaluate your sample in the same manner as the brass plate or Plexiglas.

3. Polish a classmate's teeth, using different polishing materials, such as:
   a. Toothpaste
   b. Silex
   c. Tin oxide
   d. Whiting
   e. Pumice
   f. Various brands of commercial prophy pastes

   Notice the consistency, tendency to splatter, and grit. Have the "patient" report to you on the differences in grit, taste, and texture.

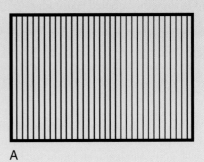

A

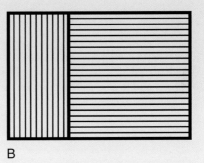

B

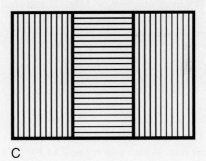

C

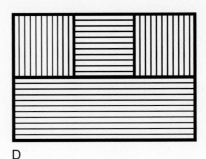

D

Review Questions

Question 1. Which type of abrasive looks like a grayish-black sand and is sometimes called "corundum"?

a. Tin oxide
b. Garnet
c. Pumice
d. Emery
e. Tripoli

Question 2. Which type of abrasive is produced from volcanoes and is used in the laboratory and on restorative materials, such as gold, amalgam, and gold foil?

a. Aluminum oxide
b. Pumice
c. Zirconium silicate
d. Sand

Question 3. Which abrasive is used as a slurry to polish amalgam restorations and is also called calcium carbonate?

a. Silex
b. Whiting
c. Pumice
d. Aluminum oxide

Question 4. When an abrasive on a dental restorative material is used, the abrasive action must be _____ the surface you are abrading.

a. Harder than
b. Softer than
c. Equal to
d. Any abrasive material will be effective

Question 5. All of the following factors affect the rate of abrasion except one. Which one is the EXCEPTION?

a. Pressure
b. Speed
c. Size of particle
d. Bonded and coated abrasives

Question 6. The process of producing the final shape and contour of a restoration is termed:

a. Cutting
b. Abrasion
c. Polishing
d. Finishing

Question 7. An example of a "vehicle" to be used with powders would be:

a. Rubber cups
b. Felt cones
c. Glycerin
d. Prophy brushes

Question 8. Polishing involves using a series of finer and finer abrasives. It can also be accomplished by using the same abrasive material in a progression of larger to smaller grit.

a. The first statement is true; the second statement is false.
b. The first statement is false; the second statement is true.
c. Both statements are true.
d. Both statements are false.

Question 9. During routine polishing with pumice, _____ μm of the fluoride-rich layer can be removed.

a. 1 to 2
b. 3 to 4
c. 5 to 6
d. 7 to 8

Question 10. The recommended prophylaxis pastes possess the properties of:

a. High polish and high abrasion
b. Low polish and high abrasion
c. Low polish and low abrasion
d. High polish and low abrasion

Question 11. Which of the following is harder than enamel?

a. Pumice
b. Amalgam
c. Composite
d. Gold alloy

Question 12. Air powder polishing is designed to remove:

a. Biofilm
b. Biofilm and stain
c. Calculus and stain
d. Plaque and calculus

Question 13. **The most frequently used abrasive in dentifrices is:**

a. Carbonates

b. Pumice

c. Silica

d. Phosphates

Question 14. **Which of the following abrasives would most likely be found in a polishing agent for esthetic restorations?**

a. Pumice

b. Calcium carbonate

c. Diamond powder

d. Emery

Question 15. **Mrs. Smith presents for her prophylaxis appointment after a year, rather than the 6-month prescribed time. She has tobacco stain on the lingual surfaces of her natural teeth, two gold alloy crowns, and several esthetic restorations. Which combination of cleaning/polishing agents should be chosen?**

a. Traditional prophy paste, tin oxide, and a polishing agent for esthetic restorations

b. Pumice, traditional prophy paste, and a polishing agent for esthetic restorations

c. Traditional prophy paste, pumice, and tin oxide

d. Silex, tin oxide, and a traditional prophy paste

Tooth Whitening

Michele R. Sweeney, R.D.H., M.S.D.H.

17

Objectives

After studying this chapter, the student will be able to do the following:

1. Define tooth whitening and explain the difference between vital and nonvital tooth whitening.
2. Explain the difference between intrinsic and extrinsic stains, and list examples of each.
3. Identify two chemical agents used for vital tooth whitening, and explain the process by which whitening agents whiten teeth.
4. Identify two chemical agents used for nonvital tooth whitening.
5. List the factors that affect the success of tooth whitening.
6. Compare and contrast patient-applied and professionally applied vital whitening.
7. List contraindications for both patient-applied and professionally applied tooth whitening procedures.
8. Discuss measures to prevent or alleviate tooth whitening side effects.
9. Become familiar with the statement made by the ADA on the safety and efficacy of tooth whitening.

Key Words/Phrases

amelogenesis imperfecta

calcium peroxide

carbamide peroxide

dentinogenesis imperfecta

dicalcium phosphate dihydrate

extrinsic stain

fluorosis

gutta-percha

hydrated silica

hydrogen peroxide

intrinsic stain

laser whitening

neutral sodium fluoride

nightguard vital whitening

nonvital tooth

potassium nitrate

power whitening

precipitated calcium carbonate

reversible pulpitis

root canal

sodium perborate

sodium percarbonate

tetracycline staining

tooth whitening or tooth bleaching

vital tooth

vital tooth whitening

walking bleach

Introduction

Teeth that are naturally discolored or have become stained can be treated with a whitening agent. Depending on the cause of the discoloration or the type of stain, one of several whitening techniques may be used. The procedure is often referred to as **tooth whitening or tooth bleaching**.

A nonvital tooth is treated differently than a vital tooth. A **nonvital tooth** gives no response to temperature change or electrical stimulus. The pulp in this tooth is no longer living, hence the term "nonvital." The pulp cavity within a nonvital tooth may contain necrotic pulp, no pulp, or an inert material placed when an endodontic procedure known as a **root canal** was completed.

The terminology used when vital teeth are treated is **vital tooth whitening**. A **vital tooth** (a tooth with living pulp tissue) can be whitened in the dental office by the dental team or at home by the patient. When the whitening treatment is done at home by the patient, it is frequently called **nightguard vital whitening** because the whitening agent is applied to the teeth inside a custom tray resembling a nightguard appliance. A trayless tooth whitening system is now available. Trayless systems use flexible, adhesive, polyethylene strips that are coated with a whitening agent. Tooth whitening is a cosmetic procedure and the most frequently performed of all cosmetic dental procedures. A patient's perception regarding his or her appearance is critical in determining whether tooth whitening is sought and/or accepted. The dentist and dental hygienist may be satisfied with the results of a prescribed whitening treatment, but the patient may or may not be satisfied, again depending on his or her perception.

I. Treatment Options: Restoration or Whitening

A. Restoration

Occasionally, tooth whitening fails to achieve the desired cosmetic result. When the discoloration or stain is severe, restoration of the tooth may be the treatment of choice. Full crowns, either all porcelain or porcelain bonded to metal, require a significant amount of tooth removal from all surfaces. Facial veneers, either porcelain or composite, are a more conservative restorative option because less tooth removal is required. In some clinical situations, restoration of teeth may not be the preferred treatment because of the need to conserve tooth structure. A treatment plan may include whitening of some teeth and restoration of others. When restoration of teeth is planned in conjunction

with whitening, whitening is usually accomplished first so that the esthetic restorations can then be matched to the resulting shade of the whitened natural teeth. An immediate relapse in the whitening effect occurs immediately after the treatment is completed. For this reason, esthetic restoration of teeth should be delayed for 2 weeks after the completion of tooth whitening.

Restorative treatment that involves bonding to enamel, such as facial veneers, must be delayed for a minimum of 2 weeks after whitening is completed, because recently whitened tooth enamel produces a weaker bond to restorative materials.

B. Whitening

Whitening is the most conservative treatment option for the esthetic improvement of discolored or stained teeth. No tooth structure is sacrificed in the preparation of vital teeth for whitening. In the treatment of nonvital teeth, an opening into the pulp chamber, either from the lingual surface of anterior teeth or from the occlusal surface of posterior teeth, is necessary. Many factors potentially affect the outcome of the whitening procedure. The success of the procedure depends on the following factors:
- Cause or type of discoloration or stain
- Degree or intensity of discoloration or stain
- Whitening agent selected
- Strength of the whitening agent
- Length of exposure of the tooth to the whitening agent
- Whitening technique
- Vitality of the tooth
- Presence of a restoration in the tooth

II. Causes of Tooth Discoloration

A. Nonvital Teeth

A tooth with a necrotic pulp or one that has been endodontically treated has a tendency to darken with the passage of time. Significantly darkened teeth should be noted during clinical examination, and the cause of darkening should be investigated.

An injury to a tooth may cause the pulp tissue to become necrotic, with no sign or symptom of necrosis other than a noticeable darkening of the tooth. The decomposition of pulp tissues, especially the hemoglobin of the red blood cells, produces a dark stain that penetrates the dentinal tubules.

After a tooth has been diagnosed as nonvital, appropriate endodontic treatment must be performed. The most common endodontic procedure is root canal therapy. When a root canal procedure is performed, the contents of the pulp cavity, including both the root canal(s) and the coronal pulp chamber, are removed. The pulp chamber and root canal(s) are then filled with an inert material, such as **gutta-percha** (a natural resin). The entire procedure is performed under aseptic conditions and usually requires multiple appointments. After a nonvital tooth has been successfully treated, a full crown is usually recommended to strengthen the tooth. If an endodontically treated tooth is not restored with a crown, a nonvital whitening treatment may be performed to lighten the color (shade) of the darkened tooth.

B. Vital Teeth

Teeth are naturally white and bright, with a translucence that contributes to their brightness. Teeth vary in color or shade from person to person, and as teeth age, they also darken. Some patients may ask if the natural shade or color of their teeth can be changed to improve their appearance. Whitening may be an effective treatment option for the esthetic improvement of healthy natural teeth.

C. Stain

Both vital and nonvital teeth are subject to staining. There are two types or classifications of stain: extrinsic stain and intrinsic stain.

1. Extrinsic Stain
   An **extrinsic stain** occurs on the surface of the tooth. Causes of extrinsic staining include foods and drinks, such as coffee and tea, and tobacco, both smoked and smokeless. Some extrinsic staining can be removed, at least partially, by the patient using a toothbrush and dentifrice. Some dentifrices are formulated and marketed to aid in extrinsic stain removal, but they have limited effectiveness in removing severe staining. Extrinsic staining that is resistant to removal by the patient may be removed with scaling and polishing by the dentist or dental hygienist. Extrinsic stains that are resistant to complete removal can be effectively removed by whitening treatments. Whitening treatments are more effective against extrinsic than against intrinsic stains.

2. Intrinsic Stain
   An **intrinsic stain** occurs within tooth structures (enamel or dentin).
   a. *Posteruptive Stain*
      Some intrinsic stain occurs after the tooth erupts. Causes for this type of stain include the following:
      1. Amalgam restorations
         Stains caused by silver amalgam cannot be successfully removed by the whitening process.
      2. Caries
         Caries should be removed and the tooth restored before whitening is attempted.

3. Endodontic treatment (root canal therapy)
   Stains resulting from endodontic treatment can be successfully whitened.
b. *Preeruptive Stain*
   Other intrinsic stains occur before tooth eruption, when the teeth are in the formative or calcification stage. These stains include the following:
   1. Tetracycline Stain
      Tetracycline antibiotics that are ingested during tooth calcification may cause an intrinsic **tetracycline staining** of both dentin and enamel. Tetracycline binds chemically with the hydroxyapatite crystals of dentin and enamel. When tetracycline-stained dentin or enamel is exposed to a black (fluorescent) light, the tetracycline crystals produce a fluorescent glow. Under natural and artificial light, tetracycline stains appear as gray or brown stains of varying intensity, usually occurring in horizontal bands within the tooth. Tetracycline-stained teeth are difficult to whiten. The milder the staining, the more successful is the result.
   2. Fluorosis
      High levels of fluoride (>1 ppm) consumed from the drinking water during tooth formation and calcification may cause staining known as **fluorosis**. Fluoride-containing dentifrices and mouthwashes are potential sources of excessive systemic fluoride. Parents should be cautioned to supervise children who use a fluoride dentifrice or mouthwash to prevent accidental or intentional swallowing. In its milder form, fluorosis appears as white spots in the enamel, with no pitting. In more severe cases, fluorosis causes brown spotting and pitting of the enamel. Teeth with fluorosis are difficult to whiten. The milder the fluorosis, the more successful is the result.
   3. Dentinogenesis Imperfecta and Amelogenesis Imperfecta
      Dentinogenesis imperfecta and **amelogenesis imperfecta** are inherited conditions that result in defective dentin and enamel formation, respectively. Whitening will not significantly improve the appearance of teeth that are affected by dentinogenesis or amelogenesis imperfecta.

III. Whitening Agents

A. Hydrogen Peroxide

Hydrogen peroxide (H_2O_2) is a strong oxidizing agent that readily decomposes into water and oxygen. The decomposition of hydrogen peroxide

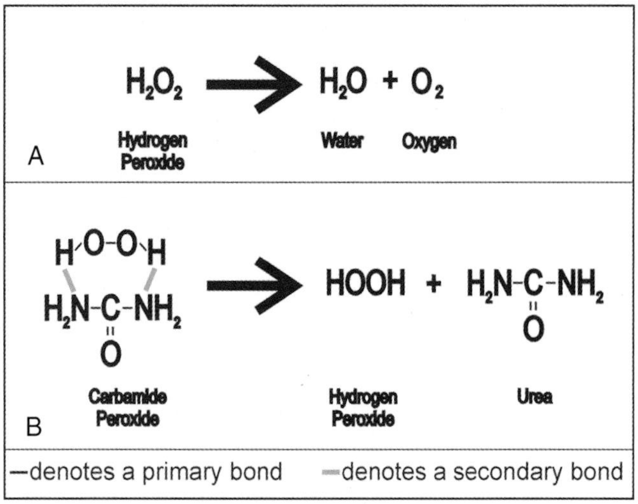

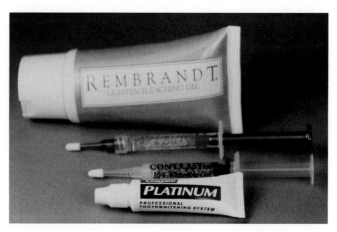

A
$$H_2O_2 \rightarrow H_2O + O_2$$
Hydrogen   Water   Oxygen
Peroxide

B
$$H\text{-}O\text{-}O\text{-}H$$
$$H_2N\text{-}C\text{-}NH_2 \rightarrow HOOH + H_2N\text{-}C\text{-}NH_2$$
        $\overset{\|}{O}$ $\overset{\|}{O}$

Carbamide   Hydrogen   Urea
Peroxide   Peroxide

—denotes a primary bond   ‒denotes a secondary bond

FIGURE 17.1. Decomposition of hydrogen peroxide. **A.** Hydrogen peroxide, a strong oxidizing agent, breaks down into water and oxygen. Oxygen reacts with the pigments in both extrinsic and intrinsic stains, producing the bleaching effect. **B.** Carbamide peroxide, a weaker oxidizing agent, breaks down into hydrogen peroxide and urea.

releases free radicals of oxygen that react with pigments in both extrinsic and intrinsic stains, producing the whitening effect. Free radicals of oxygen contain an unpaired electron and, therefore, are highly reactive. *Figure 17.1A* illustrates the decomposition of hydrogen peroxide into water and free radicals of oxygen.

Hydrogen peroxide can penetrate enamel and dentin and may produce a **reversible pulpitis**, which is a temporary inflammation of the pulp tissue. Tooth sensitivity resulting from pulpitis is the most frequently reported side effect of the whitening process. Precautions must be taken to protect the patient's eyes, face, and intraoral soft tissues (lips, cheeks, and tongue), as well as the patient's clothes from hydrogen peroxide solutions.

Hydrogen peroxide is applied to the teeth in either a liquid or a gel form and in strengths varying from 5% to 35%. *Figure 17.2* shows an example of a hydrogen peroxide tooth whitening agent (Zoom, Discus Dental).

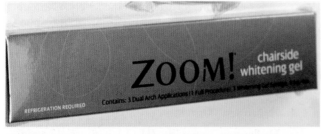

FIGURE 17.2. Zoom chairside hydrogen peroxide whitening agent. (Discus Dental).

FIGURE 17.3. Carbamide peroxide whitening gels.

B. Carbamide Peroxide

Carbamide peroxide ($CH_6N_2O_3$) is a complex (secondary bonds) of two molecules, urea and hydrogen peroxide. It is applied to the teeth in either a liquid or a gel form and in strengths varying from 10% to 20%. *Figure 17.3* shows examples of a carbamide peroxide gel (Rembrandt; Dent Mat, Santa Monica, CA) and paste (Colgate Platinum; Colgate Palmolive, New York, NY).

Carbamide peroxide decomposes into urea and hydrogen peroxide. Hydrogen peroxide then breaks down into water and oxygen (*Fig. 17.1B*). A 10% carbamide peroxide solution is equivalent to 3% hydrogen peroxide, whereas a 15% solution is equivalent to 5% hydrogen peroxide. Carbamide peroxide products are more stable (longer shelf life) than are hydrogen peroxide products. Most carbamide peroxide whitening gels contain Carbopol (BF Goodrich, Richfield, OH), which is a thickening agent that increases adhesion of the gel to the tooth, thereby prolonging exposure to the whitening agent.

C. Sodium Perborate

Sodium perborate is another weak oxidizing agent. It is sometimes used together with hydrogen peroxide to whiten nonvital teeth. Sodium perborate is the active ingredient in many household fabric bleaches, which are designated as being safe for colors.

IV. Whitening Techniques

A. Nonvital Whitening

Prior to the whitening procedure, a nonvital tooth endodontic treatment must be completed. The canal is opened by removal of the gutta-percha. Two methods can be used to attain bleaching: a power (heat- and light-activated) whitening or a walking bleach method.

The power whitening is done similarly to the vital tooth bleaching. Once the pulp chamber is cleared of debris, a bur may be used to clear the canal. The canal is sealed and the tooth is isolated with a resin dam. An in-office heat-, light-, or laser-activated bleaching material may be applied to the coronal surface of the tooth. Once activated and whitening is attained, the canal may be filled with an esthetic restorative material. Research has shown that bond strength of materials is weakest immediately after bleaching. With the weak bond postbleaching, esthetic restorations must be placed at least 7 days after the whitening procedure, preferably after 2 weeks.

Nonvital **walking bleach** is a second method of lightening endodontically treated teeth. Sodium perborate mixed with 35% hydrogen peroxide or one of the commercial in-office bleaches is placed in the cleared canal. The canal is packed with a cotton pellet and sealed with zinc phosphate or IRM. The endodontic patient will retain the bleach within the canal for 3 to 7 days; at that time, the patient will be reevaluated for results. The method can weaken the bond between tooth surface and esthetic restorations. Therefore, restorations must be done no sooner than 7 days after bleaching. Walking bleach can also increase free radical formation in the root canal of a nonvital tooth and lead to external resorption. Because of these side effects, the walking bleach method is not done as frequently.

B. Vital Whitening

Since the introduction of an effective patient-applied technique in 1989, tooth whitening has grown rapidly in popularity. Two whitening techniques are most popular:
- A professionally applied, in-office technique
- A patient-applied (at-home), professionally supervised technique. Over-the-counter whitening products are also available to the public. Some of these are not recommended; however, because they are used without professional supervision. These are discussed later in this section.
- As with any treatment modality, case selection is an important factor in determining a successful outcome. When vital teeth are to be whitened, the time that is required to achieve the desired result will vary with the technique that is chosen as well as with the type and degree of stain or discoloration. It would be difficult to say that one whitening technique is superior to another in terms of the final result that is achieved.

- It is important to note that the results achieved with any tooth whitening technique are not permanent. Some degree of relapse can be expected. Retreatment may be necessary as early as 6 months after initial treatment. For most patients, a retreatment frequency of every 2 years can be expected.

1. **Professionally Applied, In-Office Whitening**
   The professionally applied, in-office whitening technique is often referred to as **power whitening**. As power whitening uses higher concentrations of hydrogen peroxide (15–35%), all soft tissues and eyes must be protected. Teeth to be whitened are isolated with a rubber dam or a paint-on liquid resin dam. Often, a light- or heat-activated method of accelerating the bleaching process is utilized, but their effectiveness has been questioned.

   The paint-on resin dam (e.g., Liquid Dam or Pulpdent Kool-Dam) has become popular and is replacing the use of the conventional rubber dam. The paint-on resin dam may be autocure or light cure. When using a paint-on resin dam, the gingiva, tongue, and facial mucosa are protected with a coat of a petroleum-based lubricant. *Figure 17.4* illustrates proper isolation for the power whitening procedure. In addition, the patient's eyes are protected with appropriate safety glasses.

   Hydrogen peroxide is usually supplied in a gel form and delivered to the teeth from a syringe. The hydrogen peroxide is then activated with heat using a variety of lights, some being resin-curing lights. Many in-office bleaching products have a chemical added to absorb light and warm the bleaching material. To avoid damage to the vital pulp, care must be taken not to apply too

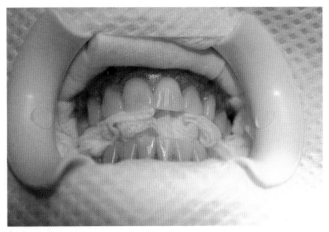

FIGURE 17.4. Patient isolated with retractors, cotton rolls, gauze, and paint-on resin dental dam awaiting power (light-/heat-activated) whitening procedure.

much heat to the teeth. In addition, the teeth must not be anesthetized with local anesthesia because this would prevent the patient from responding to painful stimulation produced by excessive heat.

2. Laser Whitening

Laser whitening utilizes a laser beam, either argon or carbon dioxide, that is applied to the teeth to activate the whitening agent. In addition to activating the whitening agent, the argon laser interacts directly with dark stains to neutralize them, but it becomes less effective in directly neutralizing stains as the tooth whitens.

Laser whitening is the most rapid whitening technique that is currently available; however, extra caution must be exercised. Both the patient and the dental team must wear special safety glasses to protect the eyes from the energy of the laser beam. Laser whitening is usually completed in one appointment. Laser whitening must be used with caution. Compared to other lights used to activate bleach, the laser is the only one that can increase intrapulpal temperature and cause dental pulp necrosis. Lasers should never be used at full power for vital bleaching.

Whitening enhancement swabs, an aqueous cleaning technology and product of GRINrx Corporation, have been introduced as a pre-bleaching procedure used to clean and remove stains prior to the power whitening procedure. The system combines the elements of time and action with solvents, surfactants, chelators, and saponifiers. The material elements are available in a convenient swab. The tooth is swabbed to remove debris and stain, enhancing the overall whitening procedure. Some evidence suggests that the procedure hydrates the tooth before the bleaching procedure that subsequently dehydrates tooth structure.

3. Patient-Applied, Professionally Supervised Whitening

Either hydrogen peroxide or carbamide peroxide may be used in the patient-applied, professionally supervised technique. Results of patient-applied whitening depend primarily on the strength of the whitening agent and the length of the treatment.

a. Hydrogen Peroxide

Hydrogen peroxide gels in strengths varying from 2% to 10% are dispensed by the patient into custom-made resin trays. The trays are worn over the teeth for multiple treatment sessions of 30 minutes each. The resin trays are commonly made by the dental

hygienist. This procedure includes making alginate impressions, fabricating gypsum casts, and trimming the tray. Chapter 31, Vital Tooth Whitening: Patient-Applied, Professionally Supervised Clinical and Laboratory Procedures, provides a step-by-step procedure to fabricate resin trays for the patient-applied, professionally supervised technique.

Another whitening technique in this category was introduced by Procter and Gamble (Cincinnati, OH) in 2000. Crest "Whitestrips" are available to the patient both over the counter and professionally; the difference between the two products is the strength of the hydrogen peroxide contained in the strip. The strips adhere to the facial surfaces of the anterior teeth. No tray is needed. The Whitestrips contain anywhere from 3% to 14% hydrogen peroxide and are worn twice a day for 30 minutes each. *Figures 17.5* and *17.6* illustrate professional whiten strips and their application.

Whitestrips Supreme are professional whiten strips from Proctor and Gamble containing the highest concentration of peroxide. The hydrogen peroxide concentration is 14%. Whitestrips Supreme is only available via a dental professional. The 14% strips

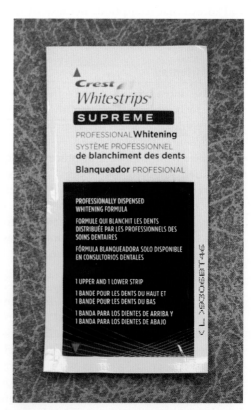

FIGURE 17.5. Individual Crest Whitestrip Packet containing upper and lower strip.

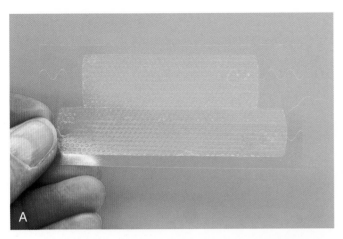 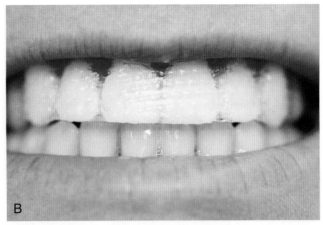

FIGURE 17.6. **A.** Crest Professional Whitestrips removed from packet. **B.** Whitestrip in place on maxillary surfaces.

are applied in the same manner as the lower concentrations. Strips are applied over the facial smile line of the dentition's upper and lower arches and worn for 30 minutes twice per day. The concentration allows these strips to work faster. The patient should be monitored by their dentist throughout the procedure.

Hydrogen peroxide in 6%, 10%, and 15% concentrations are also available from Ultradent in the Opalescence product, Go. The product is a patient-applied tray infused with hydrogen peroxide. The trays are designed to adapt and fit snugly to the teeth. The patient seats the tray on the teeth and purses the lips to draw in and form the tray around the dentition. Depending on the concentrations, the trays remain in place 60 to 90 minutes for those with 6% hydrogen peroxide, 30 to 60 minutes for those with 10% hydrogen peroxide, and 15 to 20 minutes for those with 15% hydrogen peroxide. Patients should discontinue use if sensitivity occurs. *Figure 17.7* includes photographs of the package, trays, the trays in place, and after removal of the supporting outer green tray.

b. *Carbamide Peroxide*
Carbamide peroxide gel in strengths from 10% to 22% is dispensed by the patient into custom-made resin trays. The trays are worn during the day for multiple treatment sessions of 2 hours each. Alternatively, the patient may choose to wear the trays for 8 hours while sleeping.

In February 2008, the American Dental Association (ADA) issued a statement on the safety and effectiveness of tooth whitening products. Dentist-dispensed and

over-the-counter whitening products are eligible for the Seal of Acceptance on the product packaging indicating ADA approval, as shown in Figure 1.1. Since the section for professionally applied products was discontinued from December 31, 2007, professionally applied bleach whiteners are not eligible for the ADA Seal.

c. *Professional Whitening and Stain-Removing Swabs*
Power Swabs Corporation introduced as a prebleaching cleaning product, Power Swabs, to clean and remove stains at home (*see Figure 17.8*). Use is described on the manufacturer's Web site. The detergent technology using solvents and other ingredients claims to enhance bleaching and reduce sensitivity. The swab can be dentist dispensed for touch-up enhancement. In the future, the convenient swab may find its way into hospitals, restaurants, and cafes as an alternative to tooth brushing.

4. Over-the-Counter Whitening Products (Patient-Applied, Unsupervised Whitening)
a. *Crest Whitestrips*
To date, the only over-the-counter product with demonstrated safety and efficacy is Crest Whitestrips. The over-the-counter strips are identical to the professional strips, except that they contain a less concentrated whitening agent (3–7% hydrogen peroxide gel). They are applied to the facial surface of the anterior teeth twice daily for 30 minutes each.

b. *Whitening Dentifrices*
The effect of whitening dentifrices is achieved primarily through the mechanical removal of extrinsic stain by an abrasive. Common abrasives include **hydrated silica, precipitated**

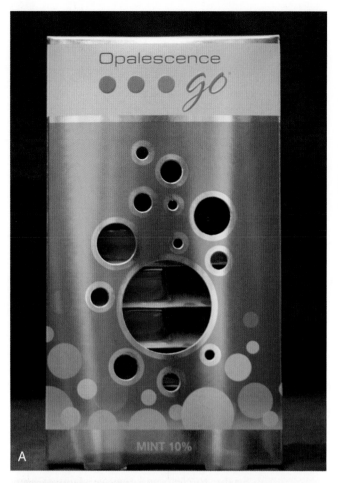

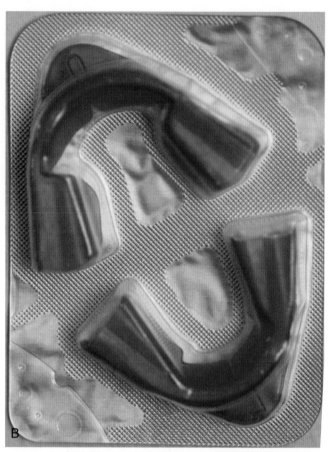

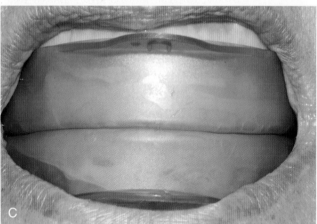

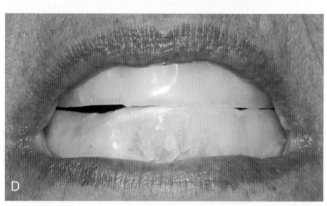

FIGURE 17.7. **A.** Opalescence Go Package. **B.** Trays. **C.** Placement of both the supporting green and the clear H$_2$O$_2$ prefilled tray in place. **D.** Adapted clear tray after patient removes the outer green tray.

calcium carbonate, and **dicalcium phosphate dihydrate**. Some whitening dentifrices contain a peroxide that also contributes to the whitening effect. Among the peroxides are hydrogen peroxide, **calcium peroxide**, and **sodium percarbonate**.

Whitening dentifrices, although somewhat effective in maintaining whitened teeth, are not as effective as whitening agents applied in the office or by the patient in a tray or on a strip. Examples of whitening dentifrices are shown in *Figure 17.9*.

c. Additional Products
With consumer demand at an increasingly high level, many additional whitening products are available. Chewing gum, floss, mouth rinses, pens, flexible waxlike strips, and even bleaching trays with light systems

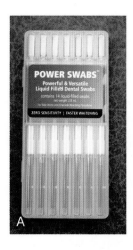

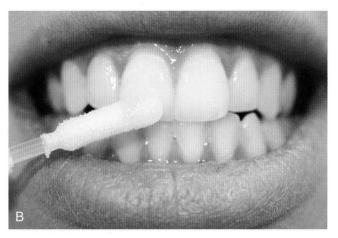

FIGURE 17.8. Power Swabs. **A.** Package. **B.** Self-application *to central incisor.*

claim to whiten or brighten the dentition. Listerine has a whitening pen available over the counter. The pen is a whitening product dispensed from a swab for hard-to-reach tooth surfaces. Suggested application is one to three times daily up to 2 weeks. Many of the products do not have any solid scientific studies to substantiate their whitening capabilities or their safety to the dentition. Dental hygienists and patients must be aware that many of these products do not have ADA approval.

V. Side Effects of Whitening

Tooth sensitivity and gingival irritation are the most frequently reported side effects of whitening. Both side effects are transient, usually lasting no more than a few days after treatment is discontinued.

A. Gingival Irritation

Gingival irritation may occur when a whitening agent exudes out of the tray or when accidentally leached onto the tissue during a power whitening procedure. Care must be taken to protect the gingival tissues completely with a conventional rubber or paint-on resin dam during in-office procedures. With patient-applied trays, the tray should be trimmed to produce a scalloped border that ends on the teeth rather than on the gingiva.

B. Tooth Sensitivity

Tooth sensitivity occurs either from pressure by a tray that is too rigid or from the whitening agent itself. If the whitening agent alone is suspected, tooth sensitivity is effectively treated by discontinuing treatment and, if necessary, topical application of either **neutral sodium fluoride** or **potassium nitrate**. The desensitizing agent can be applied in the whitening tray for 30 minutes twice daily until sensitivity is controlled.

Use of a potassium nitrate toothpaste 2 weeks prior to and during bleaching has been documented as an effective method of preventing sensitivity during the whitening process. An increase in intrapulpal temperature during heat-, light-, or laser-activated bleaching may result in reversible pulpitis. Lasers should be used at the lowest setting for bleaching to avoid pulpal necrosis.

C. Enamel Breakdown

With the high demand for whitening, products offered at spas and mall kiosks often contain chlorine dioxide, which can cause enamel damage. Staining, pitting, and enamel loss have been documented with the use of this agent. Patients must be made aware of the use of chlorine dioxide as an ingredient and its potential harm.

D. Potential Side Effects

Any bleaching procedure using peroxides will produce free radicals. Free radicals have been linked with cancers. With time, more severe consequences may be discovered with long-term overuse and abusive bleaching procedures. Patients with other

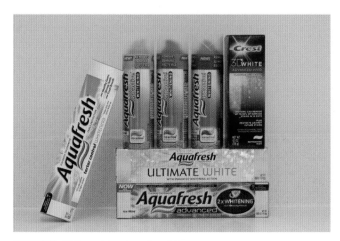

FIGURE 17.9. Whitening dentifrices.

risk factors for oral cancer, tobacco, and excessive alcohol use should be cautioned to carefully follow instructions.

VI. Concerns for the Dental Hygienist

Patients tend to rely on recommendations and advice from their dental hygienist. With the increasing demand for tooth whitening from the dental professional, the hygienists must educate their patients about the procedure. Patients must be informed of both contraindications and side effects of whitening. Studies have shown that patients experience less sensitivity when the whitening procedure is done with dental supervision.

A. Contraindications for Whitening

Patients should not bleach if:

1. The patient is unwilling to replace anterior restorations after the bleaching. Patients with esthetic anterior restorations must be informed that whitening will not change the appearance (shade) of those restorations.
2. Enamel is cracked or hypoplastic.
3. Carious lesions are present.
4. Cervical abrasions, sensitive recession areas, or tooth sensitivity is found.
5. Undergoing radiation or chemotherapy. NO use of light-activated systems.
6. Diagnosed with melanoma. NO use of light-activated systems.
7. Using photosensitive drugs or photosensitive herbal remedies. NO use of light-activated systems.
8. If nonvital tooth was extensively restored. Nonvital teeth are inherently weaker and the bleach creates an even weaker tooth structure so only nonvital teeth with minor restorations should be considered for nonvital bleach.
9. Amalgam stains in dentinal tubules must not undergo nonvital bleaching since the product will not whiten those areas.

B. Factors to Consider When Tray Whitening

1. Tooth sensitivity may be prevented with the use of a dentifrice containing potassium nitrate 2 weeks prior to, during, and after the whitening procedure.
2. Gingival sensitivity may be prevented by using scalloped trays. Patients must not dab more than one dot of bleaching material to the facial surfaces of the tray. More material does not result in faster bleaching. Apply and wipe any bleach from gingival surfaces.

3. Gingival sensitivity may warrant discontinuing the procedure for 1 to 2 days. If sensitivity remains upon resuming the procedure, see your dental professional.
4. Reversible pulpitis may occur. Patients may need to discontinue whitening for 1 to 2 days or see their dentist if sensitivity continues.
5. Sensitivity can be reduced by use of neutral sodium fluoride or potassium nitrate twice daily for 30 minutes in nightguard tray.
6. Remind patients using over-the-counter systems to search for products with the ADA seal of approval.

C. Factors to Consider When Power Whitening

1. Gingival sensitivity or irritation may occur. Use of a vitamin E oil may soothe the tissues.
2. Prophylactic use of nonsteroidal anti-inflammatory drugs may prevent effects of reversible pulpitis before and after the procedure.
3. Patient should avoid foods that stain (tea, coffee, mustard, red sauces) for 24 to 48 hours.
4. Use of neutral sodium fluoride or potassium nitrate twice daily for 30 minutes can help reduce sensitivity.
5. Additional nightguard bleaching can enhance power bleaching procedure; do not use if gingival irritation or tooth sensitivity occur.
6. Mouth rinses, dentifrices, and nightguard bleaching can be used to maintain whitening or for touch-up of whitening.
7. Dentist must be notified if sensitivity lasts more than 2 days after the whitening procedure.

D. Overbleaching

Overbleaching one's dentition could be a sign of body dysmorphic disorder (BDD). BDD is a disorder where one is never satisfied with their looks. Just as this disorder applies to shapes and body sizes, the disorder now includes tooth whiteness. Patients who whiten become obsessed with the color and the words "too light" or "too white" does not seem to be in their vocabulary. Although dental hygiene professionals are not psychiatrists or psychologists, they must try to identify such patients. Recognizing a patient's obsessive need to overbleach and prevent further abuse may save the dental health of that patient. Be aware of those patients already using an at-home whitening procedure and seeking higher strength peroxides. Evaluate the dentition for an overly white and chalky look. Advise these patients of dental health consequences such as sensitivity, pain, and pulpal necrosis.

Summary

Tooth whitening has become the most popular esthetic procedure and the most requested dental procedure. Teeth can be whitened in the office by the dentist or staff (dental hygienist) or at home by the patient. To enhance safety of whitening, professional supervision is recommended. Side effects of whitening include tooth sensitivity and gingival irritation, which are usually mild and abate within a day or 2 after treatment is discontinued. Patients must be made aware that pulpal necrosis could occur in rare cases. Any bleaching procedure using peroxides could produce free radicals. Free radicals have been linked to cancers. With time, more severe consequences may be discovered with long-term use, overuse, and abusive bleaching procedures. The dental hygienist plays an important role in identifying who may benefit from whitening and those who may be harmed by whitening. All dental professionals should be familiar with the ADA's Statement on Effectiveness and Safety of Tooth Whitening Products.

Learning Activities

1. Find a coffee or tea cup that is stained inside from use. Fill the cup one-quarter full with 3% hydrogen peroxide, which can be found on the shelf of your local pharmacy. Let the cup stand uncovered for 24 hours. Empty the cup, and rinse with cool water. Note the difference in the appearance of the bleached and unbleached inner surfaces of the cup.

2. Hard-boil two white eggs, and brew a cup of strong tea. Completely immerse both eggs in the tea, and let them stand for 24 hours. Remove both eggs from the tea, and note the dark stain. Place one egg in a cup half-filled with 3% hydrogen peroxide, and let it stand for 24 hours. Remove and dry the egg, and compare the whitened egg to the tea-stained egg.

3. Visit the household cleaning products section of a grocery store. Select several fabric bleaching products, including laundry detergents with bleach. Read the ingredients list on the labels. Which ingredients are responsible for the bleaching effect that is claimed for the product? Is there one common ingredient in most of the "color safe" products?

4. Visit the dental products or health and beauty area of a drug or grocery store. Make note of the number and variety of products claiming tooth whitening. How many have an ADA Seal?

Review Questions

Question 1. The term "nonvital" may be used to describe a tooth that has:

a. Been treated with a root canal procedure

b. A necrotic pulp

c. No pulp tissue in the pulp cavity

d. All of the above

Question 2. Which of the following esthetic tooth treatments requires no removal of tooth structure?

a. Nonvital tooth whitening

b. Vital tooth whitening

c. Facial veneer

d. Porcelain-bonded-to-metal crown

Question 3. Which of the following statements is the most accurate?

a. Hydrogen peroxide is more stable than carbamide peroxide

b. Carbamide peroxide is used in the nonvital tooth whitening technique known as a walking bleach

c. Hydrogen peroxide decomposes into water and free radicals of oxygen

d. Carbamide peroxide is most often applied to teeth as a gel at a 35% concentration

Question 4. Which of the following variables is not a factor in the success of a vital tooth whitening treatment?

a. Number of teeth to be treated

b. Strength of the whitening agent

c. Type and intensity of discoloration or stain

d. Length of exposure of the tooth to the whitening agent

Question 5. Teeth with a moderate degree of _____ are the most difficult to successfully whiten.

a. Extrinsic food and beverage stain

b. Yellow intrinsic discoloration

c. Extrinsic tobacco stain

d. Tetracycline stain

Question 6. Which of the following statements is NOT true regarding tooth sensitivity from vital tooth whitening?

a. It is a common side effect

b. It is not reversible

c. It can be treated by topical application of potassium nitrate

d. It may be caused by a tray that is too rigid

Question 7. Which of the following is the most common esthetic procedure in dentistry?

a. Facial veneer

b. All-porcelain crown

c. Porcelain-bonded-to-metal crown

d. Tooth whitening

Question 8. Brushing with a potassium nitrate–containing dentifrice before and after bleaching is advised. During power bleaching, a patient must be anesthetized.

a. The first statement is true; the second statement is false.

b. The first statement is false; the second statement is true.

c. Both statements are true.

d. Both statements are false.

Question 9. When should a bleached tooth be restored with a composite restoration?

a. Immediately

b. 1 to 2 days

c. 3 to 4 days

d. 1 to 2 weeks

Question 10. All of the following are contraindications to light-activated bleaching procedures EXCEPT:

a. Use of photosensitive drugs

b. History of melanoma

c. Undergoing radiation therapy or chemotherapy

d. Previous use of nightguard bleaching system

Question 11. An aqueous cleaning technology used in prewhitening and touch-up whitening is dispensed in a:

a. Gel

b. Liquid

c. Strip

d. Swab

Question 12. Dental professionals should be aware that a statement on safety and effectiveness of whitening products is available through the:

a. Whitening product manufacturers

b. SDS

c. ADA

d. ADHA

Oral Appliances

Christine Nathe, R.D.H., M.S.

Objectives

After studying this chapter, the student will be able to do the following:

1. List the different oral appliances used in dentistry.
2. Describe the reasons for the use of oral appliances.
3. Name the different thermoplastic materials used in the fabrication of oral appliances, and discuss the properties of these materials.
4. Explain the steps involved in fabricating an oral appliance.
5. Describe the proper maintenance of oral appliances.
6. Prepare a script or dialogue that may be used for patient education regarding oral appliances.

Key Words/Phrases

athletic mouthguard
custom-made mouthguard
fluoride custom trays
mouth-formed guard
obstructive sleep apnea
oral appliances
stock mouthguard
thermoplastic
thermoset
vacuum former
whitening tray

Introduction

Oral appliances are made from a variety of materials: thermoplastic polymers, thermoset polymers, wires, bands, and other prefabricated parts. Thermoplastic materials have an advantage over other types of materials in that they are easily used to construct an oral appliance. They simply are heated and molded into the desired shape. Thermoplastic materials are increasingly used in the dental office to serve a variety of needs.

As dental hygienists, it is our responsibility to inform the patient of the need for an oral appliance, the care that is required to maintain it, and any possible side effects. **Oral appliances** currently available to patients include athletic mouthguards, whitening trays, fluoride custom trays, orthodontic appliances, nightguards, periodontal stints, space maintainers, and appliances for the treatment of obstructive sleep apnea (OSA) and snoring as well as nonnutritive (thumb) sucking. These appliances, along with their purposes, are listed in Table 18.1. Two different oral appliances are illustrated in *Figures 18.1* and *18.2*.

Some oral appliances, such as athletic mouthguards and custom fluoride trays, are relatively easy to make in the laboratory area of a typical dental practice. This chapter discusses several types of oral appliances and provides a summary of the fabrication procedure for fluoride trays and mouthguards.

TABLE 18.1. The Purpose of Oral Appliances

Appliance	Purpose
Appliances for nonnutritive sucking habits	To help stop the habit of sucking thumb/fingers
Athletic mouthguards	To prevent orofacial injury
Whitening trays	To hold whitening solution in close proximity to dentition to "whiten teeth"
Fluoride custom tray	To hold prescription fluoride gel trays in close proximity to dentition; to decrease the occurrence of demineralization and increase remineralization
Orthodontic retainers	To stabilize teeth after movement
Nightguards	To alleviate tooth surface wear
Periodontal stints	To hold anesthetic and antiseptic materials after periodontal surgery and/or to hold gingival flaps during surgery
Snoring/sleep apnea appliances	To advance the mandible, which will decrease airway obstruction during sleep, thus alleviating snoring and mild-to-moderate cases of sleep apnea
Space maintainer	To temporarily hold teeth in position
Tooth positioners	To provide minor tooth movement

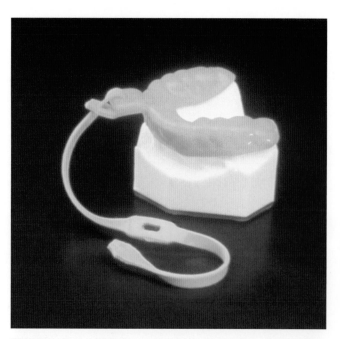

FIGURE 18.1. Athletic mouthguard. (Courtesy of Great Lakes Orthodontics, Ltd.)

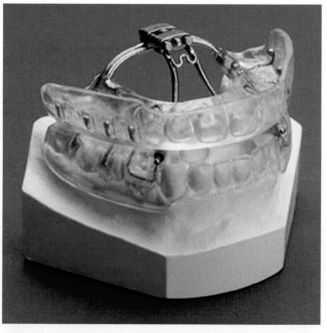

FIGURE 18.2. Klearway appliance for the treatment of snoring and obstructive sleep apnea. (Courtesy of Great Lakes Orthodontics, Ltd.)

I. Types of Oral Appliances

A. Athletic Mouthguards

An **athletic mouthguard** is a removable oral appliance that protects the teeth and surrounding tissues during contact sports (see Figs. 1.12, *18.1*, and *18.3*). The athletic mouthguard, which is sometimes referred to as a mouth protector, provides protection against injuries to the teeth and supporting structures by absorbing energy. The force of the blow is spread over many teeth, and contact between maxillary and mandibular teeth is prevented. The mouthguard is dually capable of realigning and repositioning the jaws so that the condyles of the mandible do not contact the soft tissues of the joints, thus avoiding injury to these areas. Mouthguards are used to prevent orofacial trauma during contact sports and other recreational activities.

1. Advantages

Research has shown a significant decrease in injuries when a mouthguard is used. Injuries that can be decreased by wearing an athletic mouthguard include tooth avulsion, fractured teeth, gingival and/or mucosal injuries, jaw fractures, neck injuries, and concussions.

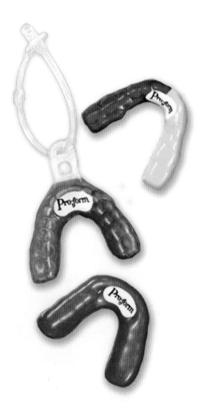

FIGURE 18.3. Athletic mouthguard. (Courtesy of Dental Arts Lab, Inc.)

2. Popularity

Mouthguards have been used since the 1950s. Many athletic associations, including the National Collegiate Athletic Association (NCAA), mandate their use. Interestingly, most professional sports do not require the use of mouthguards, but most professional athletes wear them voluntarily. The use of mouthguards by these professionals is an excellent example of a health promotional activity.

3. Wide Application

Mouthguards are recommended for a variety of contact sports and recreational activities. These are listed in Table 18.2.

TABLE 18.2. American Dental Association Recommended Activities for Use of Athletic Mouthguards

Acrobatics

Baseball

Basketball

Bicycling

Boxing

Equestrian events

Field events including discus, pole vault, and shot put

Field hockey

Football

Gymnastics

Handball

Ice hockey

In-line skating

Lacrosse

Martial arts

Racquetball

Rugby

Skateboarding

Skiing

Skydiving

Soccer

Softball

Squash

Surfing

Volleyball

Water polo

Weight lifting

Wrestling

4. Encouraging the Use of Mouthguards

Many patients are unaware of the necessity for wearing an athletic mouthguard when playing contact sports or enjoying recreational activities. Dental hygienists are responsible for educating patients on the importance of the athletic mouthguard and the need to use it in all situations. Research suggests that the earlier a child starts wearing a mouthguard during amateur sports, the higher the compliance rate will be when he or she plays in more organized, competitive sports. In fact, younger, inexperienced children are more likely than older athletes to sustain orofacial injuries. Therefore, the importance of wearing a mouthguard is greater for these young participants.

5. Types

Three types of athletic mouthguards exist.

a. The **stock mouthguard** is available in different sizes. It is not custom-made, nor is it preferred (because of poor fit and excess bulk).

b. A **mouth-formed guard**, which is generally referred to as a "boil-and-bite" style, can be heated in water and then placed in the mouth. The athlete bites into the guard, and an inexact fit is produced. This type of mouthguard can become distorted and does not accommodate an individual athlete's unique oral features.

c. The most effective mouthguard is the **custom-made mouthguard**. This type of mouthguard is custom-fabricated and fits precisely over the individual athlete's dentition. Because it is more comfortable and better fitting, compliance is increased; therefore, the custom-made mouthguard is better at reducing injuries. This type of mouthguard does need to be replaced, however, when changes occur to the athlete's dentition. See Table 18.3 for information on ideal mouthguard properties.

B. Fluoride Custom Trays

Fluoride custom trays are ideal for patients who have a high prevalence of dental caries or high caries risk (*see Fig. 18.4*). These trays are custom-made to fit the particular individual's dentition so that all tooth surfaces are covered with fluoride gel. Furthermore, these trays can be fabricated in the dental office by using the method described later in this chapter.

1. Qualifying Conditions

Use of fluoride custom trays is indicated for the following oral conditions:

- A high incidence or risk of dental caries, including rampant enamel or root caries
- Xerostomia

TABLE 18.3. Ideal Mouthguard Properties

To provide adequate protection, a mouthguard should:

- Be properly fitted to the wearer's mouth and accurately adapted to his or her oral structures
- Be made of resilient material approved by the U.S. FDA and cover all remaining teeth on one arch, customarily the maxillary
- Stay in place comfortably and securely
- Be physiologically compatible with the wearer
- Be relatively easy to clean
- Have high-impact energy absorption and reduce transmitted forces upon impact

Adapted from American Dental Association. Using mouthguards to reduce the incidence and severity of sports-related oral injuries. J Am Dent Assoc. 2006;137(12):1712–1720.

- Overdentures
- Hypersensitivity
- Radiation therapy

2. Compatible Gels

Types of fluoride gels that may be placed in the custom-made tray include

- Acidulated phosphate fluoride (0.5%)
- Sodium fluoride (1.1%)
- Stannous fluoride (0.4%)

3. Increasing Awareness

Dental hygienists should educate patients about the causes of dental caries and the role that fluoride plays in prevention of demineralization and the remineralization of teeth.

4. Other Uses

Although not thoroughly studied, these trays have been used for the treatment of dentin hypersensitivity by using desensitizing agents instead of fluoride. Remineralization is the

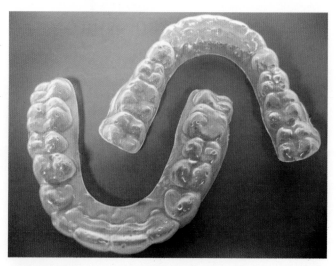

FIGURE 18.4. A fluoride custom tray. (Courtesy of Dental Arts Lab, Inc.)

process of restoring mineral ions to the tooth structure. There are calcium phosphate, arginine, and potassium nitrate products available that advertise that they may aid in the remineralization process when placed in a custom tray. These are used for caries prevention and dentinal hypersensitivity.

C. Orthodontic Appliances (Tooth Positioners)

Orthodontic appliances may be used to correct overbites, overjets, spacing problems, and slight malocclusions. Several types of thermoplastic orthodontic appliances are used. During the final stages of orthodontic treatment, tooth positioners are used to attain the final, precise position of the teeth. In cases involving only minor movements of the dentition, an oral appliance such as the Invisalign system (Align Technologies, Inc., Santa Clara, CA) can be used (*Fig. 18.5*).

During fabrication of both types of appliances, the teeth on the study model are removed. They are repositioned into their proper alignment with a hard baseplate wax used to hold the teeth in place. An impression of the corrected study model is then taken, and both a cast and an oral appliance are fabricated from this second impression. The patient may need to wear the appliance at night and possibly during the day as well.

Other orthodontic appliances include retainers and active appliances. They are fabricated from wires, bands, and thermoset resins. Several were discussed in Chapter 13, Specialty Materials.

D. Nightguards

Nightguards are prescribed for patients with bruxism. The function of the nightguard is simply to absorb the forces of clenching, thereby alleviating wear on the dentition. It is more cost-effective to periodically replace the appliance than to repair the damage to the dentition. Most patients will need to wear a nightguard only during sleep, but in extreme cases, it may also be worn during the day (*Fig. 18.6*).

E. Space Maintainers

A space maintainer is a temporary appliance that is used when primary teeth have been lost prematurely (Fig. 13.11F and G). The purpose of this appliance is to prevent the adjacent teeth from drifting and closing the space before the eruption of the succeeding, permanent teeth. Thus, crowding and the need for orthodontics are reduced. Both removable and fixed space maintainers are available.

F. OSA/Snoring Appliances

Oral appliances are also currently being used to treat **obstructive sleep apnea** (OSA) and snoring. OSA is thought to be caused by a reduced upper airway size and altered upper airway muscle

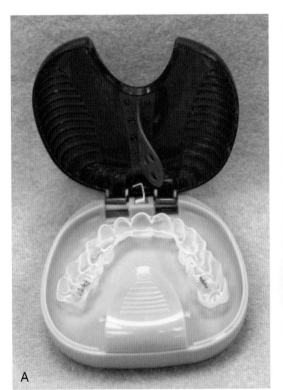
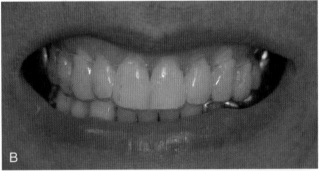
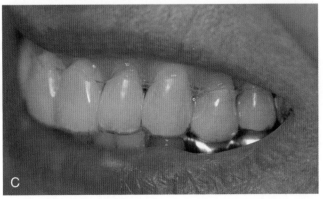

FIGURE 18.5. Invisalign appliance. **A.** Appliance in storage case. **B.** Appliance in place. **C.** Lateral view.

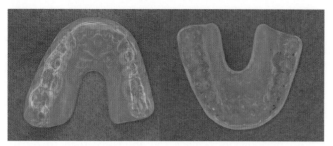

FIGURE 18.6. Nightguard. (Courtesy of Dr. James Foor, Morgantown, WV.)

activity. Positive airway pressure (PAP) remains the most common and effective treatment for sleep disordered breathing. However, there are more than 100 FDA-approved appliances currently on the market and do essentially the same thing. The goal is to advance the mandible and move the tongue forward, thus reversing some of these conditions. Patients with mild to moderate OSA and/or snoring wear this oral appliance during sleep hours. Some of these different appliances are referenced in the "Supplemental Readings" link on thePoint. Research suggests that these appliances have no significant effect on the periodontium and rarely have a permanent effect on occlusion.

G. Whitening Trays

Recently, great emphasis has been placed on cosmetic dentistry and patients are increasingly interested in whitening their teeth, which was discussed in detail in Chapter 17, Tooth Whitening. Figure 31.10 shows a **whitening tray** designed for patient application at home. Whitening trays appear very similar to fluoride trays. The whitening process can sometimes create sensitivity to a few or more teeth. There are two methods to prevent or lessen this: desensitizing agents may be added to the whitening products, or patients may use topical fluoride in the trays before and after using whitening agents. Chapter 31, Vital Tooth Whitening: Patient-Applied, Professionally Supervised Clinical and Laboratory Procedures, addresses the fabrication of whitening trays.

H. Acrylic and Bis-Acryl (TRIAD) Appliances

Acrylic and bis-acryl materials are used for custom trays, provisional bridges, and denture relines and repairs. Bis-acryl appliances closely resemble traditional acrylic appliances. Both materials are considered to be thermoset polymers. The TRIAD system from Dentsply International uses light-activated polymerization and results in a faster curing time. Also, no methyl methacrylate monomer odor or hazard is involved. The TRIAD system, as shown in *Figure 18.7*, can also be used to fabricate orthodontic retainers and nightguards.

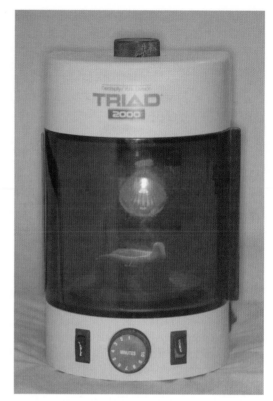

FIGURE 18.7. TRIAD 2000 visible light curing unit.

Fabrication of a custom impression tray using the TRIAD system is explained in Chapter 29, Fabrication of a Custom Impression Tray.

II. Materials Used in Fabrication

A. Definition

A variety of thermoplastic materials are used for the production of oral appliances. These are illustrated in *Figure 18.8* and listed in Table 18.4.

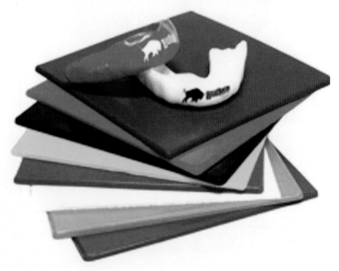

FIGURE 18.8. Thermoplastic materials. (Courtesy of Buffalo Dental Manufacturing Co., Inc.)

TABLE 18.4. Use of Thermoplastics	
Material	**Application**
Polycarbonates	Temporary crowns and bridges
	Orthodontic retainers
Polyethylene	Mouthguards
	Tooth positioners
	Nightguards
	Space maintainers
	Fluoride custom trays
	Stints
Polypropylene	Temporary crown and bridge molds
Polystyrenes	Custom impression trays
	Denture bases
Polyvinyl chloride	Splints
	Dual laminates
	Temporary removable partial denture (Flipper)
	Ortho retainers

The term **thermoplastic** implies that a polymer softens on heating and then hardens into the final shape upon cooling. This is a desirable property for an oral appliance because the final shape can be individualized for each case by using a study model. Occasionally, thermoset materials are used instead of thermoplastic materials for oral appliances. **Thermoset** materials are molded and then polymerized in the final shape. They are resistant to change when heated. Thermoplastic and thermoset polymers are discussed in Chapter 5, Direct Polymeric Restorative Materials.

B. Types

Most of the plastics that are used in the fabrication of simple oral appliances are thermoplastics. Polyethylene, polyvinyl chloride, polypropylene, polystyrenes, and polycarbonates comprise the majority of the thermoplastic materials that are used in the fabrication of oral appliances. In particular, polyethylene is used for the majority of oral appliances that may be made by the dental hygienist.

C. Properties

Each thermoplastic material has a specific major polymer component. Individualizing the addition of other components can affect the processing characteristics, physical properties, and the end performance. These are desirable properties because oral appliances are made for a variety of uses.

III. Fabrication of an Oral Appliance

This summary of the basic fabrication technique applies to most of the oral appliances that dental hygienists may fabricate "in-house." For a more complicated oral appliance, the hygienist may need to contact a laboratory. Construction of many oral appliances utilizes a vacuum former as shown in Figure 31.6. The vacuum former both heats (to soften the sheet material as shown in *Fig. 18.8*) and then molds the material onto a cast using a vacuum or suction through the cast.

The cast must show characteristics specific to the individual dentition, such as gingival margins and tooth anatomy, and must maintain occlusal relationships. Because it is porous, plaster is recommended for the model. Therefore, it is easier to create suction directly through the model. When using a suction type of vacuum former, drill a hole in the palatal or lingual area of the model to allow suction into these vacuum pockets.

After a model has been poured and trimmed, turn on the heating element of the **vacuum former** and preheat the machine for 2 to 3 minutes. The fabrication then proceeds as follows:

1. Select the appropriate thermoplastic material indicated for the particular appliance.
2. Spray the model and frame with a silicone spray to reduce sticking. Place the selected thermoplastic material into the frame, and latch it shut. Raise the frame to the heater, and allow the material to heat.
3. Each material has different thermal properties, so heating times will vary between plastics.
4. Let the material heat and sag. Thin materials will sag only a small amount (0.25–0.5 inch), and thicker materials, such as mouthguard material, will sag a greater distance (0.5–1.0 inch) before they are ready. Thus, the further the material slumps, the thinner it becomes.
5. After the material has been heated and slumped, lower the frame onto the model, and switch on the vacuum former. For the best adaptation, allow the suction to run for 20 to 30 seconds. For further adaptation, use a wet paper towel, and press the material around the model while the vacuum motor is still on.
6. Allow the material to cool on the model. Cooling times will vary between materials. To speed the cooling process, place both the molded plastic and the model in cold water.
7. Remove the appliance from the model.
8. Trim the appliance by using crown and bridge scissors for thinner materials and an acrylic bur for thicker and harder materials.

TABLE 18.5. Appropriate Technique for Finishing Appliance

Oral Appliance	Technique
Athletic mouthguard	Remove palatal area from model.
	Trim around the central frenum and lateral frena.
Whitening trays	Trim material along gingival margin.
Fluoride custom trays	Trim material along gingival margin.

9. Finish the appliance by using the appropriate technique described in Table 18.5. When trimming the appliance, the gingival margin should be replicated so that it fits properly and retention is ensured.

10. A criteria sheet for a whitening tray is included in Appendix 2. As mentioned previously, construction of a whitening tray is presented in Chapter 31, Vital Tooth Whitening: Patient-Applied, Professionally Supervised Clinical and Laboratory Procedures.

IV. Maintenance of an Oral Appliance

The dental literature suggests daily rinsing and brushing of appliances with a soft-bristled, wet toothbrush. Some oral appliances are supplied with brushes that can be used.

Professional cleaners are also available for soaking appliances. Cleaners generally are available for specific appliance materials.

Some oral appliances, particularly the "boil-and-bite" and stock appliances, should not be cleaned in hot water. This could lead to distortion.

With proper construction and maintenance, the custom-made oral appliance should last its recommended useful life, which is usually a minimum of 2 years.

Summary

Oral appliances are frequently used for a variety of reasons, ranging from treating OSA to whitening the teeth. Dental hygienists should be able to discuss with patients the reasons for using oral appliances and the proper procedures for maintaining oral appliances.

Thermoplastic materials are used in the fabrication of most oral appliances and usually require a cast of the patient's dentition. Dental hygienists should be familiar with the maintenance of each appliance and specific oral hygiene care for each patient.

 Learning Activities

1. Before fabricating an oral appliance for a student partner, practice on a study model. This provides time to learn the proper technique without encountering problems with model inconsistencies.

2. Fabricate an oral appliance on a student partner with close faculty supervision to clinical competency before completing appliances on patients.

3. Participate in role-playing activities regarding patient education for an athletic mouthguard, whitening tray, and fluoride custom tray.

4. Divide the class into several groups of approximately three to five students each, and assign an area high school to each group to research the following. Have the groups present their findings to the class.
   • The sports that require mouthguards
   • The kind of mouthguards used
   • If any injuries have occurred with their use
   • Any other comments coaches or players provide regarding mouthguards

Review Questions

Question 1. The purpose of wearing an oral appliance for OSA is to modify the position of upper airway structures so that:

a. The airway is enlarged
b. The airway is reduced
c. Collapsibility is reduced
d. Both a and c
e. Both b and c

Question 2. Patients wearing an oral appliance during sleep have NOT demonstrated a/an:

a. Increase in periodontal diseases
b. Decrease in periodontal diseases
c. Frequent occurrence of periodontal abscesses
d. Change in periodontal health

Question 3. Athletic mouthguards may prevent a concussion. However, they must be worn correctly and consistently.

a. The first statement is true; the second statement is false.
b. The first statement is false; the second statement is true.
c. Both statements are true.
d. Both statements are false.

Question 4. Nightguards are worn to:

a. Prevent dental caries
b. Alleviate tooth surface wear
c. Provide minor tooth movement or stabilization
d. Temporarily hold teeth in position

Question 5. Dental professionals fabricate stock mouthguards. Custom-made mouthguards can be purchased at most athletic and drug stores.

a. The first statement is true; the second statement is false.
b. The first statement is false; the second statement is true.
c. Both statements are true.
d. Both statements are false.

Question 6. Thermoplastic materials will _____ on heating and _____ on cooling.

a. Soften, reharden
b. Harden, soften
c. Harden, stay hard
d. Soften, melt

Question 7. Patients may clean oral appliances with a soft-bristled, wet toothbrush. No commercial products are available in which to soak oral appliances.

a. The first statement is true; the second statement is false.
b. The first statement is false; the second statement is true.
c. Both statements are true.
d. Both statements are false.

Question 8. Mouth protectors can be:

a. Custom-made
b. Stock
c. "Boil and bite"
d. All of the above

Question 9. Space maintainers are used to:

a. Alleviate bruxism
b. Hold the tongue in proper position
c. Temporarily hold teeth in position
d. Alleviate OSA

Question 10. Athletic mouthguards should be properly fitted, stay in place comfortably, be made of resilient material approved by the U.S. Food and Drug Administration, and:

a. Be physiologically compatible with the wearer
b. Have a fresh scent
c. Increase the amount of force placed on the occlusion
d. Be worn on the mandibular arch

Question 11. When fabricating an oral appliance, which of the following oral anatomical structures should be necessarily replicated?

a. Sulcus
b. Periodontal ligament
c. Gingival contours of the teeth
d. Soft palate

Question 12. Fluoride custom trays are recommended for which of the following patients?

a. Elderly patient with severe periodontal disease
b. Three-year-old patient with early childhood caries
c. Adult patient undergoing head or neck radiation therapy
d. Adolescent patient with severe halitosis

Instruments as Dental Materials—Care and Maintenance*

Andrea Warzynski, R.D.H., M.Ed.

Objectives

After studying this chapter, the student will be able to do the following:

1. Explain the basic differences between carbon steel and stainless steel instruments.
2. Discuss the processes of passivation and electropolishing.
3. Summarize the problems or conditions that can affect instruments, including corrosion, rust, pitting, spotting, and stains.
4. Explain why it is important to inspect instruments.
5. Explain the reasons for sharpening instruments, and determine the appropriate time and frequency of sharpening.
6. Discuss the cleaning of instruments, both immediately after use and when timely cleaning is not possible.
7. Recall the advantages and disadvantages of the four methods of sterilizing instruments.
8. Design an instrument maintenance schedule or cycle that could be used routinely in a private practice office setting.

Key Words/Phrases

carbon steel instruments

corrosion

electropolishing

passivation

pitting

rust

spotting

stainless steel alloy

tarnish

---

*Note: The information in this chapter is provided courtesy of Hu-Friedy Manufacturing Co., Inc.

Introduction

The previous chapters have discussed dental materials such as gypsum, cements, and impression and restorative materials, all of which are typically used in a dental practice. Other dental materials that are important to the dental hygienist but often overlooked are those that constitute dental instruments. It is a rare workday for a dental hygienist when a dental instrument goes unused. A hygienist's instruments are some of the most important items necessary to fulfill his or her professional responsibility.

Dental instruments represent a significant financial investment. For this reason alone, it would benefit the student to have a clear understanding of the materials from which they are made and what is necessary to keep them in good working condition. The amount of care that is given to dental instruments directly affects the lifetime of those instruments. The longer an instrument lasts, the greater return it yields on the financial investment.

This chapter addresses the composition, undesirable conditions, inspection, and care of instruments.

I. Composition of Instruments

Dental instruments are usually made of either carbon steel or stainless steel alloys. Some instruments have resin handles.

A. Carbon Steel Alloy

Carbon steel instruments are known for their hardness and ability to hold sharp, cutting edges. They are more sensitive than stainless steel instruments to chemicals, are susceptible to corrosion, and require special handling.

B. Stainless Steel Alloy

Major components of **stainless steel alloy** include iron, chromium, and nickel. The amount of carbon in a stainless steel alloy is directly related to the alloy's hardness and ability to hold a sharp, cutting edge. The addition of chromium enhances corrosion resistance, and nickel improves the mechanical properties of the metal. The problems with stainless steel instruments are discoloration, constant necessity of sharpening, and corrosion when exposed to certain chemicals. Some instruments are made with two kinds of stainless steel. One is hard and maintains a sharp edge; this is used to make the cutting edge or tip. The second is more resistant to corrosion and is welded or soldered to the first to form the handle.

The carbon in the alloy, which is necessary for hardness and a sharp edge, is the culprit that causes corrosion or rusting. Instrument manufacturers reduce surface corrosion by using two processes:

1. Passivation
   Passivation is a chemical process that creates a thin layer of chromium oxide on the surface of the instrument. This layer is transparent but tough, and it protects the underlying metal. After passivation, the instrument is much less likely to corrode.

2. Electropolishing
   Electropolishing produces a smooth, highly polished finish. A highly polished surface is less likely to corrode. Electropolishing is an efficient method for polishing complex shapes.

C. EverEdge 2.0 Technology

EverEdge 2.0 is the newest and most advanced scaler developed by Hu-Friedy Mfg. Co., Inc. EverEdge Technology was introduced about 10 years ago. This technology in metallurgy, heat treatment, and cryogenics is used in the manufacturing of instruments enabling their blades to stay sharper significantly longer when compared to other instruments. Recently, EverEdge 2.0 instruments have been developed. These instruments are designed to stay sharper even longer than the original EverEdge instruments. These instruments are not coated, but the long-lasting wear is present throughout the entire instrument tip. If the instrument stays sharper longer, there is less sharpening required and less hand fatigue. An EverEdge 2.0 instrument is illustrated in *Figure 19.1*.

D. Resin Handles

Some instruments may have resin handles. Inside the resin is a full-length, steel inner core for added strength and tactile sensitivity. The handles may have grooves and knurling to increase rotational control and to provide a light (but secure) grasp. Resin instruments and items require specific care.

E. Separation of Stainless Steel and Carbon Steel Instruments

Stainless steel and carbon steel instruments should be kept separate throughout the cleaning and sterilization process. If processed together, the carbon steel instruments may create cross-corrosion on the stainless steel instruments.

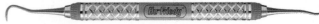

FIGURE 19.1. An EverEdge 2.0 scaling instrument. (Courtesy of Hu-Friedy Mfg. Co., Inc.)

Carbon steel instruments should be thoroughly dried before sterilization to prevent rusting or corrosion. Use of a protective rust inhibitor solution is recommended before sterilization.

II. Problems of Instruments

A. Forms of Corrosion

1. Corrosion
Corrosion is a process in which a metal is changed to a metal oxide. A common example is when iron is changed to iron oxide, or rust. Corrosion occurs because the metal oxide is the lower-energy form of the metal. Corrosion is increased in a warm, wet environment, such as in the mouth or an autoclave. An example of a corroded curette tip is shown in *Figure 19.2B*.

2. Tarnish
Tarnish is a chemical or electrochemical attack on a metal surface. Many times, corrosion starts as a surface discoloration called tarnish. If tarnish is a continuous film, it will protect the metal from the environment (like paint on metal) and prevent corrosion. Many films on metals are transparent and unseen, but they may still protect the surface from corrosion. If the film is not continuous and the surface not protected, corrosion may proceed, and loss of material will occur.

3. Galvanic Corrosion
Corrosion in a wet environment, such as saliva, is an electrochemical process called galvanic corrosion. Galvanic corrosion is the same process that produces electricity in a battery. In a battery, two dissimilar metals cause a current to flow. Corrosion may be caused by two dissimilar metals in contact, such as carbon steel and stainless steel, or by the same metal existing in two different environments. The two environments could differ in humidity, pH, oxygen concentration, or other chemical concentrations. As corrosion proceeds, the material is lost. The instrument or object becomes discolored and weakened.

Corrosion does not always occur uniformly over a metal surface. Many times, corrosion aggressively attacks small areas. As a result, surface staining and pitting occur. The base of a pit in a metal restoration or an instrument may have a different pH and oxygen concentration compared to the rest of the surface. The different environments at the base of the pit and the surface will encourage corrosion. Corrosion will continue in the pit, and the pit may become deeper and deeper. Therefore, removing pits and other surface defects by polishing reduces corrosion.

4. Galvanism
When two dissimilar metals are present in the mouth, galvanic corrosion may occur. Sometimes, this is called oral galvanism. The closer the two metals are physically, the greater the likelihood of galvanism. Several authors have stated that one should not place an amalgam restoration in contact with a gold crown, and vice versa. Galvanism is the alleged reason. However, such adjacent restorations frequently occur in patients with little or no ill effect on either restoration. Galvanism has been blamed for numerous health problems, but without a scientific basis.

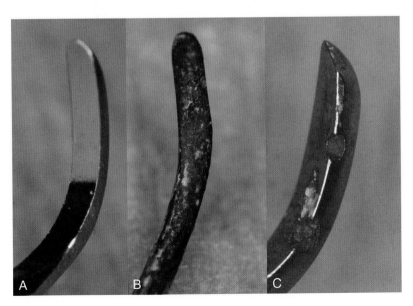

FIGURE 19.2. Photographs of **A.** a well-maintained instrument, **B.** a corroded curette tip, and **C.** a pitted instrument. (**C.** Courtesy of Hu-Friedy Mfg. Co., Inc.)

TABLE 19.1. Hu-Friedy Troubleshooting Guide for Instruments[a]

Problem	Cause	Prevention
Spotting	• Insufficient rinsing after ultrasonic cleansing	• Rinse thoroughly under a steady stream of water for 30 seconds.
	• Insufficient drying after ultrasonic cleaning	• Rinse with hot water. Optional: Dip cassettes in alcohol after rinsing.
	• Not changing ultrasonic solution	• Solution should be changed at least once a day.
	• Sterilizer has not been cleaned	• Sterilizers should be cleaned weekly. Use only distilled water for reservoir.
Rust	• Corrosion from carbon steel instruments spreads to stainless steel instruments.	• Separate stainless steel and carbon steel. • For carbon steel instruments: Dip in rust-inhibiting solution as suggested by sterilizer manufacturer.
Pitting	• Chemical attack on instruments	• Rinse and dry instruments thoroughly. • Use approved cleaning and sterilization solutions only.

[a]Courtesy of Hu-Friedy Mfg. Co., Inc.

5. Preventing Corrosion

In dentistry, we protect metallic restorations and instruments from corrosion by using two techniques.

a. The first technique is to make restorations with noble metals. Noble metals do not corrode; but they are expensive—too expensive to use for instruments.

b. The second technique is to use metals that form a tough, adherent oxide layer on the surface. This is called passivation, and it protects the metal surface from the environment. Stainless steel works this way. Unfortunately, the chromium oxide layer that protects stainless steel can break down in the presence of chloride ions. It is important to rinse off chloride-containing cleaning agents before sterilizing instruments. Residual cleaning chemicals can attack the protective film; instruments may then corrode, rust, stain, and pit.

6. Pitting

Pitting is caused by a chemical and electronic attack on surfaces. Pitting is localized corrosion, and it is prevented by:

• Rinsing instruments thoroughly after use
• Avoiding long exposure to chlorides and acids
• Avoiding detergents with high pH
• Not mixing metals in ultrasonic cleaners

An example of pitting is shown in Figure 19.2C.

7. Spotting

Slow or improper drying leaves mineral deposits that cause **spotting**. To prevent this, check the operation of the autoclave, and use chloride-free solutions for sterilizing, disinfecting, rinsing, and cleaning.

8. Summary

Table 19.1 summarizes several of the instrument problems discussed above.

B. Stains

Stains can either be deposited onto the instrument, as in the case of spotting caused by contaminated water in the autoclave, or develop from within the alloy, as in the case of rust. Identifying the source of the stain is important in solving instrument staining problems. Most stains occur during the sterilization cycle. Possible causes of stains include

• An inadequately maintained sterilizer
• Instrument contact with harsh detergents and chemicals
• Processing dissimilar metals together during cleaning and sterilization cycles

C. Rust

Rust is iron oxide that forms when iron or steel alloys corrode. Rust can be black, brown, or reddish in color. Severe rust appears as pits in the surface or as blisters, which eventually flake off the surface.

1. Without proper care, dental instruments may corrode. Rust, in the form of stains and pits, may appear on instruments as a result.

2. Rust can also be deposited on instruments when water containing dissolved rust evaporates, leaving behind a rust stain. This process is similar to what happens when drinking glasses are left to air-dry after washing, resulting in water spots.

3. If solid rust is suspended in the water of an autoclave, it can be deposited on instruments during sterilization. A properly maintained autoclave with clean water will minimize this problem.

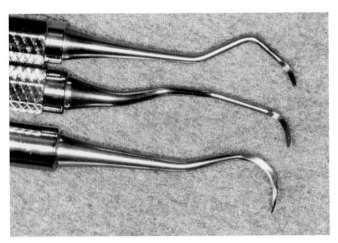

FIGURE 19.3. Photograph of two curettes and a scaler in optimum condition.

III. Instrument Inspection

In every dental hygiene practice setting, a regular routine should be established for inspecting instruments between uses. The purpose of instrument inspection is to determine aging of the instruments or other compromising conditions. Several instruments in optimum condition are shown in *Figure 19.3*. Instruments should be inspected for the following conditions:
- Corrosion
- Pitting
- Discoloration
- Broken, loose, or bent tips or components
- Cracked handles
- Dull or oversharpened edges
- Damaged blades

IV. Re-tipping

Instrument re-tipping services are available from many sources. However, having new tips inserted into an old instrument handle involves risks.

A. Detachment

The handle may develop small cracks when the tip is removed, creating a weakened point of attachment. Repeated re-tipping increases the chance for cracked handles to develop and the possibility of the tip to fall out during treatment.

B. Contamination

Small cracks in the handle may collect debris and interfere with proper sterilization.

C. Imbalance

Re-tipping often results in an unbalanced instrument.

D. Wear Rates

Stainless steel blades may vary from lot to lot. Therefore, the cutting edge may wear at a faster rate and dull more easily.

V. Sharpening Instruments

A. Why Sharpen Instruments?

Instruments should be kept sharp and true to their original design so that quality care may be provided to the patient. Properly sharpened and maintained instruments make dental procedures easier for both patient and clinician. The additional benefits of sharp instruments include the following:

1. Reduced Clinician Fatigue
   Fewer strokes and less pressure per stroke are needed when the blade is sharp. This is less demanding on the clinician's hand, muscles, and tendons.

2. Improved Removal of Calculus
   As you may have experienced by now, a dulled, or blunt cutting edge is difficult to control because it will slip and slide off the tooth surface. It is incapable of cleaving under a deposit to remove it. Instead, it slides over the outer surface, which results in burnished calculus. A sharp instrument will remove the entire deposit, as shown in *Figure 19.4*.

3. Less Chair Time
   Sharp instruments decrease chair time for patient and clinician.

4. Improved Tactile Sensitivity
   A sharp edge allows the clinician to feel the deposit more easily.

5. Less Patient Discomfort
   Fewer strokes and less pressure will be needed in the same area, thus increasing overall patient comfort.

B. When Should Instruments Be Sharpened?

The safest time to sharpen instruments is after sterilization, immediately before use. This requires the availability of a sterile stone that can be used for additional chairside sharpening and then sterilized with the instruments. Do not wait until an instrument is seriously dull and ineffective before sharpening it. Maintain instruments daily on a regular schedule to protect your financial investment.

The maintenance cycle, as shown in *Figure 19.5*, represents a maintenance routine that can be easily adapted to your own practice setting. Sterilization should be done again after sharpening if electric

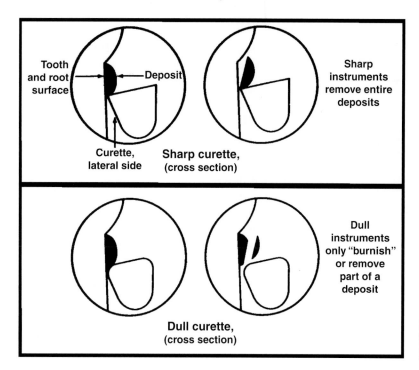

FIGURE 19.4. Sharp (*top*) versus dull (*bottom*) instruments for removal of calculus. (Courtesy of Hu-Friedy Mfg. Co., Inc.)

honing equipment is used. The honing stone and its plastic mounting cannot be sterilized because the plastic portion would melt in the autoclave. Therefore, sterilized instruments would no longer be sterile with use of a honing machine.

C. How Often Should Instruments Be Sharpened?

You can answer this question by looking at your appointment book and asking three simple questions:

1. How many times a day did I, or will I, use a specific instrument?

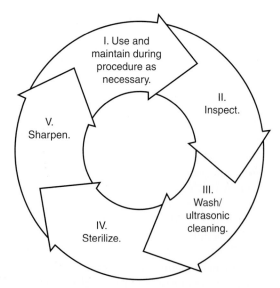

FIGURE 19.5. Instrument maintenance cycle. (Courtesy of Hu-Friedy Mfg. Co., Inc.)

2. What degree of difficulty did I, or can I expect to, encounter while using this instrument?
3. For what procedures did I, or will I, use the instrument?

Using the answers to these three questions, you will be able to design the most effective sharpening schedule for your own day-to-day requirements.

D. Sharpening Devices

Several manufacturers have developed sharpening devices that eliminate the margin of error that may occur in the traditional freehand method of sharpening. Each device operates differently and it would be important to follow the written instructions carefully so that instruments are not damaged. They range in expense from a few to several hundred dollars. One such device is pictured in *Figure 19.6*.

VI. Cleaning of Instruments

When cleaning instruments, special gloves that protect the skin from possible puncture wounds are recommended.

A. After Patient Care

Before they are sterilized, all instruments should be cleaned (ultrasonic cleaning is recommended) with a noncorrosive, low-sudsing detergent. Enzymatic cleaners maximize cleaning for surgical and periodontal instruments by digesting blood proteins, tissues, and other debris faster than ordinary cleaners. These specific cleaners also eliminate the need for hand scrubbing, which decreases

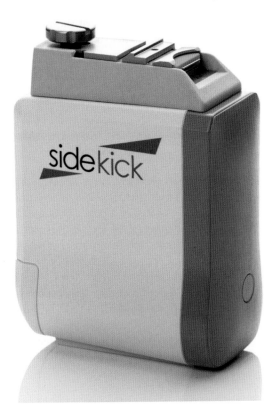

FIGURE 19.6. Hu-Friedy's "Sidekick" sharpening device. (Courtesy of Hu-Friedy Mfg. Co., Inc.)

the risk of hand injuries and the spread of contamination because of splatter. Phenols, glutaraldehyde, and iodophors are contraindicated for resin instruments.

B. When Timely Cleaning Is Not Possible

If the instruments cannot be cleaned immediately, place them in a presoak solution. Dried debris can result in instrument staining and inadequate sterilization. The presoaking liquid should completely cover the instruments.

VII. Sterilization of Instruments

Proper sterilization can extend the life of instruments and keep the need for costly replacements to a minimum. Sterilization of instruments may be accomplished by using the following methods.

A. Steam Autoclave

Steam autoclaving is regarded as most effective for destroying pathogenic organisms or vegetative forms. It is achieved at 270°F and 27 pounds per square inch (psi) for at least 6 minutes; this is for a station-type autoclave (rapid steam heat) only. Check with autoclave manufacturers for

correct cycle times. Cycle time should be closer to 15 minutes depending on whether the unit is hot or cold at the start of the cycle. Also, times for both ultrasonic cleaning and sterilizing differ if instruments are bagged or are in cassettes. Use of a steam autoclave is recommended for resin instruments.

B. Unsaturated Chemical Vapor

Unsaturated chemical vapor is effective for all metal instruments. It is best suited for carbon steel instruments, however, because chemical vapors contain less water, which causes rust and corrosion in certain instruments, compared to other sterilization methods. It is achieved at 270°F and 20 to 40 psi for at least 20 minutes. Disadvantages include odor and the need for ventilation.

C. Dry Heat

Dry heat sterilization is achieved when the internal temperature of the unit is maintained at 320°F for approximately 2 hours (temperatures >350°F may cause premature instrument failure). This method is used for items that will not withstand compressed steam conditions. Less corrosion occurs with this method, and tips and cutting instruments stay sharper.

D. Chemical Solutions

Several chemical solutions are available for sterilization. However, the American Dental Association and the Centers for Disease Control and Prevention recommend their use only for materials that cannot withstand a heat sterilization process. These solutions are not recommended for sterilization of metal dental instruments. To be effective, the solution must come in direct contact with an organism for the appropriate length of time for that organism to be destroyed. This length of time may extend to several hours.

E. How Should Instruments Be Packaged for Sterilization?

There are various methods that can be used to package instruments for sterilization. One method is to place instruments into a paper pouch after they have been run through the ultrasonic bath, rinsed, and dried. This method requires the hygienist to handle the instruments multiple times, which will increase the risk of a puncture wound or potential damage to the instrument.

Another method is the use of sterilization cassettes. This method has many benefits for the sterilization process and chairside procedures. Cassettes come in a variety of shapes and sizes

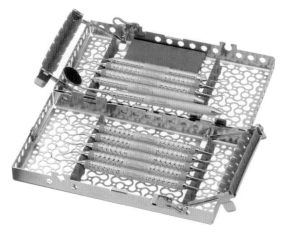

FIGURE 19.7. Sterilization cassette for hand instruments and sharpening stone. (Courtesy of Hu-Friedy Mfg. Co., Inc.)

to fit the needs of a specific procedure or office setting. The use of cassettes can increase organization by keeping sets of instruments neatly and safely bound together from the start of a procedure throughout the sterilization process. The cassettes can be closed and locked in the operatory, placed directly into the ultrasonic bath, rinsed, dried, wrapped, and placed directly into the autoclave. This method will decrease the handling of instruments, reducing the potential for a puncture wound or the loss or breakage of an instrument. Efficiency can also be increased by using cassettes that are big enough to fit a complete set of dental hygiene instruments including a sharpening stone, as shown in *Figure 19.7*. This will decrease the time spent looking for a specific instrument in another package or trying to find a sharpening stone while

the patient is in the chair. All of these benefits can increase the life of the instruments and make for a more organized clinical environment.

VIII. Sterilization, Care, and Maintenance of Special Instruments

A. Magnetostrictive and Piezoelectric Tips

1. Sterilization

After proper cleaning, it is recommended to sterilize magnetostrictive and piezo tips in an instrument cassette or a paper pouch in a steam autoclave. *Figure 19.8A* and *B* illustrates sterilization cassettes for magnetostrictive tips and piezo handpieces.

For magnetostrictive tips, use of the following is unacceptable and/or not recommended: chemical vapor sterilization, cold liquid/chemical sterilants, rapid heat transfer, phenols, chlorides, sulfates, and surface disinfectants. For piezo tips, do not expose to phenols, iodophors, or dry heat sterilization.

2. Care and Maintenance

To maintain magnetostrictive tips, manufacturers' directions should be followed that include flushing the waterlines before use and between insert placements. Scaling efficiency for both piezo and magnetostrictive instrumentation is diminished with worn tips. Inferior performance and poor water delivery can result from worn, damaged, bent, or altered tips. It is recommended that inserts be checked at least monthly for signs of wear.

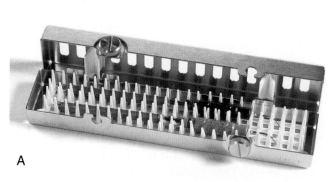

A

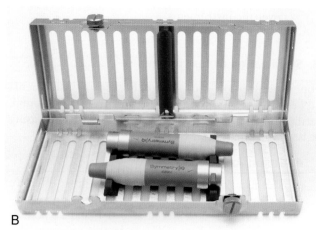

B

FIGURE 19.8. Sterilization cassettes for **A.** magnetostrictive tips and **B.** piezo handpieces. (Courtesy of Hu-Friedy Mfg. Co., Inc.)

B. Implant Instruments—Sterilization and Care

As we have learned in our clinical and instrumentation courses, typical dental hygiene instruments cannot be used on dental implants. Special probes, scalers, and curettes have been developed to measure pockets and remove deposits without affecting the titanium implant surface. You may have these special instruments in your student instrument kit.

Most of these implant probes and instruments are designed for one use, or short-term use. Hu-Friedy's Colorvue Probe Tips should be replaced after 30 uses. Their scaler and curette tips are made of an unfilled resin material and are disposed after each patient use. A variety of probes and scaling instruments can be seen in *Figure 19.9*.

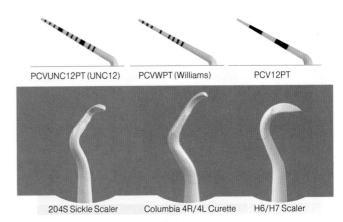

PCVUNC12PT (UNC12)   PCVWPT (Williams)   PCV12PT

204S Sickle Scaler   Columbia 4R/4L Curette   H6/H7 Scaler

FIGURE 19.9. A variety of implant probes and scaling instruments. (Courtesy of Hu-Friedy Mfg. Co., Inc.)

Summary

Dental instruments are also considered to be a dental material. Because a dental hygiene student invests a significant amount of money for his or her instruments, it is beneficial to have a good understanding of instrument care and maintenance.

Dental instruments are made of carbon steel alloy or stainless steel alloy. Some instruments may have resin handles. Surface corrosion of stainless steel instruments may be reduced during manufacturing by passivation and electropolishing. Stainless steel instruments should be kept separate from carbon steel instruments during cleaning and sterilization so that cross-corrosion does not occur. The problems of instruments such as corrosion, tarnish, galvanic corrosion, pitting, spotting, stains, and rust are discussed in this chapter.

Instruments should be inspected for a variety of conditions. The purpose of inspection is to determine aging or other compromising conditions. Re-tipping of instruments is not recommended because of the risk of detachment, contamination, imbalance, and wear.

Instruments should be sharpened to reduce clinician fatigue, improve calculus removal, save time, improve tactile sensitivity, and increase patient comfort. The safest time to sharpen instruments is after sterilization and before use. An instrument maintenance cycle is recommended.

All instruments should be cleaned before sterilization; ultrasonic cleaning is recommended. If timely cleaning is not possible, a presoak solution should be used. Methods to sterilize instruments include steam autoclave, unsaturated chemical vapor, dry heat, and chemical solutions. Not all methods are appropriate for all instruments. The recommended method for each instrument composition (resin, carbon steel, and stainless steel) is discussed in this chapter.

Proper care and maintenance of instruments enhances their function. This, in combination with clinical expertise, will result in quality care for patients.

Learning Activities

1. Divide into small groups, and examine used instruments. Look for the conditions discussed in the chapter. Review the causes and prevention of these conditions.

2. With gloves, select some extracted teeth with calculus (or paint on artificial calculus), and scale them with both sharp and dull instruments. Discuss any differences between the two. Note and discuss the following: hand fatigue, ease of calculus removal, and tactile sensitivity.

Review Questions

Question 1. A uniform corrosive attack that produces a film or surface layer on the metal is termed:

a. Corrosion
b. Tarnish
c. Electrochemical corrosion
d. Concentration cell corrosion

Question 2. A beneficial chemical process in manufacturing that creates a thin layer of chromium oxide on the surface of the instrument to protect it from corrosion is called:

a. Manufacture of alloy
b. Electroplating
c. Passivation
d. Electropolishing

Question 3. The standard protocol for chemical vapor sterilization is:

a. 270°F at 27 psi for at least 6 minutes
b. 320°F for approximately 2 hours
c. 270°F at 20 to 40 psi for at least 10 minutes
d. 270°F at 20 to 40 psi for at least 20 minutes

Question 4. Risks are involved when re-tipping instruments. One of these risks is frequent breakage between the shank and tip.

a. The first statement is true; the second statement is false.
b. The first statement is false; the second statement is true.
c. Both statements are true.
d. Both statements are false.

Question 5. To determine when the instruments should be sharpened, this chapter provides _____ questions to ask when looking over the appointment book so that an effective sharpening schedule may be developed.

a. 2
b. 3
c. 4
d. 5

Question 6. The major components of stainless steel alloy are:

a. Tin, chromium, and nickel
b. Iron, silver, and nickel
c. Iron, aluminum, and nickel
d. Iron, chromium, and nickel

Question 7. The major disadvantage of using noble metals for the fabrication of instruments is:

a. Cost
b. Corrosion
c. Wear rate
d. Pitting

Question 8. The dry heat method of sterilization is used when:

a. Ventilation is not adequate
b. Items cannot withstand temperatures greater than 270°F
c. Items cannot withstand compressed steam conditions
d. Items are needed for the next patient

Question 9. Which of the following sequence of steps is correct for the instrument maintenance cycle?

a. Use and maintain, sharpen, sterilize, inspect, wash/ultrasonic clean
b. Sharpen, inspect, use and maintain, sterilize, wash/ultrasonic clean
c. Use and maintain, inspect, wash/ultrasonic clean, sterilize, sharpen
d. Use and maintain, inspect, wash/ultrasonic clean, sharpen, sterilize

Question 10. The name of the procedure that produces a smooth, highly polished finish on an instrument is:

a. Passivation
b. Electropolishing
c. Heat treatment polishing
d. Cryogenic polishing

Infection Control and Safety in the Dental Office

20

Carol Spear, B.S.D.H., M.S. and Linda Bagby, B.A., B.S.

Objectives

After studying this chapter, the student will be able to do the following:

1. Describe safety and risk in terms of common hazards in everyday life and work in a dental office.
2. Appreciate the necessity of recommended vaccines for dental health care providers.
3. Be cognizant of emerging diseases and the precautions necessary for their prevention.
4. Define and appreciate the practice of standard precautions in dentistry.
5. Identify the types of personal protective equipment (PPE) that must be used for the practice of dentistry in the operatory and laboratory.
6. Explain the criteria for selection of PPE during dental procedures.
7. Determine the methods of sterilization or disinfection that can be used to decontaminate each type of instrument or item in the dental operatory or laboratory.
8. Practice appropriate sterilization monitoring when processing dental instruments and devices.
9. Evaluate surface disinfectants that may be used in the dental office.
10. Recall the methods that may be used to prevent cross-contamination during distribution of dental supplies.
11. Describe effective ways to manage contamination caused by aerosols and splatter.
12. Discuss safe handling and disposal of sharp items contaminated with blood or saliva.
13. Appreciate the significance of an office exposure control plan and protocol for managing exposure to blood-borne pathogens.
14. Describe the infectious, physical, and chemical hazards in a dental office.
15. Recognize office and laboratory housekeeping practices that contribute to infection control and safety.

Key Words/Phrases

AMMI guidelines

Bacillus subtilis

biological indicators (BIs)

biological monitoring

challenge pack

class I, IV, and V chemical indicators

critical objects

Ebola

ergonomics

erythema

exam gloves

exposure control plan

Geobacillus stearothermophilus

ground fault circuit interrupter (GFI)

Harvoni

hepatitis B

hepatitis C

high-efficiency particulate air (HEPA) masks

high-level disinfectants

hydrophilic

influenza

intermediate-level disinfectants

internal indicator strips

lipophilic

low-level disinfectant

measles, mumps, rubella (MMR)

mechanical/digital, chemical, and biological indicators

nitrous oxide

(continued)

Key Words/Phrases (continued)

noncritical objects

Occupational Safety and Health Administration (OSHA)

overgloves

personal protective equipment (PPE)

risk

safety

Safety Data Sheet (SDS)

semicritical objects

Spaulding Classification of Inanimate Objects

spray, wipe, spray

standard precautions

surgeon's gloves

tetanus, diphtheria, pertussis (Tdap)

time-weighted average (TWA)

unit dose

universal precautions

urticaria

utility gloves

varicella (chickenpox)

Introduction

What kind of health and safety issues could be involved in working at a dental office? In general, a dental office is a very safe place to make your livelihood. However, some hazards do require that you take precautions to minimize the risk of accident or injury, either to yourself or to those around you.

I. Definitions

A. Risk

Risk is the probability of harm. All of us take chances in everyday life. Do you wear your seat belt? Some people enjoy the thrill of risk taking. Others do not and hence avoid it.

B. Safety

Safety is the opposite of risk; it is the probability of no harm. In reality, nothing is completely safe. People are injured in car accidents every day. Lightning strikes. Bees sting. Some days, it even seems that trouble comes looking for us. In fact, there is a real chance (albeit very, very small) that an airplane will fall from the sky and kill us when we are "safe" in our bed at night. (And you thought passing the next dental materials exam was your biggest worry!) We can reduce the hazards of work and play by using common sense, avoiding excessive risk, and using safety equipment. This chapter discusses many of the risks that are present in the dental office and the ways to reduce the likelihood of harm.

II. Ionizing Radiation

Ionizing radiation, such as that produced by X-ray machines, could potentially involve some risk if it is not handled properly. Precautions for the safe use of ionizing radiation are normally addressed in radiology classes and are not covered in this text.

III. Infection Control

Some of the potential risks in a dental office involve exposure to infectious agents borne in bodily fluids, such as blood or saliva. Taking precautions to protect oneself from these fluids and from those objects contaminated by these fluids will minimize risk to infections.

In 2003, the Centers for Disease Control (CDC) released *Guidelines for Infection Control in Dental Health-Care Settings–2003*, which is a comprehensive overview of infection control. In March 2016, the CDC released the document *Summary of Infection Prevention Practices in Dental Settings*. The 2016 document does not replace the 2003 document but summarizes it with a series of handy checklists for the dental care provider. It also contains relevant CDC recommendations since 2003.

The Standard for Occupational Exposure to Bloodborne Pathogens by **the Occupational Safety and Health Administration (OSHA)** mandates the practice of "**universal precautions**" in dentistry when a potential exists for exposure to blood-borne pathogens in the dental operatory and laboratory. In 1996, guidelines were issued for precautions for contact with blood and other bodily fluids, including secretions (except sweat) and excretions. These guidelines include and supersede universal precautions and are referred to as standard precautions. **Standard precautions** require that the same infection control procedures for any given dental procedure or task must be followed for each patient and that all patients and materials must be treated as potentially infectious. Therefore, standard precautions should be used.

A. Recommended Vaccines and Precautions for Emerging Diseases

Health care workers (HCWs) are often at risk for exposure to diseases and spreading diseases. Therefore, HCWs should make sure that they are up-to-date with the following vaccines.

1. **Hepatitis B:** 3-dose series (first dose, second dose 1 month later, and third dose 5 months after second dose). To ensure immunity, obtain serologic testing for antibodies 1 to 2 months after third dose. If antibodies are not detected, undergo a second 3-dose series.

2. Influenza: 1 dose annually

3. Measles, Mumps, Rubella (MMR): If born in 1957 or later with no serologic evidence of immunity or vaccine, the HCW should obtain 2 doses of MMR 4 weeks apart.

4. Varicella (Chickenpox): If no proof of immunity, vaccination, or history of chickenpox, obtain 2 doses of vaccine 4 weeks apart.

5. Tetanus, Diphtheria, Pertussis (Tdap): After an initial dose of the vaccine, obtain a tetanus and diphtheria every 10 years thereafter.

6. Hepatitis C: At the time of this writing, there is no vaccine for hepatitis C. **Harvoni** is a recently developed medication for hepatitis C but is extremely expensive.

There are emerging diseases of which the HCW constantly should be aware. One such disease is the highly contagious **Ebola** virus. Though not typically found in the United States, it was prevalent in West Africa in 2014. A person infected with the virus is not contagious until symptoms appear from 2 to 21 days. Symptoms include fever, muscle pain, diarrhea, bleeding and often death. Because of the seriousness of the outbreak of the disease in West Africa, the CDC recommends that prior to any treatment, patients should be asked if they have travelled outside of the United States within the previous 21 days. If a patient is suspected of having had contact with the virus or has any symptoms of the disease, dental treatment must be avoided and specific CDC guidelines must be followed.

B. Personal Protective Equipment and Barriers

Dental health care providers and patients may be exposed to a variety of infectious diseases. The use of **personal protective equipment (PPE)** and physical barriers between the body and the source of contamination will inhibit transmission of the infections and reduce the likelihood of harm from chemical and physical hazards. Under its Bloodborne Pathogen Standard, OSHA requires that the dental care provider wear appropriate PPE (gloves, masks, eye protection, and clothing) during all patient care activities involving contact with saliva and blood. The PPE should not be worn out of the clinical treatment area or room. An example of a dental care provider wearing PPE is shown in *Figure 20.1.*

1. Gloves

Appropriate gloves must be worn for each specific dental task that involves direct contact with blood or saliva and when handling items that may be contaminated with these bodily fluids.

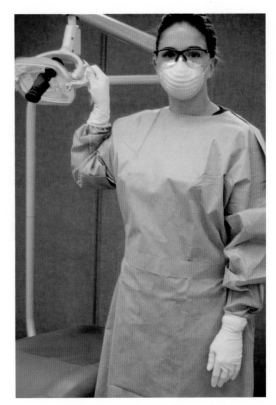

FIGURE 20.1. Dental care provider wearing required eye protection, gloves, mask, and cover gown.

Types of gloves include sterile surgeon's gloves, nonsterile exam gloves, overgloves, and utility gloves, as shown in *Figure 20.2.*

Sterile **surgeon's gloves** are recommended for use during invasive procedures, which include surgery and involved periodontal scaling. They are the most expensive type of gloves because of their sterility and the high degree of quality control used during their manufacture. In addition, they are available in actual sizes (i.e., 6, 6½, 7, 7½, etc.).

Nonsterile **exam gloves** may be worn for examination and nonsurgical procedures that are not invasive and when handling most contaminated objects (instruments, impressions, and dental appliances). They are not subject to the same quality control standards as sterile surgeon's gloves. Exam gloves are available in sizes ranging from extra small to extra large and as both ambidextrous and right/left sided. In 2016, a glove manufacturer has provided half-size exam gloves (i.e., small, small 1/2, etc.). Exam gloves are the suggested gloves for use by dental personnel during most procedures.

Overgloves are thin copolymer or plastic "food handler" gloves that may be worn over nonsterile exam gloves when it is necessary

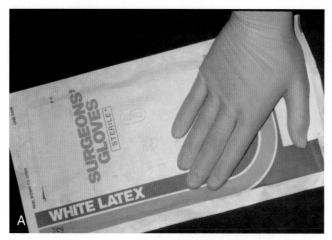
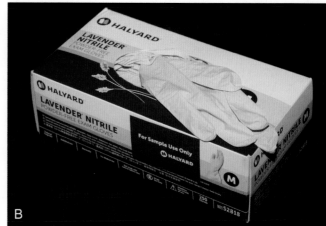
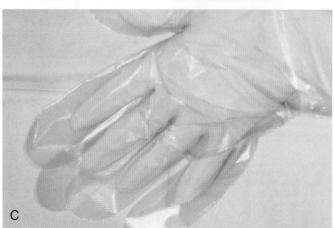
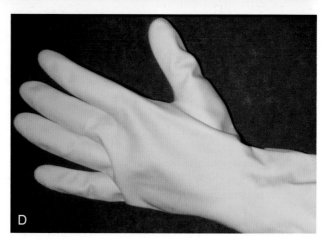

FIGURE 20.2. Types of gloves. **A.** Sterile surgeon's glove. **B.** Nonsterile nitrile exam gloves. **C.** Overglove. **D.** Utility glove.

to touch objects not in the oral cavity, such as patient charts, during patient treatment. However, it is difficult to don overgloves without contaminating the exam gloves. In most instances, therefore, a better alternative is to remove exam gloves and then replace them with new gloves when resuming patient treatment. Overgloves are discarded after use on each patient.

Utility gloves are heavy, nonsterile, puncture-resistant gloves that should be worn during cleaning and processing of contaminated instruments, cleaning and disinfecting of contaminated surfaces, and handling of chemicals. They must be cleaned and disinfected after each use.

Gloves used for treatment (exam and surgeon's gloves) are available in both natural latex and synthetic materials, such as vinyl, nitrile, and neoprene. In addition, they may be powdered or powder-free. Both exam and surgeon's gloves must be changed for each patient—or more often if the texture of the glove is modified during use.

2. Hand Washing

Use of gloves during patient treatment does not preclude hand washing. Prior to nonsurgical dental procedures, hands should be washed for at least 15 seconds, rinsed, and dried thoroughly before donning and after removing gloves. Do not wash the gloves because wicking and breakdown of composition may occur. Use of an antimicrobial handwash is preferable, although a milder cleanser may be used if the dental operator experiences skin irritation from the hand-cleansing agent. Avoid long fingernails or wearing rings under treatment gloves. This may contribute to holes or tears in gloves, and they can harbor bacteria because of inadequate cleaning of hands during hand washing. Fungal infections may also occur under rings or artificial nails because of retained moisture.

In October 2002, the Centers for Disease Control and Prevention added to its hand hygiene recommendations an endorsement of 60% to 95% alcohol-based (ethyl alcohol preferred) products for hand cleaning. These products are available as foams, gels, or rinses, and they are applied to the hands and rubbed for at least 15 seconds until the agent is dry. These products are not appropriate, however, when hands are visibly contaminated or soiled. They also must be used and stored away from high temperatures because they are highly flammable.

3. Preventing or Managing Latex Irritation
   An awareness of hypersensitivity to latex or other irritants by either the patient or the operator is extremely important so that allergic reactions can be avoided.

   a. *Latex Allergy in Dental Staff*
      Gloves worn to protect the hands may cause skin problems. In one study, 15% of dental students developed nonallergic irritation or contact dermatitis from disposable latex gloves that were commonly worn. Sometimes, this results from the talc or cornstarch with which many gloves are dusted, and in some cases, prolonged exposure may result in either immediate or delayed hypersensitivity reactions. Immediate hypersensitivity is indicated by **urticaria** (hives) and **erythema** (redness) at the points of contact with the skin minutes after the exposure. The severity of this immediate hypersensitivity may range from a rash to systemic reactions, even including life-threatening bronchospasm, hypotension, anaphylaxis, and death. Contact dermatitis, which occurs from 6 to 72 hours after exposure, is the manifestation of delayed hypersensitivity. If hypersensitivity develops, a nonlatex glove made of synthetic material should be worn. However, it is important to determine if a true latex allergy exists; therefore, one should see an allergist and get an accurate diagnosis.

   b. *Latex Allergy in Patients*
      An awareness of latex allergy in patients is extremely important. This knowledge should be gained before beginning any dental treatment by questioning the patient during the medical history review. Risk factors for latex allergy include a history of allergies, multiple surgeries, and frequent contact with latex. For treatment of a patient with known latex allergy, schedule the patient early in the day to minimize exposure to airborne latex powder and residue. In addition, those involved in direct patient care must wear nonlatex gloves, and other dental personnel should wear powder-free gloves. During the dental procedure, avoid the use of any latex-containing items. Common dental products that may contain latex are listed in Table 20.1.

TABLE 20.1. Latex Dental Products

Ambu bags
Elastic waistbands and wristbands
Gloves
Mask neck/ear loops
N_2O/O_2 analgesia masks
Orthodontic elastics
Rubber dams
Prophy cups
Syringe tips

4. Facial Masks and Shields
   A mask must be worn by the dental operator during any treatment in which splatter or aerosol is created. The mask should be changed for each patient because its outer surface becomes contaminated either with splatter and aerosol or from the operator touching the mask during dental procedures. Likewise, the mask should be changed during treatment of one patient if it becomes wet from exhaled air and, thus, ceases to act as a filter.

   Face masks are available in various styles, as shown in *Figure 20.3*. Acceptable face masks are composed of synthetic material that filter out small particles and bacteria that contact the mask. Standard masks are not intended to protect health care providers against inhalation of highly infectious aerosols, such as those containing *Mycobacterium tuberculosis*. In such instances, **high-efficiency particulate air (HEPA) masks** must be worn. These masks are designed to filter out small particles and are more form-fitting to the face. It may be necessary to check respiratory fit (no leakage around the mask) in cases where complete filtration is required.

   A complete face shield, as shown in *Figure 20.4B*, protects the face from splatter, but not from aerosol, because of the potential for suction of aerosol up under the shield. Therefore, a mask must be worn under a face shield. If worn, a shield must be cleaned and disinfected between use with each patient.

5. Eye Protection
   Protective eyewear with side shields must be worn by the dental care provider during any patient treatment or procedure in which aerosol, splatter, or projectiles may be generated. This is not only for protection against infectious disease agents but also for protection against objects and chemicals that could damage the eyes.

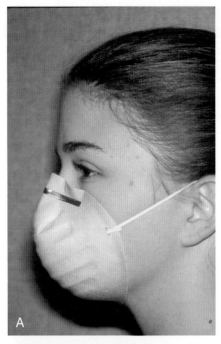

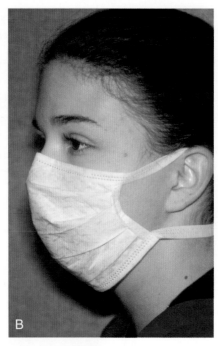

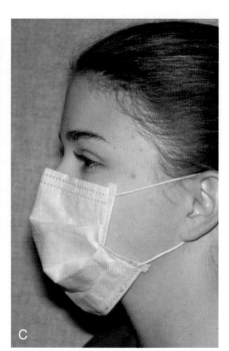

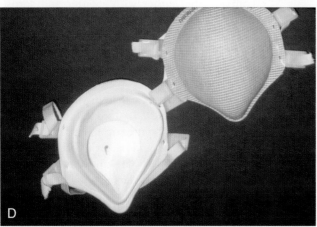

FIGURE 20.3. Standard face masks are available in various styles. **A.** Preformed cone. **B.** Soft, with head and neck ties. **C.** Soft, with elastic over-the-ear loops. **D.** Front and back of HEPA mask, which is more efficient, thicker, and more formfitting than standard masks.

a. *Hazards*

Hazardous chemicals, such as acids, stannous fluoride, disinfectants, and silver nitrate, can be splashed into the eyes. Ultrasonic and high-speed equipment create a spray of aerosols during use; particulates from broken teeth, amalgam, calculus, pumice, gold, or pieces of burs can be expelled from the mouth at speeds of nearly 60 mph. In the laboratory, personnel are exposed to hazards from rotary equipment, such as grinders; hazardous chemicals, such as disinfectants and developers; and high temperatures. To minimize the consequences of a chemical splash, eye wash equipment should be readily available, especially in the laboratory.

b. *Equipment*

Most potential injuries of these types can be avoided if appropriate eye protection is worn. Acceptable eyewear can include safety glasses with side shields, a face shield, or goggles, as shown in *Figure 20.4*. Corrective lenses can be incorporated in safety glasses. The American National Standards Institute has issued guidelines for selecting eye protection.

c. *Patient Protection*

When being treated in a reclining position, the patient not only is exposed to the same hazards as the dental personnel but also is at risk from instruments, syringes, or materials that drop from the practitioner's hand or off of the delivery tray. Although not mandated, protective eyewear should also be worn by the patient. Unless disposable glasses are provided to the patient, eyewear should be cleaned and disinfected between each use.

d. *Curing Light Hazards*

Today, dental personnel also face eye hazards from several types of light: ultraviolet (UV) light, visible blue light, and lasers. Especially

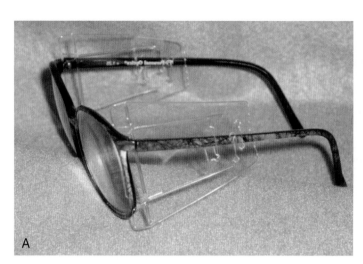
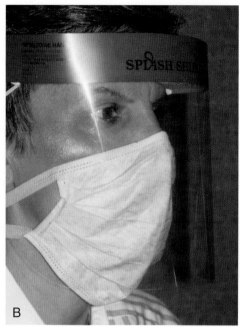

FIGURE 20.4. Protective eyewear. **A.** Glasses with side shields. **B.** Face shield.

wavelengths between 320 and 400 nm, UV light can cause cataracts and retinal damage. At one time, UV light was used to activate addition polymerization, but visible blue light (400–500 nm) has now replaced UV light in dental polymerization applications. Although blue light is not inherently hazardous, the high intensity of curing lights can cause injuries to the retina. Protective equipment recommended by manufacturers includes safety shields or specially tinted glasses. The ADA is a good source for information on the efficiency of these protective filters.

e. *Lasers*

When lasers are used, it is important not to direct the laser at any nontarget tissue, especially the eyes, or toward any reflective surface. Special eye protection is required for both the operator and the patient. This eye protection must be matched to absorb the specific wavelength of the laser that is used. Nonreflective instruments and personnel shields are available for use with lasers. Signs are also required in any area where a laser is being used.

6. Protective Attire

Protective attire is the outer layer of clothing worn over underlying clothes. The type and characteristic of protective clothing depends on the exposure that is anticipated. A convenient approach is to use disposable gowns with long sleeves, a high neck, and sufficient length to cover street clothes. This outerwear

may be disposable or reusable, and it includes uniforms, clinic jackets, lab coats, and gowns. By OSHA mandate, contaminated reusable attire cannot be laundered at home; it must be laundered in the office or by a commercial laundry service. Protective clothing should be changed daily (or sooner, if it becomes visibly soiled or wet) and should be worn only in the clinical area.

C. Instrument Sterilization and Surface/ Equipment Disinfection

1. Degree of Decontamination

The degree of decontamination of a dental instrument or equipment depends on its risk of transmitting infection or disease. To determine which method of decontamination to use, categorize the object as critical, semicritical, or noncritical according to the **Spaulding Classification of Inanimate Objects**.

2. Critical Objects

Critical objects must be heat sterilized in steam, dry heat, or saturated chemical vapor. This category includes items that may penetrate or touch broken mucous membranes or skin. Examples include all instruments, handpieces, and burs. Before packaging for sterilization, all instruments must be cleaned either ultrasonically or by scrubbing. If instruments cannot be cleaned immediately after use, they should be immersed in a holding solution containing enzymes to help break down protein and keep debris from drying. Follow the manufacturer's guidelines for cleaning and preparing handpieces for sterilization. Store sterile instruments in their sterile wraps, and unwrap them just before use. If a device has no manufacturer's guidelines for cleaning and sterilization, it should be treated as a single-use item and may not be reprocessed for patient use.

3. Semicritical Objects

Semicritical objects include items such as radiographic film holders, shade guides, and mouth props that contact, but do not penetrate, mucous membranes. Heat or chemical liquid sterilization **(high-level disinfectants)** is required for these objects. Heat sterilization is preferred, although chemical liquid sterilization may be necessary for items that may be damaged by heat. Liquid chemicals for sterilization include glutaraldehyde, hydrogen peroxide, and peracetic acid. The long sterilization time (6–10 hours), potential for corrosion, and maintenance of sterility during storage are disadvantages of liquid chemical sterilization.

4. Noncritical Objects

Noncritical objects are those items that do not come in contact with mucous membranes but that are touched or contaminated during dental treatment. These items include the dental unit, switches, handles, radiographic tube heads, the dental chair, and plaster bowls and spatulas.

Intermediate-level disinfectants should be used for the disinfection of noncritical objects. Acceptable disinfectants are those that are registered with the U.S. Environmental Protection Agency (EPA), tuberculocidal, and virucidal. These disinfectants must be virucidal against both lipophilic and hydrophilic viruses. **Lipophilic** viruses, which are enveloped by lipids, are much easier to kill than are **hydrophilic** viruses, which are coated with protein. Properties of acceptable surface disinfectants are summarized in Table 20.2.

Acceptable surface disinfectants include hydrogen peroxide, citric acid, iodophors, phenols, quaternaries, sodium hypochlorite and sodium bromide, and chlorine. Products for surface disinfection are summarized in Table 20.3. Because of their instability, some of these disinfectants must be mixed fresh daily; however, some are premixed and have a 2-year shelf life. You should inquire about all the aforementioned features before selecting the product that is most appropriate for use in your office.

TABLE 20.2. Properties of Acceptable Surface Disinfectants

Property	Type of Microorganism Destroyed
Tuberculocidal	*Mycobacterium tuberculosis*
Lipophilic	Hepatitis B virus
	Human immunodeficiency virus
	Herpes simplex virus
	Herpes zoster virus
	Influenza virus
Hydrophilic	Adenovirus
	Rotavirus
	Coxsackievirus
	Poliovirus

Low-level disinfectants are actually detergents or cleaning agents. Some disinfectants contain detergents, but many do not. This information must be obtained from the manufacturer of the disinfectant. The cleaning agent, whether it is a component of the disinfectant or a separate product, must be used during the initial step in the process of disinfecting surfaces.

Surface disinfectants may be applied by sprays or wipes (see examples in *Fig. 20.5*). Application from bottled surface disinfectants involves a **spray, wipe, spray** procedure. The initial spray may be completed with a cleaning agent or a disinfectant that contains a detergent. The surface is then wiped (cleaned), usually with a disposable paper towel. This is followed by a final, light spray with the surface disinfectant, after which the surface is allowed to air-dry for the time recommended by the manufacturer. The spray, wipe, spray procedure is shown in *Figure 20.6*. If disinfectant wipes are used, use one soaked wipe to first clean the surface. Then, use a new wipe to disinfect the surface and let it air-dry for the time recommended by the manufacturer (usually 5–10 minutes).

5. Sterilization Monitoring

To ensure that sterilization of instruments and devices has occurred, sterilizers should be monitored with a combination of **mechanical/ digital, chemical, and biological indicators**. Mechanical or digital monitoring involves monitoring gauges or displays during the operation of the sterilizer.

In accordance with the **Association for the Advancement of Medical Instrumentation**

TABLE 20.3. Surface Disinfectant Reference Chart—2011

Category	Active Ingredient
Accelerated hydrogen peroxide	Hydrogen peroxide in an aqueous solution
Phenolics (dual) water-based	Phenylphenol and benzylchlorophenol or tertiary amylphenol
Phenolics (dual) alcohol-based	Tertiary amylphenol and/or phenylphenol + ethyl alcohol or isopropyl alcohol
Quaternaries dual or synergized plus alcohol	Diisobutylphenoxyethoxyethyl dimethylbenzyl ammonium chloride; isopropanol or ethanol; alkyl dimethyl benzyl ammonium chloride
Quaternary ammonium; no alcohol	Alkyl dimethyl benzyl ammonium chloride; EDTA
Sodium hypochlorite	Sodium hypochlorite in an aqueous solution
Sodium bromide and chlorine	NaBr and NaCl

Important Information:
Numerous disinfectant products are available. However, all products to be used as disinfectants on precleaned surfaces must be registered with the U.S. EPA. It is important to read the label for specifics on shelf life and use. Some disinfectant agents degrade certain materials.

This resource is based on information from http://www.osap.org/page/SurfDisinfec2010. OSAP is a nonprofit organization, which provides information and education on dental infection control and office safety. For more information, please call 1-800-298-6727. Organization for Safety & Asepsis Procedures (OSAP), 3525 Piedmont Rd., Bldg. 5, Suite 300, Atlanta, GA 30305, www.osap.org, (410) 571–0003. Fax: (404) 264–1956, Email: office@OSAP.org.

(AMMI) Guidelines, external and internal chemical indicators are available and consist of heat or chemical sensitive ink impregnated on strips, instrument pouches, or tape. **Internal indicator strips** must be placed inside the package/cassette with instruments and indicator is visible from outside the packaging.

The AMMI has established classifications (I–V) for Chemical Indicators. The classifications of most importance are the following:

Class I—external indicators in the form of tape or printed packaging that distinguish between a processed and an unprocessed item

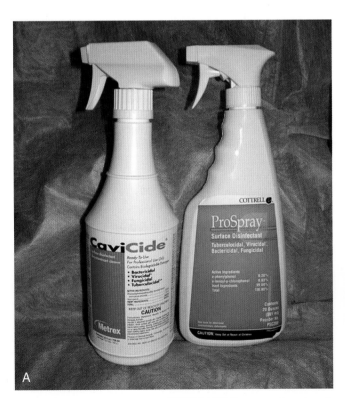

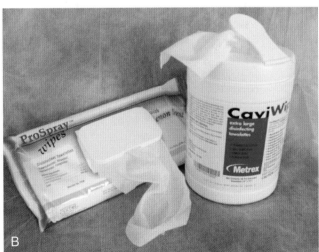

FIGURE 20.5. Examples of surface disinfectant. **A.** Sprays. **B.** Wipes.

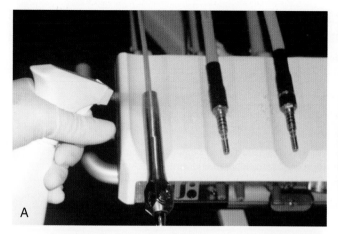

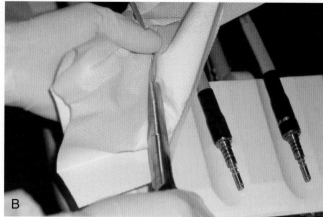

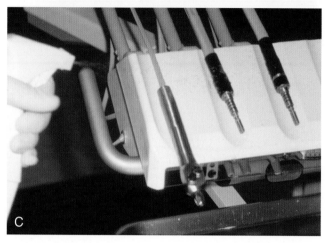

FIGURE 20.6. Surface disinfection includes a "spray, wipe, spray" procedure. **A.** The initial spray, **B.** cleaning by wiping, and **C.** the final spray with a disinfectant.

Class IV—multivariable indicators placed inside packaging and designed to react to two or more of the critical variables for sterilization (pressure, time, and temperature)

Class V—integrating indicators that measure all critical variables for sterilization and which are placed in the same type of packaging **(challenge pack)** as that of the items being processed in the sterilizer load.

Biological monitoring is the use of bacterial spores or indicators to test the ability of the sterilization cycle to kill highly resistant microorganisms. **Biological indicators (BIs)** are available as self-contained vials of spores of either *Geobacillus stearothermophilus* for steam autoclaves or chemiclaves or *Bacillus subtilis* for dry hear sterilizers. The BI is placed in a challenge pack and then placed in the sterilizer along with the items to be sterilized. After the sterilization cycle is complete, the vial is tested for spore growth. This can be done with in-house kits or by mail-in kits with professional labs. In-house kits are more efficient because they provide results in as little as 24 hours. Do not use any items processed from a failed biological spore test. As per CDC guidelines, biological monitoring must be conducted at least weekly, as well as every time an implant is sterilized.

D. Protective Barriers

An effective way to maintain surface disinfection is to cover cleaned and disinfected surfaces with disposable protective barriers. This involves proper placement of a surface cover before there is an opportunity for contamination of the surface after disinfection, as shown in *Figure 20.7.* Surface covers should be impervious to fluids, and they include clear plastic wrap, bags, or tubes. These plastic covers are available in preformed shapes that fit over specific items or as plain sheets that must be wrapped around items. Choose the type of barrier that is most economical and appropriate for your office.

Use of protective barriers on surfaces does not preclude surface disinfection; rather, these barriers are used in combination with it. If you choose to use protective barriers, clean and disinfect surfaces at the beginning of the workday and then cover these surfaces with clean barriers between patient treatments. Remove contaminated barriers with gloved

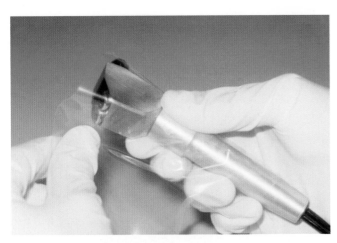

FIGURE 20.7. Protective barriers or covers may be placed over surfaces after they are disinfected and before there is an opportunity for contamination.

hands, and replace clean barriers carefully so that the disinfected surfaces are not contaminated. Use of protective barriers is especially advocated for surfaces that contain buttons, knobs, and crevices.

E. Other Infection Control Issues

1. Distribution of Supplies and Materials
   Numerous supplies and materials are used for patient care, and their proper storage and distribution should be of primary concern so that cross-contamination is avoided. Examples include gauze, cotton rolls, articulating paper, prophy paste, impression materials, and other restorative materials.
   a. *Bulk Supplies*
      To avoid contamination of supplies stored in bulk, sterile retrievers (forceps) must be provided for aseptic removal of items. Extreme care must be taken by all office personnel when obtaining these items.

   b. *Kits*
      Kits of restorative materials, such as dentinal bonding systems that are used at chairside on more than one patient, must be cleaned and disinfected between each patient. The box may be covered with a clean barrier for each patient; however, any bottles or tubes that are contaminated must be disinfected before being returned to the box or cabinet for storage.
   c. *Unit Dose*
      Many types of supplies or materials can be supplied as a **unit dose**, as shown in *Figure 20.8A*, so that cross-contamination can be avoided. This is accomplished by packaging small amounts of materials or supplies in individual packets for use on individual patients. Unit dosing can be more expensive, but it is very effective in the prevention of cross-contamination and also reduces labor costs.

2. Use of Disposable/Single-Use Items
   Disposable items are usually manufactured from inexpensive materials, such as plastics, and are designed to be disposed of after use. Examples include the saliva ejector, evacuation tip, air/water syringe tip, impression trays, and prophy angles (*see Figure 20.8B*). Other items include treatment gloves, cover gowns, surface covers, facial masks, and anesthetic syringe needles. Use of disposable items also reduces labor costs.

   It is important to properly dispose of these items after use. Avoid any attempt to clean, sterilize, or disinfect them for reuse.

F. Managing Aerosol and Splatter

Aerosol and splatter that are generated and propelled from the patient's oral cavity during dental treatment create the potential for microbial

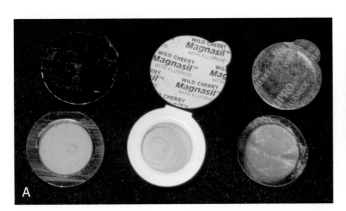
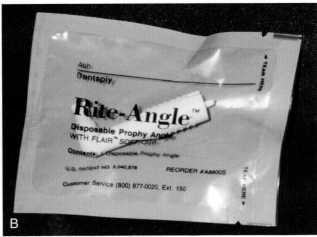

FIGURE 20.8. **A.** Unit-dosed prophy paste. **B.** Disposable prophy angle.

contamination of the dental operator and the adjacent environmental surfaces. The amount of aerosol and splatter can be controlled, however, by using the following practices.

1. Dental Dam and High-Speed Evacuators
Whenever possible, use a dental dam (rubber dam) to reduce the amount of saliva at the operative site. Simultaneous use of high-speed evacuation along with a dental dam provides optimum reduction of dental aerosol and splatter.

2. Pretreatment Mouth Rinse
Provide the patient with a pretreatment mouth rinse, such as an American Dental Association (ADA)-approved mouth rinse containing chlorhexidine gluconate or essential oils. These significantly reduce the number of microorganisms that may escape in splatter or aerosol.

3. Pretreatment Toothbrushing
A simple but effective way to reduce the potential for microbial contamination from aerosol and splatter is to have the patient brush his or her teeth with an ADA-approved dentifrice before any treatment begins.

G. Safe Handling and Disposal of Sharp Items Contaminated with Blood or Saliva

1. Sharps Containers
Extreme safety precautions should be followed when handling any sharp instrument, orthodontic wire, anesthetic needle, irrigating syringe, or other item that may be contaminated with blood-borne pathogens. These precautions include avoiding punctures or cuts during the use of these sharp items and proper disposal of these items into hard "sharps" containers. These containers must be placed at the dental unit or in the lab and must be readily accessible (i.e., not under sinks or in enclosed cabinets). An example of a "sharps" container is shown in *Figure 20.9.*

2. Recapping Needles
Recapping of anesthetic needles should never be performed as a two-handed technique. The two-handed technique greatly contributes to needlestick accidents. One of the following practices can greatly reduce the potential for accidental needlesticks: the one-handed scoop technique, use of a barrier cap-holding device, or use of a disposable self-capping "safe" syringe (*Fig. 20.10*). The safe syringe has a retractable sheath that covers the needle before use and retracts over the barrel of the syringe when in use. The sheath slides back over the needle after the injection is completed.

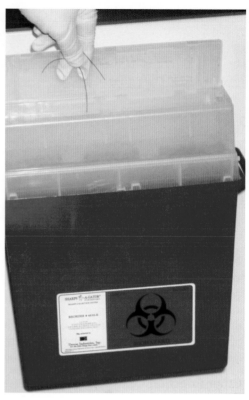

FIGURE 20.9. Dispose all sharp items into a hard "sharps" container.

H. Office and Laboratory Housekeeping Practices

To minimize the potential for infection of the dental care provider by cross-contamination, the following housekeeping practices should be observed.

1. Eating and Cosmetics
Do not eat, drink, apply cosmetics or lip balm, or place or remove contact lenses in the treatment area, dental laboratory, or sterilization and radiograph-processing area. Use disposable tissues rather than handkerchiefs.

2. Food Storage
Do not store food or drink in refrigerators or freezers that are also used to store dental products or other potentially infectious or hazardous materials.

3. Separate Contaminated Items
Keep two separately designated areas in the laboratory for receiving contaminated items and for storing or handling clean or sterile items.

4. Infectious Wastes
All infectious wastes must be disposed of according to local, state, and federal regulations. As a general rule, blood-soaked items as well as hard and soft tissue are considered to be infectious

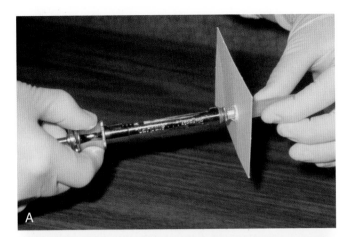

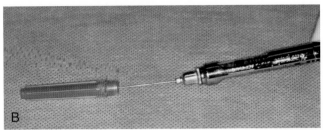

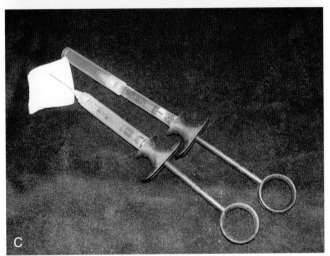

FIGURE 20.10. Two acceptable methods for recapping needles. **A.** Use of a barrier cap-holding device. **B.** A one-handed scoop technique. **C.** Self-capping "safe syringe."

waste and must be placed in appropriately marked biohazard infectious waste containers (boxes, plastic bags) and disposed by specified agencies. The sharps container in *Figure 20.9* is also an infectious waste container and displays the biohazard symbol.

I. Exposure Control Plan

The dental office or laboratory must have a written **exposure control plan** that includes all steps necessary to prevent exposure to blood-borne pathogens for each dental procedure that is performed. The plan must also include the protocol to follow if exposure to a blood-borne pathogen occurs. You must familiarize yourself with the exposure plan, and you should review it at least annually. Someone in the office should be designated to update this plan each year.

IV. Physical Hazards

Many common sense things can be done to minimize possible accidents. Arrange the work area to allow enough room for people to pass and safely get around each other and any equipment.

A. Trips, Slips, Hits, and Spills

1. Floors

Use no-skid absorbent rugs at doorways and in areas likely to get wet, such as near the sink. Use only low matte rugs because wrinkled throw rugs can be the cause of trips, especially for the elderly. Mobile equipment often has cords and tubes that can also be a trip hazard; keep these out of traffic areas. Spills on smooth floors are an important concern as well and should be cleaned up as soon as possible. Some powders used in dentistry, such as plaster and acrylic powders, can make a smooth floor very slippery.

Cabinet drawers and doors should not be left open, especially in a high-traffic area. An open cabinet drawer or door can cause an injury. A lower drawer, left open, can be a trip hazard. One can walk into an open upper cabinet door when looking down or hit one's head when rising after bending over.

2. Patients

When patients have been reclined for an appointment, it is a good idea to sit them up when giving them postoperative instructions.

If they stand up immediately after they are moved to an upright position, fainting or light-headedness may occur. Raising patients to an upright position for a few minutes will reduce such problems. For some patients, it is advisable to have them turn in the dental chair and sit with their feet on the floor for a few additional minutes. One may want to stand near certain patients in a supportive position should they feel light-headed when they stand up. In addition, one must move the operatory light and other equipment out of the patient's way to avoid head injuries. Patients with impaired vision are a special concern; if necessary, they should be escorted into and out of the dental operatory.

B. Lifting Injuries

Back injuries are a major problem in many types of work. Although this may not be a frequent problem in the dental office, boxes of files, disinfectant, or developing solution may be heavy. The general rule is to bend the legs instead of the back when lifting heavy items. This may include patients who may need help to get in or out of the chair.

C. Lathes

It is very easy to get loose items tangled in the rapidly spinning parts of a lathe and other equipment. Be sure to contain long hair securely, and do not use the lathe while wearing loose jewelry, ties, scarves, or loose-fitting gloves. These loose items can get caught and drag the hand—or, worse, the head—into the rapidly spinning shaft or cutting device. Eye protection is a must when a lathe is being used, and a mask is also recommended.

D. Model Trimmers

When a model trimmer is used, it is important to make sure that a slip will not result in a finger or a hand being thrust into the cutting disk. Use a "palm rest," where the palm of the hand rests on the front of the table of the model trimmer (see Chapter 28, Fabrication and Trimming of Study Models). The fingers should hold the cast in the area most distant from the cutting disk. Use flexure of the fingers to push the cast toward the cutting disk rather than pushing the cast with an unstable hand or fingers. If the flexure method is used and the part of the hand that is pushing slips off the cast, the fingers will only straighten and extend over the cast, not into the cutting disk.

E. Burns, Scalds, and Fires

1. Sterilization Equipment
Removing items from a hot autoclave has been the cause of numerous burns and scalds. Be sure that items have adequately cooled before taking them out of an autoclave, or use heat-resistant gloves. Follow the manufacturer's directions for opening an autoclave or other heat sterilization equipment. Remember, hot items do not look different from cold items.

2. Personal Protection Equipment
Loose-fitting gloves are a hazard when a lighter is used to heat an instrument or light a Bunsen burner. If the tip of the glove extends into the flame, it will melt onto the finger. Lighters with extended tips are available for lighting grills and candles. These are much safer to use than the typical disposable lighter. Also, use only flame-resistant or flame-retardant disposable cover gowns.

3. Flammables
Many of the chemicals used in dentinal bonding systems are flammable. Luckily, they are packaged in small containers and are used in very small quantities. They do not present a great hazard.

Acrylic monomers are also flammable but are packaged and used in much greater quantities. Do not use them around open flames, and clean up any spills immediately. Acrylic monomers and any alcohol that is used as a fuel should be properly stored. Do not leave an open flame unattended. It is important to know where the fire extinguishers are located, and all employees should know how to use them. Smoke detectors should also be present. Remember, if a fire should occur, the first priority is to get people to safety, not to fight the fire.

4. Oxygen
Oxygen is used in every dental office that uses nitrous oxide. Oxygen should be present in the emergency kits in a dental office. If one remembers that fire requires oxygen, the danger of pure oxygen is obvious. If an oxygen leak occurs in any equipment, a spark could mean disaster. Also, the metal tanks that are used to supply oxygen and nitrous oxide are heavy and need to be securely fastened in place. If they were to fall over, serious injury could occur. Any tank of compressed gas could become a missile if the tank falls and the valve breaks off.

5. Electric Handpieces
The FDA has received several reports of patients being burned by overheated electric handpieces. While it is less likely for a hygienist's patient to be anesthetized and unaware of the high temperature, care must be taken when using these rotary devices. Proper maintenance and the use of lower-speed settings should minimize this risk of patient injury.

F. Electrical Hazards

1. Outlets Near Sinks

To minimize the chance of electrocution, current standards for electrical safety require that outlets near a sink incorporate a **ground fault circuit interrupter** (**GFI**, or GFCI), either in the outlet itself or in the electrical box. Should equipment plugged into a GFI outlet become immersed in water, the resulting short circuit would trigger the GFI. Electricity is then rapidly cut off to the circuit so that anyone touching the item would avoid serious injury. Keep portable electrical equipment away from sinks to minimize the hazard of the equipment falling into water.

2. Maintaining Equipment

When performing maintenance on equipment, such as replacing a bulb in a curing unit, it is important to unplug the unit. Repairing or maintaining equipment that is plugged into an electrical outlet presents a significant risk and should be avoided. Depending on the nature of the task, it may be wise to unplug some equipment during cleaning.

3. Pacemakers

Pacemakers may be affected by an electromagnetic field that is given off by some dental equipment. Electrosurgery and ultrasonic units should not be used on patients with an older, "unshielded" pacemaker. If the patient or the patient's doctor cannot ensure that use of such equipment is safe for the patient with a pacemaker, do not use this equipment.

G. Hearing Protection

1. Harmful Noise Levels

For many years, noise from dental equipment has been suspected of contributing to hearing loss. Dental professionals as a group experience hearing losses. Many studies of the dental environment have been done, but the results have been contradictory. In the dental office, exposure to noise should be controlled in accordance with OSHA standards. The occupational exposure limit is given in terms of an 8-hour, time-weighted average of 85 decibels (dBA). Harmful noise levels can be encountered from a variety of sources, many of them not work-related. Examples of noise sources that have been measured to generate sound levels above 85 dBA include a vacuum cleaner, lawn mower, car radio, hair dryer, and TV commercials. To protect hearing from all sources, the U.S. EPA specifies that exposures should not average more than 70 dBA during a 24-hour period.

2. Protection

The susceptibility to hearing loss varies from person to person. Noise-induced hearing loss is subtle and, eventually, irreversible. Usually, it first affects a higher frequency range than is normally used in conversation, so it may go unnoticed for some time. To determine if a person has a hearing loss, he or she can be tested by an audiologist. Measurements of noise levels in the dental office can be made by hearing conservation companies. Hearing protection, in the form of ear plugs or ear covers, can be effective in reducing exposure, but it may also affect a dental practitioner's ability to converse with a patient. Some practitioners have earplugs connected by a cord that they can hang around their neck when talking but are easily available for use when needed. With all the noises present both in and out of work, it may be prudent to take preventive measures to reduce exposure to excessive noise from any source.

H. Respiratory Hazards

1. Aerosols, Dusts, Allergies, and Asthma

In the dental office, there is the potential for injury to the respiratory system from a number of different sources, including infectious agents. Occupational asthma, pneumoconiosis (an example is silicosis), and chronic bronchitis may occur from the inhalation of fine particles into the respiratory tract. Some of the dusts generated in a dental office can include amalgam, asbestos, beryllium-containing alloys, cobalt, enamel, dentin, gold, gypsum, pumice, and silica. Various size particles and aerosols are produced from grinding and polishing techniques, and some of the fine particles may be suspended in the air for hours or even days if adequate ventilation is not present. Spray disinfectants are another source of aerosol. They may irritate the respiratory system or aggravate asthma. Lasers also produce aerosols of tissue debris that may be infectious.

2. Allergic Sensitization

Exposure to acrylic dusts has been related to allergic sensitization of the respiratory tract. Occupational asthma has occurred from exposures to persulfates (found in many plastics), stainless steel, nickel, cobalt, chromium, tungsten carbide, formaldehyde, solvents such as toluene, oil of orange, xylene, and various epoxy compounds. The respiratory hazards of mercury are considered in a later section.

3. Protection

To minimize the distribution of these particulates and aerosols, a high-velocity vacuum system with filters should be used. The practitioner should also wear a mask that is capable of filtering out these particles and eye protection. The types of masks currently worn to protect from infectious material (for particles 1–2 μm in diameter) will not filter out many of the dusts and aerosols that have been noted. Masks designed to filter out respirable dusts are available and are recommended, especially for use when grinding composite materials and porcelain.

In general, the use of volatile materials and the performance of activities that produce dusts and aerosols should be carried out in an area that is equipped with proper dust collection equipment. In the operatory, good general ventilation is also essential. Although standards may not be specified for operatories, those for laboratories would probably be appropriate. A rate of six air exchanges per hour is recommended. To minimize energy costs, replacement air could be heated with an air-to-air heat exchanger, which can usually be incorporated into the existing furnace/air-conditioning system.

I. Dermal Hazards

The skin on the hands of a dental care provider can be subject to many different types of abuse.

Irritants can include soaps and detergents, germicides, adhesives, essential oils, filling materials, metals, organic solvents, and radiograph-processing chemicals.

1. Allergic Contact Dermatitis

Allergic contact dermatitis can be caused by a number of dental materials. Examples include acrylic monomers (among them, methyl methacrylate), ethylene glycol dimethacrylate, eugenol, bisphenol A (an epoxy resin compound), and disinfectants. Acrylic monomers and glutaraldehyde can penetrate latex and polyvinyl chloride gloves. See the Safety Data Sheet, as shown in *Figure 20.11*, or contact the product's manufacturer for information on appropriate alternatives.

2. Latex Gloves

As previously discussed, gloves that are worn to protect the hands may be the cause of problems. Latex sensitivity should be considered when any dermal irritation occurs on the hands. Powderless latex gloves cause fewer problems than powdered gloves.

3. Ultrasonic Cleaners

Manuals for ultrasonic cleaners warn users to not place fingers or hands in the bath of an

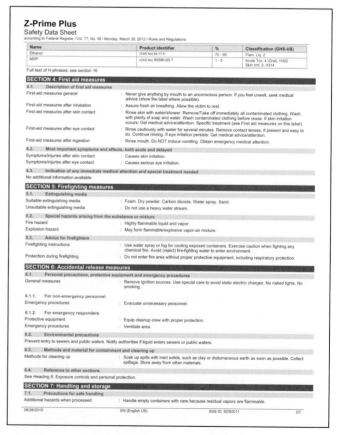

FIGURE 20.11. Two of seven pages of an SDS for a bonding primer. (Courtesy of BISCO Dental Products, Schaumburg, IL.)

operating unit. Surprisingly, it is difficult to find any research identifying hazards from the device itself. One sound reason to avoid reaching into an ultrasonic cleaner, on or off, is the irritating nature of cleaning solution in the unit. It is recommended gloves or instruments are used to retrieve items in an ultrasonic cleaner.

J. Musculoskeletal Problems

Although it does not directly relate to dental materials safety, another health concern for dental care providers is that of musculoskeletal disorders. Recent studies have shown a large increase in the number of occupationally related disorders involving the musculoskeletal system, particularly among dental hygienists. These disorders are also known as cumulative motion trauma, repetitive motion disorders, and/or cumulative trauma disorders. They result from repetitive insults to the muscles, bones, and related structures. Musculoskeletal disorders can occur in any part of the body, but the areas most often noted as being problematic for dental care providers are the lower back, neck, shoulders, arms, wrists, and hands. Carpal tunnel syndrome is a disturbingly common problem and is discussed in most dental hygiene texts.

1. **Ergonomics**

   Dental professionals can be at risk for injuries because of the nature of their work. Experts in **ergonomics** (also known as biomechanics or human factor engineering) seek to assess the best way for a person to perform a task. Ergonomics takes into consideration the physical dimensions and capabilities of the human body as well as the optimal design of equipment and the work area to promote the comfort and efficiency of the worker.

   Following are recommendations for improved musculoskeletal health.

2. **General Recommendations**
   a. Good lighting is important to avoid eyestrain. Good light and the use of magnification will reduce slouching over the patient and associated problems.
   b. Use good posture. Keep the back and neck in line without tipping forward or twisting.
   c. Use a chair that provides good lumbar support and has a seat width that allows for shifting and movement. The height of the seat should be adjusted so that the feet can be flat and the thighs parallel to the floor. Casters on the chair should make it easy to move without twisting.
   d. Get up and move around between patients. This gives a break to the muscles used during

sitting and takes the pressure off some of the discs between the vertebrae.
   e. Ask patients to change their head position instead of leaning or twisting for a better view or work angle.
   f. Use indirect vision with a dental mirror to view hard-to-see areas of the mouth. Avoid leaning and twisting to use direct vision.
   g. Do exercises that promote flexibility and strengthen the hand, back, abdominal, hip, and leg muscles.
   h. Consider limiting off-the-job activities that contribute to musculoskeletal problems. These include certain sports, excessive computer use, and repetitive finger activities, such as knitting or crocheting.

3. **Hand and Wrist Recommendations**
   a. Use gloves that fit well.
   b. Use a neutral hand position and finger rests. Less pressure will be exerted on the median nerve in the wrist if flexion and extension can be minimized.
   c. Lower the vibration components when using vibratory instruments. Vibration can contribute to carpal tunnel syndrome.
   d. Rest and exercise hands. Stretch the hands when changing instruments and between patients.

4. **Instrument Recommendations**
   a. Use the proper instrument for the task.
   b. Use lightweight and evenly balanced instruments. Consider using hollow instruments.
   c. Choose instruments with a textured grip. They are easier to hold and require less "pinching" when in use.
   d. Larger-diameter instruments, when being used, also minimize the need to pinch.
   e. Keep the cutting edges of instruments sharp to make them effective with a minimum amount of force and fewer deliberate strokes. This recommendation is discussed in more detail in Chapter 19, Instruments as Dental Materials—Care and Maintenance.

5. **Preventing Injuries**

   Having a coworker watch or videotape you while you work can be helpful. Another person can often spot potential ergonomic problems that are overlooked when the dental care worker is concentrating on patient care. At present, OSHA is working with organized dentistry to address ergonomic issues in the workplace. Even without such a standard, dental professionals should take steps to prevent musculoskeletal disorders and the discomforts they cause.

V. Chemicals

The term "chemical" may sound scary to many people. We do not want chemicals in our water or our food. On the other hand, water is a chemical, and most foods are a complex mixture of many chemicals. (Try reading the label on a cereal box.) Here, we are interested in the hazardous chemicals and materials in the dental office. We need to know what chemicals we are using and how to avoid injury from them.

A. Safety Data Sheets (formerly Materials Safety Data Sheets)

Manufacturers usually send a **Safety Data Sheet (SDS)** with products that meet the OSHA definition of a hazardous material. An SDS is shown in *Figure 20.11*. The SDS lists the hazards of the material, precautions that should be employed when the material is used, and procedures to be followed during emergencies. If you do not have an SDS for a particular product, call the manufacturer or check online. All dental personnel should know where the SDSs are stored. They should be available to be read by anyone who might come in contact with the material in question.

The information in an SDS is for worker safety as directed by OSHA. Only hazardous chemicals are included. Chemicals added to a product that are "generally recognized as safe" are not detailed in the SDS, nor are they listed as ingredients in a product unless directed by the FDA. Many additives that flavor or sweeten are not listed on professional dental products' labels or package inserts. This lack of information can be a problem for patients or personnel with unusual allergies or metabolic problems. Obtaining complete information from a manufacturer about all ingredients in a professional product such as a fluoride gel or prophy paste can be difficult. Manufacturers regard such information as proprietary. What is the dental professional to do? We must assess patient risk on an individual basis and provide the best treatment possible.

B. Labels

It is very important that chemicals be properly labeled. The name of the chemical and other important information should be on each and every chemical container. Hazardous chemicals must not be stored in the same refrigerator as food.

C. Disinfectants

Disinfectants can be very irritating to the skin. Many disinfectants are corrosive; that is, they can cause a chemical burn if they come in contact with bare skin. Some disinfectants may penetrate some types of glove material; it is important to pay attention to the manufacturer's instructions for handling a material. Some disinfectants may react with other chemicals used in the office. Avoid such mixing, unless it is known to be safe.

D. Mercury

Mercury is used in the making of dental amalgams, as discussed in Chapter 6, Amalgam. For many years, concern has been raised about the hazards to patients and dental professionals from exposure to mercury. Mercury was observed to be related to neurological problems even before *Alice in Wonderland* was published in the 1860s. The "Mad Hatter" character was based on hat makers of the time who became "mad" from their use of inorganic mercury salts to soften fur to make felt hats.

1. Mercury Toxicity
   Most forms of mercury can be toxic. The degree of toxicity is related to the chemical form of mercury. Organic forms, such as methyl mercury, are particularly hazardous. These forms are not used in dentistry. Inorganic mercury salts are toxic and are also not used in dentistry. The mercury in dental amalgam is an intermetallic compound and has very low or no toxicity. The most hazardous form of mercury in the dental office is metallic or elemental mercury. In this "quicksilver" form, it becomes volatile, especially if heated. When mercury vapor is inhaled, most is absorbed through the lungs. If liquid mercury or freshly mixed amalgam is handled without gloves, it can be absorbed through the skin. Chronic mercury toxicity affects the central nervous system. In addition, muscle tremors, mouth inflammation, irritability, and decreased kidney function can result from chronic exposure to unsafe levels of mercury. Acute mercury poisoning affects the kidneys.

2. Dental Personnel
   Studies have found some dentists to have elevated mercury levels in their blood and urine compared to nondentists. Some dentists have demonstrated early signs of neurological damage. Their offices were found to have poor mercury hygiene habits. Mercury was spilled when reusable amalgam capsules were not handled properly.
   Spilled mercury will roll off countertops, hide within cracks in tile floors, or be absorbed by carpets. Precapsulated amalgam has reduced the need to handle mercury and greatly simplified mercury hygiene. It is very important that

mercury spills be cleaned immediately. Spill kits are available specifically for mercury. Amalgam alloy (the powder) will absorb and react with mercury. The ADA has published guidelines for mercury hygiene. If good mercury hygiene is practiced in a dental office, then exposure and risk of toxicity are greatly reduced. In fact, this risk is small when compared to the risk posed by infectious agents.

E. Nitrous Oxide

Nitrous oxide (also known as laughing gas) is used as an analgesic in some dental offices. Exposure of dental personnel to nitrous oxide most often occurs during its administration to the patient (if protective measures are not used). Some effects that have been associated with exposure to high levels of nitrous oxide include spontaneous abortion and reduced fertility. Other effects include neurologic, hematologic, immunologic, liver, and kidney problems as well as certain kinds of malignancy. Most data supporting the relationship between nitrous oxide exposure and the occurrence of these problems were obtained before the use of protective measures had been widely implemented.

1. Reproductive Problems

   The use of scavenging equipment seems to lessen the risk of spontaneous abortion. In a study published in 1995, women who worked in offices where they were exposed to unscavenged nitrous oxide for 3 hours or more per week had a substantially higher rate of spontaneous abortion than an unexposed group. Those women who worked in offices using scavenging equipment showed no significantly different rate of spontaneous abortion compared to unexposed women. Another study showed that men as well as women were affected by exposure to the gas. Male dentists exposed to high levels of nitrous oxide were also subject to reduced fertility. The mechanism(s) by which nitrous oxide produces these effects is still being investigated.

2. Exposure

   Debate exists regarding how much exposure is too much. As of the writing of this chapter, OSHA has not issued regulations about exposure to nitrous oxide. The National Institute of Occupational Safety and Health (NIOSH), the group that researches the hazards of materials and makes recommendations to OSHA, has recommended limiting exposures to a **time-weighted average (TWA)** level of 25 ppm for dental personnel. A TWA measures the average exposure to a chemical over a period of time, and NIOSH has publications giving advice on practical ways to reduce exposures for dental personnel.

3. Measures to Reduce Exposure to Nitrous Oxide

   a. Check and maintain the delivery system to prevent leaks. Any leaks must be repaired before the equipment is used again.

   b. Employ a scavenging system to reduce the amount of waste gas that is released in the room. Vent the system to the outdoors.

   c. Make sure the scavenging system's mask fits the patient.

   d. Monitor periodically to determine exposure levels. Commercially available monitoring devices can be used to estimate personnel exposure.

   e. Use local exhaust near the patient's mouth to capture excess nitrous oxide.

   f. Ensure good room ventilation. The supply and exhaust vents should be well separated to prevent intake of contaminated air.

F. Disposal of Chemicals

Some chemicals can be poured down the drain. For many chemicals, however, it is illegal to do so because they may harm the environment. Proper disposal is required. Unused materials and chemicals may need to be disposed as hazardous waste. Some, such as amalgam scrap, can be recycled. Radiology wastes, such as developer, film (Ag), and lead foil, can also be recycled. Unfortunately, it is beyond the scope of this text to cover this subject in detail.

VI. Emergencies

Emergencies can happen even in the safest and most conscientious dental office. It is important to know what to do in the event of a medical emergency, fire, or other accident. Some state boards require first aid and cardiopulmonary resuscitation training for dentists and dental hygienists. Such training should be considered for all dental personnel. Phone numbers for emergency services, such as "911," local hospitals, poison centers, etc., should be posted by the phone. Emergency exits and escape routes should be posted as well. Emergency lighting and fire extinguishers should be properly maintained. There is no substitute for training in the event of an emergency. Remember, the most likely person to have a heart attack in the dental office is the dentist. First aid kits, emergency drug kits, and emergency equipment, including an AED (defibrillator), should be properly maintained or restocked.

Children in the dental office could be described as trouble waiting to happen. They should not be allowed in office and laboratory areas. They should not be left unsupervised in the clinic or waiting rooms while a parent or sibling receives treatment. The waiting room should be childproofed in the same manner as a home. Unused electrical outlets should be covered. Toys should not have small parts that may cause choking. Children should not be allowed to climb on the furniture and disrupt the waiting room. An area with entertainment such as books and puzzles should be provided for young children. Many "kids' videos" are enjoyed by both children and adults.

VII. Putting Risk in Perspective

By now, you might be thinking, "Wow! There are a lot more hazards in this job than I realized. It might be safer to be a stunt double or a rodeo clown!" It is true that many safety issues need to be considered in the dental profession. However, it is also important to remember that the existence of a risk does not automatically result in an injury or an illness.

We face many potential hazards all the time in our daily lives. We routinely cook our food, drive our cars, cut our lawns, and so on without giving too much thought about the risks we take in doing these activities. Most of the time, our daily activities do not result in accidents because we take the necessary precautions to avoid problems as a natural part of performing the task. In general, what are the precautions to be taken to reduce your risk of injury or illness in the dental office?

- Keep yourself informed. Learn about hazards and how to protect yourself. Some information has been provided under specific topics in this chapter, but research continues. Professional groups often are aware of the latest studies and may be a good source of information.
- Use proper procedures and equipment to minimize the chances of injury.
- Be prepared to deal with accidents or emergencies.
- At least annually, or more frequently if problems arise, do a self-audit. Take the time to examine what you are doing, and consider if it could be done better or more safely, not only regarding your own safety but also that of your patients and coworkers.

VIII. Acknowledgment

The authors thank Dr. Daniel Della-Giustina, Professor of Industrial and Management Systems Engineering at West Virginia University, for his review of this chapter.

Summary

Standard precautions must be followed for each patient. By OSHA mandate, dental care providers must wear appropriate gloves, mask, eye protection, and clothing during patient care activities involving saliva and blood. Patient treatment gloves are available in a variety of materials. Use of gloves does not preclude hand washing.

Facial masks are available in various styles and should be changed for each patient. For protection against inhalation of highly infectious aerosols, HEPA masks must be worn. Protective eyewear with side shields must be worn during procedures that may generate aerosol, splatter, or projectiles.

Dental instruments and equipment are categorized as critical, semicritical, or noncritical to determine the required method for decontamination. Intermediate-level disinfectants should be used for disinfecting noncritical items. Acceptable surface disinfectants are registered with the U.S. EPA. They are tuberculocidal and kill both lipophilic and hydrophilic viruses. An effective way to maintain surface disinfection is to cover the cleaned and disinfected surface with protective barriers.

Precautions must be taken to avoid punctures when handling sharp objects. Housekeeping practices must also be followed to protect the patient and dental care providers from cross-contamination. Each dental office and laboratory must have a written exposure control plan that includes the necessary steps to prevent exposure to blood-borne pathogens. This plan must be updated annually and be reviewed by all dental care workers in the facility.

Physical hazards in a dental office include the typical trips and falls that are risked in everyday life. Injuries from chemicals and equipment are also a concern. Flammable materials and oxygen increase the risk of fire, and autoclaves can be another cause of burns. Latex gloves, disinfectants, and other chemicals can cause skin problems. Ergonomics, for obvious reasons, are a particular concern for dental hygienists. Proper posture, lighting, and instrumentation reduce the likelihood of musculoskeletal problems. Chemicals should be properly stored and labeled. Mercury and nitrous oxide are known hazards in the dental office, but following proper procedures will reduce their risk. Preparations should be made to handle emergencies.

Learning Activities

1. Observe a student in the clinic. Make notes detailing proper and improper ergonomic practices.

2. Observe a student in the clinic. Look for errors in infection control procedures.

3. Make an inventory of the items in a cabinet of clinical supplies. Note which are hazardous materials.

4. Make a list of your daily activities, and note the procedures and equipments that are used to reduce risk.

Review Questions

Question 1. By OSHA mandate, the dental care provider must wear appropriate PPE (glove, mask, eye protection, and clothing) during patient care involving contact with blood and saliva. This PPE should be worn only in the clinical treatment area.

a. The first statement is true; the second statement is false.

b. The first statement is false; the second statement is true.

c. Both statements are true.

d. Both statements are false.

Question 2. Which type of patient care glove is recommended for noninvasive intraoral procedures?

a. Sterile surgeon's

b. Nonsterile exam

c. Copolymer "overgloves"

d. Utility gloves

Question 3. Hands should be washed before putting on and after removing gloves. If not visibly soiled and for nonsurgical procedures, hands may be cleaned by applying an alcohol-based solution and rubbing the hands for 15 seconds until the agent is dry.

a. The first statement is true; the second statement is false.

b. The first statement is false; the second statement is true.

c. Both statements are true.

d. Both statements are false.

Question 4. Which type of protective glove should be worn when hand scrubbing contaminated instruments before sterilization?

a. Exam gloves

b. Overgloves

c. Utility gloves

d. Sterile surgeon's gloves

Question 5. What type of PPE must be worn while treating a patient with a highly infectious disease, such as tuberculosis, spread by aerosol?

a. Full face shield with a standard mask

b. Full face shield

c. HEPA mask

d. Standard face mask

Question 6. Anesthetic needles, orthodontic wire, irrigation needles, and anesthetic cartridges must not be discarded in the regular trash. These items must be discarded in appropriately labeled cardboard boxes or plastic bags.

a. The first statement is true; the second statement is false.

b. The first statement is false; the second statement is true.

c. Both statements are true.

d. Both statements are false.

Question 7. All of the following chemicals are acceptable surface disinfectants except one. Which one is the EXCEPTION?

a. Phenols

b. Iodophors

c. Chlorine

d. Quaternaries

e. Glutaraldehydes

Question 8. An acceptable surface disinfectant must be tuberculocidal and kill both hydrophilic and lipophilic viruses. Hydrophilic viruses are much harder to kill than lipophilic viruses.

a. The first statement is true; the second statement is false.

b. The first statement is false; the second statement is true.

c. Both statements are true.

d. Both statements are false.

Question 9. According to Spaulding's Classification of Inanimate Objects, critical items are those items that may penetrate soft tissue or bone. These items must be sterilized by heat or high-level disinfection.

a. The first statement is true; the second statement is false.
b. The first statement is false; the second statement is true.
c. Both statements are true.
d. Both statements are false.

Question 10. Surface disinfection occurs after an intermediate-level disinfectant is sprayed onto a surface and allowed to air-dry. Disinfection, however, is not effective unless the surface is first cleaned.

a. The first statement is true; the second statement is false.
b. The first statement is false; the second statement is true.
c. Both statements are true.
d. Both statements are false.

Question 11. What is the recommended time to be serologically tested for antibody response after receiving the 3-dose series of hepatitis B vaccine?

a. 1 to 2 days
b. 1 to 2 weeks
c. 1 to 2 months
d. 1 to 2 years

Question 12. According to CDC guidelines, how often should biological monitoring of sterilizers be conducted?

a. At least weekly
b. At least monthly
c. For every sterilizer load
d. Only if the sterilizer is malfunctioning

Question 13. Safety equipment in the dental office should include the following EXCEPT:

a. A fire extinguisher
b. GFI outlets
c. Steel-toed shoes
d. Neoprene (rubber) gloves
e. Eye protection

Question 14. Health care workers have exhibited health problems from exposure to the following EXCEPT:

a. Mercury
b. Disinfectants
c. Latex gloves
d. Nitrous oxide
e. Fluorescent lighting

Question 15. Several chemicals used in the dental office penetrate latex gloves. Information on the proper protective gloves may be found in the SDS.

a. The first statement is true; the second statement is false.
b. The first statement is false; the second statement is true.
c. Both statements are true.
d. Both statements are false.

Question 16. Which of the following does not contribute to musculoskeletal problems?

a. Poor lighting
b. Poor posture
c. Indirect vision
d. Repetitive motions

Question 17. The most hazardous form of mercury encountered in a dental office is:

a. Mercury vapor
b. Liquid mercury
c. Dental amalgam
d. Amalgam scrap

Disinfection of Impressions, Dentures, and Other Appliances and Materials

Ashlee Sowards, R.D.H., M.S.D.H., T.T.S. and
Carol Spear, B.S.D.H., M.S.

21

Objectives

After studying this chapter, the student will be able to do the following:

1. Describe an effective infection control protocol for handling impressions and dental appliances that are transferred between the following:
   - Dental operatory and the dental laboratory within the dental office
   - Dental operatory and an outside commercial laboratory
2. Discuss and demonstrate the procedure for disinfecting dental impressions.
3. Explain and demonstrate the procedure for disinfecting dentures and other dental appliances after they have been processed or adjusted.
4. Describe and apply the infection control protocol that must be followed when grinding or polishing dentures and other appliances.
5. Review the preferred method (or methods) of sterilizing or disinfecting instruments or items used during manipulation of dental materials and prostheses.

Introduction

The primary goal of infection control is to prevent cross-contamination between patients and dental care providers. Because impressions or appliances contaminated by saliva or blood are often transported to and from in-office or remote dental laboratories, the potential for cross-contamination exists. Therefore, when these items are being handled, an infection control protocol must be explicitly communicated among and observed by the office staff as well as between the office and any remote dental laboratory. The Occupational Safety and Health Administration (OSHA) regulates the transportation of contaminated items between the dental office and dental laboratory. All items must be properly packaged and labeled.

Such an infection control protocol should include guidelines for the proper handling and disinfection or sterilization of impressions, dentures, appliances, and the equipment or materials used during the processing of these items. Attention must also be given to the personal protective equipment that is worn when handling these items and to the physical layout of the laboratory (see Chapter 20, Infection Control and Safety in the Dental Office).

Acceptable disinfectants include glutaraldehydes, iodophors, sodium hypochlorite, synthetic phenols, dual or synergized quaternaries, and sodium bromide and chlorine. However, all impression materials are not compatible with all disinfectants. Use of quaternaries or sodium bromide and chlorine for disinfecting impressions and prostheses is not found in the literature; however, if you select either of these chemicals for use as such in your dental office or laboratory, test it on samples of materials to check for compatibility. In addition, glutaraldehydes should never be sprayed because they are extremely toxic as aerosols.

I. Disinfection of Impressions

A. Personal Protective Equipment

Wear protective eyewear, an outer cover gown with long sleeves, a mask, and gloves when handling a contaminated impression until it has been disinfected.

B. Rinse the Impression

Immediately after an impression is taken in the dental operatory, rinse it under running water to remove any saliva or blood (*Fig. 21.1*). This step is essential for optimum disinfection of the impression.

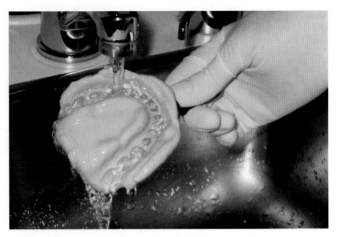

FIGURE 21.1. Rinsing an impression with running water.

C. Disinfection Techniques

Once the impression has been rinsed and shaken to remove excess water, it must be disinfected. This may be accomplished by immersing the impression in or spraying it with an acceptable disinfectant (Table 21.1). Always refer to the manufacturer's recommended disinfection technique for a particular material.

1. Disinfection of an Impression by Immersion
   Disinfection by immersion is preferred over disinfection by spraying. Spraying may not be as effective because constant contact of the disinfectant with all surfaces of the impression cannot be assured.
   a. Place the rinsed impression into a zippered plastic bag containing appropriate disinfectant (*Fig. 21.2*). Expel air to ensure contact of the entire impression with disinfectant. Seal bag.
   b. Exposure time to a disinfectant should be that which is recommended by the manufacturer of the product. Polyether and hydrocolloid impression materials may be adversely affected by disinfectants; therefore, limit their immersion time to no more than 10 minutes.
   c. Remove the impression from the disinfectant.
   d. Rinse the impression with running water, and shake to remove excess water.

2. Disinfection of an Impression by Spraying
   a. Spray the rinsed impression and impression tray with an acceptable disinfectant (*Fig. 21.3*).
   b. Seal the sprayed impression in a zippered plastic bag for the disinfection time recommended by the manufacturer.
   c. Remove the impression from the sealed bag.
   d. Rinse the impression with running water, and shake to remove excess water.

TABLE 21.1. Recommended Disinfectants for Impression Materials*ᵃ*

Impression Material	Glutaraldehydes	Iodophors	Sodium Hypochlorite (1:10 Dilution)	Synthetic Phenols
Alginate	No	Yes	Yes	Yes
Silicone	*ᵇ*Yes	Yes	Yes	Yes
Polyether	*ᵇ*Yes	Yes	Yes	Yes
Polysulfide	*ᵇ*Yes	Yes	Yes	Yes
Zinc oxide–eugenol (ZOE) paste	*ᵇ*Yes	Yes	No	No
Compound	No	Yes	Yes	Yes
Reversible hydrocolloid	No	Yes	Yes	Yes
Wax bites	No	Yes	No	Yes

aBite registrations are made of various materials and should be disinfected with the same chemical that is used on the impression. Incompatibility between materials and disinfectants, as well as between the same materials of different companies, may exist.
bUse only if another disinfectant is not readily available.
Adapted from Merchant VA. Infection control in the dental laboratory environment. In: Molinari JA, Harte JA, eds. Practical Infection Control in Dentistry. 3rd ed. Philadelphia, PA: Lippincott Williams & Wilkins; 2010:251–258; Miller CH, Palenik CJ. Infection Control and Management of Hazardous Materials for the Dental Team. 4th ed. St. Louis, MO: Mosby; 2010:208–209.

D. Pour the Impression

Once the impression has been disinfected, it may be poured with the desired gypsum product or sent to a lab.

II. Chairside Adjustments

For chairside adjustments of appliances, use a sterile handpiece, a sterile rag wheel, and unit dose of abrasive for polishing. Abrasive impregnated rubber points as shown in Figure 16.7 are an alternative. This eliminates the need to disinfect the prosthesis during handling. Handpieces and rag wheels will need to be resterilized after completion of the chairside adjustment.

A. Clean the Prosthesis or Appliance before Disinfecting

1. Brush the prosthesis with an unused toothbrush or denture brush, or clean it in an ultrasonic unit.

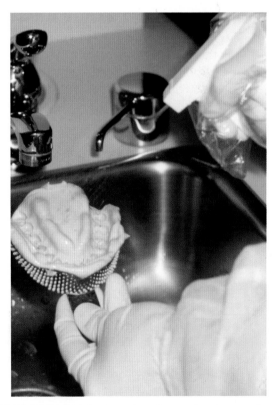

FIGURE 21.3. Disinfection of an impression by spraying and then immediately sealing it in a plastic bag for the manufacturer's recommended disinfecting time.

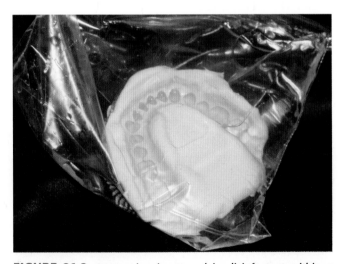

FIGURE 21.2. Impression immersed in disinfectant within a zippered plastic bag.

TABLE 21.2. Disinfection of Dentures and Other Appliances*a*

Prosthesis	Glutaraldehydes	Iodophors	Sodium Hypochlorite (1:10 Dilution)	Synthetic Phenols
Complete dentures	No	Yes	Yes	Yes
Removable appliances	No	Yes	No	Yes
Fixed prostheses	Yes	Yes	No	Yes

aFollow manufacturers' recommendation for disinfection, but limit exposure time of metal-containing prostheses to 10 minutes.
Adapted from Merchant VA. Infection control in the dental laboratory environment. In: Molinari JA, Harte JA. Practical Infection Control in Dentistry. 3rd ed. Philadelphia, PA: Lippincott Williams & Wilkins; 2010:255–256.

2. To avoid cross-contamination during ultrasonic cleaning, place the appliance in a zippered plastic bag or sterile glass beaker that contains fresh ultrasonic cleaning solution. Then, place the closed bag or beaker into the ultrasonic solution in the unit's holding tank.

3. Rinse the prosthesis after cleaning, and shake to remove excess water.

4. Use air abrasion only on cleaned and disinfected prostheses.

B. Disinfect the Cleaned Prosthesis

1. Place the prosthesis in a zippered plastic bag containing an acceptable disinfectant (Table 21.2) for the disinfection time recommended by the manufacturer. Immersing a metal prosthesis in a hypochlorite solution may damage the metal; therefore, use one of the other suggested disinfectants.

2. Spraying the prosthesis with a disinfectant and then sealing the sprayed appliance in a zippered plastic bag for the exposure time recommended by the manufacturer is an alternative disinfection method. However, the American Dental Association recommends immersion in disinfectant rather than spraying.

C. Rinse the Prosthesis

Thoroughly rinse the prosthesis as soon as it is removed from the disinfectant. Disinfectant remaining on the appliance tastes very bad and may cause tissue irritation.

D. Store the Prosthesis

Store the disinfected prosthesis in a clean, zippered plastic bag containing a mixture of mouthwash and water, or water alone. Never allow the prosthesis to be stored in a dry environment.

III. Disinfecting Dentures and Other Appliances

Dental appliances that have been worn by the patient must be cleaned and disinfected before repairs or adjustments are made in the dental laboratory. Likewise, dental prostheses must be cleaned and disinfected in the dental laboratory before they are returned to the dental office for patient try-in. Handle contaminated appliances with gloved hands, and return disinfected dental prostheses to the patient with clean, gloved hands.

IV. Infection Control Protocol for Grinding or Polishing Dentures or Other Appliances

Laboratory work may be performed on items or materials that have been used or worn by the patient. However, these items or materials must first be disinfected. Manipulation of these materials still requires following an infection control protocol:

• Make certain the ventilation system in the room is properly functioning.

• During operation of the dental lathe (*Fig. 21.4*), wear protective eyewear and a mask. See Chapter 20, Infection Control and Safety in the Dental Office regarding the safe use of a lathe.

• Clean and disinfect the dental lathe at least once daily.

• Use sterile rag wheels and stones as well as fresh pumice and pan liners for each prosthesis.

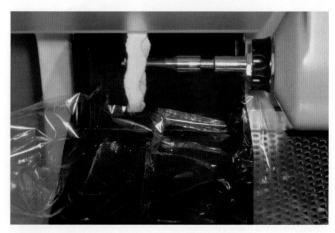

FIGURE 21.4. Dental lathe with sterile rag wheel attached and a single-use liner.

V. Sterilization/Disinfection of Items Used during Manipulation of Dental Materials and Prostheses

All items that come in contact with oral tissues or touch objects that contact oral tissues must be heat sterilized. These items include metal impression trays, burs, rag wheels and disks, metal spatulas, and glass mixing slabs.

Other items that do not come in direct contact with oral tissue may be disinfected or, if disposable, discarded. Sterilization and disinfection are presented in detail in Chapter 20, Infection Control and Safety in the Dental Office.

Remember, before an item can be successfully sterilized or disinfected, it must first be cleaned of all bioburden.

Summary

Because many impressions or appliances contaminated with saliva or blood are often transported to and from in-office or remote dental laboratories, the potential for cross-contamination exists. Therefore, an infection control protocol must be observed by the office staff and between the office and remote dental laboratory.

Personal protective equipment must be worn when handling contaminated impressions and dental prostheses.

Impressions must be rinsed, shaken to remove excess water, and then immersed or sprayed with an acceptable disinfectant.

Appliances worn by the patient must be cleaned and disinfected before adjustments are made in the dental laboratory. Likewise, dental prostheses must be cleaned and disinfected in the laboratory before they are sent to the office for patient try-in.

When grinding or polishing dentures or other appliances on a dental lathe, use sterile rag wheels and stones as well as fresh pumice and pan liners for each prosthesis. Wear protective eyewear and a mask, and make certain that the room is properly ventilated.

Metal impression trays, burs, rag wheels and disks, metal spatulas, and glass mixing slabs must be heat sterilized. Other items should be disinfected or, if disposable, discarded.

Learning Activities

Divide students into pairs, and have each pair observe and critique the infection control protocol for the situations that follow.

1. Handling an impression before pouring a model. Each student can take an impression of another student's dentition and pour the models.

2. Polishing an appliance in the laboratory after adjustments have been made and preparing it for return to the patient. This can be a mock situation because appliances from actual patients may not be readily available.

Review Questions

Question 1. **Immediately after an impression is taken, it must be rinsed under running water to remove saliva or blood. This step is essential before the impression can be disinfected.**

a. The first statement is true; the second statement is false.

b. The first statement is false; the second statement is true.

c. Both statements are true.

d. Both statements are false.

Question 2. **Chairside adjustments of appliances may be performed with a unit dose of abrasive, a sterile handpiece and bur, and a sterile rag wheel for polishing. This eliminates the need for disinfecting the appliance before handling.**

a. The first statement is true; the second statement is false.

b. The first statement is false; the second statement is true.

c. Both statements are true.

d. Both statements are false.

Question 3. All but one of the following steps must be performed when disinfecting a removable dental appliance before making laboratory adjustments. Which one is the EXCEPTION?

a. Handle a contaminated appliance with gloved hands

b. Clean ultrasonically by placing the appliance directly into the solution in the ultrasonic unit holding tank

c. Rinse the appliance under running water

d. Shake to remove excess water

e. Disinfect the appliance by spraying it with, or immersing it in, an acceptable disinfectant and then allowing contact for the time specified by the manufacturer.

Question 4. In the laboratory, when polishing dentures that have been worn by a patient, it is not necessary to use a sterile rag wheel. This is because the dentures will be disinfected before and after any adjustment is made.

a. Both the statement and the reason are correct.

b. Neither the statement nor the reason is correct.

c. The statement is correct, but the reason is not.

Question 5. After chairside adjustments are made to a dental prosthesis, it is cleaned, disinfected, rinsed, and stored. The recommended storage method is:

a. Placement of the prosthesis back on patient's stone cast

b. An individualized, plastic, closed container for each patient, similar to those used for overnight soaking

c. A zippered plastic bag containing mouthwash and water

d. A zippered plastic bag containing sterile water

Question 6. The primary goal of infection control when handling and disinfecting impressions, dentures, and appliances is to:

a. Protect the patient from the laboratory personnel

b. Protect the laboratory personnel from the patient

c. Prevent cross-contamination

d. Prevent contamination of equipment in the dental laboratory

Question 7. Disinfection by immersion is preferred over disinfection by spraying. The most important reason is because:

a. Office personnel don't have the necessary time available to spray thoroughly

b. The spraying procedure must be performed twice, with 10 minutes in between

c. Constant contact of the spray with all surfaces of the impression cannot be assured

d. The aerosol produced is usually toxic

General Rules for Handling Dental Materials

22

Objectives

After studying this chapter, the student will be able to do the following:

1. Give reasons why correct dispensing, timing, and mixing of materials are important.
2. Discuss the difference in setting times of dental materials in the oral cavity and on the instrument tray.
3. Summarize the recommended guidelines for light-activated dental materials.

Introduction

A dental hygienist must understand the composition, use, physical properties, and manipulation techniques for commonly used dental materials. This will promote office efficiency, economy of materials, and quality care for the patient. Based on this understanding, a few general rules should be followed to ensure success in the manipulation and application of these dental materials.

I. Follow the Manufacturer's Directions

A. It is very important to read, understand, and follow the directions that accompany dental materials. One should not only read the directions but also understand why each step is performed in the manner directed by the instructions.

B. Office personnel should save copies of directions for the materials used in that office. It is recommended that these copies be kept in a file, hard copy, or digital. Thus, if the directions for a kit are lost, a copy will be readily available. Most manufacturers have directions available online.

C. When a new material is purchased, practice using the new material at least once before using that material clinically. Check the "feel" of the new product; how does it compare to other products?

D. Store materials in a cool dry place. The shelf life of many materials is lengthened by refrigeration. On the other hand, some materials will gel or mixtures will separate if they are refrigerated. See manufacturers' directions for proper storage.

II. Mixing and Setting Times

A. Use a clock that has a second hand or displays seconds to time etching, mixing, setting, and other important time spans. This applies to the clinic and to the laboratory.

B. The mouth is a warm environment. Therefore, materials set faster when in the mouth than on the instrument tray or countertop. If a material is set on the instrument tray, it is set in the mouth. Exceptions to this rule are materials that set by cooling, such as impression compound, and light-activated materials.

C. The setting of some materials is also accelerated by the humidity of the mouth.

III. Dispensing Materials

A. Dispense materials properly, as directed by the instructions. Recap tubes and bottles after dispensing materials. Volatile solvents will evaporate from open containers. The chemical composition of the material will then change; performance will suffer.

B. Dispense equal lengths, not equal volumes, of pastes.

C. Dispense consistent drops. Allowing the drop to run onto a mixing pad before it turns into a separate drop and falls from the dispensing tip will result in inconsistent drops. Inconsistent and incorrect powder/liquid ratios result from this type of dispensing method. The powder/liquid ratio is an important determinant of properties.

D. Fluff powders if recommended by the manufacturer. Alginate powder should be tumbled periodically to fluff the powder; it is not necessary to fluff alginate for every impression.

E. Do not dispense materials too early; allowing them to sit out unused may be detrimental, especially if the humidity is high.

IV. Mixing

A. Mix dental materials aggressively. They are not alive; they cannot be harmed. After mixing alginate, your arm should be tired.

B. The setting rate of some materials is affected by the mixing technique that is used.

C. When mixing cements, force the powder into the liquid.

V. Light-Activated Materials

A. You can undercure, but you cannot overcure, light-activated materials.

B. Maintain a space between the tip of the curing light and the oral tissues. Some light tips become quite warm and may overheat the tooth or soft tissues.

C. Light-activated materials will begin to set in ambient room light. They should not be dispensed ahead of time and left exposed. Therefore, light-activated materials need to be protected from light if not used immediately.

VI. Contamination

Contamination by oral fluids is bad for all materials. This concept applies to adhesive restorative materials as well as nonadhesive restorative materials. It is critical to keep teeth clean and, sometimes, dry when using adhesive materials.

Summary

Following and saving the manufacturer's directions when using any dental material will enhance the quality of patient care. Manipulation factors, such as proper dispensing, correct mixing, adequate curing, and avoiding contamination, will promote successful use and service of the dental material.

 Learning Activities

1. Develop a list of dental materials commonly used in your clinic. Which of the general rules presented in this chapter apply to these materials?

2. Can you locate the manufacturer's directions for the materials listed in learning activity #1?

 Review Questions

Question 1. When dispensing paste/paste dental materials, equal _____ are usually the proper method for proportioning the two pastes.

a. Weights
b. Volumes
c. Lengths
d. Loads

Question 2. It is important to read the directions that accompany a dental product. It is more important to understand the dispensing, mixing, and handling of a dental material.

a. The first statement is true; the second statement is false.
b. The first statement is false; the second statement is true.
c. Both statements are true.
d. Both statements are false.

Question 3. All of the following statements are true except one. Which one is the EXCEPTION?

a. Practice using new materials at least once before using clinically
b. Setting of some materials is accelerated by the humidity of the mouth
c. Dental materials set slower in the mouth than on the bracket tray
d. For cement, powders should be forced into the liquid when mixing

Question 4. Dental materials should be mixed:

a. Slowly and deliberately
b. In large increments, every 5 seconds
c. In small increments, every 5 seconds
d. Aggressively

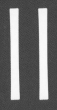

Laboratory and Clinical Applications

Mixing Liners, Bases, and Cements

23

Objectives

After performing the laboratory/clinical exercises in this chapter, the student will be able to do the following:

1. Describe the use or purpose of the following materials:
   - Calcium hydroxide
   - Zinc phosphate
   - Glass ionomer
   - Zinc oxide–eugenol (ZOE)
   - Temporary cement
2. Demonstrate the proper mixing technique for the materials listed above, and then, evaluate the mix according to the criteria stated in this chapter.
3. Recall the approximate mixing and setting times for the liners, bases, and cements discussed in this chapter.
4. Clean the cement spatula or mixing instrument and slab with the appropriate cleaning agent before the material sets.

Key Words/Phrases

obtundent

exothermic

Introduction

The various cements, bases, and liners used in restorative dentistry are discussed in detail in Chapter 7, Dental Cements. The discussion covers the use, composition, and physical as well as chemical properties of each material. As stated earlier, these materials can be used as base or lining agents, luting materials, or permanent or temporary restorations. This chapter focuses on the manipulation of some of these commonly used materials.

I. Purpose

Mixing of cements, bases, and liners is not a procedure that the dental hygienist typically performs on a routine basis. However, the hygienist may be asked by the dentist to mix these materials if the dental assistant is absent. This situation would include using them as a temporary restoration. Step-by-step instructions for measuring and mixing some of the commonly used cements, bases, and liners serve as the basis for this chapter.

II. Calcium Hydroxide Base/Liner Material

A. Use

Calcium hydroxide may be used for pulp capping and as a base/liner under other dental restorative materials in deep preparations.

B. Protective Properties

Calcium hydroxide serves as a protective barrier between tooth tissues (dentin and pulp) and acid-containing cements and restorative materials.

C. Measuring

1. The items necessary for mixing calcium hydroxide base/liner material are listed in Table 23.1.
2. Dispense small but equal amounts on a paper mixing pad, as shown in *Figure 23.1*.

D. Mixing

1. Mix thoroughly with a cement spatula or the crook of a small, ball-pointed instrument until

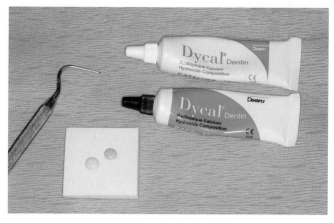

FIGURE 23.1. Calcium hydroxide dispensed on a paper mixing pad.

a uniform color is achieved. A completed mix of calcium hydroxide is shown in *Figure 23.2*.
2. Mixing should be completed within 10 seconds.
3. The criteria for a correct mix of calcium hydroxide are listed in Table 23.2.

E. Application

Use the tip of the ball-pointed instrument to place the mixed material on the floor of the cavity preparation. Avoid placing the mixed material on walls and margins, and avoid placing it in large amounts.

F. Setting

1. The setting time of mixed calcium hydroxide is 2 to 3 minutes on the mixing pad at normal room temperature.
2. The setting time for a pulp capping or base/liner will be greatly decreased in the mouth because of the moisture of dentin.

TABLE 23.1. Armamentarium for Mixing Calcium Hydroxide Base/Liner Material

Paper mixing pad

Mixing instrument

Calcium hydroxide base and catalyst

2 × 2 gauze

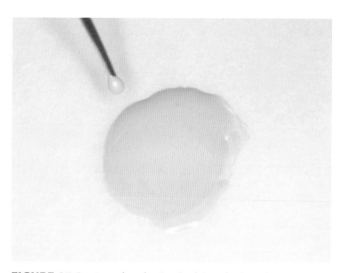

FIGURE 23.2. Completed mix of calcium hydroxide.

TABLE 23.2. Evaluation Criteria for Mixing Calcium Hydroxide Material

1. An appropriate amount is dispensed.
2. Mixing occurs within 10 seconds.
3. Completed mix is uniform in color.

III. Zinc Phosphate Cement

A. Use

As discussed in Chapter 7, Dental Cements, zinc phosphate cement is used to lute inlays, crowns, bridges, orthodontic bands, and other appliances to tooth structure. It can also be used as a base material under restorations.

B. Related Information

Remember that when the powder and liquid are mixed, an **exothermic** (heat-releasing) reaction occurs, as discussed in Chapter 7. To dissipate the heat of this reaction:
1. A large portion of the glass slab must be used during mixing.
2. The powder must be added in small increments.
3. The mixing time must extend to 1.5 to 2 minutes.

C. Measuring, Mixing, and Application for Luting Consistency

1. The items necessary to mix zinc phosphate cement are listed in Table 23.3.
2. This technique is described in detail, along with illustrations, in Chapter 7.
3. The number of drops of liquid and scoops of powder that are required can be found in the directions provided by the manufacturer.
4. Forcibly mix the powder into the liquid by increments. A figure-8 motion is frequently used, as shown in *Figure 23.3*. Sometimes, a back-and-forth stropping motion is used.
5. The mixing time is usually 15 seconds for each increment.

TABLE 23.3. Armamentarium for Mixing Zinc Phosphate Cement

Zinc phosphate powder

Zinc phosphate liquid

Liquid dispenser

Powder scoop

Cement spatula

Glass slab

Solution of bicarbonate of soda (optional)

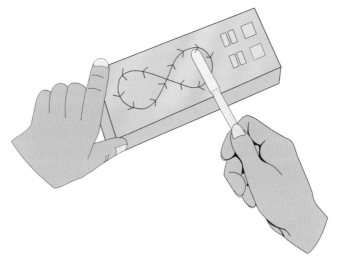

FIGURE 23.3. The Figure-8 mixing technique for a dental cement.

6. Remember that for correct luting consistency, the cement should form a "1-inch string" between the spatula and the slab, as shown in Figure 7.6E.
7. The Skill Performance Evaluation sheet for mixing zinc phosphate cement to a luting consistency is located in Appendix 2.

D. Measuring, Mixing, and Application for Base Consistency

1. The difference between luting consistency and base consistency is that a higher powder/liquid ratio is used for base consistency. This means that fewer drops of liquid will be needed to mix the cement for a base consistency. The specific amounts to be used are provided by the manufacturer.
2. The powder is also divided into increments for base consistency, but this may include the division of one powder increment into yet smaller increments.
3. The mixing time is approximately the same as that for luting consistency (1.5–2 minutes).
4. The completed mix should be thick, putty-like, and able to be rolled into a ball.
5. The base consistency for zinc phosphate is shown in Figure 7.6F.
6. The Skill Performance Evaluation sheet for mixing zinc phosphate cement to a base consistency is located in Appendix 2.

E. Setting

The setting time for both consistencies of zinc phosphate cement is between 5 and 9 minutes.

F. Cleanup

Tap water is used to clean the spatula and glass slab before the cement sets. If the mix has set on the spatula and slab, the instruments can be cleaned by soaking them in a solution of bicarbonate of soda (baking soda) and water.

Tips for the Clinician

Calcium Hydroxide Liner/Base

- Mix until a homogeneous color is obtained.
- Wipe the mixing instrument clean with a gauze before applying material to the cavity preparation.

Zinc Phosphate Cement

- Mix using a large area of the slab to dissipate the heat.
- When finished, clean the slab and spatula immediately with soap and water.

Glass Ionomer Cement

- When dispensing the liquid, take the necessary time to make precise, uniform drops.
- Mixing time is short, usually 45 seconds or less.

Zinc Oxide–Eugenol (ZOE) Cement

- Use firm pressure with the flat face of the spatula when incorporating powder.
- Enough powder has been incorporated for a base consistency when the mix "flakes" from the spatula when pressing on the cement.

Temporary Cement

- Mix until a homogeneous color is obtained.

IV. Glass Ionomer

A. Use

Glass ionomer cement may be used as a base, a luting agent, or a restorative material. As a luting agent, it is used to permanently cement crowns, bridges, and orthodontic bands. As a base, it is used as a thermal insulating material in deep cavity preparations.

B. Related Information

As discussed in Chapter 7, Dental Cements, glass ionomer cements are high in strength and low in solubility. Compared to other cements, they are also relatively kind to the pulp. They chemically bond to tooth structure, and they release fluoride ions into enamel and dentin, which is believed to reduce recurrent decay. It is for these reasons that this cement has become so popular.

C. Dispensing Systems

Glass ionomer may be dispensed in three ways:

1. Powder/Liquid Systems
   Examples of powder and liquid are shown in Figures 7.7A and *23.4*. This chapter focuses on the powder/liquid systems.

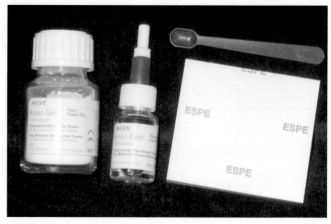

FIGURE 23.4. Glass ionomer cement: powder, liquid, dispensing scoop, and paper pad.

2. Disposable Capsules
   The capsule form of glass ionomer cement is illustrated in Figure 7.7B. This capsule is mixed in an amalgamator, similar to the way in which an amalgam capsule is mixed. Specific directions for mixing are provided by the manufacturer.

3. Paste/Paste Systems
   Paste/paste systems are now being marketed. One such dispensing device is pictured in *Figure 23.5*. Pressing the lever dispenses the proper ratio of each paste. The material is mixed as in other paste/paste systems until a homogeneous color is obtained. This material may come with an auto-mix tip similar to those used with impression materials.

D. Measuring and Mixing for Luting Consistency

The items necessary to mix a powder/liquid glass ionomer cement are listed in Table 23.4.

1. Measure the Powder
   a. Shake the jar of powder to "fluff" the contents.
   b. Fill, but not pack, the dispensing scoop.
   c. Remove the scoop from bottle by sliding it against the plastic lip in the neck of the bottle, as shown in *Figure 23.6*. This action will eliminate excess powder.
   d. Place one scoop of powder on the paper mixing pad.

2. Measure the Liquid
   a. Hold the bottle vertically when dispensing the liquid so that precise and uniform drops will be produced, as shown in *Figure 23.7*.
   b. Dispense appropriate number of drops of liquid.

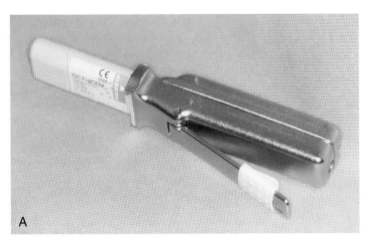

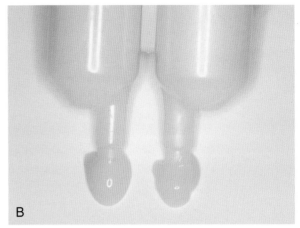

FIGURE 23.5. **A.** Dispenser for a paste/paste glass ionomer material. **B.** Paste materials being dispensed.

3. Mix the Powder and Liquid
To mix, the powder should be added to the liquid in one portion. The typical luting consistency is such that the material stretches 0.5 inch between the spatula and slab, as shown in *Figure 23.8*.

4. Mixing Time
Mixing time ranges between 15 and 30 seconds. Refer to the manufacturer's instructions.

5. Immediate Use
The cement must be used while glossy. When the surface becomes dull, the setting reaction has begun, and the mix should be discarded.

6. Skill Performance Evaluation Sheet
The Skill Performance Evaluation sheet for mixing glass ionomer luting cement is located in Appendix 2.

E. Measuring and Mixing for Base Consistency

1. For bases and liners, a different glass ionomer product is employed with a higher powder/liquid ratio.

2. The powder and liquid are usually measured and mixed in the same manner for base consistency as that described earlier for luting consistency.

3. The mixing time for base consistency ranges between 15 and 30 seconds. Specific directions for mixing are provided by the manufacturer.

F. Setting

The setting time for both consistencies of glass ionomer is usually 7 minutes.

G. Cleanup

The spatula can be cleaned with soap and water before the cement has set.

H. Light-Activated Glass Ionomer Materials

Light-activated glass ionomer materials are typically used as a base or restorative material. They may be a powder/liquid system in bottles or in capsule form. The manufacturer's directions should be followed for mixing.

TABLE 23.4. Armamentarium for Mixing Glass Ionomer Cement

Glass ionomer powder
Glass ionomer liquid
Dispensing scoop
Liquid dispensing tip
Treated paper pad
Cement spatula

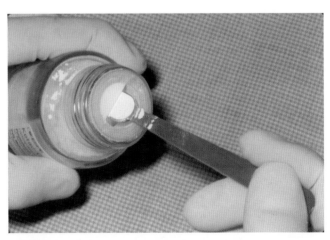

FIGURE 23.6. Eliminating excess glass ionomer powder from the scoop.

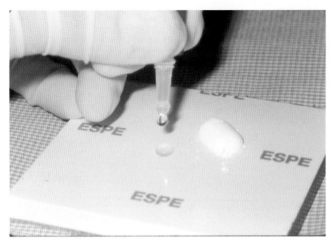

FIGURE 23.7. Measuring glass ionomer liquid.

V. Zinc Oxide–Eugenol (ZOE) Cement

A. Use

Zinc oxide–eugenol (ZOE) cement is one of the least irritating dental materials, and it may be used for several purposes:

1. To cement a temporary crown while a permanent one is being fabricated
2. To create an insulating base under permanent restorations
3. To provide a sedative or **obtundent** (soothing agent) filling for sensitive teeth

B. Protective Properties

As an insulating base, ZOE cement will protect the pulp from thermal trauma. It also has a sedative and soothing effect on the dental pulp; for this reason, it is used as a temporary restoration before a permanent one is placed.

C. Measuring

1. The items necessary to mix ZOE cement are listed in Table 23.5.

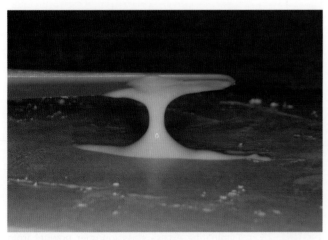

FIGURE 23.8. Proper luting consistency of glass ionomer cement.

TABLE 23.5. Armamentarium for Zinc Oxide–Eugenol (ZOE) Cement
Zinc oxide powder
Powder scoop
Eugenol
Eye dropper
Glass slab or treated paper pad
Cement spatula
2 × 2 gauze sponges
Isopropyl alcohol

2. Using the measuring scoop provided by the manufacturer, place one scoop of powder on a glass slab or treated paper pad. The product, scoop, and slab are illustrated in *Figure 23.9.*
3. Dispense two drops of eugenol liquid by holding the dropper perpendicular to the glass slab. The drops should not touch the powder, but they should be placed near it. The measured powder and liquid are shown in *Figure 23.10.*

D. Mixing Technique for a Base/Temporary Restoration Consistency

1. While holding the spatula in a "flat" position, draw approximately half the powder into the liquid.
2. Using a small portion of the mixing surface, spatulate the powder and liquid in a quick motion with the flat side of the spatula. The mixing technique is illustrated in *Figure 23.11.*
3. Continue to incorporate small portions of powder by deliberately "pressing" the powder into the mix with the spatula. The mix must be thick, putty-like, and almost "crumbly."

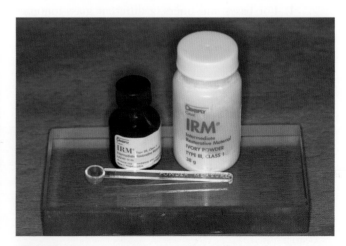

FIGURE 23.9. Zinc oxide and eugenol (IRM), measuring scoop, and glass slab.

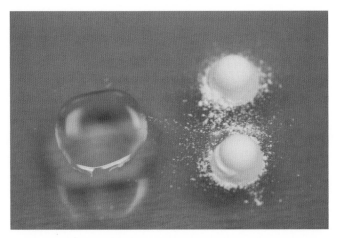

FIGURE 23.10. Zinc oxide and eugenol measured for a base or temporary restoration.

4. The mix should be completed in 1.5 minutes.
5. The Skill Performance Evaluation sheet for mixing ZOE cement to a base/temporary consistency is located in Appendix 2.

E. Application

1. Gather the cement into one mass on the slab.
2. The cement may be rolled with the fingers to form a ball.
3. Any suitable flat-bladed instrument, such as a plastic filling instrument (PFI), may be used to carry portions of the cement to the cavity preparation. The fingers or instrument may first be dipped into some extra powder to prevent the mixed cement from sticking.

F. Setting

The setting time is between 2.5 and 3.5 minutes in the mouth.

G. Cleanup

The slab and spatula may be cleaned with isopropyl alcohol and 2 × 2 gauze sponges.

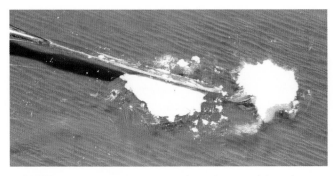

FIGURE 23.11. Mixing of zinc oxide and eugenol for a base or temporary restoration.

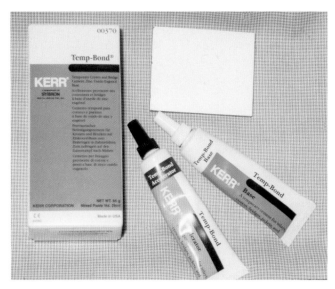

FIGURE 23.12. Base and accelerator of a temporary cement.

VI. Temporary Cement

A. Use

Temporary cement may be used in trial cementing of permanent restorations or in cementing of temporary crowns, bridges, or splints.

B. Properties

Temporary cements have high flow, which permits the restoration to be easily seated. They are strong enough to withstand the stresses of mastication, yet they allow the restoration to be easily removed when desired.

C. Measuring

The components of temporary cement are a base and a catalyst, which are supplied in two tubes. An example of this material is shown in *Figure 23.12*.
1. The items necessary to mix temporary cement are listed in Table 23.6.
2. Squeeze equal lengths from each tube onto a paper mixing pad, as shown in *Figure 23.13*.

D. Mixing

1. Thoroughly mix the pastes within 30 seconds.
2. Mix the pastes in a small area until a homogeneous color is obtained.

TABLE 23.6. Armamentarium for Mixing a Temporary Cement

Cement spatula

Paper mixing pad

Temporary cement base and catalyst

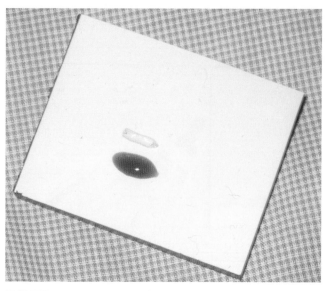

FIGURE 23.13. Equal lengths of temporary cement pastes dispensed on a paper mixing pad.

3. Material should form a string when stretched from the mixing pad. The mixing procedure is illustrated in *Figure 23.14*.
4. Criteria for the correct mix of a temporary cement are listed in Table 23.7.

E. Application

Spread a thin layer of cement over all areas of the restoration that will contact the preparation.

F. Setting

The setting time is approximately 2 minutes in the mouth.

VII. Resin Composite Cements

Composite cements are the material of choice for all-ceramic crowns and veneers. They are paste/paste systems

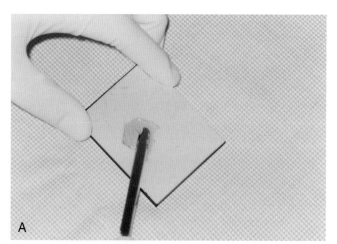

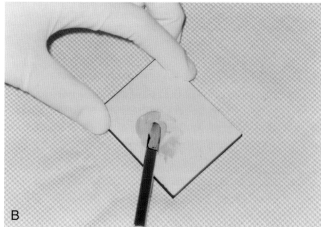

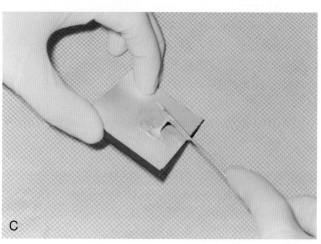

FIGURE 23.14. Mixing procedure for a temporary cement. **A** and **B.** Mixing. **C.** Proper luting consistency.

TABLE 23.7. Evaluation Criteria for Mixing Temporary Cement

1. An appropriate amount is dispensed.
2. Mixing occurs within 30 seconds.
3. Completed mix is uniform in color.
4. Cement makes a string between slab and spatula.

Precautions

Calcium Hydroxide Liner/Base

- Humid conditions will accelerate the setting reaction.

Zinc Phosphate Cement

- Do not cool the slab beyond the dew point. Condensation will adversely affect the mix and the setting time.
- It is critical to mix the cement slowly, in increments, to dissipate heat.
- Make sure the bottles are always properly closed to prevent absorption of moisture.

Glass Ionomer Cement

- The mix must be used while it is glossy.

Zinc Oxide–Eugenol (ZOE) Cement

- For a base consistency, it is important that enough powder is incorporated. Otherwise, the mixture will be "sticky" and difficult to place.

Temporary Cement

- Humidity will accelerate the setting of ZOE-based materials.

Composite Cement

- It is important to follow the manufacturer's directions for the bonding system and use of the cement.

that are used with a bonding system as shown in Figure 7.9. They typically come as two tubes or a dispensing system similar to that shown in *Figure 23.5B*. The material is mixed as with other paste/paste systems until a homogeneous color is obtained. These materials may come with an auto-mix tip as shown in Figure 7.9B. When using composite cements, it is important to follow the manufacturer's instructions for both the cement and the bonding system. Isolation from oral fluids is critical. The mixed material is applied to the inside of the crown and the restoration is seated on the prepared tooth. It is important to remove the excess cement when it reaches a "doughy" consistency; again follow the manufacturer's directions. If the cement is allowed to set to a brittle mass, removal of excess material can be very difficult.

Summary

Each of the various cements used in dentistry has its own uses, mixing and setting times, mixing techniques, and characteristics of a proper mix. Proper handling will result in the optimum properties for each material.

Calcium Hydroxide Liner/Base

- Dispense small, but equal, amounts on the paper pad.
- Use an appropriate instrument to mix the components in 10 seconds.
- Apply material with a clean instrument. Avoid using large increments.

Zinc Phosphate Cement (Luting and Base Consistencies)

- Dispense the manufacturer's recommended amounts of liquid and powder for the desired consistency.
- Divide into appropriate increments.
- Mix using a large portion of the slab.

- Add powder in small increments.
- Mixing time ranges from 1.5 to 2 minutes (usually 15 seconds per increment).
- Luting consistency: material forms a 1-inch string between the slab and the spatula.
- Base consistency: thick, putty-like, and will roll into a ball.

Glass Ionomer Cement

- Measure the powder by "fluffing" the container and then sliding the scoop against the lip of bottle to eliminate excess powder.
- Measure the liquid by holding the bottle vertically to get precise, uniform drops.
- Powder is added to the liquid in one or two portions. Mixing time is usually 30 to 45 seconds.
- Luting consistency: Mix should form a 0.5-inch string between the slab and the spatula.

Zinc Oxide–Eugenol (ZOE) Cement (Base and Temporary Restoration)

- Measure the powder and the liquid according to manufacturer's directions.
- Draw half the powder into the liquid.
- Spatulate using the flat of the spatula and a small portion of the slab surface.
- Continue adding small portions of powder by "pressing" it into the mix.
- Mixing should take approximately 1.5 minutes to complete.
- The finished mix should appear thick, putty-like, and almost "crumbly."

Temporary Cement

- Squeeze equal lengths from each tube onto the paper pad.
- Thoroughly mix to a homogeneous color.
- Material should form a string when stretched from the pad.
- Apply the material to the entire surface to be luted.

Composite Cement

- Dispense equal amounts and mix to a homogenous color.

Review Questions

Question 1. Which of the following dental cements is significantly accelerated by humidity during mixing?

a. Calcium hydroxide
b. ZOE
c. Both
d. Neither

Question 2. Which dental cement is used to calm an irritated dental pulp?

a. Calcium hydroxide
b. ZOE
c. Zinc phosphate
d. Glass ionomer

Question 3. Which dental cement is mixed slowly to dissipate the heat of the setting reaction?

a. Calcium hydroxide
b. ZOE
c. Zinc phosphate
d. Glass ionomer

Question 4. Which dental cement should be applied before its glossy appearance becomes dull?

a. Calcium hydroxide
b. ZOE
c. Zinc phosphate
d. Glass ionomer

Question 5. Cleanup of the mixing slab and cement spatula are best accomplished before the material sets. After cement materials set, they are easily cleaned by soap and water.

a. The first statement is true; the second statement is false.
b. The first statement is false; the second statement is true.
c. Both statements are true.
d. Both statements are false.

Question 6. Which dental cement is typically used with a dentin bonding system?

a. Resin composite
b. ZOE
c. Zinc phosphate
d. Glass ionomer

Application and Removal of the Rubber Dam

Rebecca Thomas, B.S.D.H.

Objectives

After performing the laboratory/clinical exercises in this chapter, the student will be able to do the following:

1. List the indications and contraindications for placing the rubber dam.
2. Describe the purpose of the rubber dam armamentarium (rubber dam, rubber dam clamp, punch, etc.).
3. Summarize the steps for placement and removal of the rubber dam.

Key Words/Phrases

aspirating

isolating

ligature

septum

winged clamps

wingless clamps

Introduction

Basic, step-by-step instructions for application and removal of the rubber dam are discussed in this chapter. In most cases, one of two placement techniques is routinely used: the one-step method, in which the dam and clamp are placed simultaneously or the two-step method, in which the clamp is placed on the anchor tooth and the dam material is then stretched over the clamp. In this chapter, the one-step method will be the technique of choice.

Clinical success of rubber dam isolation (exposure of selected teeth) is determined by the placement and retention methods of the clinician. Problems with rubber dam placement are often the result of torn rubber dam material, improper hole size and placement, or inadequate tautness of frame placement.

The rubber dam is usually placed after local anesthesia has been administered and while waiting for that anesthetic to take effect. Proper rubber dam placement can be achieved by a clinician in 3 to 5 minutes or, with a team approach, within 2 minutes.

I. Purpose and Indications

Proper isolation during technique-sensitive dental procedures is important but is also sometimes difficult to achieve. The purpose of rubber dam placement is to improve the overall quality of dental treatment. Indications for rubber dam placement are moisture control, visibility, patient protection, and patient treatment.

Rubber dam placement allows the clinician to achieve a dry field by **isolating** the tooth (or teeth) indicated for treatment from oral fluids and other oral tissues (lips, cheeks, tongue, and gingiva). This protects the patient from swallowing or **aspirating** (drawing into the lungs) debris and dental objects that are used during the procedure. It also protects the tissues from irritating materials used for the procedure such as acids for etching enamel.

II. Contraindications

Rubber dam placement is contraindicated for patients who are claustrophobic, suffer from severe asthma, or have trouble breathing through their nose. Other contraindications include patients with teeth that are not fully erupted as the clamp may not be stable and patients who cannot tolerate the clamp without anesthesia.

III. Procedure

The success of rubber dam placement is dependent on the technique and skill of the clinician. The items needed for rubber dam placement are listed in Table 24.1.

TABLE 24.1. Armamentarium for Placing the Rubber Dam

Clamps

Floss

Forceps

Frame

Ink pad

Ligatures

Mirror

Plastic filling instrument (PFI)

Punch

Rubber dam material

Scissors

Stamp

A. Choosing the Rubber Dam Material

Selection of the rubber dam material is based on the clinician's preferences regarding size, color, and thickness. Traditional dam material was latex rubber. Nonlatex rubber dams are necessary for those patients or operators with a latex hypersensitivity. Nonlatex dams are becoming popular. The most common size is the precut, 6- × 6-inch square, which is used for isolation of posterior teeth in the permanent dentition. Another common size is the precut, 5- × 5-inch square, which is used for primary dentition or anterior applications. A continuous roll of rubber dam material is available as well, and the choice of colors ranges from pastels to browns and greens. The color is used to contrast the tooth, making the treatment field more visible.

The rubber dam is also available in thicknesses (gauges) of thin, medium, and heavy. The medium rubber dam is widely used because of its ease of handling and resistance to tearing. The armamentarium, less the rubber dam stamp and ink pad, is shown in *Figure 24.1.*

B. Preparing the Rubber Dam Material

1. Stamp the Material

   The rubber dam stamp has markings for the average permanent and primary dentitions. The use of the stamp allows several sheets of dam material to be marked in advance. A rubber dam stamp and stamped dam are shown in *Figure 24.2.*

2. Punch the Holes

   Next, holes are punched into the rubber dam to correspond to the teeth that are to be isolated. The rubber dam punch usually consists of a rotating punch plate that allows holes of five or

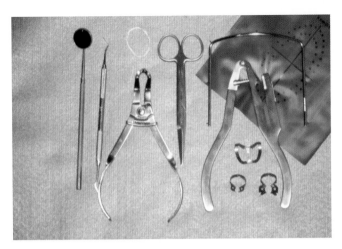

FIGURE 24.1. The basic rubber dam armamentarium.

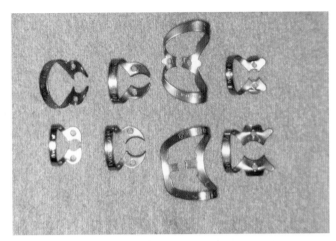

FIGURE 24.3. An assortment of rubber dam clamps: winged clamps (*right side*), wingless clamps (*left side*), and "butterfly-shaped" clamps (*middle*) used to isolate anterior teeth and the buccal of some posterior teeth (*see Fig. 24.8*).

six different sizes and a metal point (punch) that creates the holes. The larger holes are used for posterior teeth, the smaller holes for premolars and canines, and the smallest holes for incisors. Correct hole size plays a critical role in successful tooth isolation.

3. **Prepare the Clamp (Retainer)**

The clamp is prepared by threading floss through the facial hole and then tying a knot. This prevents the clamp from being aspirated should it spring free and allows for quick retrieval. The clamp is used as an anchor for the dam material and to retract the gingiva. Both **winged clamps** (clamps with extra projections) **and wingless clamps** (clamps without projections) are available, as are different shapes and sizes to fit the primary and permanent teeth. These are illustrated in *Figure 24.3*. The extra projections of winged clamps allow the dam and the clamp to be applied simultaneously. These are shown in *Figure 24.4*. When wingless clamps are used, they

are applied first to the tooth, and the rubber dam is then stretched over the clamp and the tooth.

C. Placement of the Rubber Dam

1. Check the patient's record and medical history for documentation of the area that needs to be isolated and for potential contraindications. Inform the patient of the procedure and the steps involved in placing the rubber dam.

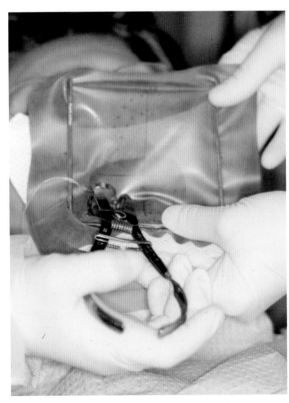

FIGURE 24.4. The placement of the rubber dam, clamp, and forceps for a mandibular tooth.

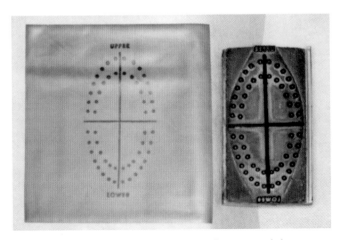

FIGURE 24.2. A rubber dam stamp and a stamped dam.

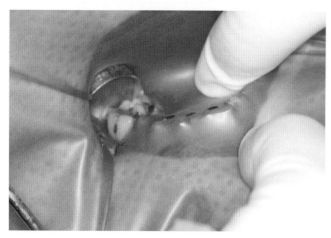

FIGURE 24.5. Once the anchor tooth is clamped, the last-punched hole is placed first for easier orientation when placing rubber dam over the rest of the teeth.

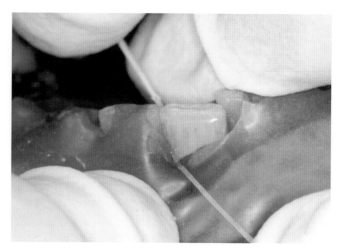

FIGURE 24.6. Flossing of the dam septum past tooth contact areas.

2. Prepare the rubber dam by stamping and punching the correct holes that will be needed for isolation.
3. Stretch the dam material over the bow and wings of the clamp.
4. Place the rubber dam napkin on the patient. This is used to absorb moisture and to reduce latex hypersensitivity.
5. Place the forceps in the clamp, and position it so that the bow of the clamp is at the distal of the anchor tooth. The forceps are held so that the beaks are directed toward the occlusal surface of the tooth (for a maxillary anchor tooth, the palm of the hand will be up; for a mandibular anchor tooth, the palm of the hand will be down). *Figure 24.4* illustrates clamp application for a mandibular tooth.

6. Place the clamp on the designated anchor tooth. The clamped anchor tooth is distal to the tooth that will be receiving treatment. Check for proper fit when placing the clamp from the lingual to the facial, and keep the clamp stabilized with the index finger while releasing the forceps. Make sure that "all four corners" of the clamp are seated on the tooth, not on the gingiva.
7. Place the frame on top of the rubber dam. The dam is stretched and hooked onto the projections of the frame. Make sure the dam is smooth and free of tears.
8. Place the last-punched hole of the dam over the tooth on the opposite side of the anchor tooth, as shown in *Figure 24.5*. This allows the operator to easily locate the remaining holes for the remaining teeth.

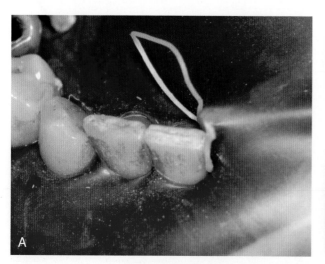

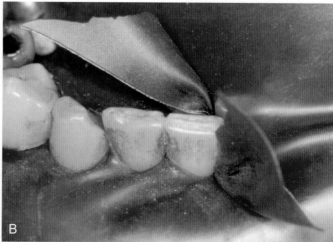

FIGURE 24.7. Two types of ligatures. **A.** Dental floss. **B.** Small corner of the rubber dam.

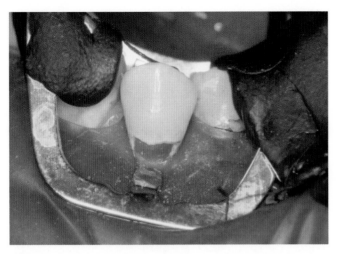

FIGURE 24.8. A "butterfly-shaped" clamp used to isolate the gingiva of the buccal surface of a lower canine.

9. Once the punch holes are positioned, stretch the dam **septum** (the dam membrane between the punched holes) and floss its leading edge between each of the remaining teeth. Continue to floss the remainder of the septum into the gingival embrasures. This is shown in *Figure 24.6.*

10. Place a **ligature** (a binding) at the opposite end of the anchor tooth to stabilize the dam. This can be done by using floss or a piece of dam material, as shown in *Figure 24.7.*

11. Invert the rubber dam around the necks of the isolated teeth, using the plastic filling instrument (PFI) (beaver tail). Imagine the dam being tucked into the sulci of the isolated teeth. This provides a well-sealed field. If possible, gently use the air syringe to assist with the inversion and to thoroughly dry the area.

12. A variety of special-use rubber dam clamps are available. The use of a "butterfly-shaped" clamp (#212) is shown in *Figure 24.8.* Such clamps are used to retract the gingiva and isolate facial surfaces of the teeth.

13. Readjust the frame if necessary.

D. Evaluate Rubber Dam Placement

Assess the rubber dam placement using the Skill Performance sheet in Appendix 2.

E. Removal of the Rubber Dam

The items needed for removal of the rubber dam are listed in Table 24.2. Removal of the dam may be done while the patient is seated in an upright or a supine position.

1. Remove the ligature that is stabilizing the rubber dam.

2. Remove the clamp with the forceps.

TABLE 24.2. Armamentarium for Removing the Rubber Dam

Scissors

Rubber dam forceps

Explorer

Floss

3. Before removing the rubber dam, each septum is cut with scissors. The dam is stretched to the facial and a finger is placed gingival to the teeth. This is to protect the gingival tissue and to guide the scissors, as shown in *Figure 24.9.*

4. Pull the rubber dam occlusally to remove it from the interproximals. Remove the dam and the frame as one unit.

5. Use an explorer in the interproximal areas to inspect and remove any remaining pieces of the rubber dam. Retention of dam fragments will cause gingival irritation.

6. Inspect the removed rubber dam against a contrasting background to make sure that all dam septa are intact (distinct circular openings), as shown in *Figure 24.10.*

7. Thoroughly rinse and evacuate the treatment area.

8. Massage the gingiva around the clamped tooth to increase circulation.

F. Evaluate Rubber Dam Removal

Assess the rubber dam removal using the Skill Performance sheet in Appendix 2.

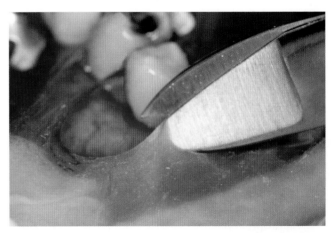

FIGURE 24.9. The rubber dam is stretched when interproximal areas are being cut.

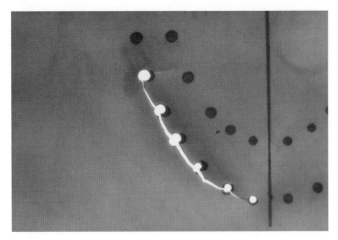

FIGURE 24.10. Inspection of the removed rubber dam against a white background.

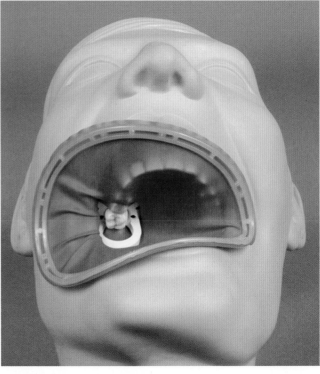

FIGURE 24.11. The Insti-Dam in place on a mannequin to demonstrate the frame's flexibility. (Courtesy of Zirc Company, Buffalo, MN.)

IV. Other Types of Rubber Dams

Insti-Dam (*see Fig. 24.11*) is a preframed rubber dam setup. The flexible frame includes the rubber dam material with a prepunched hole. The Insti-Dam reduces the number of steps in the application and removal of the rubber dam.

Tips for the Clinician

- The rubber dam should cover the upper edge of the lip but should not cover the nose.
- All the interproximal gingiva should be covered.
- Make sure the clamp is secure and stable.
- Check for leakage and torn dam material.

Precautions

- Inadequate stability of the clamp may result in the clamp "springing" off the tooth.
- Clinicians and patients should wear eye protection during the entire procedure.
- Ligate the clamp with floss so that if the clamp should "spring" free, it can quickly be retrieved.
- During removal of the rubber dam, cut the septa very carefully, using a fulcrum, to avoid injury to the gingival tissue.

Summary

Placement
1. Select appropriate rubber dam material (size, color, etc.).
2. Prepare the rubber dam appropriately (correct hole size, hole distance, clamp ligation).
3. Carefully seat the clamp.
4. Floss the rubber dam between contact areas where appropriate.
5. Invert the rubber dam around the necks of the teeth.
6. Ligate the last tooth in the exposed sequence.

Removal
1. Remove the clamp from the anchor tooth.
2. Cut the rubber dam septa with scissors.
3. Remove the rubber dam material and the frame as one unit.
4. Inspect the interproximals for rubber dam material.
5. Inspect the removed rubber dam.
6. Rinse and evacuate the oral cavity.
7. Massage the gingiva.

Review Questions

Question 1. The most common size of rubber dam material is:

a. 5- × 5-inch square
b. 6- × 6-inch square
c. 4- × 4.5-inch square
d. None of the above

Question 2. The armamentarium for removing the rubber dam is:

a. Scissors
b. Rubber dam forceps
c. Floss
d. Explorer
e. All of the above

Question 3. What is the position of the tooth receiving treatment in relationship to the anchor tooth?

a. The treatment tooth is distal to the anchor tooth.
b. The anchor tooth is the same as the treatment tooth.
c. The treatment tooth is mesial to the anchor tooth.
d. The anchor tooth is in the opposite quadrant of the treatment tooth.

Question 4. Indications for rubber dam placement include all of the following except one. Which one is the **EXCEPTION?**

a. Visibility
b. Patient protection
c. Patient with severe asthma
d. Moisture control

Question 5. Which clamp is used for isolation of the facial surfaces of anterior and some posterior teeth?

a. Winged clamps
b. Wingless clamps
c. Butterfly-shaped clamps

Pit and Fissure Sealants

25

Objectives

After performing the laboratory/clinical exercises in this chapter, the student will be able to do the following:

1. Discuss the factors determining the success of a sealant.
2. List the indications and contraindications for applying a sealant.
3. Describe the acceptable, but different, methods for preparing the enamel surface for a sealant.
4. Summarize the steps of applying a sealant.
5. Evaluate a placed sealant regarding proper isolation, coverage, and defects.
6. Explain the importance of recall visits for sealant maintenance.
7. Professionally speak to the parent of a child who is in need of sealants. Include in the discussion the rationale, procedure, time involved, and prognosis.

Key Words/Phrases

air abrasive polishing

micropores

Introduction

The basic steps for pit and fissure sealant application are discussed in this chapter. It is always important to review—and to follow—the manufacturer's directions for the application and storage of a particular sealant material.

Clinical success of sealants is determined by proper placement and retention. The most common reasons for sealant failure are inadequate isolation and subsequent contamination. The dentist must choose a sealant material based on the following properties:

- Autopolymerizing (chemical cure) or visible light-cure sealants. Examples of light-activated sealant kits are provided in *Figure 25.1.*
- Fluoride-releasing or nonfluoride-releasing sealants.
- Clear, tinted, or opaque sealants.
- The composition, properties, and mechanism for retention of bonding resins are discussed in Chapter 4, Adhesive Materials.

I. Purpose and Indications

Pit and fissure sealant material will literally flow into the deep pit and fissured areas on occlusal surfaces and seal them from bacterial activity. *Figure 25.2* illustrates a magnified occlusal surface exhibiting several deep pit and fissure areas. Sometimes, the fissure is shaped in an "I" formation that is very narrow but has a bulbous base. The formation is too narrow to accommodate toothbrush bristles. The "I"-shaped fissure can be seen in *Figure 25.3.* The American Dental Association Council on Scientific Affairs has determined that sealants are indicated for patients with the following conditions: an elevated risk for caries, incipient caries within enamel in pit and fissure areas, or existing pits and fissures anatomically susceptible to decay.

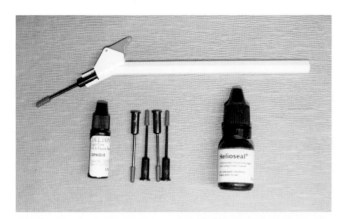

FIGURE 25.1. Examples of light-activated sealants. **Top.** Dispenser with unidose Delton sealant. **Bottom,** *left to right.* Bulk Delton sealant, unidose Delton sealant, and bulk Helioseal.

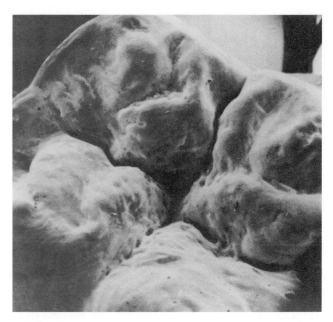

FIGURE 25.2. Magnified occlusal surface showing deep pit and fissure areas. (Reproduced from Gwinnett AJ. The bonding of sealants to enamel. *J Am Soc Prevent Dent.* 1973;3:21, with permission.)

II. Contraindications

Pit and fissure sealants are contraindicated on tooth surfaces having frank caries or on surfaces that have well-coalesced pits and fissures.

III. Procedure

The clinical success of a pit and fissure sealant is dependent on the meticulous technique of the clinician. The items needed to place sealants are listed in Table 25.1.

A. Surface Preparation

The clinician may use one of the following methods to prepare the enamel surface for sealant application. Research has found them all to be acceptable.

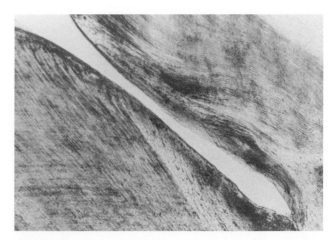

FIGURE 25.3. "I"-shape fissure, very narrow with a bulbous base. (Reproduced from Gwinnett AJ. The bonding of sealants to enamel. *J Am Soc Prevent Dent.* 1973;3:21, with permission.)

TABLE 25.1. Armamentarium for Placing Sealants

Mirror

Explorer

Cotton pliers

Sealant resin

Etchant (phosphoric acid)

Gauze

Low-speed handpiece

Curing light with shield

No. 6 or 8 round bur or a green or white stone

Dry angles or rubber dam setup

Air/water syringe tip

Saliva ejector

High-speed suction

Bristle polishing brush

Articulating paper

Floss

Pumice

Cotton rolls and Garmer holder

Posterior scaler

1. Bristle brush or rubber cup and low-speed handpiece with plain pumice and then rinse for 10 seconds.
2. Bristle brush with water.
3. Etchant only (no surface preparation) for patients with good plaque control.
4. **Air abrasive polishing** (prophy jet; sodium bicarbonate particles propelled by compressed air in a water spray) or very light air abrasion with aluminum oxide.

B. Isolation

Isolation may be accomplished in two ways.

1. Rubber Dam

    The rubber dam method is recommended when more than one tooth in the quadrant is to be sealed. If a rubber dam is not utilized, as in mentioned in Cotton Roll Application and Dry Angle (Triangular Cotton) Isolation below, assistance from an auxiliary is highly recommended.

2. Cotton Roll Application

    Use the saliva ejector and a Garmer holder for cotton rolls for the mandibular arch (*Fig. 25.4A* and *B*).

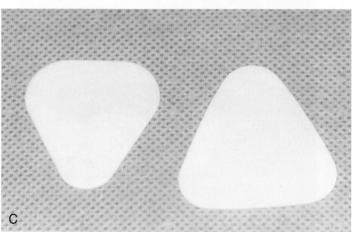
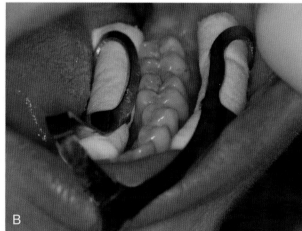
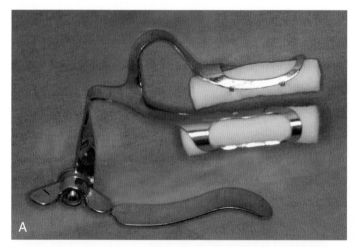
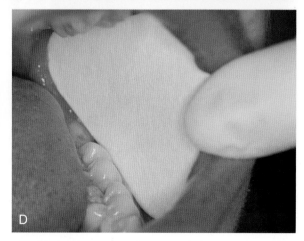

FIGURE 25.4. **A.** Right-side Garmer cotton roll holder. **B.** Cotton roll holder in use. **C.** Dry angles. **D.** Dry angle in use.

3. Dry Angle (Triangular Cotton) Isolation
Triangular cotton isolation, as shown in *Figure 25.4C* and *D*, can also be used in conjunction with either method.

C. Dry the Tooth or Teeth Thoroughly

Make sure the air/water syringe does not leak water or oil because this will interfere with formation of the "enamel tags" or "micropores" during the etching process. These **micropores** are minute, microscopic openings in the enamel surface, as shown in Figure 4.3. Dry the area for at least 10 seconds and inspect for caries.

D. Apply Etchant

1. Application time is 15 to 20 seconds.
2. If using a liquid etchant, apply with a brush. An enamel etchant material is a gel or liquid composed of 37% phosphoric acid.
3. If using a gel etchant, apply and then leave undisturbed. Gel etchants are illustrated in *Figure 25.5*. Etchant gel clinically applied to a premolar is shown in *Figure 25.6*.

E. Thoroughly Rinse

1. If using an etching gel, rinse for at least 30 seconds. If using a liquid etchant, rinse for 10 to 15 seconds.
2. Use high-speed evacuation during the rinse procedure.

F. Dry the Tooth or Teeth Again

Each tooth should be thoroughly dried again for 15 to 30 seconds.

G. Evaluate the Etched Surface

1. An adequately etched surface will have a dull, chalky white, opaque appearance.

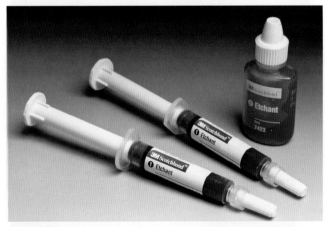

FIGURE 25.5. Gel etchants, syringe delivery, and dispenser bottle for use with a brush/applicator. (Courtesy of 3M Dental Products Division.)

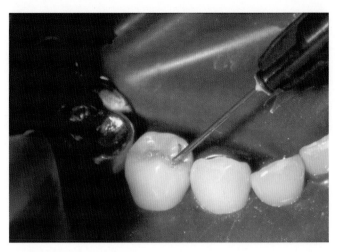

FIGURE 25.6. Clinical application of gel etchant applied to a premolar.

2. If this appearance is not evident, re-etch the surface by using the same procedure. *Figure 25.7* illustrates a properly etched premolar.

H. Apply a Primer from a Dentinal Bonding System: Optional

1. Primers from dentinal bonding systems can help the sealant wet a surface contaminated with moisture after etching. A dry surface is preferred, but saliva control and moisture condensation are always a concern. Primers usually contain alcohol or acetone. They combine with water and evaporate as one, taking the water off the surface.
2. Self-etching primers may also be used; some replace the usual phosphoric acid etching step. They should be covered with sealant.

I. Apply the Sealant to the Tooth Surface

1. Sealant may be applied by:
   a. Using the applicator provided by the manufacturer. If applying sealant by this method,

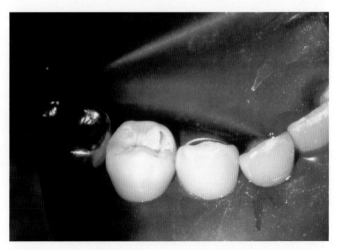

FIGURE 25.7. Etched premolar appearing chalky white.

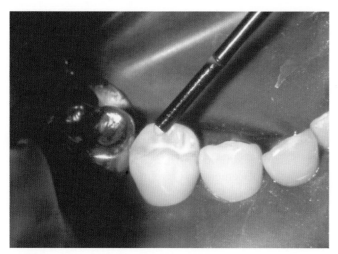

FIGURE 25.8. Sealant material applied to a premolar with an applicator tip.

allow the material to flow ahead of applicator tip, as shown in *Figure 25.8.*
  b. Using a small brush.
  c. Using an explorer.
2. Remove excess amounts of material, and attempt to eliminate any bubbles occurring within the sealant.
3. Extend the sealant material along inclined planes of cusps.
4. Don't forget the pits and fissures on the buccal of mandibular and lingual of maxillary molars.

J. Polymerize the Sealant

1. Light-Activated Sealants
   a. Use amber eyewear or light shields during the curing process.
   b. Hold the tip of the curing light as close as possible to the tooth surface.
   c. Curing time is 20 seconds, but an additional 5 to 10 seconds are recommended for each surface.
   d. Some products change color when properly light-activated.
2. Chemically Activated Sealants
   a. Measure the drops, and mix. One mix will seal two teeth.
   b. Once the sealant is applied, do not disturb the material during the curing process.
   c. Use residual material in mixing well to determine the setting time (~2 minutes).

K. Occlusal Adjustment

1. Unfilled sealants will wear easily, and occlusal adjustment at the time of placement is usually unnecessary.

2. Occlusal adjustment when filled sealants are being used requires articulating paper and either a # 6 or # 8 round bur or a green or white stone.
   a. After using articulating paper, note any markings on the sealants.
   b. Remove any markings with a stone or bur.

Precautions

- For sealant retention, it is critical that the area be free of moisture during the entire placement procedure.
- Eye protection is necessary.
- During curing, use of a light shield is required.
- Before placing etchant, be certain that the tip of the syringe is securely attached and the etchant flows freely.

L. Evaluate the Sealant

1. Visually and tactilely (with an explorer) inspect the sealant for:
   a. Complete coverage of all pits and fissures
   b. Absence of voids, bubbles, and defects (overmanipulation of sealant material before curing can incorporate air into the sealant)
2. Attempt to dislodge the sealant with an explorer. If successful, replace the sealant immediately, using a "dry, 10-second re-etch, rinse, dry, seal" sequence.
3. Use floss between the interproximals of all sealed teeth and those adjacent to sealed teeth. If cured sealant material has closed the interproximal space, it can be reopened by removing the material with a scaler and/or floss.

M. Evaluate the Sealant Placement Procedure

Assess the sealant placement by using the Skill Performance Evaluation sheet in Appendix 2.

N. Follow-Up Evaluation

During recall examinations, the dental hygienist will need to reevaluate sealed tooth surfaces for sealant loss, exposure of voids, and possible caries. This is done both visually and tactilely. If a sealant is partially lost, attempt to dislodge the remaining material with an explorer. If this portion remains intact, simply etch the adjacent enamel and sealant and then apply additional sealant.

IV. Self-Etching and Fluoride-Releasing Sealants

A. Self-Etching Sealants

Self-etching sealants have reappeared on the market. These were one step, one material products. These products were not successful and most have disappeared. Current self-etching sealant products are usually a system that utilizes a self-etching primer or adhesive. These systems may not etch with phosphoric acid. There may be a prescribed time for the material to sit on the tooth before light-curing. The system may not be easier or quicker than the process described in this chapter.

B. Fluoride-Releasing Sealants

Many dental materials contain fluoride. Some materials release more fluoride than others. Glass ionomer products release many times more fluoride than polymer-based products such as dentinal

bonding systems, composites, and sealants. Clinical research has yet to demonstrate improved caries inhibition by fluoride-releasing sealants.

Tips for the Clinician

- Light-cure sealants provide more working time for the clinician than autocure sealants.
- Having additional assistance for this procedure makes placement and retention more effective.
- To avoid the incorporation of bubbles, drag the explorer tip along all pits and fissures before curing.

Summary

1. Cleanse the tooth surface(s).
2. Isolate the selected teeth from moisture.
3. Dry teeth for 10 seconds and inspect for caries.
4. Etch for 15 to 20 seconds.
5. Rinse: for liquid etchants, 10 to 15 seconds; for etching gels, 30 seconds.
6. Thoroughly dry, 15 to 30 seconds.
7. Evaluate the etched surface.
8. Apply sealant according to the manufacturer's directions.
9. Polymerize the sealant.
10. Evaluate the sealant for coverage, retention, and absence of voids and bubbles.
11. Check/adjust occlusion and adjacent interproximal spaces.

 Review Questions

Question 1. Dental sealants are effective in _____ dental caries.

a. Reversing
b. Restoring
c. Preventing
d. Proliferating

Question 2. Properly etched and dried enamel appears:

a. Shiny and pale
b. Chalky white
c. Dull gray
d. Chalky gray

Question 3. After placement, the sealant should be checked for:

a. Hyperocclusion of occlusal contacts
b. Interproximal contacts bonded together
c. Both
d. Neither

Question 4. Liquid etchants should be rinsed for _____ to _____ seconds, and gel etchants for at least _____ seconds.

a. 10 to 15; 20
b. 10 to 15; 30
c. 5 to 10; 30
d. 5 to 10; 20

Question 5. Filled sealants may need adjustment on the occlusal surfaces. This may be done only by using articulating paper and a #6 or #8 round bur.

a. The first statement is true; the second is false.
b. The first statement is false; the second is true.
c. Both statements are true.
d. Both statements are false.

Amalgam Placement, Carving, Finishing, and Polishing

Meg Zayan, R.D.H., M.P.H., Ed.D., and Michael J. Meador, D.D.S.

26

Objectives

After performing the laboratory/clinical exercises in this chapter, the student will be able to do the following:

1. Describe, understand, and explain the sequence of steps for the placement and carving of a dental amalgam restoration.
2. Name the instruments and materials used for placement of dental amalgam restorations.
3. Explain the rationale for amalgam finishing and polishing.
4. Recall the benefits of properly finished and polished amalgams.
5. List two indications for finishing and polishing amalgams.
6. Discuss the possible results of poor amalgam placement and carving.
7. Assess an amalgam restoration to determine whether it needs replacement or finishing and polishing.
8. Differentiate between the procedures of amalgam finishing and amalgam polishing.
9. Explain the importance of temperature control and related factors during finishing and polishing.
10. Evaluate a well-finished and polished amalgam according to the criteria provided in this chapter.

Key Words/Phrases

amalgam finishing
amalgam polishing
burnishing
cavosurface margin
condense
contact area
flash
matrix band
matrix retainer
open margin
overextension
overhang
premature contact
submarginal area

Introduction

The procedures discussed in this chapter (or portions thereof) may not be included in the dental hygienist's scope of practice in all states. Procedures that a dental hygienist may legally perform are listed in each state's practice act.

Proper placement of dental amalgam is essential to the long-term success of the amalgam restoration. Modern amalgams are strong and hard enough to support most chewing forces and are versatile enough for restoring lesions in almost all teeth. Care must be taken and attention to detail must be observed when placing and carving these restorations. It is important not to become discouraged when following your "learning curve" to become proficient. Repetition, learning the handling characteristics, and persistence will allow you to become confident and skilled in this phase of restorative dentistry.

Amalgam finishing and polishing is an integral part of the patient's treatment plan in the prevention of periodontal and dental disease, and it should be routinely performed by the dental hygienist. Finished and polished amalgams are less prone to plaque retention and have a greater resistance to tarnish and corrosion than unpolished amalgams. Traditionally, finishing and polishing should be performed at least 24 hours after amalgam placement. This allows the amalgam alloy to set completely before being exposed to the abrasives of polishing. Spherical fast-setting amalgams, which could be finished and polished shortly after placing and carving, are the exception. Spherical amalgams are discussed in Chapter 6, Amalgam. For previously placed amalgams, finishing and polishing may be started as soon as the procedure is indicated.

TABLE 26.1. Armamentarium for Amalgam Condensation and Carving
Rubber dam, frame, clamps (retainers), and punch forceps
Amalgam carrier and well
Matrix bands, retainer, and wedges
Amalgam condensers: large and small
Carvers: discoid/cleoid, Hollenback, proximal carver, and large spoon excavator
Burnishers; ball burnisher, acorn burnisher, and football burnisher
Explorer and mirror
Articulating paper
Finishing strips

I. Procedure for Condensing Amalgam

Proper placement of an amalgam restoration results in a well adapted, void-free, and anatomically correct replacement of lost tooth structure. An example of the armamentarium for amalgam condensation and carving is shown in Table 26.1.

A. Matrix Band Placement

Proper amalgam condensation requires a three-dimensional "form" or box with only one surface or side open. A class II restoration has at least two surfaces open and therefore lacks the box-like shape for proper condensation. A **matrix band** is a thin strip of material that is placed around the tooth to establish the missing sides of the box and allows adequate condensation of amalgam (see *Fig. 26.1A*). The **matrix retainer** holds the band in a loop and tightens the band around the tooth.

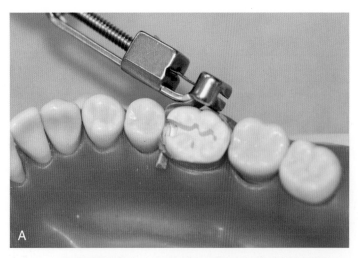

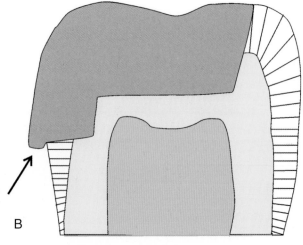

FIGURE 26.1. A. Properly wedged matrix band tightened with a matrix retainer. **B.** An amalgam overhang that can result when a matrix band is not properly adapted.

1. Select appropriate matrix band and matrix retainer. Matrix bands are available in a variety of shapes (universal, bicuspid, molar), different thicknesses (0.002, 0.0015, and ultrathin 0.001 gauge), and flexibilities (regular or dead soft).
2. Burnish matrix band on countertop prior to placement to create a more curved/anatomical form.
3. Place matrix band and firmly wedge. Burnish the band to the adjacent tooth to assure good adaption of the proximal contact of the restoration.
4. Check the proximal box to make certain that the band is adapted with no area for the amalgam to escape, which could cause an overhanging margin (see *Fig. 26.1B*).

B. Mix (Triturate) Amalgam According to Manufacturer's Specification

Mix the amalgam in the amalgamator according to the manufacturers' directions, usually included as a package insert. Different triturators have different mixing time and speed recommendations.

C. Technique for Amalgam Condensation

1. After mixing, place the triturated material in the amalgam well.
2. Use amalgam carrier to pick up the amalgam and transfer to the preparation; see *Figure 26.2*.
3. Place increments and condense the material after each placement; see Figure 6.4A–D. Use the appropriately sized condenser to **condense**, push to compact the amalgam toward the floor of the preparation and also laterally into the line angles and proximal box. Use firm, overlapping condensing strokes (larger condensers need greater pressure); see *Figure 26.3A* and *B*.
4. Working from the floor of the preparation, continue to place and condense increments until the preparation is overfilled by approximately 1 mm.

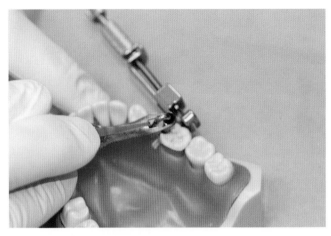

FIGURE 26.2. Placing the first increment of amalgam into the preparation with an amalgam carrier.

Use a larger condenser to condense the overfilled preparation. This ensures complete coverage of the margins of the cavity preparation for proper carving and to remove excess mercury.
5. Using a burnisher to precarve the overfilled amalgam as shown in *Figure 26.4* will also help bring mercury to surface. **Burnishing** pushes and adapts the material contiguous to the margins to eliminate voids. Burnish mesiodistally and faciolingually forming the major grooves of the occlusal anatomy. The condensing phase should take approximately 2½ to 3½ minutes.

II. Procedure for Carving Amalgam

Carving of the amalgam begins immediately after burnishing. Use sharp instruments.

A. Marginal Ridge and Contact Area

1. Use an explorer to carve the amalgam adjacent to the matrix band forming the occlusal

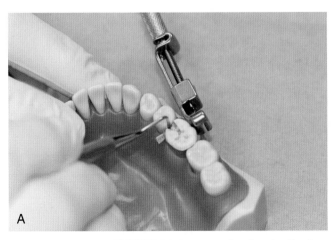

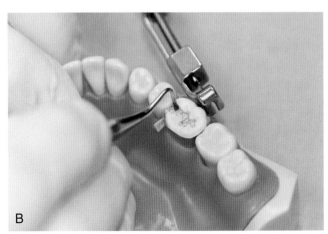

FIGURE 26.3. **A.** Condensing the first increment. **B.** Condensing subsequent increments.

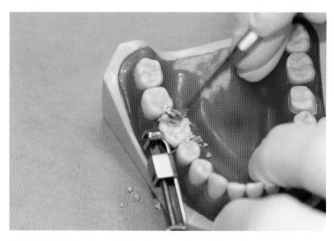

FIGURE 26.4. Burnishing the condensed amalgam.

embrasure. Keep the tip of the explorer against the band surface and move the explorer from the buccoproximal margin toward the lingual, stopping at the center of the box. Repeat the procedure, this time from the linguoproximal margin to the center, as shown in *Figure 26.5A* and *B*.

2. Such carving defines the contact area and the marginal ridge. The marginal ridge of the restoration and the marginal ridge of the adjacent tooth should be at the same level. Usually, the **contact area** is in the middle of the mesial or distal surface or the restoration.

B. Occlusal and Proximal Anatomy

1. Use the discoid/cleoid to carve the occlusal surface. Keep the edge of the carver blade perpendicular to the margins. Rest part of the blade of the carving instrument on the enamel adjacent to the restoration, and use a pulling stroke to carve with the margins of the preparation; see *Figure 26.6A* and *B*. Do not allow the tip of the carving instrument to pass the center of the prepared cavity; see *Figure 26.6C*. Carve occlusal margins so that there is no feathered overextension of amalgam or "step-down" at the margin, such as that shown in *Figure 26.7A*. Take care to create a smooth, continuous surface from the enamel to the restoration.

2. Develop occlusal grooves to complete the restoration's anatomy. These are distinct, but not necessarily deep grooves. When an occlusal groove needs to be deepened, the side of the carver should not make contact with the amalgam at the preparation margin; see *Figure 26.6D* and *26.8*.

3. Carving the mesial and distal pits and triangular fossa is important for correct development of the occlusal anatomy. The crest of the marginal ridge is the base of the triangle, and the facial and lingual supplemental grooves in the restoration form the two sides of the triangular fossa that meet in the mesial or distal pit. When carving the triangular ridges, keep the blade of the carver angled in harmony with slope of the cusp.

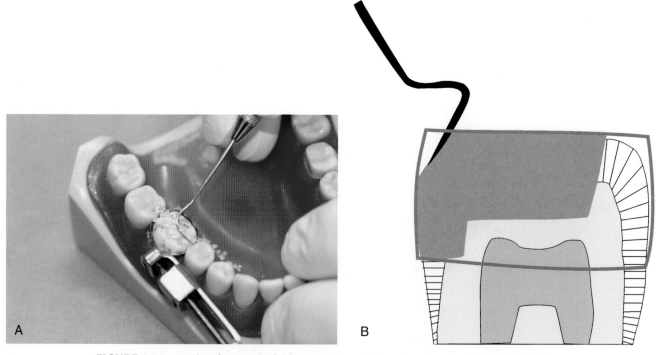

A   B

FIGURE 26.5. Carving the marginal ridge. **A.** Picture. **B.** Drawing of carving the marginal ridge.

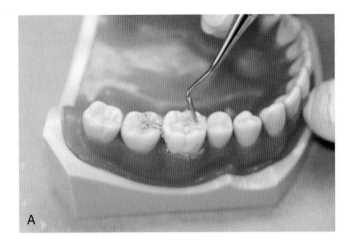

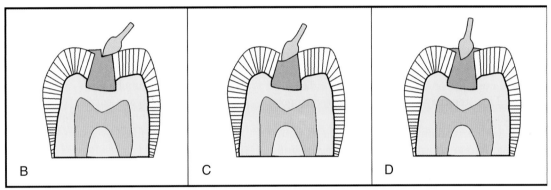

FIGURE 26.6. **A.** Carving the margin. **B.** The carving instrument properly rests on the tooth creating a flush margin. **C.** The carver does not rest on the tooth and is placed too far toward the opposite margin resulting in a step at the margin. **D.** The carver does not rest on tooth structure leaving flash on the occlusal surface.

4. Refine proximal contour with a Hollenback carver or proximal carver. Use a series of shaving strokes occlusally from the cavity proximal corners. Use only minimal pressure with the shaving stroke. Blend the proximal margins to the occlusal margins. Keep part of the blade resting on adjacent enamel. At this time, the carver can be used to adjust the marginal ridge height and shape, occlusal embrasures, and the rounding of the marginal ridge. Use carvers to remove any excess amalgam from the cervical area.

5. Use the tip of a carver or explorer to remove any flash remaining in the occlusal grooves of the tooth.

6. Burnishing after carving will smooth hard to polish occlusal grooves of the restoration.

7. Examine the restoration for proper marginal adaption, anatomy, and contours; see *Figure 26.9.*

C. Check and Adjust Occlusion

1. To check occlusion, have the patient bring his/her teeth together lightly, check for a shiny area on the restoration and remove the premature contact with a carver.

2. Check the occlusion again with articulating paper. Have patient lightly tap teeth together,

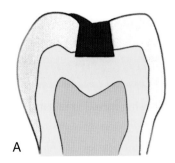
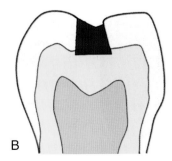
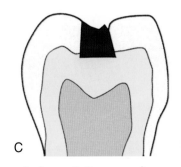

FIGURE 26.7. Results of poor carving. **A.** Overextension or flash. **B.** Submarginal area. **C.** Open margin.

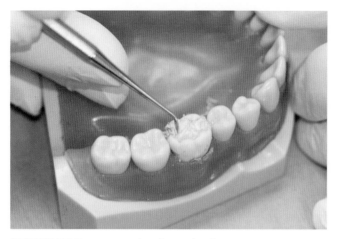

FIGURE 26.8. Accentuating the occlusal anatomy.

carve prematurities until any contact with the restoration occurs simultaneously with other centric contacts on the tooth and the adjacent teeth. This step may need to be repeated to get even contact.

3. Next, with articulating paper, have the patient to make lateral and protrusive movements and reduce any interferences present.

D. Examine the Restoration

Double-check the interproximal for amalgam debris, rubber dam material, or overhangs. Remove any overhangs or debris. Check interproximal contact visually to make sure that no light passes through the contact. Hold the mirror on the lingual and facial aspects of the teeth and check at different angles. Then check with dental floss, making sure there is resistance when the floss passes through the contact area.

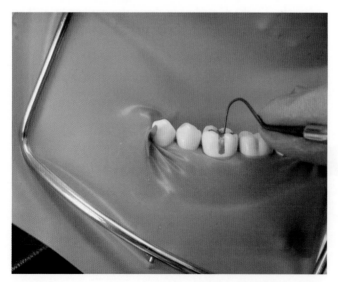

FIGURE 26.9. Examining for marginal discrepancies.

E. Postoperative Instructions

1. Instruct patient not to chew on the new restoration for at least 2 hours.
2. If patient was given anesthesia, remind him/her to be careful not to bite a lip or tongue.
3. Inform the patient that he or she may experience postoperative sensitivity to hot or cold for a few days.
4. If the patient feels that occlusion (bite) is too high after anesthesia wears off, have him/her contact the office for occlusal adjustment.
5. Have the patient schedule a return appointment after 24 hours to finish and polish the restoration.

F. Summary for Condensing and Carving Amalgam

1. Select and place appropriate matrix band and matrix retainer.
2. Triturate amalgam.
3. Use amalgam carrier to place amalgam into preparation and condense using increments until overfilled by 1 mm.
4. Burnish.
5. Carve marginal ridge with explorer to establish embrasure and marginal ridge height.
6. Remove matrix band.
7. Carve occlusal surface using discoid/cleoid carver.
8. Develop mesial/distal pits and the triangular fossa.
9. Use Hollenback carver to refine the proximal and gingival margins—the Hollenback may also be used to refine or to deepen the occlusal grooves and anatomy.
10. Check the interproximal contacts, the occlusion, and make any necessary adjustments.
11. Give the patient postoperative instructions and dismiss with an appointment to return for polishing the restoration.

Tips for the Clinician

- Stabilize the mandible with the nondominant hand when condensing an amalgam restoration in the lower arch.
- Condense the amalgam in all three dimensions.

Precautions

- Do not handle freshly mixed amalgam with bare hands.
- Make sure to properly adapt and wedge the matrix band.

III. Purpose of Finishing and Polishing

The primary purpose of finishing and polishing amalgams is to produce a restoration that can be easily cleaned by the patient, thereby promoting an improved oral environment. Additional benefits of finishing and polishing amalgams are listed below.

A. Benefits of Finishing and Polishing

The following conditions result from proper finishing and polishing:
1. Smooth and flush cavosurface margins
2. Recreation of defined anatomy
3. Decreased plaque retention
4. Healthier surrounding tissue
5. Higher resistance to tarnish and corrosion
6. Increased longevity of the restoration
7. Improved esthetics

B. Methods by Which These Benefits Are Achieved

These benefits are achieved by properly smoothing the cavosurface margins, reconstructing functional anatomy, and creating an amalgam surface that is both smooth and free of voids. It is necessary to obtain a smooth surface and achieve a high gloss. If only a high gloss is achieved through the polishing sequence, the remaining irregularities will tend to corrode faster than a smooth surface. Ultimately, this will not prolong the life of the restoration.

IV. Indications for Finishing and Polishing

Ideally, all amalgam restorations should be finished and polished 24 hours after placement. Realistically, however, this may not happen. Previously existing amalgam restorations, as well as "newer" ones, should be finished and polished to correct various problems or conditions incurred during placement. These problems are often a result of incorrect condensing, poor carving, moisture contamination, natural expansion, or wear. In all these cases, plaque has a greater chance of accumulating on the restoration's surface, which creates a higher risk for recurrent caries.

A. Typical Problems with Amalgam Restorations

1. **Overhang**

   An **overhang** is an excess amount of amalgam that extends beyond the cavosurface margin, and it is caused by improper placement of the matrix band or wedge during amalgam condensation (*Fig. 26.1B*). An overhang increases susceptibility to decay and periodontal disease.

2. **Anatomy**

   Functional anatomy is not created during placement. A lack of functional anatomy increases the risk for plaque and food debris retention.

3. **Contact**

   Interproximal contact is not created. Open contact areas are susceptible to the lodging of food debris and can cause decay and periodontal disease.

4. **Tarnish**

   Tarnish is a removable surface film or discoloration on the amalgam. It does not affect the internal integrity of the restoration.

5. **Corrosion**

   Corrosion is a surface or subsurface chemical deterioration that occurs on or within an amalgam restoration. Corrosion is discussed in detail in Chapter 19, Instruments as Dental Materials: Care and Maintenance.

6. **Fracture**

   A bulk fracture can occur in the amalgam restoration. Bulk fractures are a common result of recurrent caries and a lack of support to part of the restoration. A fractured restoration that remains in place can be a source of sensitivity, leakage, and recurrent caries.

7. **Results of Poor Carving**

   a. *Overextension or Flash*

   Overextension or **flash** are terms used when a thin ledge of amalgam extends beyond the cavosurface margin, as illustrated in *Figure 26.7A*.

   b. *Submarginal Area (or Deficient Margin)*

   A **submarginal area** results when the margin is overcarved, creating a deficiency of amalgam, as shown in *Figure 26.7B*. An internal wall of the preparation is exposed.

   c. *Open Margin*

   An **open margin** is created as a result of poor condensation or when an opposing cusp fractures an overextended portion of amalgam. An illustration of an open margin is shown in *Figure 26.7C*.

B. Amalgam Restoration Assessment

During patient assessment, all amalgam restorations must be carefully evaluated to determine if amalgam finishing and/or polishing is indicated. As listed in Table 26.2, some amalgam restorations should not be finished and polished but replaced instead.

V. Amalgam Finishing and Polishing Considerations

Amalgam finishing and polishing can be considered as two separate procedures or as two steps in a single process. During **amalgam finishing**, marginal irregularities are removed, and all areas of roughness are smoothed.

TABLE 26.2. Determining Factors for Finishing and Polishing Versus Replacement

Finish and Polish Restoration	Replace Restoration
• Overhangs	• Open contact
• Lack of functional anatomy	• Excessive corrosion
• Tarnish	• Amalgam fracture
• Overextension	• Open margin
• Premature occlusal contacts	• Recurrent decay

During **amalgam polishing**, the surface is smoothed to a high luster by using a sequence of abrasives (from fine to most fine). Whenever an amalgam restoration is finished, polishing is then performed; for those restorations not indicated for finishing, polishing may be done alone. The abrasives used during finishing are coarser than the milder abrasives that are used during polishing.

During the finishing and polishing procedures, it is essential that the dental hygienist avoid generating any heat within the amalgam restoration. Because of the high thermal conductivity of amalgam, excessive heat could injure the pulp and cause pain to the patient. Also, when heat is generated above 140°F (60°C), mercury from the amalgam restoration may be released to the surface, resulting in a dull, cloudy appearance. Excessive heat generation may also produce increased susceptibility to breakdown and corrosion. Therefore, use of water from a syringe as a coolant during these procedures is recommended. After each step, when burs or abrasives are changed, the area should be thoroughly rinsed, dried, and evaluated. Factors that affect the rate of abrasion must also be considered; these are discussed in Chapter 16, Polishing Materials and Abrasion.

VI. Procedure for Amalgam Finishing

A. Evaluate the Restoration

1. Surfaces
   Visually examine the amalgam surfaces for functional anatomy and defects. Functional anatomy includes cusps, cusp ridges, the central groove, and the buccolingual groove. Defects include surface pitting and wear facets.

2. Margins
   Using a sharp explorer in a zigzag motion, determine if the cavosurface margins have any excessive discrepancies (*Fig. 26.9*). The **cavosurface margin** is the area formed by the cavity wall and the external tooth surface. Remember that a rough margin is a poor predictor of recurrent decay, as explained in

Chapter 6, Amalgam. Rough surfaces along the margin encourage plaque accumulation, which may result in a greater susceptibility to dental caries. The patient's risk for caries must also be considered.

3. Occlusion
   Evaluate the patient's occlusion.
   a. *Use Articulating Paper*
      Insert articulating paper along the occlusal surface and have the patient tap his or her teeth together.
   b. *Determine Intensity*
      Observe all markings to determine if they have the same intensity.
   c. *Reduce Premature Contacts*
      Occlusal contacts are registered by using articulating paper. **Premature contacts** are areas where the amalgam has been undercarved. These will register as darker areas when they are checked with articulating paper.
   d. *Check Areas of Equal Intensity*
      Once again, use articulating paper to check occlusal markings for equal intensity.

4. Proximal Area
   a. Check proximal contacts with dental floss. The dental floss should resist passing through the contact. Remember, an open contact serves as a precursor to food impaction.
   b. Using dental floss and an explorer, check for overhangs.

B. Discuss the Procedure with the Patient

1. Rationale
   Explain the rationale of amalgam finishing and polishing, and review the steps of the procedure.

2. Sensations
   Inform the patient of any sensations that he or she may experience during the process, especially those of finishing burs with a low-speed handpiece.

C. Gather the Necessary Equipment

Select instruments based on the restoration and the clinician's preference. An example of an equipment listing is shown in Table 26.3.

D. Isolate the Area with Cotton Rolls or a Rubber Dam

Rubber dam isolation is presented in Chapter 24, Application and Removal of the Rubber Dam. Cotton roll isolation is described in Chapter 25, Pit and Fissure Sealants.

TABLE 26.3. Armamentarium for Finishing and Polishing Amalgam Restorations

Mouth mirror

Articulating paper

Explorer

Slow-speed handpiece

Contra angle or prophy angle

Air/water syringe

Saliva ejector or high-speed suction

Rubber dam setup or cotton rolls

Finishing burs

Abrasive stones and discs

    Green stone (silicone dioxide)

    White stone (aluminum oxide)

    Finishing discs (zirconium silicate)

Hand instruments

    Dental file

    Gold knife

    Amalgam knife

Dental floss or tape

Finishing strips

Polishing supplies

    Rubber points and cups

      Brown points or cups

      Green points or cups

      Yellow-banded green points or cups

      OR

    Two dappen dishes

    Pumice and water

    Tin oxide and alcohol/mouthwash

Polishing cups (unwebbed)

Brushes (tapered and wheel)

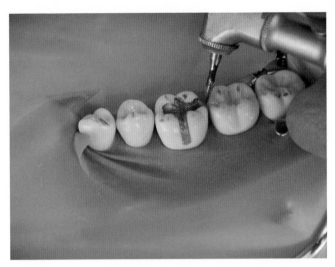

FIGURE 26.10. Finishing bur used to smooth amalgam in the proximal area.

E. Smooth Proximal Areas if Necessary

This may be done by using hand instruments or finishing burs, discs, and strips.

1. Hand Instruments
   a. Use a finishing knife and/or a dental file at the gingival and proximal margins to remove overhangs.
   b. Use short, overlapping, shaving strokes to prevent the amalgam from fracturing.

2. Finishing Burs
   a. A flame-shaped bur is recommended when the area is easily accessible.
   b. Care must be taken to prevent damage to the contact area or the gingival papilla (*Fig. 26.10*).

3. Finishing Discs
   a. *Selection*
      Discs come in varying sizes and grits. Select a size that is easily adaptable to the proximal surface.
   b. *Technique*
      Use short, overlapping strokes, and move diagonally across the cavosurface margins.
   c. *Sequence*
      Discs are used in a sequence of more abrasive to less abrasive grits.
   d. *Embrasures*
      When you are using discs in embrasure areas, take care not to damage the contact area or papilla.

4. Finishing Strips
   a. Use fine or medium finishing strips after using discs, burs, knives, or files.
   b. Position the strip such that it is both on the tooth and the amalgam, and move it in a back-and-forth motion.
   c. Avoid the contact area when using finishing strips, and use caution in areas of the interdental papilla and surrounding tissue. Wider strips may be cut lengthwise in half to make narrow strips.

F. Remove Occlusal Excess and Eliminate Flash

1. With Burs or Stones
   Use a round finishing bur or a green stone to remove excess material and irregularities from the occlusal surface, grooves, and the cavosurface margin (*Fig. 26.11*).

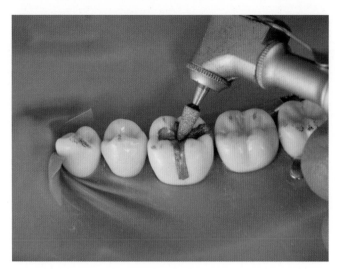

FIGURE 26.11. Green stone used to remove excess material and irregularities.

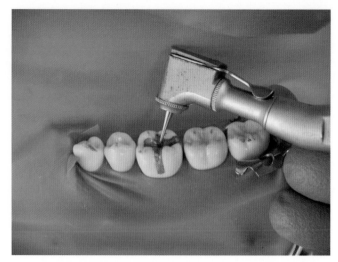

FIGURE 26.12. Defining anatomy by using a small round bur.

2. Sequence

Begin with the largest finishing bur that will adapt to the surface, and progress to smaller and less abrasive finishing burs.

3. Technique

Adapt the side of the bur or stone to the margin, contacting both the tooth and the amalgam, as shown in *Figure 26.11*.

4. Direction of Rotating Bur or Stone

Rotate the bur or stone from the amalgam to the tooth to avoid fracturing the amalgam margins.

5. Direction of Stroke

Always begin at the center of the restoration, and work toward the cavosurface margin.

6. Pitted Areas

Use a pointed white stone on tarnished and pitted areas.

G. Define the Occlusal Anatomy

1. With moderate pressure, define the occlusal anatomy using a small round finishing bur or the tip of a green or white stone. *Figure 26.12* illustrates this procedure using a small round bur.

2. Refer to existing teeth as a guide for anatomic definition.

H. Smooth Cavosurface Margins and the Occlusal Surface

1. Use a large round or a flame-shaped finishing bur to smooth the occlusal surface and cavosurface margins.

2. Change to a smaller round or a flame-shaped finishing bur to further smooth grooves and cusp slopes.

3. Reduce small areas of enamel (submarginal areas) or amalgam (overextensions) at the cavosurface margin by using a white stone.

4. The restoration should now appear smooth and shiny. Minute scratches may be present but may not be visible to the unaided eye.

I. Smooth Facial and Lingual Surfaces

1. Use a flame-shaped finishing bur or finishing discs, which vary in size and grit, to define and smooth the facial and lingual surfaces.

2. Adapt the bur along the cavosurface margin, contacting both the tooth and the amalgam in the same manner as illustrated in *Figure 26.6B* but for the facial and lingual surfaces.

3. Use caution when adapting the bur or discs near the gingival margin, especially if near the cementum.

4. When using discs, first use a coarser one, such as garnet, and progress to one having a finer abrasive, such as a cuttle.

5. If developmental grooves are part of the restoration, use a round or flame-shaped bur to define these.

J. Evaluate the Finishing Procedure

Assess the finishing procedure by using the criteria listed in Skill Performance Evaluation sheet in Appendix 2. *Do not proceed to the polishing procedure until these criteria have been met.* Polishing will not accomplish a smooth surface unless each step during the finishing process has been successfully accomplished.

VII. Procedures for Two Methods of Amalgam Polishing

A. Pumice and Tin Oxide Slurries

This method is accomplished by using a rubber cup, brush, and wheel brush.

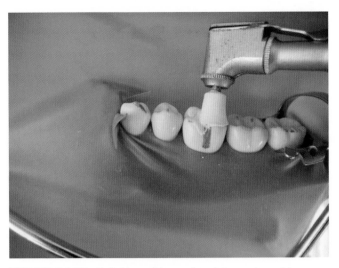

FIGURE 26.13. Polishing with pumice slurry and a rubber cup.

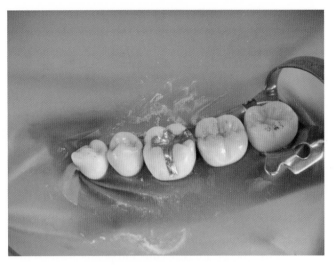

FIGURE 26.15. Finished and polished restoration.

1. Prepare a slurry mix of pumice and water in a dappen dish.
2. Polish all surfaces of the restoration with a brush or cup and plentiful pumice slurry (*Fig. 26.13*). Remember, the pumice does the polishing; the cup only moves the pumice. A smooth satin finish, which will exhibit a dull appearance, is accomplished.
3. Polish the proximal surface with medium and fine polishing strips.
4. Rinse and dry the tooth.
5. Prepare a wet mixture of tin oxide and alcohol in a dappen dish. Water or mouthwash is an acceptable substitute for alcohol.
6. Polish all surfaces of the restoration with a new clean cup or brush and the tin oxide slurry.
7. An optimal final step may include using a soft wheel brush in a straight handpiece with tin oxide. Continue to polish the amalgam until the tin oxide begins to dry and a high luster is achieved (*Fig. 26.14*).
8. Rinse and dry the tooth.

9. Assess the polished amalgam by using a mouth mirror, explorer, and the Skill Performance Evaluation sheet in Appendix 2. *Figure 26.15* illustrates an amalgam restoration that has been finished and polished.

Tips for the Clinician

- Effective lighting allows for ease in evaluating surface irregularities.
- The sequence of steps is crucial. Do not proceed to the next step until the previous step is completed.
- The polishing points and cups technique is less messy than the slurry technique.

B. Rubber Cups and Points Impregnated with Abrasive Particles

1. Colors
   Abrasive-impregnated rubber cups and points are supplied in three colors: brown, green, and yellow-banded green. Each color denotes a different degree of abrasiveness. In some instances, they are referred to as "brownies," "greenies," and "super greenies."

2. Use
   The cups are designed for use on the proximal surfaces, and the points are used on the occlusal surface. They are often used interchangeably, provided that the dental hygienist properly adapts them to the amalgam surface. They should be operated at a relatively low speed with light, intermittent strokes under wet conditions.

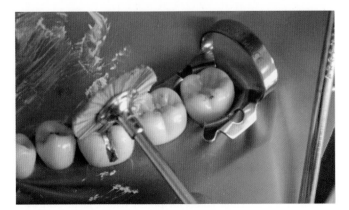

FIGURE 26.14. Polishing with a soft wheel brush.

3. **Advantages**

   The cups and points polish restorations quickly and tend to be less messy than the use of two slurries of different abrasive agents.

4. **Disadvantages**

   Both the cups and points wear quickly from use and autoclaving. Eventually, a metal shank is exposed that will scratch the amalgam surface. The greatest disadvantage, however, is heat production. The amalgam surface MUST NOT be heated above 140°F by the polishing procedure. Heat is generated rapidly with the use of abrasive-impregnated rubber cups and points.

5. **Procedure for Use**

   a. Brown abrasive cups and points are used first to produce an initial, smooth satin finish. Polish the occlusal, the proximal, and then finally the facial and lingual surfaces. Use of a brown polishing point on the occlusal surface is pictured in *Figure 26.16.*

   b. The green cups and points are used in the same manner as the brown cups and points. After use, examine to determine if a smooth, shiny finish has been achieved.

   c. A yellow-banded green cup or point is used as the final step. These cups and points are used in the same manner as the brown and green cups and points. *Figure 26.17* illustrates the use of a yellow-banded green point. Examine the surface to determine if a smooth, lustrous polished finish has been achieved.

   d. Rinse and evacuate debris.

   e. Assess the polished amalgam by using a mouth mirror, explorer, and the Skill Performance Evaluation sheet in Appendix 2. The amalgam should appear smooth and

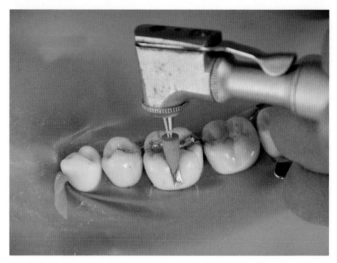

FIGURE 26.17. Yellow-banded green point adapted to the occlusal surface.

highly polished, and it should have a lustrous shine. There should be no damage to the adjacent tooth structure. A final amalgam polish with use of brown, green, and yellow-banded green points can be seen in *Figure 26.18.*

Precautions

- Heat can be generated rapidly on the tooth during amalgam finishing and polishing.
- Aerosols are frequently created when polishing with pumice and tin oxide.
- Cups and points wear quickly from use and autoclaving. An exposed metal shank will scratch the amalgam surface.

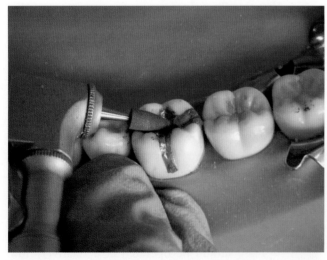

FIGURE 26.16. Brown polishing point adapted to the occlusal surface.

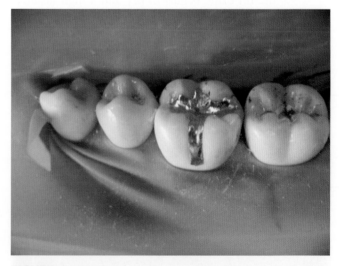

FIGURE 26.18. Final amalgam polish with use of abrasive-impregnated polishing points.

Summary

At each patient recall appointment, amalgam restorations should be evaluated for finishing and polishing. If indicated, this procedure may be performed during the recall visit, or it may be scheduled as a separate appointment. Research has documented the long-term benefits of finishing and polishing amalgam restorations. When an amalgam restoration is properly placed, carved, finished, and polished, the patient will have less plaque retention and, subsequently, a lower incidence of periodontal disease and caries. In addition, finishing and polishing may increase the lifetime of the restoration as well as patient satisfaction.

Finishing

1. Evaluate the restoration (margins, occlusion, proximal areas).
2. Discuss the procedure with the patient.
3. Isolate the area with cotton rolls or a rubber dam.
4. Smooth the proximals if necessary (with files, burs, discs, strips).
5. Remove occlusal excess, and eliminate flash (with burs or stones).
6. Define the occlusal anatomy (with burs or stones).
7. Smooth cavosurface margins and occlusal surface.
8. Smooth facial and lingual surfaces.

Polishing

Slurry Method

1. Prepare slurries of tin oxide and pumice.
2. Polish all surfaces with pumice and cup or brush.
3. Polish proximals with medium and fine polishing strips.
4. Rinse and dry tooth.
5. Polish all surfaces with a clean cup or brush and tin oxide slurry.
6. Rinse and evacuate debris.

Polishing Points and Cups Methods

1. Use brown abrasive cups and points to polish occlusals, proximals, and then facial and lingual surfaces.
2. Use the green cups and points in the same manner.
3. Produce the final polish with a yellow-banded green cup or point.
4. Rinse and evacuate debris.

 ## Learning Activities

1. In the dental materials or oral anatomy laboratory, observe existing amalgams on extracted teeth.

2. During patient assessment, evaluate amalgam restorations with an explorer and mouth mirror to determine if the amalgams should be finished and/or polished.

3. Evaluate patient amalgams to determine if any amalgams have already been finished or polished.

4. In the dental materials laboratory and on a typodont tooth with an existing cavity preparation, place and carve an amalgam. After 24 hours have elapsed, practice finishing and polishing the restoration.

 ## Review Questions

Question 1. **A metal matrix band and retainer would most likely be used to place a class _____ restoration.**

a. I
b. II
c. III
d. IV
e. V

Question 2. **When condensing a dental amalgam, the tip of the condenser _____ the amalgam into the cavity preparation.**

a. Shears
b. Pushes
c. Pulls
d. Rotates
e. Flows

Question 3. Which of the following polishing agents is used intraorally to give a high luster to amalgam restorations?

a. Alumina
b. Tin oxide
c. Zirconium silicate
d. Flour of pumice

Question 4. An operator is polishing an amalgam and inadvertently overheats it. The overheating may likely cause the following except one. Which one is the EXCEPTION?

a. Pulpal injury
b. Release of mercury
c. A dull appearance to restoration
d. Decreased susceptibility to corrosion

Question 5. What occurs when a metal becomes tarnished?

a. The surface becomes pitted
b. The surface is discolored
c. The surface becomes scratched
d. Mercury has risen to the surface

Question 6. During amalgam finishing and polishing, coarser abrasives should be followed by finer abrasives. This allows for larger scratches in the amalgam surface to be reduced to less defined scratches.

a. The first statement is true; the second statement is false.
b. The first statement is false; the second statement is true.
c. Both statements are true.
d. Both statements are false.

Question 7. Ideally, amalgam restorations should be finished and polished after:

a. 1 week
b. 24 hours
c. 2 hours
d. The initial set

Question 8. Polishing amalgam reduces the likelihood that tarnish and corrosion will occur because it:

a. Helps to create a smooth, homogeneous surface that resists tarnish and corrosion
b. Brings excess mercury to the surface to aid in preventing tarnish and corrosion
c. Increases the likelihood for galvanic currents to occur
d. Forces free mercury to the base of the cavity preparation

Question 9. You are utilizing an explorer in a zigzag motion to examine an amalgam on tooth #18. As you explore the buccal cavosurface, you note a deficient amount of amalgam in several areas. Your explorer catches only as you move from restoration to the tooth. This marginal discrepancy is best described as a (an):

a. Submarginal area
b. Open margin
c. Flash
d. Overextension

Question 10. When finishing the occlusal surface of an MOD restoration, care must be taken to:

a. Reduce all occlusal contact with opposing tooth
b. Reduce both marginal ridges slightly
c. Maintain the original anatomy of the restoration
d. Produce a high luster of the amalgam surface

Question 11. Finishing and polishing amalgams improves all of the following except one. Which one is the EXCEPTION?

a. Marginal deficiencies
b. Surface tarnish
c. Marginal flash
d. Excessive corrosion

Question 12. When polishing amalgams, green and brown points and cups are utilized to:

a. Remove gross irregularities from the amalgam surface
b. Remove bulky contact area
c. Polish the amalgam to achieve high surface luster
d. Prepare the surface for finishing burs

Taking Alginate Impressions

M. Suann Gaydos, R.D.H., M.S.D.H.

27

Objectives

After performing the laboratory/clinical exercises in this chapter, the student will be able to do the following:

1. Select the appropriate tray for the patient by using the criteria listed in this chapter.
2. Prepare the impression trays with rope wax, including the palatal area of the maxillary tray.
3. Discuss the aspects of patient preparation for alginate impressions.
4. Demonstrate proper mixing of the alginate as well as loading, seating, and removal of the tray to obtain acceptable alginate impressions.
5. Evaluate the impression by using the criteria listed in this chapter, and determine if the impression is acceptable.

Key Words/Phrases

homogeneous

mandibular tori

maxillary exostosis

setting time

study casts

study models

working time

Introduction

Use of alginate impression material is the most common method for obtaining diagnostic casts. It is pleasant tasting, inexpensive, and easy to manipulate. It also adequately records details of the patient's oral structures. **Study models** or **study casts** are positive reproductions of the patient's dental arches and surrounding tissues. They are important visual aids in diagnosis and treatment planning for a patient, and they also serve as an important part of the patient's permanent record. In addition, diagnostic study models are useful as pretreatment and posttreatment records for patients who undergo extensive restorative or orthodontic treatment, fabrication of vital bleach trays, and bruxism splints. Taking (or making) alginate impressions is a procedure that is included in the scope of practice in most states for both dental hygienists and dental assistants.

I. Purpose

The purpose of taking an alginate impression is to make an accurate reproduction of the maxillary and mandibular arches and adjacent tissues. Study models constructed from alginate impressions can be used for planning patient treatment and can serve as part of the patient's permanent record.

II. Selection and Preparation of the Tray

A. Perforations

Impression trays are usually perforated so that the alginate will flow through the holes when the tray is seated on the dental arch. These perforations act as a retentive mechanism to keep the set alginate from separating from the tray upon removal.

B. Available Varieties

Impression trays are available in a variety of sizes and materials. Disposable (or single-use) trays are usually made of plastic, and autoclavable (permanent) trays are made of stainless steel.

C. Proper Tray Selection

Before taking the impression, one should conduct an oral exam to assess the maxillary and mandibular arch for its width, length, or presence of **mandibular tori** or **maxillary exostosis** (harmless overgrowth of bone). If tori/exostosis is present, a wider or larger tray will be necessary for patient comfort. The empty tray should be seated in the patient's mouth to determine the correct fit. Each tray should

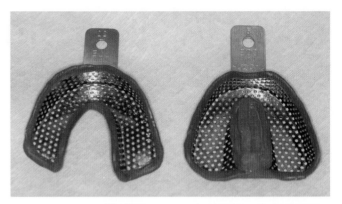

FIGURE 27.1. Beading wax placed around tray peripheries and in the maxillary palatal area.

1. Extend facially to include all teeth as well as the musculature and vestibule.
2. Extend distally approximately 2 to 3 mm beyond the last tooth in the arch to include the retromolar area.
3. Provide a 2- to 3-mm depth of alginate beyond the occlusal surface and incisal edge.
4. Be comfortable for the patient.
5. Some metal trays can be adapted to the patient by bending the sides of the tray.

D. Sterilization

Trays that have been "tried" or "used" for taking the impression should be sterilized before they are returned to storage.

E. Adding Wax to the Tray

After the impression trays have been selected, rope (beading) wax can be molded around the periphery of the tray. This protects the tissues from injury, extends the tray, and may aid in the retention of alginate material within the tray.

F. Adding Wax to the Palatal Area

The maxillary tray may also have rope wax placed in the palatal area of the tray to support the alginate in a high vault and to avoid trapping air. *Figure 27.1* illustrates rope wax placed on tray peripheries and the palatal area.

III. Preparation of the Patient

A. Explain the Procedure

Ask the patient if he or she has had impressions taken in the past. If not, explain the procedure. Advise the patient that the material has the consistency of mashed potatoes or pudding when first placed in the mouth and will then change to a rubberized material, much like silly putty. The patient should follow the directions of the clinician during the procedure. Instruct the patient that the setting time is 3 to 4 minutes depending on the use of fast- or regular-set material and that the tray cannot be removed before this time period. Instruct the patient not to talk but, rather, to raise his or her hand to signal any needs or discomfort.

B. Guard against Spills

Place a napkin on the patient to protect his or her clothing. Give the patient a tissue or paper towel should excessive salivation occur.

C. Minimize Gagging

To minimize the chance of gagging or vomiting, have the patient breathe through his or her nose while seated in an upright position. The gag reflex is stimulated when material touches the posterior third of the tongue, so avoid touching the tongue with either the tray or material overflow. Material overflow can possibly be removed using the end of the mirror and a high-speed evacuation tip.

D. Dental Appliances

Have the patient take out all removable dental appliances such as full or partial dentures, orthodontic retainers, and so on. Cover the gingival areas of fixed bridges and other fixed appliances with rope wax to prevent alginate from locking under crowns and pontics, which causes tearing and distortion of the impression on removal.

E. Rinse

Ask the patient to rinse with mouthwash to reduce the amount of bacteria, debris, and saliva. The result is a more accurate impression.

F. Sequence

It is recommended that the mandibular impression be taken first to familiarize the patient with the procedure as well as with the taste and consistency of the alginate material.

IV. The Alginate Impression

Alginate material is available in regular-set and fast-set products. The regular-set material has a **setting time** of approximately 3 to 4 minutes, whereas the fast-set material will set (or gel) in approximately 1 to 2 minutes. The **working time**, or the time that it should take to mix the alginate, is 1 minute.

A. Mixing the Alginate

1. You will need the necessary equipment listed in Table 27.1.
2. If the bulk form of alginate is used, shake or "fluff" the can, as discussed in Chapter 8, Impression Materials. Both bulk and unit packaging are illustrated in *Figure 27.2*. Wait 30 seconds to allow the "dust" to settle before opening the lid.

TABLE 27.1. Armamentarium for Taking Alginate Impressions
Impression trays
Rope (beading) wax
Rubber mixing bowl
Alginate spatula
Alginate powder
Measuring scoop for alginate
Water measurer
Tap water
Disinfecting solution
Mouthwash
Infection control attire
Air/water syringe
Gauze

3. Using the calibrated water measure, which is marked and provided by the manufacturer, place one measure of water for each scoop of alginate powder into the flexible rubber bowl. Use three "measures" of water for most preweighed alginate packets (three scoops). The cooler the water, the more working time you will have; however, the consistency of the mix will be thinner. With warmer water, the working time is decreased.

4. For bulk alginate, use the measuring scoop provided. Measure the amount of alginate powder needed for the impression as directed by the manufacturer's instructions. Add the alginate to the bowl containing the water. For preweighted packets, tear or cut open the packet and empty into the bowl.

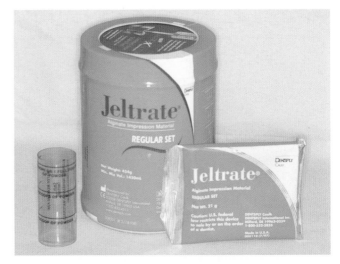

FIGURE 27.2. Alginate in bulk and packet form; water measure on left.

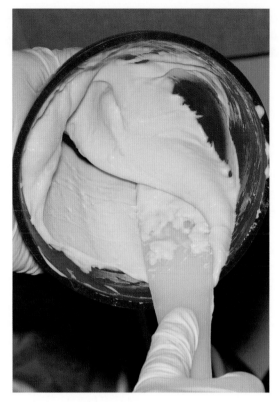

FIGURE 27.3. Spatulation of the alginate impression material.

5. Holding the bowl in one hand and the spatula in the other, gently stir to wet the alginate powder with the water.

6. Once the powder and water have been incorporated, start to rotate the bowl in the palm of one hand, and vigorously press the spatula flat against the bowl with the other. This spatulation method is pictured in *Figure 27.3*.

Incorporate the powder and water thoroughly to create a **homogeneous** mix—one that has a smooth consistency. At the completion of

spatulation, the alginate will become "creamy," similar to the consistency of peanut butter.

7. With the spatula, gather the alginate material into one mass in the bowl.

B. Filling the Tray

Load the alginate material onto the spatula. With the spatula in one hand and the tray in the other, begin to place the alginate in the tray.

1. Mandibular Tray
   a. *Load the Tray*
   Begin loading the tray from one then the other facial aspect of the tray, as shown in *Figure 27.4A*. Continue to deposit material filling the anterior of the tray, as shown in *Figure 27.4B*.
   b. *Eliminate Trapped Air*
   Using the tip or the end of the spatula, press the material into the tray so that any trapped air in the alginate is released.

2. Maxillary Tray
   a. *Load the Tray*
   Begin loading the tray from the posterior aspect of the tray, pushing the alginate anteriorly, as shown in *Figure 27.5A*. Add material in the anterior region and fill the tray to its periphery, as shown in *Figure 27.5B*.
   b. *Eliminate Trapped Air*
   Using the tip or the end of the spatula, press the material into the tray so that any trapped air between the tray and the alginate is released.

3. Moisten and Smooth the Alginate
   Using a fingertip moistened with tap water, smooth the alginate material, and make a slight indentation in the surface, as shown in *Figure 27.6*. This will help in placing the tray over the teeth correctly and in preventing the

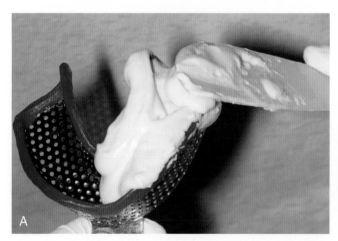
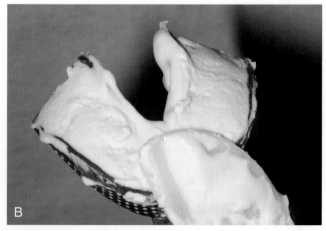

FIGURE 27.4. Loading the mandibular tray with alginate impression material. **A.** Loading from the facial aspect. **B.** Loading and contouring the anterior of the tray.

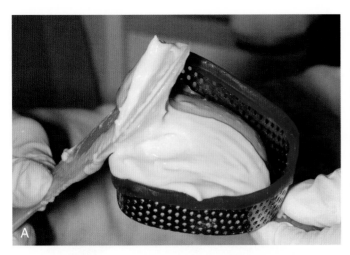

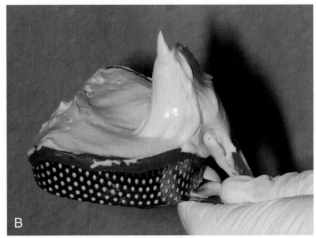

FIGURE 27.5. Loading the maxillary tray with alginate impression material. **A.** Loading from the posterior aspect. **B.** Loading from the anterior aspect.

formation of air bubbles. Excessive water may prevent bonding of the material placed in the tray to the material on the occlusal surfaces of the teeth, as will be discussed later.

C. Seating the Impression

1. Mandibular Arch
   a. The operator should be in a 7-o'clock position (5 o'clock for left-handed operators) to the side and in front of the patient.
   b. The chair should be raised for easy access to the patient. Adjust the headrest so that the occlusal plane is parallel to the floor. This patient and operator position is illustrated in *Figure 27.7.*
   c. Using a 2 × 2 piece of gauze or the air syringe, dry the patient's teeth as thoroughly as possible to remove excess saliva before seating the impression tray. This will help to increase the accuracy and detail of the impression.

d. Ask the patient to open his or her mouth. Using the index finger and thumb of one hand, retract the patient's cheek. Some dental professionals prefer the use of a mouth mirror for cheek retraction since it is thinner than a finger and may ease placement of the tray. Rub a small amount of alginate material over the occlusal and interproximal surfaces of the mandibular teeth with the index finger of the other hand. This additional alginate material helps reduce air bubbles in the impression.

e. Grasp the handle of the impression tray so that the tray and the alginate are facing downward. Rotate the tray into the mouth by using the front of the tray to retract the near cheek and your free hand to retract the far cheek. Once the tray has been inserted, straighten it so that the tray handle is in line with the patient's midface.

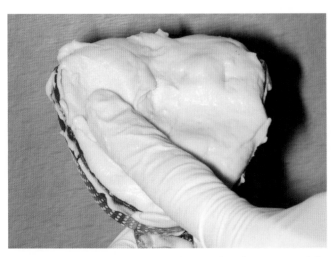

FIGURE 27.6. Moistening and indenting the alginate material.

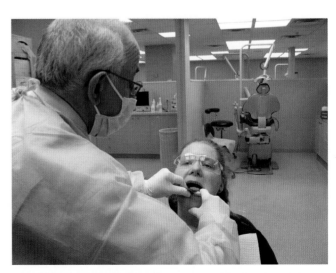

FIGURE 27.7. Operator and patient positioning for taking an impression of the mandibular arch.

f. Note the position of the anterior teeth in relation to the tray. Using the index fingers of both hands, press the tray downward, lightly and evenly, over the mandibular arch until resistance is felt. The lip should lap over the front of the tray, and the alginate should extend into and fill the labial periphery. Excess alginate material will flow out of the perforations as well as into the vestibular and lingual areas. Once the tray has been properly seated, use the index fingers to manipulate the patient's cheeks and release air from the vestibular areas. This will help to create a more detailed anatomy in the facial vestibular area.

g. Ask the patient to raise his or her tongue to the roof of the mouth and move it from side to side. Have the patient close his or her mouth to relax the tongue and cheek muscles, and then carry the tray in a downward direction. This will help to create a more detailed anatomy in the lingual and facial areas.

h. Instruct the patient to breathe normally through his or her nose. If gagging occurs, seat the patient in the most upright position, and ask the patent to lean slightly forward.

i. Keep the tray in place until the alginate is completely set (2–3 minutes after gelation). Alginate material usually sets within 3 to 4 minutes depending on which type of alginate is used (fast or regular set), room temperature, body temperature, water temperature, and consistency of the mix. Because body temperature is higher than room temperature, the alginate material sets faster in the mouth than the remaining alginate in the bowl. Setting a timer to the material's set time (found in the container's packaging) will eliminate guess work on remaining time.

2. Maxillary Arch

a. Operator position when taking this impression should be from the side and back of the patient. This patient–operator position is frequently referred to as 11 o'clock (1 o'clock for left-handed operators) and is shown in *Figure 27.8.*

b. As with the mandibular arch, use a 2 × 2 piece of gauze or the air syringe for drying the patient's teeth as thoroughly as possible to remove excess saliva before seating the impression tray.

c. Ask the patient to open his or her mouth. Using the index finger and thumb or mouth mirror, again retract the patient's cheek, and rub a small amount of alginate on the occlusal

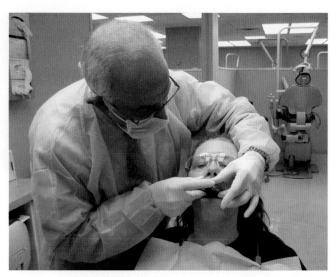

FIGURE 27.8. Operator and patient positioning for taking an impression of the maxillary arch.

and interproximal surfaces of the maxillary teeth to possibly eliminate air bubbles in the impression.

d. The impression tray and the alginate material should be facing upward.

e. Turn the tray slightly to one side, placing the tray in the patient's mouth. Insert the tray by rotating it into the mouth as previously described. Once the tray is inserted, straighten it so that the tray handle is in line with the midface of the patient.

f. Begin to apply light and even pressure upward until resistance is felt. Seat the impression tray in the posterior region, and then seat it toward the anterior, allowing the alginate to flow over the molars. Retract the front of the upper lip as the tray is seated, as shown in *Figure 27.9.* This will allow any excess alginate and air to be expressed through the front of the tray, minimizing the chance of air voids and patient gagging.

g. Instruct the patient to breathe through his or her nose and to lean slightly forward, with the head down toward the chest. This will help to minimize the gagging reflex.

h. Set a timer according to the material's set time (found in the container's packaging) and hold the tray in place until the alginate is completely set (2–3 minutes after gelation).

D. Removing the Impression Tray

1. Mandibular Tray

a. Use the fingers of one hand to retract the corner of the mouth and allow air to enter the vestibule.

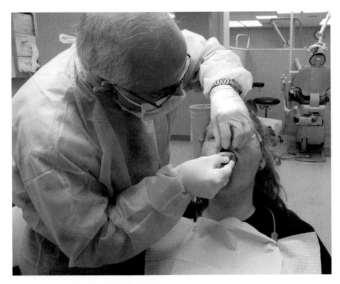

FIGURE 27.9. Seating of the maxillary impression.

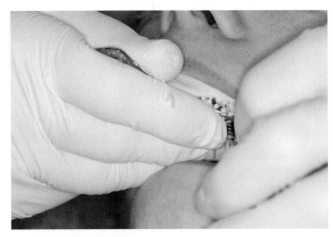

FIGURE 27.10. Removal of the maxillary impression tray.

b. To remove the tray, place the middle and index finger under the tray handle. The thumb sits on top of the handle and tray, between the tray and the opposing anterior teeth to protect the opposing teeth during the tray removal. The free hand should be used to stabilize the mandibular arch during tray removal to decrease injury to the temporomandibular joint. Use a firm, sideways lifting motion to remove the impression. The impression tray should flip free, with the alginate material held securely in the impression tray.

c. If the tray does not release, a suction seal has been created. To break this seal, place the index finger of one hand under the periphery of the posterior portion of the tray on either the right or left side. The tray should now be easy to remove.

d. Assess the impression by using the Skill Performance Evaluation sheet in Appendix 2.

2. Maxillary Tray

a. With the fingers of one hand, retract the corner of the mouth to allow air to enter the vestibule.

b. To remove the tray, grasp the tray handle with the thumb on top of the handle and the middle and index fingers between the tray and the opposing teeth, as shown in *Figure 27.10*. Break the seal and use a downward, sideways flipping motion to remove the impression. The tray should remove easily, with the set alginate secured in the impression tray. The free hand should stabilize the head during tray removal.

c. Assess the impression by using the Skill Performance Evaluation sheet in Appendix 2.

3. Postremoval Procedures

a. After an impression procedure, ask the patient to rinse with water or mouthwash to remove any excess alginate.

b. Remove any alginate that may be remaining on the teeth or in the interproximal spaces by using an explorer or floss.

c. Before dismissing the patient, have the patient rinse again. Use a moistened towel to remove any alginate on the face or lips.

d. Be sure to return any removable dental appliances to the patient.

E. Disinfecting the Impression

1. Gently rinse the alginate impression under cool tap water to remove any debris that may be remaining in the impression.

2. Gently shake off any excess water.

3. Spray the entire impression (top and bottom) with an Occupational Safety and Health Administration–approved disinfecting solution.

4. Place the impression in a headrest cover or plastic bag.

5. Disinfection is usually complete in 10 minutes depending on the disinfectant used.

6. Rinse again with water, shake dry, and place in a clean headrest cover or plastic bag.

7. If the impression(s) cannot be poured immediately, store them in an area with 100% humidity.

Precautions

- Wear a mask when fluffing the alginate.
- Remember that the impression is contaminated with saliva and should be properly handled and disinfected.

Tips for the Clinician

- Fluff the alginate container before dispensing alginate into the bowl.
- Do not overfill the tray.
- The patient should be in an upright position when taking the alginate impression.
- Do not clean the mixing bowl immediately. Use the alginate remaining in the bowl as an indicator for setting time. If the alginate in the bowl is set, then the material in the mouth is also set.
- If taking impressions for both arches, take the mandibular impression first to get the patient accustomed to the procedure.

Summary

1. Discuss the procedure with the patient.
2. Select the proper tray by inserting an empty tray in the patient's mouth.
3. Prepare the trays by adding wax to the periphery and palatal areas if needed.
4. Have the patient rinse with mouthwash.
5. Mix the alginate following the manufacturer's directions, and fill the tray.
6. Smooth the alginate with a moistened finger.
7. Take a mandibular impression from the 7-o'clock position.
8. Take a maxillary impression from the 11-o'clock position.
9. With a quick motion, remove the impressions 2 to 3 minutes after gelation.
10. Properly disinfect the impression.
11. Pour the impression as early as convenient.

 ## Review Questions

Question 1. When preparing the patient for an impression, the operator should:

a. Explain the procedure to the patient
b. Place a napkin on the patient to protect his/her clothing
c. Place the patient in the upright position
d. Have the patient remove all removable appliances
e. Have the patient rinse with antibacterial mouthwash
f. All of the above
g. a, b, and d only

Question 2. When taking a maxillary impression, a right-handed operator should be standing in which position?

a. 12:00
b. 7:00
c. 11:00
d. 9:00

Question 3. When mixing alginate impression material:

a. Add the water to the powder
b. Add the powder to the water
c. Add the powder and water together, at the same time
d. Either water or powder can be added in any sequence

Question 4. All of the following statements are true about the "working time" of alginate material except one. Which one is the EXCEPTION?

a. Working time begins when water and powder come together
b. Cooler water increases working time
c. Warmer water decreases working time
d. Working time begins when the impression is seated

Question 5. The typical mixing time for alginate is _____ and the setting time for regular-set material is _____.

a. 1 minute; 1 to 2 minutes
b. 1 minute; 3 to 4 minutes
c. 3 to 4 minutes; 1 minute
d. 1 to 2 minutes; 1 minute

Fabrication and Trimming of Study Models

28

Objectives

After studying this chapter, the student will be able to do the following:

1. Demonstrate the following laboratory procedures:
   - Use a gypsum product to pour a study model from an impression.
   - Trim the study model on the model trimmer.
2. Differentiate between the two methods of diagnostic cast/study model fabrication.
3. Describe, in order, the cast cuts that are used to trim a study model for patient consultation and dental treatment planning.
4. Explain the laboratory safety procedures and necessary equipment for use in the laboratory mandated by the Occupational Safety and Health Administration.
5. Critique the completed study model for acceptable cuts.

Key Words/Phrases

diagnostic cast

diagnostic model

study model

Introduction

The composition, properties, and uses of gypsum materials are discussed in Chapter 9, Gypsum Materials. **Study models (diagnostic models** or **diagnostic casts**) are defined as "a positive replica of the dentition and surrounding structures used as a diagnostic aid and/or base for construction of orthodontic appliances or prosthetic devices."

Because a dental hygienist is legally permitted to perform these procedures, competency is expected in the associated knowledge and skills. These procedures are commonly performed in the practice of dentistry to gather information concerning the patient's dentition and to establish an accurate diagnosis. As with all skills, however, "practice makes perfect." Most people must continue to practice to be consistently competent. Therefore, do not be discouraged if your first attempt is not exact.

During any process, each step is important to the quality of the final outcome. If a flaw is present in step one, that flaw will be reproduced throughout the entire procedure and be present in the final product. The ability to self-critique to make adjustments or repeat the step is critical for obtaining satisfactory results. The procedural steps for these techniques are detailed in this chapter.

I. Purpose/Indications

The purpose of this chapter is to apply previously learned information and acquire the necessary skills to prepare esthetically pleasing and useful study models. The process of pouring an alginate impression, preparing a base for the model, separating the model from the impression, and trimming the model, is described in the following pages. It is also important that these skills are practiced both safely and effectively; therefore, compliance with Occupational Safety and Health Administration (OSHA) guidelines is mandatory.

II. Construction of a Study Model

Several laboratory techniques for fabricating study models are acceptable. The armamentarium is listed in Table 28.1. This chapter presents two of these techniques: one using a "double-pour" and another using a "single-pour" of the impression.

A. Using a Double-Pour Technique

A two-stage pour will prevent distortion and provide an adequate base for reproduction of the oral structures. The double-pour technique involves two separate mixes and, thus, two separate setting times.

TABLE 28.1. Armamentarium for Constructing Study Models

Equipment and Supplies

Plaster bowl

Plaster spatula

Gypsum material

Vibrator

Ruler

Lab knife

Wax Spatula

Protractor (optional)

Boxing wax (optional)

Beading wax (optional)

Wet/dry sandpaper (optional)

Maxillary and mandibular impressions

Scale

Graduated cylinder

Pencil

Pink baseplate wax

Model trimmer

Glass or acrylic slab

Infection control and safety

Protective eyewear

Lab jacket or clinic gown

Gloves

1. First-Stage Pour
   a. Measure 100 to 150 g of the dental stone or other gypsum depending on the size of the impression. Regardless of the material, follow the manufacturer's directions.
   b. Measure the correct quantity of the corresponding water, and pour it into your plaster mixing bowl. Pour the powder into the liquid.
   c. Spatulate (stir) the mixture for 30 seconds with a stropping motion. Pressing the spatula against the side of the bowl helps to remove air bubbles from the mixture.
   d. Place the mixing bowl on the vibrator, and compress the sides of the bowl. Bubbles should rise to the surface and break. Remove the mixing bowl from vibrator.
   e. Place the impression on the vibrator. Starting at one corner and using a wax spatula, "deliver" a small amount (pea size) of the mix into the mold distal to the last molar (*Fig. 28.1A*). Allow this material to flow into the impression under vibration, filling the impression of the most distal tooth in the quadrant.

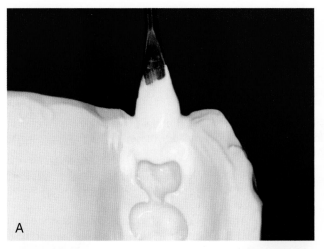

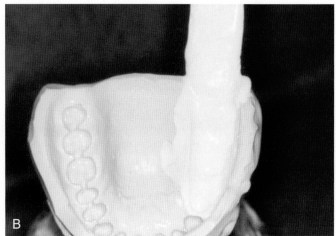

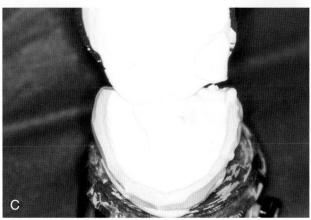

FIGURE 28.1. Pouring an impression. **A.** A small amount of gypsum material is added distal to the most posterior molar. **B.** Larger increments are added with the plaster spatula. **C.** After the teeth are filled, the remaining gypsum material is poured to fill the impression.

f. Repeat the previous step until the impression is filled, adding the new material at the same location as the initial increment. The material should flow around the arch, filling one tooth at a time. The size of the increment may be increased when the material has a greater distance to flow around the arch. The plaster spatula may be used to add larger amounts of material for these final additions (*Fig. 28.1B*).

g. After all the teeth are filled, pour the remainder of the mix from the bowl into the impression (*Fig. 28.1C*). Overfill the impression with gypsum material sufficiently to cover all areas by approximately 0.25 inch.

h. Add small amounts of the gypsum material to the surface of the pour to assist in retention of the second pour (*Fig. 28.2*). Allow the impression to set facing up.

i. Allow the mix to reach the initial set (see the manufacturer's instructions). This will be several minutes after the "loss of gloss," or approximately 10 minutes after the initial pour.

2. Second-Stage Pour
   a. Make a thicker mix of gypsum product (100–150 g) to serve as a base to support the first pour.
   b. Make a paddy of gypsum material approximately 1 inch thick in a shape resembling the size of the impression tray, and place it on a glass or acrylic slab or a surface that will not absorb water or stick to the mix (*Fig. 28.2*).

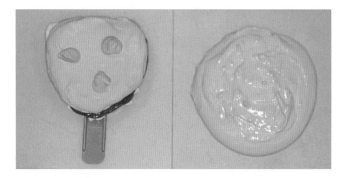

FIGURE 28.2. Alginate impression poured with dental stone. The paddy serves as a base for the alginate impression.

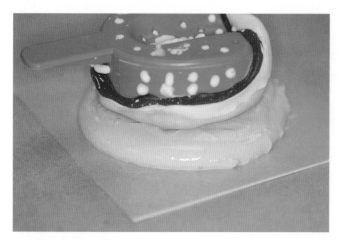

FIGURE 28.3. Inverted set impression on the dental stone paddy.

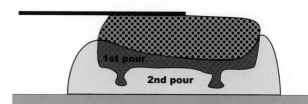

FIGURE 28.5. Cross section of the poured alginate impression inverted onto the gypsum paddy (base).

mounds of gypsum added to the first pour "interlock" into the base to provide a stronger finished product.

c. Invert the poured impression onto the paddy. Do not apply pressure to the inverted impression tray or allow the impression to sink closer than 0.5 inch to the surface. Do not allow the gypsum material to overlap outside the tray (*Fig. 28.3*).

d. Blend the two gypsum mixes together with the plaster spatula to create a continuous connection of the two mixes (*Fig. 28.4*). While holding the handle of the impression tray, use the spatula to shape the sides of the stone around the first pour. Avoid placing the wet gypsum material from the base onto the impression tray because this would create a mechanical lock that is difficult to separate when set. Be certain that the handle of the impression tray and the occlusal surface of the teeth are parallel with the slab to promote a base of uniform thickness. A cross section of the base and impression is illustrated in *Figure 28.5*. Note how the additional small

e. After loss of gloss, trim the excess stone base with a laboratory knife to approximately ¼ inch from the outer border of the impression (*Fig. 28.6*). This will develop the sides and base area of the cast, thus requiring minimal use of the model trimmer.

f. Wait 45 to 60 minutes after the beginning of the second pour to separate the cast from the impression. Carve away gypsum material and alginate exposing the edge of the tray.

g. To begin tray removal from the cast, place the laboratory knife on the edges of the periphery of the tray, and slightly twist the knife to pry apart the adhering alginate and gypsum materials (*Fig. 28.7*). Repeat this procedure around the periphery of the tray.

h. When the margins of the tray are free of the cast, use an upward, pulling motion to facilitate the separation (*Fig. 28.8*).

i. If the tray does not freely separate from the cast, determine the location of the obstruction on the periphery, and carefully remove it with a laboratory knife.

j. Avoid rocking the impression tray back and forth or side to side. This may cause the teeth to fracture.

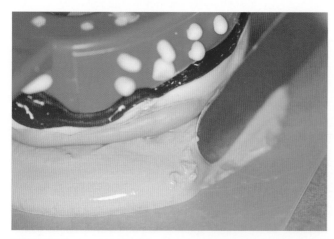

FIGURE 28.4. Adapting the dental stone base material to the set stone in the impression tray.

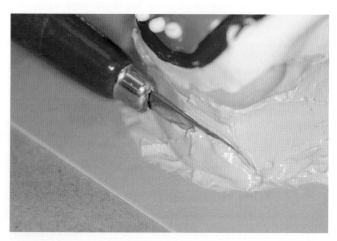

FIGURE 28.6. Trimming the excess dental stone with a laboratory knife after loss of gloss.

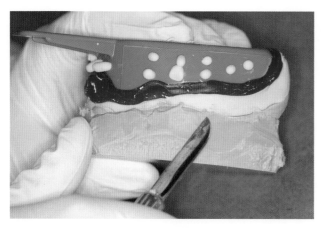

FIGURE 28.7. Separating the cast from the impression tray with the laboratory knife.

  k. Trim the base and sides of the cast on the model trimmer. Use of the model trimmer is discussed later in this chapter.

B. Using a Single-Pour Technique

  After developing skill with the double-pour technique, a single-pour technique may be used for some models or casts. In the single-pour technique, a larger amount of material is initially mixed. The impression is filled and the paddy prepared as described above. The filled impression is inverted and placed on the paddy before the material sets. Greater care is needed to prevent the impression tray from being locked into the setting gypsum material.

C. Using Boxing Wax

  Boxing wax can be used to form a mold for the base of the study model. The boxing wax completely encircles the impression tray and creates a temporary "extension" of the impression. This extension forms the mold for the base of the study model. Use of boxing wax is more common for pouring casts for dentures and other restorations.

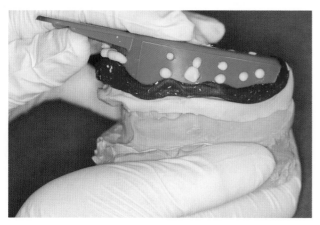

FIGURE 28.8. Using an upward, pulling motion to separate the cast from the impression.

Tips for the Clinician–Pouring an Impression

- Properly proportion and mix the gypsum product.
- Fill one tooth at a time.
- Do not lock the impression tray into the cast.
- Do not allow the material to vibrate out of the impression at the opposite end of the arch.

Precautions–Pouring an Impression

- Disinfect the impression before pouring.

III. Trimming Diagnostic Casts or Study Models

A nicely trimmed cast or study model gives the patient a professional and esthetic-looking representation of their oral tissues. It can be used during a consultation appointment to inform the patient about his or her existing oral status and the proposed plans for dental treatment. A prepared study model that is neat and accurate adds to the precise, professional content of the presentation. Study models may also serve as part of the patient's record.

  The following general directions are intended for a wide variety of clinical needs. Specific needs may require the trimming technique to be modified.

A. Cast Design and Terminology

  Note the cast's appearance and terminology in *Figure 28.9*. Note the similarities and differences

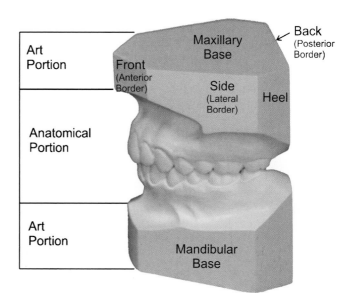

FIGURE 28.9. Cast terminology and identification of cast landmarks.

TABLE 28.2. Armamentarium for Trimming Study Models

Models or casts

Model trimmer

Pencil and ruler

Wax spatula and laboratory knife

Eye protection

Handpiece and burs

Lathe and attachments

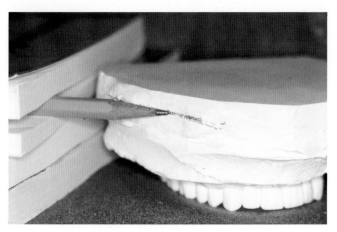

FIGURE 28.11. The base of the maxillary cast is marked parallel to the occlusal plane.

in the cuts and shapes between the maxillary and mandibular casts.

1. Bases are parallel to the occlusal plane.
2. The backs are perpendicular to the bases.
3. The sides and heels are trimmed even.
4. The anterior of the upper cast has a point at the midline, but the anterior of the mandibular cast is rounded.

B. Preparation for Trimming

1. Assemble the necessary materials and equipment, which are listed in Table 28.2.
2. Don appropriate personal protective equipment.
3. Make sure the casts have set for a minimum of 30 minutes, and then separate the casts from the impressions. If the casts are dry, thoroughly wet them.
4. Remove small nodules of stone on the casts and/or residual bits of alginate with a wax spatula, particularly on the occlusal surfaces of the teeth (*Fig. 28.10*).
5. Secure hair away from your face. Remove any hanging or dangling jewelry, accessories, or clothing. Removal of rings is recommended.
6. Turn on the model trimmer. Establish a steady flow of water over the grinding wheel of the model trimmer so that it does not become clogged and will function smoothly.

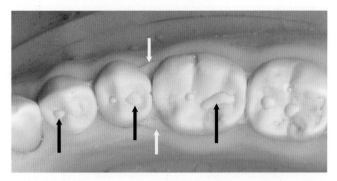

FIGURE 28.10. Blebs of dental stone (*black arrows*) and bits of alginate (*white arrows*) to be removed from the model.

7. Trim excess stone that grossly extends beyond the anatomy of interest. At this and all other steps, DO NOT TRIM AWAY CRITICAL ANATOMY!

C. Trimming Models

1. Maxillary Base
   a. *Establish a Plane for the Maxillary Model Base*
      To make the base of the maxillary model parallel to the occlusal plane, place the model occlusal surface down on a cushioned (several layers of paper towels), flat surface. If the cast is not stable when resting on the occlusal surface, rock it onto the anterior teeth and do one of the following:
      1. Using a pencil and ruler, mark the model in at least four places at an equal height around the periphery of the model.
      2. OR, use a pencil placed between the pages of a book at the needed height. Mark the model in at least four places around the periphery, as shown in *Figure 28.11*.
      3. Connect the pencil marks with a solid line as shown in *Figure 28.12A*.
      4. The base should be approximately one-third of the total model height in the anterior region.

   b. *Trim the Base of the Maxillary Model (Fig. 28.12)*
      Gently feed the maxillary cast into the grinding wheel of the model trimmer with a steady pressure to trim the base and leave a smooth, flat cut. Cut parallel to the penciled line (and the occlusal plane). Trim until the model base is approximately 0.5 to 1 inch in height at the maxillary anterior region and the base is flat. It is not necessary to trim to the pencil marks, only to trim parallel to them.

Step-By-Step Checklist for Trimming Models

1. **The Maxillary Base**
   _____ A. To make the maxillary arch parallel to the bench top, do one of the following after you have rocked the arch forward onto the anterior teeth:
   1. Use a pencil and ruler to mark the model in four places at an equal height around the periphery.
   2. Use a pencil between the pages of a book to the required height. Turn the model to mark it in at least four places (*Fig. 28.11*).
   3. The base should be approximately one-third of the total model height in the anterior region.
   _____ B. Trim the base of the maxillary model (*Fig. 28.12*).
   Place on grinding wheel and trim the base parallel to the pencil marks. The trimming goal is one flat surface. Rinse clean. Check periodically by laying trimmed surface on counter and attempt to "rock" the base from side to side. It should not have any bevels or exhibit a rocking motion.

2. **Maxillary Posterior Border (*Fig. 28.13*)**
   _____ Put both arches in occlusion and mark with a pencil the location on the maxillary cast of the most posterior anatomy that is present on either cast (so you know "how far in" to grind).
   _____ Also mark the median raphe (midline of palate) with a pencil (*Fig. 28.13A*).
   _____ Now trim the maxillary model at a right angle to the penciled midline. Grind to the marked area identifying the most posterior anatomy (*Fig. 28.13*).

3. **Mandibular Posterior Border (*Fig. 28.14*)**
   Place the base of the maxillary model on the stage of the model trimmer. Occlude the mandibular model with the maxillary (mandibular model will be on top–look closely at *Figure 28.14A*).
   _____ Trim the back of the mandibular model until it is even with the back of the maxillary model, but do not trim away any anatomy.
   _____ Both posterior sides (backs) should be flat, and the occluded models should not open when set "on end" (on posterior sides).

4. **Mandibular Base**
   _____ Keep both models in occlusion with the backs on the trimmer stage. Trim the base of the mandibular model so that it is parallel with the maxillary model (*Fig. 28.15A and B*). The combined height should be 2 to 2½ inches.
   _____ The bases of the models and the occlusal plane should be parallel to the bench top.

5. **Lateral Borders (*Fig. 28.16*)**
   _____ Trim the sides of the widest cast first from canine to the last molar (*Fig. 28.16A*). Trim parallel to the central grooves (*Fig. 28.16B*).
   _____ Next, put teeth in occlusion and trim the other arch to match (*Fig. 28.16C*).

6. **Anterior Borders (*Fig. 28.17*)**
   A. Maxillary Cast
   _____ Mark the canine eminence and the midline *on the base* portion of the model with a pencil.
   _____ Trim the anterior portion from the canine eminence to anterior midline on both sides (*Fig. 28.17A and B*). These cuts will form a point with each other and with each lateral border.
   B. Mandibular Cast
   _____ Trim the anterior portion from canine to canine following the form of the arch (*Fig. 28.17A and C*). It will be rounded in appearance.

7. **Posterior Angles**
   _____ Place the teeth in occlusion and trim the posterior angles (heels) (*Fig. 28.18*) of both casts to be even and symmetrical with the lateral and posterior sides of the casts.

8. **Finishing the Casts**
   _____ A. Trim and smooth the tongue area of the mandibular cast with a lab knife or large acrylic bur and lab handpiece
   _____ B. Trim the excess "lip" (land area) of lateral and posterior borders of both casts (*Fig. 28.19*). Do not remove the mucobuccal fold unless instructed to do so.
   _____ C. Fill in voids with a putty of matching gypsum product in the base portion of casts. Use waterproof sand paper to smooth the base; do not round or sand the edges.
   _____ D. Remove any remaining nodules or blebs of gypsum from the cast with a lab knife.
   _____ E. Check casts for symmetry.
   _____ F. Label both casts with your name (for laboratory exercises) or the patient's name (for the clinical setting) and the date.

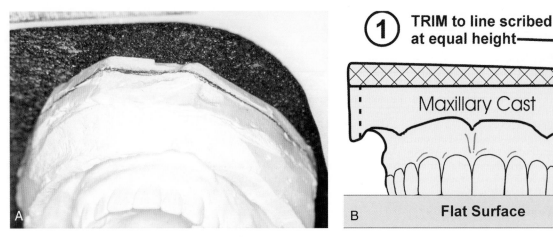

FIGURE 28.12. **A.** The base of the maxillary cast is trimmed parallel to the pencil line. **B.** Drawing showing the portion of the cast to be removed. The *cross-hatched area* indicates the material to be trimmed in this step. The *dashed lines* indicate areas to be trimmed in subsequent steps.

Evaluate the cuts by periodically placing the cast on the countertop to assess the overall cast appearance. The base should be parallel to the occlusal plane in both the anteroposterior and the lateral directions. When using the model trimmer, immediately rinse away any gypsum debris on the model.

2. Maxillary Posterior Border (*Fig. 28.13*)
   a. Occlude models with or without a wax bite. If the models will not completely occlude, trim the interfering base material. Do not trim away any anatomy of interest.
   b. With a pencil, mark the location on the maxillary cast of the most posterior anatomy of either cast: retromolar pad, hamular notch, or maxillary tuberosity. Also, on the maxillary cast, mark the midline and the median raphe with a pencil.

c. Trim the posterior surface of the maxillary model at a right angle to this line, as shown in *Figure 28.13*. Trim to the most posterior anatomy of either cast.

3. Mandibular Posterior Border (*Fig. 28.14*)
   Place the base of the maxillary model on the model trimmer table; the model is upside down. Articulate the mandibular model with the maxillary having the interocclusal bite registration wax between the teeth, if available, to avoid fracture. In other words, place the maxillary and mandibular model in occlusion and turn them upside down (maxillary now on bottom) on the trimmer table. Trim the back of the mandibular model until it is even with the back of the upper model, but do not trim away any anatomy. The backs (posterior borders) should be flat and the models should not

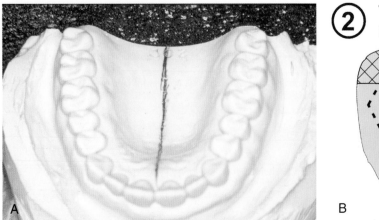

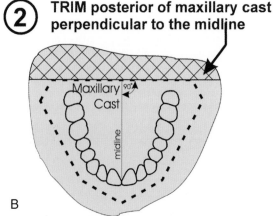

FIGURE 28.13. **A.** The posterior of the maxillary cast is trimmed perpendicular to the midline. **B.** Drawing showing the portion of the cast to be removed. The *cross-hatched area* indicates the material to be trimmed in this step. The *dashed lines* indicate areas to be trimmed in subsequent steps.

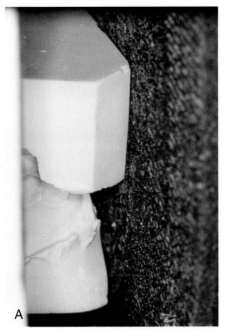
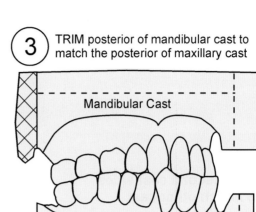

FIGURE 28.14. **A.** The posterior of the mandibular cast is trimmed to match the posterior of the maxillary cast. **B.** Drawing showing the portion of the cast removed. The *cross-hatched area* indicates the material to be trimmed in this step. The *dashed lines* indicate areas to be trimmed in subsequent steps. The models correctly sit on their posterior borders with the teeth in occlusion.

open when they are placed "on end" (posterior borders).

4. **Mandibular Base** (*Fig. 28.15*)
   Keep the upper and lower casts in occlusion with their backs resting on the trimmer table. Trim the base of the lower cast so that it is perpendicular to the backs of both casts and parallel to the base of the upper cast and occlusal plane. The combined height of both models should be approximately 2 to 2.5 inches. When finished, the bases of the occluded models and the occlusal plane should be parallel to the benchtop and the bases flat.

5. **Lateral Borders** (*Fig. 28.16*)
   Trim the sides of the widest cast first, from the canine to the last molar. Trim parallel to the central grooves of the teeth. With teeth in occlusion, trim the lateral borders of the opposing cast to match those of the first cast trimmed. When finished, the lateral borders of both casts should be flat and flush with each other.

6. **Anterior Borders** (*Fig. 28.17*)
   a. *Maxillary Cast*
      With a pencil, mark the canine eminence and the midline on the base portion of the model to

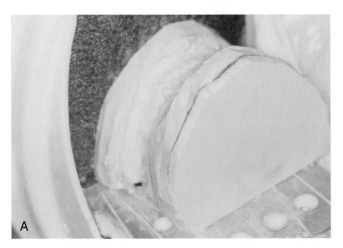
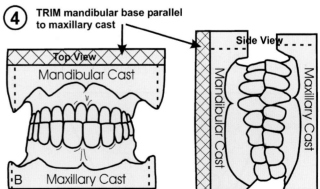

FIGURE 28.15. **A.** The posterior of the mandibular cast is trimmed perpendicular to posterior of the maxillary and mandibular casts. **B.** Drawing showing the portion of the cast to be removed. The *cross-hatched area* indicates the material to be trimmed in this step. The *dashed lines* indicate areas to be trimmed in subsequent steps.

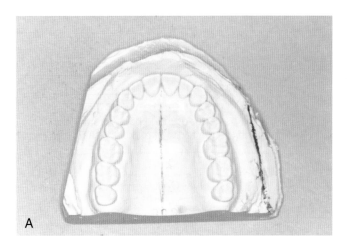

A

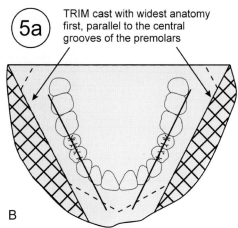

5a TRIM cast with widest anatomy first, parallel to the central grooves of the premolars

B

5b **TRIM second cast sides to match other cast**

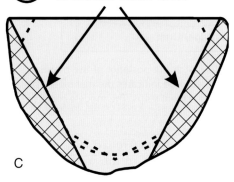

C

FIGURE 28.16. **A.** The sides of the casts are trimmed parallel to the central grooves of the teeth. **B** and **C.** Drawings showing the portion of the cast removed. The *cross-hatched area* indicates the material to be trimmed in this step. The *dashed lines* indicate areas to be trimmed in subsequent steps.

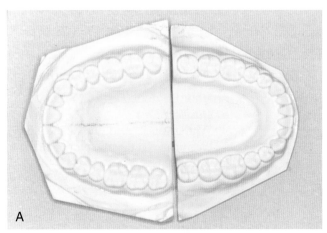

A

6a TRIM anterior of cast to be symmetrical canine to canine

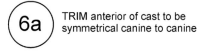

Maxillary Cast

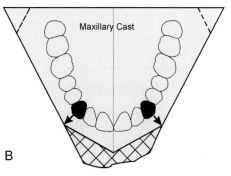

B

6b **TRIM anterior region canine to canine**

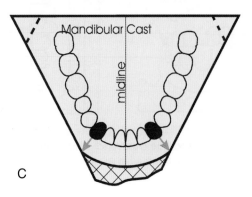

C

FIGURE 28.17. **A.** The anterior of the maxillary cast is trimmed to form a point at the midline, while the anterior of the mandibular cast is rounded. **B** and **C.** Drawings showing the portion of the cast to be removed. The *cross-hatched area* indicates the material to be trimmed in this step. The *dashed lines* indicate areas to be trimmed in subsequent steps.

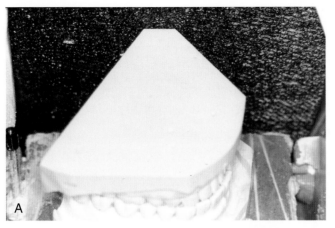
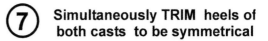
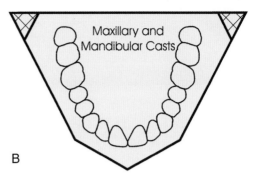

FIGURE 28.18. **A.** The heels of both casts are trimmed to form equal angles with the posterior and the sides. **B.** Drawing showing the portion of the casts to be removed (*cross-hatched areas*).

guide your cuts. Trim the anterior portion from the canine eminence to the anterior midline on both sides. These cuts will form a point with each other and with each of the lateral borders.

b. *Mandibular Cast*
Trim the anterior portion from canine to canine following the form of the arch. The result is a rounded cut.

7. Posterior Angles (*Fig. 28.18*)
With the casts in occlusion, trim the posterior angles (heels) of both casts to be even and symmetric with the lateral and posterior sides of the casts.

D. Finishing the Casts

1. Use a lab knife, handpiece, or lathe and accessories to trim and smooth the tongue area of mandibular cast. Do not remove any anatomy (lingual frenum). Preserve the lingual alveolar sulcus.

2. Trim the excess "lip" (land area) of the lateral and posterior borders of both casts, as shown in *Figure 28.19*. Do not remove the mucobuccal fold unless directed to do so.

3. Fill voids in the base portion with the proper gypsum material. Use waterproof sandpaper to smooth the base portion of the casts (*Fig. 28.20*). Do not round or sand the edges.

4. Remove any remaining nodules or blebs of stone from the casts using a small lab knife or other instrument.

5. Check the casts for a symmetric appearance where appropriate.

6. Label both casts with your name (for laboratory exercise) or the patient's name (for clinical setting) and date.

7. Assess your casts by using the Skill Performance Evaluation sheet in Appendix 2. Completed study models are shown in *Figure 28.21*.

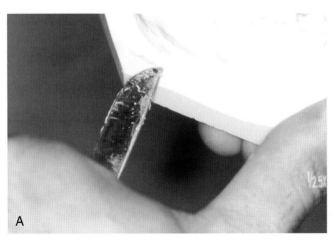

FIGURE 28.19. **A.** The land area is created by trimming the excess material above the mucobuccal fold. **B.** Drawing showing the portion of the cast to be removed.

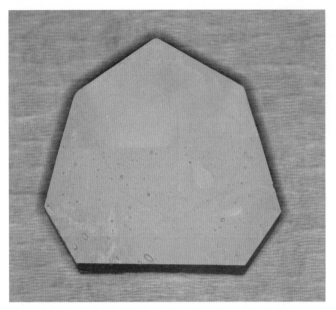

FIGURE 28.20. Pores and voids are present in the lower half of the base of this cast. In the upper half, the pores and voids have been filled and sanded for final finishing.

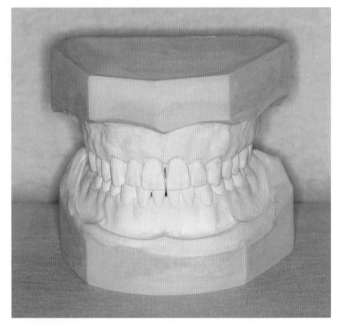

FIGURE 28.21. Trimmed and finished study models.

Tips for the Clinician–Trimming Models

- Make sure that adequate water is flowing through the model trimmer to prevent clogging.
- Rinse the trimming debris from the model immediately after using the model trimmer.
- Take care not to trim away teeth and other oral anatomy.

Precautions–Trimming Models

- Rest the palm of the hand on the trimmer's table.
- Keep fingers "tucked in" and away from rotating wheel.
- Do not use excessive force.

Summary

Pouring an Impression
1. Mix the gypsum material.
2. Fill the impressions of the teeth.
3. Fill the rest of the impression.
4. Construct a base.

5. Wait 30 to 45 minutes for the gypsum material to set.
6. Separate the model from the impression by lifting the impression upward (do not use a tipping motion).

Summary

Trimming Models
1. Trim the maxillary base parallel to the plane of occlusion.
2. Trim the posterior of the maxillary model perpendicular to its base.
3. Trim the posterior of the mandibular model even with that of the maxillary model.
4. Trim the base of the mandibular model perpendicular to the backs of both models.

5. Trim the sides parallel to the central grooves of the posterior teeth with the models in occlusion.
6. Trim the anterior of the models.
7. Trim the heels of the models while they are in occlusion.
8. Remove blebs of excess stone or plaster.
9. Fill in pores, and sand smooth.

Review Questions

Question 1. **Why would the double-pour technique be a preferred method of fabricating a cast/study model?**

a. It is the quicker method of the two
b. Prevents distortion of oral structures
c. Produces a better reproduction of oral structures
d. It is a safer technique

Question 2. **Which is the best indicator of the initial set of gypsum products?**

a. Loss of gloss
b. Loss of resilience
c. Decreased compressive strength
d. Decreased elasticity

Question 3. **The overall, combined height of both maxillary and mandibular models should be _____ inches.**

a. 1.5 to 2
b. 2 to 2.5
c. 2.5 to 3
d. 3 to 3.5

Question 4. **Listed below are the basic steps in model trimming. Starting with number 1 as the first step, identify the steps in the proper sequence using numbers 1 through 7.**

_____ Trim the posterior surface of the maxillary model perpendicular to the marked midline

_____ Trim the base of the lower cast so that it is perpendicular to the backs of both casts and parallel to the base of the maxillary cast

_____ Remove small nodules on the casts with a wax spatula

_____ Trim the lateral borders

_____ Trim the anterior borders

_____ Trim the base of the maxillary model parallel to the established plane (pencil line)

_____ Trim the back of the mandibular model until it is even with the back of the maxillary model

Fabrication of a Custom Impression Tray

29

A. Todd Walls, D.D.S.

Objectives

After performing the laboratory/clinical exercises in this chapter, the student will be able to do the following:

1. List the differences between the acrylic resin and visible light–cured (VLC) resin tray fabrication techniques.
2. Briefly describe the characteristics of an exothermic reaction.
3. Name the three purposes of an impression tray.
4. Recall the four reasons why a dentist may choose to fabricate a custom tray for a patient rather than using a stock tray.
5. Explain the purpose of the occlusal stops that are designed in a custom impression tray.
6. Discuss two methods of trimming a custom tray.

Key Words/Phrases

arbor band

burley arbor

exothermic reaction

occlusal stops

visible light–cured (VLC) resins

Introduction

Custom impression trays can be constructed of several types of resins. Autopolymerizing acrylic resins and visible light–cured resins are two types of useful materials for the production of custom impression trays, orthodontic appliances, temporary restorations, and denture fabrication. These materials are discussed in detail in Chapter 5, Direct Polymeric Restorative Materials.

Autopolymerizing resins (*Fig. 29.1*) may be formed by adding measured amounts of the monomer liquid to the polymer powder and then mixing and molding the resin into the desired shape before the initial set. When the material cools from the exothermic phase (material gives off heat) of the setting reaction, it may be removed from the die, cast, or model and then trimmed and/or polished.

The **visible light–cured (VLC) resins** are supplied in lightproof plastic packages. After the package is opened, the material is molded to the desired shape and then made rigid by exposure to high-intensity visible light in a light-curing unit.

I. Purpose

The purpose of an impression tray can be remembered by using "the 3 Cs"—to carry, control, and confine the impression material. Custom-made impression trays made from either acrylic or VLC resins are used in final impressions for crown and bridge restorations and for denture construction.

Custom rather than stock trays are used for the following reasons:

• The operator can better control the thickness of the material.
• Custom trays can accommodate any anatomic anomaly, such as large lingual tori.

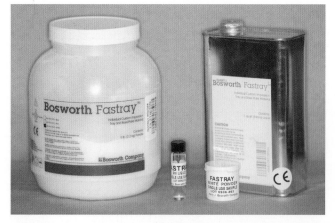

FIGURE 29.1. Tray resin powder and liquid supplied in bulk form and in single-use packaging.

• Custom trays are more stable than stock trays.
• Custom trays can be used again for the same patient.

These are accomplished best with custom impression trays. Use of custom trays is described in Chapter 8, Impression Materials. A custom tray requires a preliminary impression to produce a preliminary cast.

Tips for the Clinician

• If adding a handle to an autopolymerizing resin tray, wet the tray in the area of intended handle placement with monomer. This will enhance the bond.
• Make sure the resin is a doughy consistency before manipulating it. If the resin is a viscous consistency, it will be difficult to adapt into the shape of a tray.
• Construct the handle in the proper shape, size, and position to be functional for taking the impression.

II. Tray-Spacing Procedure (for a Dentulous Custom Tray)

For this discussion, we will assume that fabrication of a custom tray will be a laboratory exercise, with the impression being taken on a Dentoform rather than on an actual patient. For this reason, fabrication of a quadrant tray will be presented so that the subsequent impression can be easily removed from the Dentoform. In clinical practice, however, custom impression trays are usually made as a full maxillary or mandibular arch tray rather than as a quadrant tray for greater stability and ease of articulation. The VLC tray is illustrated with this technique.

Impression materials need a uniform thickness to produce the most accurate casts. The construction of a custom tray uses a blockout procedure and "occlusal stops" to accomplish this uniform thickness. These procedures are the same for both autopolymerizing and VLC resin trays. The blockout procedure adds wax to eliminate or "block out" any cast undercuts that would lock the set custom tray to the cast. The same wax provides an even space for impression material. Stops are holes in the blockout wax that result in a precise seating of the custom tray. The exact location of stops, thickness of wax, and extent of the wax and impression tray depend on the patient, impression material, and clinician's personal preferences. The following is a general technique useful for most patients. The items necessary to prepare a cast for custom tray construction are listed in Table 29.1.

    A. Coat the preliminary cast with Foilcote (Whip Mix Corp., Louisville, KY) or a similar separator material (see *Fig. 29.2*).

TABLE 29.1. Armamentarium for Custom Tray Blockout	
Stone cast of patient	Aluminum or tin foil
Laboratory knife	Foilcote
Baseplate wax	Small paint brush
Bunsen burner	

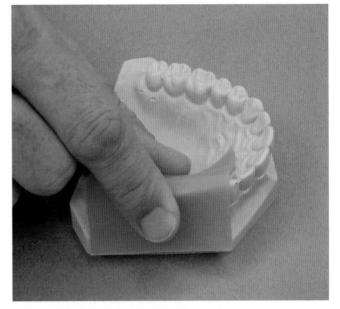

FIGURE 29.3. Adapting baseplate wax over patient's cast.

B. Using a Bunsen burner or hot water, soften a piece of baseplate wax that is approximately 2 × 3 inch in size for the quadrant tray. Be careful not to overheat the wax, as this could result in unwanted thin areas.

C. Loosely adapt the warm wax over the tooth to be restored and adjacent teeth (see *Figure 29.3*). Extend the wax onto the buccal and lingual tissues 3 to 4 mm beyond the gingival margin of the teeth. Adapt a second layer of wax on top of the first. This will give a space of about 2 to 3 mm for the impression material. Trim the excess wax with a warm dental lab knife.

D. Provide occlusal stops by cutting three 1- to 2-mm openings in the wax on the occlusal portion of two teeth, not teeth to be prepared for restoration. When preparing a full-arch custom tray, three occlusal stops should be cut in a tripodal configuration: two posterior stops and one anterior stop. The cut openings in the wax for occlusal stops are shown in *Figure 29.4*. They allow the tray material to flow into these openings and create a "bump" or a protuberance on the tissue side of the tray. When the tray is made, the tray will seat until these occlusal stops

or bumps fit onto their mating surfaces of the teeth in a stable and predictable manner. Precise seating of the tray will provide space for a uniform layer of impression material. *Figure 29.5* illustrates this result in cross section. **Occlusal stops** are pictured on the inside of a tray in *Figure 29.6*.

E. Place a layer of aluminum foil, tin foil, or foil substitute separating medium over the wax to ensure the tray material separates from the blockout after fabrication. The inside surface of the tray should not be contaminated with wax (*Fig. 29.7*). Your instructor (or future employer) will select the separating material to be used.

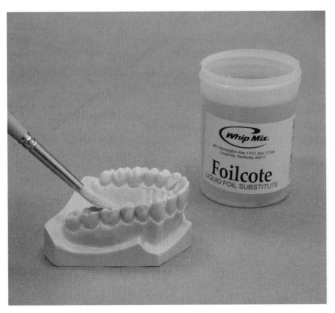

FIGURE 29.2. Stone cast coated with a separating medium.

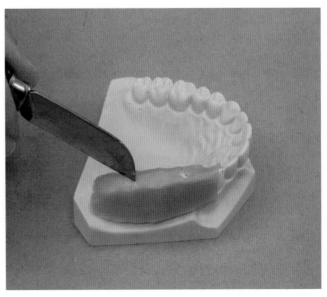

FIGURE 29.4. Adapted wax cut with openings for occlusal stops.

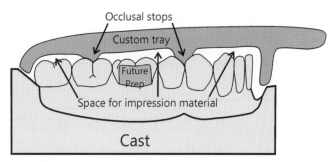

FIGURE 29.5. Cross section of tray, space for impression material, occlusal stops, and prepared tooth.

Precautions

- The monomer liquid and vapors are flammable.
- The monomer liquid will dissolve many plastic materials and penetrate some gloves.
- Frequent contact with autopolymerizing resin monomer liquid will cause skin irritation. Use of Vaseline or butyl rubber gloves will prevent this.
- Wear eye protection during the entire procedure. Monomer may splash, especially when rotary equipment is used.
- Hold the tray firmly while trimming with a dental lathe.

III. Construction Procedure for Autopolymerizing Resin Trays

The armamentarium necessary to fabricate a traditional custom tray is listed in Table 29.2.

A. Mix one unit of tray resin, or measure the powder and liquid of the bulk material with the measuring devices supplied by the manufacturer. Use a waxed paper cup as a mixing bowl. Remember that acrylic monomer is a powerful solvent and will dissolve certain plastics.

B. Stir thoroughly with a wooden tongue depressor. All liquid and powder must be homogeneously incorporated into the resin mass.

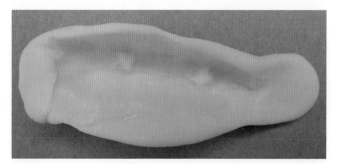

FIGURE 29.6. Untrimmed custom tray showing "stops" on the inside surface.

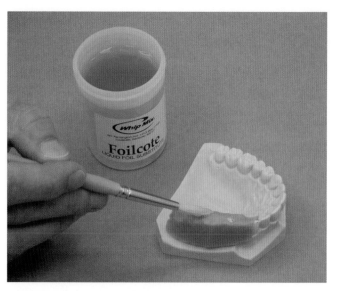

FIGURE 29.7. Painting baseplate wax and cast with a separating medium.

C. When the mixture reaches a doughy consistency (2–3 minutes), lightly coat your hands with petroleum jelly or wear gloves so that the tray resin will not stick to them while you are working.

D. Once the doughy mixture no longer sticks to the fingers when touched, remove it from the paper cup, create a short "sausage" shape with your hands, and lay it on the blocked-out area of the cast (*Fig. 29.8*).

E. Adapt the mixture over the blockout and cast while keeping a uniform thickness, and extend the tray borders to the edge of the blockout, as illustrated in *Figure 29.9*. Push the resin into the occlusal stop areas so that it contacts the cast.

F. Form a handle in the anterior portion of the tray by pressing some of the material between your thumb and forefinger. The handle must not set in a drooped position. A functional handle is shown in *Figure 29.10*.

TABLE 29.2. Armamentarium for Acrylic Custom Tray Construction

Blocked-out stone cast of patient

Waxed paper cup

Laboratory knife

Tray resin powder

Tray resin liquid

Wooden tongue depressor

Petroleum jelly or butyl rubber gloves

Dental lathe, burley arbor, and arbor band

OR

Barrel-shaped acrylic bur and laboratory handpiece

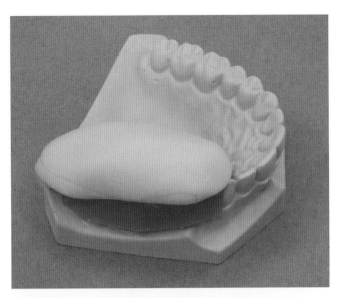

FIGURE 29.8. Initial shape of resin before adaptation.

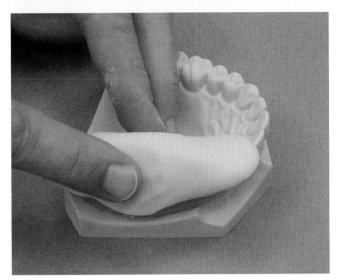

FIGURE 29.9. Tray resin adapted over wax and cast.

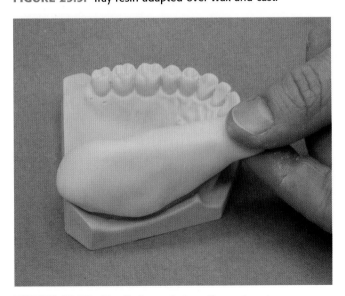

FIGURE 29.10. Handle formation on the custom tray.

G. Note the temperature of the tray as it sets (**exothermic reaction**). After the tray is almost cool, remove it from the cast. If wax sticks to either the tray or the cast, soak the wax-covered object in hot water for a few minutes, and then gently pull the wax away.

H. Tray trimming is discussed later in this chapter.

IV. Construction Procedure for VLC Resin Trays

The armamentarium necessary to fabricate a full-arch VLC resin tray is listed in Table 29.3.

A. Follow the tray-spacing procedures described earlier in this chapter to block out the cast.

B. Remove the VLC resin from its package (*Fig. 29.11*)

C. Next, adapt the resin over the blocked-out cast keeping a uniform thickness, and extend the tray borders to the edge of the blockout as illustrated in *Figure 29.12*. Push the resin into the occlusal stop areas of the cast.

D. Mold an unused piece of VLC resin into a handle shape and adapt it to the anterior of the tray as illustrated in *Figure 29.13*.

E. Paint the tray with Triad air barrier (Dentsply International, York, PA) as illustrated in *Figure 29.14*.

F. Place the cast and tray into a Triad light-curing unit and cure for 2 minutes (see Figure 18.7).

G. Remove the tray from the cast and remove all blockout materials inside the tray.

H. Paint the tissue side of the tray with Triad air barrier coating.

I. Place the tray in the curing unit tissue side up and cure for an additional 2 minutes.

J. Remove the air barrier coating by washing with soap and water.

K. Check that the tray properly seats on the cast. It should be stable, and all stops should seat accurately.

L. Proceed to the next section to trim the tray.

TABLE 29.3. Armamentarium for Acrylic Custom Tray Construction

Blocked-out stone cast of patient

Waxed paper cup

Laboratory knife

Tray resin powder

Tray resin liquid

Wooden tongue depressor

Petroleum jelly or butyl rubber gloves

Dental lathe, burley arbor, and arbor band

OR

Barrel-shaped acrylic bur and laboratory handpiece

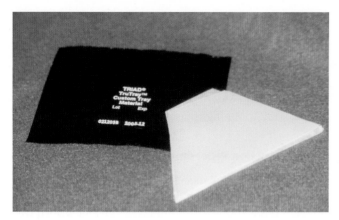

FIGURE 29.11. Visible light–cure (VLC) tray material removed from package.

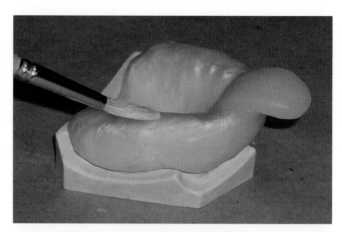

FIGURE 29.14. Painting the tray with air barrier coating.

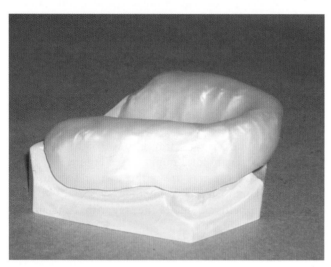

FIGURE 29.12. Visible light–cure (VLC) tray material molded onto the cast and trimmed.

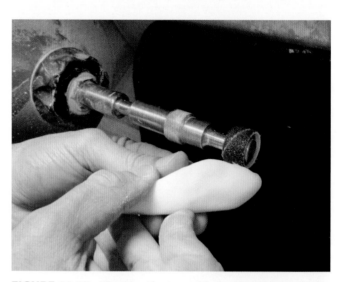

FIGURE 29.15. Trimming the tray with the dental lathe, burley arbor, and arbor band.

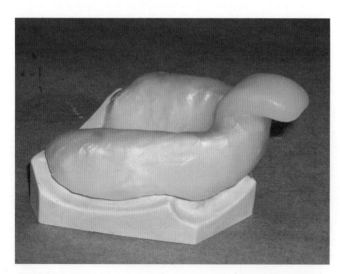

FIGURE 29.13. VLC material added to form the tray handle.

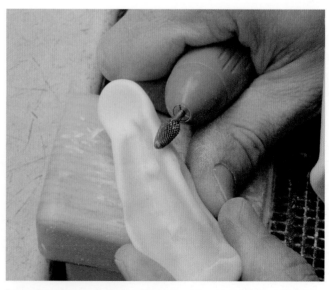

FIGURE 29.16. Trimming the tray with a handpiece and bur.

V. Trimming the Tray

A. Trim the tray to eliminate excess material and rough edges in all areas. Do this by using the dental lathe, burley arbor, and arbor band. The **burley arbor** attaches to the lathe and holds the arbor band. The **arbor band** is a 0.75-inch-wide, coarse sandpaper ring. The lathe, burley arbor, and arbor band are pictured in *Figure 29.15*.

B. During trimming, check for smoothness by rubbing all edges with a finger. If the edge feels sharp to your finger, it will be uncomfortable for the patient. Trim sharp edges so that they are smooth and rounded.

C. An alternative method of finishing the tray is to trim it with a laboratory handpiece and barrel-shaped acrylic bur. Use a palm grasp for this procedure, as illustrated in *Figure 29.16*.

D. Evaluate the custom tray by using the Skill Performance Evaluation sheet in Appendix 2.

Summary

Application of Wax Spacer
1. Coat the cast with a separating material.
2. Apply softened wax, and cut stops.
3. Reapply separating media or foil.

Tray Construction Procedure
Autopolymerizing Resin
1. Mix the resin to a homogeneous consistency.
2. Coat your hands with petroleum jelly or wear gloves.
3. When the mix reaches a doughy consistency, adapt over the blockout and form a handle.
4. When the resin begins to heat, remove the tray from the cast.
5. Remove the blockout, and reseat the tray on the cast.

Visible Light–Cure (VLC) Resin
1. Remove VLC resin from the package, and adapt it over the blockout.
2. Add the handle.
3. Paint the tray with an air barrier coating.
4. Place the resin in a curing unit for 2 minutes.
5. Remove the tray from the cast, and remove the blockout.
6. Paint the tray on the tissue side with an air barrier coating, and cure again for 2 minutes.
7. Remove barrier with soap and water.

Tray Trimming
1. Smooth the surfaces and edges with a bur or other abrasive.
2. Check the entire tray and all edges by rubbing with a finger.

Review Questions

Question 1. All of the following are true regarding custom trays except one. Which one is the EXCEPTION?

a. There is better control of the thickness of impression material with the use of a custom tray

b. Custom trays cannot accommodate anatomic features such as tori

c. A custom-made impression tray can be used again for the same patient

d. There is more stability when using a custom tray as compared to a stock tray

Question 2. The tray-spacing (blockout) procedure during custom tray fabrication should provide _____ mm of space between the cast and the tray.

a. 0.5 to 1

b. 1

c. 2 to 3

d. 4 to 6

Question 3. **What is important to do when adapting resin on the blocked-out cast?**

a. Always extend the resin over the land area

b. Extend the resin onto the tissues 3 to 4 mm beyond the gingival margin

c. Press out the resin to make it as thin as possible

d. Ensure the final thickness of the resin is at least 6 to 7 mm for rigidity

Question 4. **Which of the following is true about occlusal stops?**

a. Are needed to ensure proper seating of the custom tray

b. Should be placed on centric cusps

c. Are only needed on the maxillary arch

d. Are placed on the buccal gingiva

Question 5. **Trimming the tray can be accomplished with a dental lathe or a laboratory handpiece with a barrel-shaped acrylic bur. The tray borders should have square rough edges to ensure proper seating and impression material retention.**

a. The first statement is true; the second statement is false.

b. The first statement is false; the second statement is true.

c. Both statements are true.

d. Both statements are false.

Elastomeric Impressions

Frank Mastalerz, D.D.S.

Objectives

After performing the laboratory/clinical exercises in this chapter, the student will be able to do the following:

1. Briefly discuss the rationale for dental hygienists to learn the preparation and technique of addition silicone impression material.
2. Recall the reasons for using addition silicone impression material.
3. Explain the tray preparation that is necessary for use of addition silicone impression material.
4. Summarize the steps involved in:
   - Preparing the putty (tray) material
   - Preparing the wash (syringe) material

Key Words/Phrases

addition silicone impression material

automix gun

retraction cord

tray adhesive

Introduction

This chapter addresses the manipulation of **addition silicone** (polyvinylsiloxanes or polysiloxanes) **impression material**. This is one of the four types of impression materials discussed in Chapter 8, Impression Materials. This material commonly involves the use of an automix gun, as shown in Figure 8.14. Use of the **automix gun** eliminates hand mixing with a spatula and paper mixing pad.

I. Purpose

Addition silicone impression material is generally used as a "final impression material" for the fabrication of crowns and bridges. Dental hygienists may (or may not) take this type of impression depending on their state practice act. From time to time, however, even those who do not take this type of impression may find themselves assisting with this procedure. An advantage of this material is that it does not need to be poured immediately after the impression is taken. Its stability and accuracy make it a very popular material.

II. Procedure for the Double-Mix Putty-Wash Technique

The double-mix impression technique uses two different viscosities of impression material. One is very thick and is used in the tray. The second has a low viscosity. It is syringed on and around the tissues of interest. The tray is seated immediately after the syringe material is injected into place. Typically, the tray and syringe materials are prepared simultaneously by two people.

A. Tray Preparation (Table 30.1)

1. A plastic stock tray is selected and painted with a **tray adhesive**. This adhesive aids in retention of the impression material in the tray.

TABLE 30.1. Armamentarium for Addition Silicones

Stock tray (usually plastic)

Tray adhesive

Impression material (putty)

Cartridge gun

Impression syringe

Syringe tips

Impression cartridges (wash or light body)

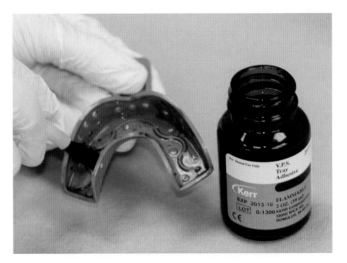

FIGURE 30.1. Stock impression tray coated with adhesive.

Use an adhesive from the same manufacturer as the impression material.

2. Be sure to coat the facial, lingual, and occlusal surfaces of the inside of the tray, as shown in *Figure 30.1*.
3. Allow approximately 10 minutes to air-dry so that the adhesive becomes tacky.

B. Preparing the Automix Gun

The automix gun is prepared by loading the cartridge and installing the mixing tip. The system must be ready to dispense material when needed.

1. Load the cartridge into the gun.
2. Twist off the sealing cap. Save the cap.
3. Dispense a pea-sized amount of material onto a paper towel by squeezing the handle. This ensures that the base and catalyst materials have not set and clogged either opening of the cartridge. Wipe the end of the cartridge.
4. Install a new mixing tip, and twist it into the locked position.
5. After use of the automix system, remove the used mixing tip, and replace the cap.

Tips for the Clinician

- Avoid wearing latex gloves when mixing the putty.
- For best results, tray and syringe materials are prepared simultaneously by two people.
- Moisture control is critical.
- It is much easier to wait and remove set material from a patient's face (or other places) than it is to remove unset material.

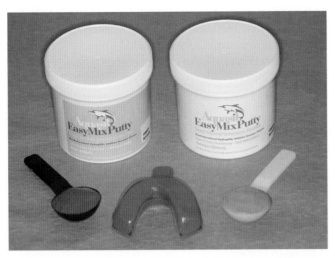

FIGURE 30.2. Top. Putty material supplied in tubs. **Bottom out-side.** scoops of base and catalyst. **Bottom center.** mixed putty in impression tray.

C. Preparing the Putty Material

1. Don plastic overgloves. Latex gloves are not used because they may inhibit the setting of the material.
2. Dispense equal volumes of the putty base and catalyst materials, using the appropriate scoops. Using the same scoop in both jars will contaminate the remaining material.
3. Knead the material with your fingertips rather than in the palm of the hand. Kneading with your palms will warm and accelerate the set of this material. A homogeneous color should be obtained in 30 seconds.
4. Roll the mix into a 3- to 4-inch-long cylinder, and place this into the tray, as shown in *Figure 30.2.*

D. Preparing the Wash Material

1. Squeeze the trigger of the automix gun to dispense an appropriate amount into the back end of the barrel of an impression syringe, as shown in *Figure 30.3*. Backfill by withdrawing the tip of the automix gun from the syringe barrel.
2. Place the plunger into the impression syringe. It is important to do this in a way that does not trap air.

E. The Impression

1. Most impressions for crown and bridge restorations use retraction cord. **Retraction cord** is a fine string that is placed in the gingival sulcus of the prepared teeth below the margins, as shown in Figure 8.6. Retraction cord pushes the gingiva away from the teeth. Many times, retraction cord is treated with a hemostatic or vasoconstrictive

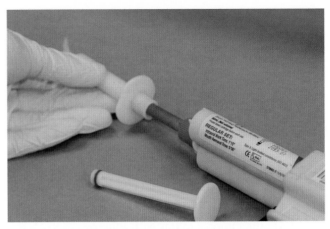

FIGURE 30.3. Filling the impression syringe from the cartridge gun.

agent to reduce bleeding and temporarily shrink the gingival tissues. Depending on the dentist's preference, the retraction cord may or may not be removed before the impression is taken. When the retraction cord is removed, the syringe material will flow into the space that the retraction cord created. This captures the fine details of the preparation's margins.

2. The syringe material is placed in the interproximal areas and over the margins and occlusal surfaces of the prepared teeth, as shown in *Figure 30.4.*
3. The previously prepared tray material is immediately placed directly over the syringe material. It is then held without motion for approximately 5 to 7 minutes (or the appropriate amount of time as specified by the manufacturer).
4. The tray is removed with a quick snap motion, rinsed, and disinfected. It is then poured or sent to a dental laboratory.
5. Assess the impression by using the Skill Performance Evaluation sheet in Appendix 2.

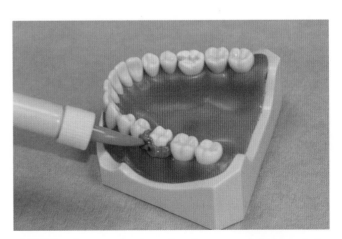

FIGURE 30.4. Application of syringe material around the preparation.

Precautions

- To avoid an accelerated set, mix the putty material with your fingertips.
- Follow the manufacturer's directions regarding used tips and cartridge caps.

- For putty material, use the designated scoops for each jar to avoid cross-contamination.
- Protect the patient's clothing when using impression materials to prevent staining.

Summary

Tray Preparation
1. Coat the impression tray with adhesive.
2. Wait for 10 minutes.

Automix Gun
1. Load the cartridge into the gun, and squeeze out material to ensure its free flow.
2. Install a mixing tip.
3. After use, follow the manufacturer's directions regarding the used tip and cartridge cap.

Putty Material
1. Don nonlatex overgloves.
2. Dispense equal volumes of putty base and catalyst.
3. Knead the material with your fingertips for 30 seconds (until a homogeneous color occurs).

4. Roll mix into a 3- to 4-inch-long cylinder, and place this into the tray.

The Impression
1. Remove the retraction cord if desired, and control moisture.
2. Place the syringe material over the margins and in the interproximal areas, and then cover the entire preparation.
3. Seat the tray directly over the syringe material.
4. Hold the tray without motion for 5 to 7 minutes.
5. Remove the tray with a quick snap motion, rinse, and disinfect.

 ## Review Questions

Question 1. The addition silicone tray material is placed over the syringe material and held in place for approximately _____ minutes.

a. 1 to 3
b. 3 to 5
c. 5 to 7
d. 6 to 8

Question 2. An advantage of addition silicone impression material is:

a. Stability
b. That it can be poured at a later time
c. Accuracy
d. All are advantages

Question 3. Addition silicone material is best prepared:

a. By a single operator
b. With two people
c. Using latex gloves
d. In a moist environment

Question 4. The putty material of addition silicone should be kneaded in the preparer's fingertips rather than in the palm of the hand because of:

a. Staining from the material
b. Difficulty in removing from hands
c. Accelerating the set of the material
d. Increasing the setting time

Question 5. The tray adhesive used in the double-mix putty-wash technique should dry in the impression tray for approximately _____ minutes.

a. 3
b. 5
c. 7
d. 10

Vital Tooth Whitening Procedures

Michele R. Sweeney, R.D.H., M.S.D.H.

31

Objectives

After studying this chapter, the student will be able to do the following:

1. List the indications and contraindications for use of the patient-applied, professionally supervised whitening technique.
2. Recall the indications and contraindications for professionally applied power whitening techniques.
3. Outline the steps in the clinical phase of patient-applied, professionally supervised vital whitening technique.
4. Identify the essential elements of home care instructions for the patient using the professionally supervised, self-applied technique.
5. Summarize the steps in construction of the whitening tray, and identify the equipment and materials used.
6. Outline the steps in the professionally applied power whitening technique. Identify the equipment and materials used.

Introduction

Delivery of the patient-applied and professionally applied "power" whitening techniques may be shared between the dentist and the dental hygienist. The critical elements of both techniques include the patient's medical history, intraoral examination, discussion of benefits and risks, informed consent, collection of data, record maintenance, detailed patient instruction, and follow-up evaluation. The hygienist may assume many of these responsibilities.

I. Purpose/Indications

Patient-applied whitening or professionally applied power whitening is generally effective on vital teeth that are affected by slight-to-moderate intrinsic staining. Yellow, orange, and light brown intrinsic stains are more receptive to whitening than are dark blue–gray and dark brown stains. White spots can be difficult to mask with whitening. Tetracycline staining becomes more difficult to treat as the degree of staining intensifies. Extrinsic stains are more easily whitened than are intrinsic stains; however, a prophylaxis may be all that is necessary to obtain the desired esthetic result.

II. Contraindications

Teeth that have been stained as a result of caries, pulpal necrosis, or endodontic therapy are not good candidates for patient-applied whitening. Stains caused by amalgam restorations also resist whitening. Teeth with sensitive root surfaces should not be whitened aggressively because of the potential for increased tooth sensitivity. A small minority of patients may be sensitive or allergic to a component in the whitening agent, and occasionally, a patient may not exhibit the degree of motivation and/or cooperation that is necessary for successful treatment. Table 31.1 lists the indications and contraindications for the use of patient-applied, professionally supervised vital whitening.

TABLE 31.1. Indications/Contradistinctions for Patient-Applied, Professionally Supervised Whitening

Indications	Contraindications
Vital teeth	Nonvital teeth
Extrinsic stain	Severe intrinsic stain
Light-to-moderate intrinsic stain	Sensitive root/dentin
Cooperative/compliant patient	Sensitivity to components of whitening agent
	Unreasonable expectations

TABLE 31.2. Indications/Contradistinctions for Professionally Applied Power Whitening

Indications	Contraindications
Vital teeth, endo treated nonvital teeth	Untreated nonvital tooth
Extrinsic stain	Severe intrinsic stain
Light-to-moderate intrinsic stain	Sensitive root/dentin
Cooperative/compliant patient	Sensitivity to whitening components
	Unreasonable expectations
	Use of photosensitive drugs/herbs
	Hx of melanoma
	Hx of chemo/radiation therapy

Professionally applied power whitening should not be used on patients with photosensitivity due to drugs or herbal supplements. Patients undergoing chemotherapy or radiation therapy must not be bleached with the power technique. Patients with a history of melanoma should avoid the power bleaching systems because of the potential exposure to harmful light sources. Severe intrinsic stains, cervical erosion/sensitivity, cracks in the enamel, caries, and anterior restorations not scheduled for replacement are also contraindications for power whitening procedures. Local anesthesia must not be used as tissues could be harmed when patient sensations are not present. Nonvital teeth may undergo professionally applied power bleaching systems. Table 31.2 lists indications and contraindications for the professionally applied power whitening.

Before whitening treatments are prescribed, the patient's medical history should be thoroughly reviewed. The procedure is contraindicated in the following patients:

- Pregnant or lactating women
- Children under the age of 18 years without parental consent
- Heavy smokers
- Patients who are sensitive to any ingredient in the whitening agent
- Anterior restorations that will not be replaced

III. Clinical Procedure—Three Patient Appointments for Professionally Monitored Patient-Applied Tray Whitening

Professionally prescribed whitening agents for patient application are available in the popular kit form, which contains all the necessary supplies for an average treatment sequence. The following is a brief description of the recommended clinical procedure for vital tooth bleaching

TABLE 31.3. Armamentarium for the Clinical Procedure for Processionally Supervised Whitening

Forms: medical history, informed consent, clinical examination, and treatment

Prophylaxis instruments

Camera: video, film, or digital

Shade guide or other color-measuring device

Written instructions

using carbamide peroxide agents. Necessary items for this procedure are listed in Table 31.3.

A. First Appointment

A summary of the clinical procedures in this section can be found at the end of the chapter.

1. Medical History

Obtain a complete medical history from the patient. Other than conditions listed above or a sensitivity or allergy to hydrogen peroxide or carbamide peroxide or other ingredients contained in the bleaching agent, there are no medical contraindications.

2. Informed Consent

An informed consent should be read and signed by the patient at this time. The **informed consent** form should briefly describe the bleaching procedure as well as the possible benefits and side effects. The informed consent should become a part of the patient's record. A sample consent form is illustrated in *Figure 31.1*.

3. Intraoral Examination

Perform a complete intraoral examination. Examine the soft tissues for lesions, which would be irritated by the tray or the bleaching agent. Examine the teeth for caries, exposed root surfaces, exposed dentin, and broken or cracked restorations as well as teeth. Any findings from this exam should be documented in the patient's record.

4. Prophylaxis

Perform a prophylaxis. Scale and polish the teeth to remove plaque, calculus, and stain.

5. White Swabs

White stain remover swabs with aqueous cleaning technology are available. The swabs known as Power Swabs, Whitening Enhancement Swabs, and GRINrx Whitening Stain Remover Swabs (Power Swabs Corporation, Beaverton, OR) may also be used to enhance bleaching. The tabs are swabbed gently over all surfaces to be whitened. The swab removes stains, prepares surface for whitening, and reduces sensitivity through its hydration properties.

6. Intraoral Photograph

Take an intraoral photograph showing both the upper and lower teeth. In this photograph, include a **shade guide tab** that is matched to the shade of the anterior teeth, *Figure 31.2A*. The tab may be positioned adjacent to the incisal edge of a central incisor. *Figure 3.4* shows a VITA shade guide. Intraoral color-measuring devices, such as the **spectrophotometer** shown in *Figure 31.2B*, may also be used to document the initial tooth color.

Informed Consent for Patient-Applied, Professionally Supervised, Tooth Whitening Treatment

The product you will apply to your teeth contains the active whitening ingredient, ***Carbamide Peroxide***. The most frequently reported side effects of peroxide tooth whitening are tooth sensitivity and irritation of the gums. Sore throat and nausea may occur if you accidentally swallow some of the product.

Patient Consent: I _____ (full name), hereby consent to treatment using a patient-applied, professionally supervised tooth whitening agent. I have been informed of the potential benefits and side effects of the treatment, and affirm that I have read and understand the instructions below.

Signed: _____

Witness: _____

Date: _____

One copy for the patient.

One copy for the patient's record.

FIGURE 31.1. Informed consent form for patient.

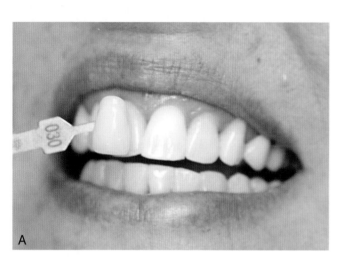
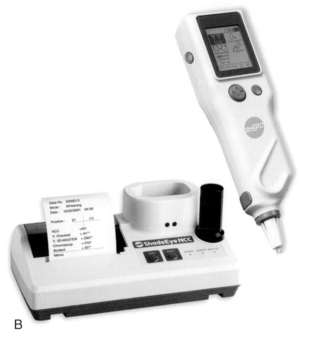

A

B

FIGURE 31.2. **A.** Photograph of anterior teeth and shade guide for color evaluation and pre-/post-op records. **B.** Photograph of an intraoral spectrophotometer, a clinical color-measuring device. (Courtesy of Shofu Dental Corp.)

7. Full-Arch Impression

Take a full-arch alginate impression of the teeth that are to be whitened. Carefully pour the impression in dental stone. The whitening tray is fabricated on the stone model before the next appointment.

B. Second Appointment

1. Test Fit

Try the custom tray in the patient's mouth, and make any necessary adjustments. *Figure 31.3*

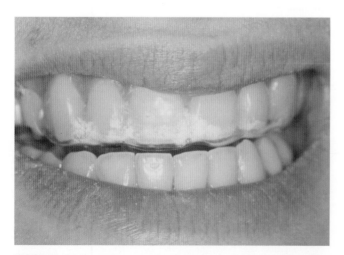

FIGURE 31.3. Custom resin whitening tray in place over the maxillary teeth.

shows a custom tray in place over the maxillary teeth. The tray should not impinge on frenal attachments.

2. Patient Instruction

Instruct the patient regarding use of the tray. The patient may wear the tray at night or during the day. When used at night, the tray is worn over the teeth while the patient sleeps. When used during the day, the tray is worn twice daily for 1 hour each. On average, initial results are achieved in 2 weeks; however, longer treatment may be required to achieve the desired result.

a. Load the tray with fresh whitening agent before each treatment. Do not fill the tray completely. Fill only the space that is created by the reservoirs in the tray; use only one dot of material per facial surface.

b. Place the tray firmly over the teeth. Wipe any excess whitening agent from outside the tray with fingers or a piece of gauze.

c. Do not swallow the excess whitening agent.

d. Remove the tray at the end of each treatment period, and rinse it with cold water.

e. Brush the teeth and rinse the mouth at the end of each treatment.

f. Store the tray in the storage box between treatments. Do not expose the tray or box to heat.

g. Record each whitening treatment with the date and the hours treated.

3. Side Effects

Describe the possible side effects, such as tooth sensitivity or soft-tissue irritation (gums, lips, or cheeks), to the patient. Instruct the patient to call the office should any side effects occur. If the teeth become sensitive, the patient should discontinue treatment until the sensitivity disappears and then begin treatment again with a reduction in the daily treatment time. Tooth sensitivity can be effectively treated with application of neutral sodium fluoride or potassium nitrate in the whitening tray twice daily for 1 hour each.

4. Written Instructions

Give the patient written instructions. These instructions should include space to record the date and length of treatment (*Fig. 31.4*).

5. Follow-up Appointment

Schedule an appointment for the patient to return when the treatment is completed. The duration of treatment may vary but usually requires 2 to 6 weeks. Whitening one arch at a time will allow the patient to better visualize the results of treatment by allowing comparison between treated and untreated teeth.

C. Third Appointment

1. Examination

Examine the patient for results of the whitening treatment. Record the total amount of treatment in hours, and note any negative side effects.

Instructions for Patient-Applied, Professionally Supervised Tooth Whitening

You should expect a gradual improvement in the whiteness of your teeth with repeated applications of the whitening product. Apply the whitening product to your teeth twice daily for one hour each application, following these directions:

- Brush and floss your teeth in the usual manner.
- Place one dot of the whitening gel on each facial surface in the custom tray.
- Place the tray securely over your teeth.
- Remove any excess gel with your toothbrush.
- Do not swallow the gel.
- After one hour, remove the tray from your teeth and rinse your mouth with plain water.
- Rinse the tray in cool water and store it in the storage box away from heat.
- Repeat the application twice daily.
- If you experience any negative side effect, discontinue use and call the office for instructions. (Telephone: _____)
- Return to the office for re-examination and evaluation at the appointed time.
- Store the whitening gel safely out of reach of small children.

Record of Treatment (patient name _____)

Make an entry each time you apply the whitening agent to your teeth. Record the date of treatment and the length of time of each treatment in hours or fraction of an hour.

Date of Treatment	Length of Treatment

FIGURE 31.4. Patient-instruction form.

2. Additional Whitening

If additional whitening is desired, dispense more whitening agent to the patient, and schedule an appointment for a follow-up examination at the end of a sufficient treatment sequence (usually 2–4 weeks).

3. Intraoral Photograph

When the desired result has been achieved, take a posttreatment intraoral photograph of the treated teeth, including a matching shade guide tab (as in the first photograph, *Fig. 31.2A*). Together with the pretreatment photograph, this photograph becomes part of the patient's record to document the results of the bleaching treatment. Alternatively, a new color measurement with an intraoral color-measuring device can be used to document the color change.

The Skill Performance Evaluation sheet for patient protocol and bleaching tray fabrication as a clinical procedure is located in Appendix 2.

IV. Laboratory Procedure—Constructing the Custom Tray

The **custom whitening tray** is made of clear vinyl resin. A stone model is produced from an alginate impression, and the custom tray is fabricated on the model. Many of the oral appliances discussed in Oral Appliances are constructed in a similar way. Necessary items for the laboratory procedure are listed in Table 31.4.

A. Make a Stone Working Model

1. Mix the dental stone and pour into the alginate impression. The impression need not be boxed, but should be poured into a horseshoe shape to avoid additional trimming.
2. Remove the model from the impression after the stone has completely set, and trim on a

---

TABLE 31.4. Armamentarium for Tray Construction

Vacuum former

Resin-curing light

Light-cure blockout resin

Small, curved scissors

Microtorch

Sheet vinyl (thickness, 0.04 inch)

Dental laboratory stone

Storage container for tray(s)

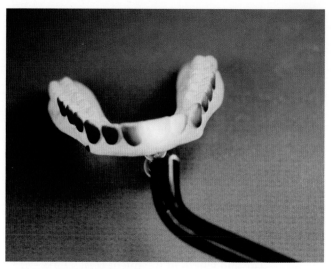

FIGURE 31.5. Blockout resin exposed to curing light (10 seconds for each tooth).

model trimmer. Keep the base small, thin, and horseshoe shaped.

B. Create a Reservoir for the Whitening Agent

1. After the model has completely dried, create a reservoir on the facial surface of the teeth to be bleached if the manufacturer of the whitening product recommends one. The **reservoir** is a space created between the tray and the teeth to hold the bleaching material. It should be no more than 1 mm thick. Carefully place light-cure **blockout resin** on the facial surface of each tooth to be whitened. Stop the material 1 mm short of the gingiva. Do not cover the incisal or occlusal surfaces, and do not fill the interproximal spaces.
2. Cure the resin on each tooth by exposing the resin to a curing light for 10 seconds (*Fig. 31.5*).

C. Vacuum Sheet Resin Over the Working Model

1. Place a 6 × 6-inch piece of **sheet resin** material in the frame of the vacuum former. Vinyl resin with a thickness of 0.04 inch makes an adequate tray.
2. Place the thoroughly dry model in the center of the vacuum former platform.
3. Heat the resin material until it sags downward approximately 1 inch below the frame. *Figure 31.6* shows the heated resin in the vacuum former frame over the stone model.
4. Turn on the vacuum, and immediately pull the frame down over the model. Vacuum for 30 seconds.
5. Allow the resin to cool, and then remove the resin-covered model from the frame.

Tips for the Clinician for Patient-Applied Whitening

Patient Instructions

- For best results, encourage patients not to smoke, eat food, or drink beverages that stain.
- Emphasize that "more is not better." Stress that the patient should follow instructions given by the dental professional.

Tray Construction

- Trim the base of the stone model as thin as possible.
- Allow the stone model to dry completely before the blockout or vacuum-forming procedures.
- Allow the resin to cool completely before attempting to trim or remove it from the model.
- A thin layer of Silly Putty (available in toy stores) can be substituted for the blockout resin. Cover all but the gingival third of the facial surfaces of the teeth to be whitened.

Precautions

Patient Instructions

- If tooth sensitivity occurs, stop treatment. Resume treatment after the sensitivity disappears (usually in a few days), but decrease the treatment time by half.

Tray Construction

- Do not look directly at the curing light when curing the blockout resin.
- The heating element and the frame that holds the resin remain hot after the vacuum have been turned off.

D. Trim the Whitening Tray

1. Trim the vinyl material with scissors, and carefully separate the tray from the model. Trim the tray again, creating a scalloped border following the gingival margins of the teeth. The tray border should end on the teeth, just gingival to the reservoir spaces. A tray being trimmed is shown in *Figure 31.7*.
2. Gently heat the cut edges of the tray with a microtorch or warm instrument (*Fig. 31.8*).
3. Immediately return the tray to the model, and with a wet finger, readapt the edges to the model (*Fig. 31.9*). Readapting with dry fingers could leave fingerprints on the tray material.

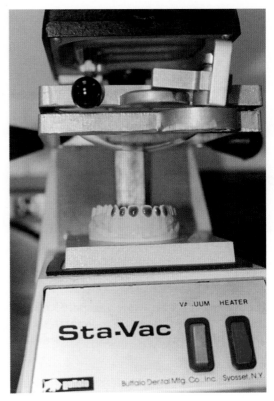

FIGURE 31.6. Stone model with facial reservoirs centered on the vacuum former. Warm resin is sagging below the frame.

4. Keep the tray on the model until it is delivered to the patient. Instruct the patient to keep the tray in the storage box and away from heat. *Figure 31.10* shows a trimmed custom bleaching tray inside its storage box.
5. Assess the tray by using the Skill Performance Evaluation sheet in Appendix 2.

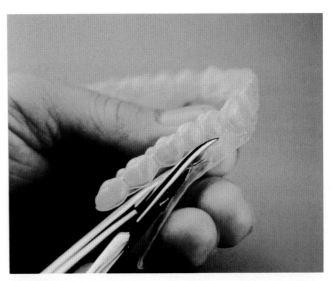

FIGURE 31.7. Trimming of the whitening tray with curved scissors.

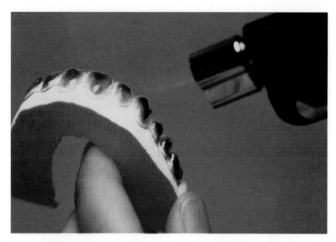

FIGURE 31.8. Edges of the trimmed tray are softened with a microtorch. (Courtesy of Ultradent Products, Inc.)

V. Clinical Procedure for Professionally Applied Power Whitening (Light-/Heat-Activated or Chemically Activated Chairside): Two Appointments

Patient demands for faster methods of whitening have created a need for clinical competence in chairside **power whitening**. Armed with higher percentages of peroxide whiteners enhanced with chemical activators and light/heating equipment, the dental team may now offer those near immediate results. Clinically the patient may be seen only once for the procedure and once for a follow-up evaluation. Now higher concentrations of hydrogen peroxide formulas enhanced with activators are available in power bleaching systems. Activators absorb light, warm the bleaching chemical, and accelerate the chemical reactions. A warmed bleaching agent is more effective. Some agents require no light. Those using lights utilize resin curing lights, violet wavelength lights, gas plasma lights, or LED lights. The following describes the clinical methods for applying those higher percentage (15–35%) hydrogen

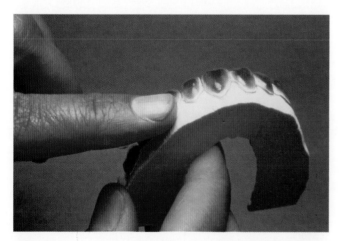

FIGURE 31.9. Warmed edges of the tray being readapted to the model with a wet finger. (Courtesy of Ultradent Products, Inc.)

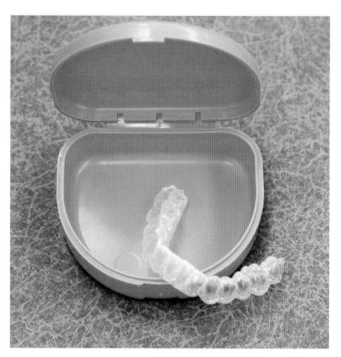

FIGURE 31.10. Custom whitening tray, trimmed, in its storage box.

peroxide whitening agents. Necessary items for this procedure are listed in Table 31.5. A summary of this section's clinical procedures can be found at the end of this chapter.

A. Whitening Appointment

1. Medical History
   Obtain or review a complete medical history from the patient. Carefully evaluate that there are no contraindications such as sensitivity to

---

TABLE 31.5. Armamentarium for Professionally Applied Light-/Heat-Activated Whitening Agents

Forms: medical history, informed consent, clinical exam, and treatment

Prophylaxis instruments

White swabs (optional)

Camera for digital pictures or video

Shade guide or other color-measuring device

Written instructions

Safety glasses for operator and patient

Gauze and cotton rolls

Cheek retractors

Sunscreen and/or vitamin E oil

Paint-on resin dam

Curing light, bleaching light

Hydrogen peroxide bleaching agent with activators

whitening agent, use of photosensitive drugs or herbs, radiation or chemotherapy, history of melanoma, caries, cracked enamel, or root sensitivity, as listed Table 31.2. The dental professional should determine if the patient is overusing whitening procedures. Review the number of times a patient has undergone whitening procedures. Proceed once medical history is cleared.

2. Informed Consent

An informed consent should be read and signed by the patient prior to the procedure. The bleaching consent should briefly describe the treatment, the benefits, and the possible side effects. Postoperative sensitivity should be emphasized more to the patient with power whitening than the other patient-applied products. Informed consent should be kept with the patient's records. A sample consent form is found in *Figure 31.11*.

3. Intraoral Examination

Patient is given a thorough intraoral exam. Soft tissues must be free of lesions or potential areas of irritation. Caries, root sensitivity, cracks, or broken restorations must not be present. Any anterior restorations that are not being replaced would negate the procedure. At this time evaluate the need for whitening. Check for already whitened teeth with chalky appearance. Patients with **body dysmorphic disorder**

(**BDD**), a psychological disorder in which one has the inability to be pleased with their body image, may insist on a procedure that is highly unnecessary.

4. Prophylaxis

Complete a prophylaxis that includes scaling, polishing and flossing to remove plaque, calculus, and stain. Remove all extrinsic stain.

5. White Swabs with Aqueous Cleaning Technology (Power Swabs, Stain-Away LLC, Farmingdale, NY)

Optionally, you may swab the surfaces to be whitened with **white swabs**. The swabs will remove stain and hydrate teeth before the whitening procedure. The swabs contain solvents, surfactants, anionic detergents, chelators, saponifiers, and effervescents. Recent studies have shown less surface damage via the use of the product. Patients report less sensitivity when white swabs are used in the preceding whitening techniques. The reduced sensitivity is thought to be the result of the hydrating capabilities of the swabs. Scientific studies are needed to determine if the swabs' hydration is effective in reducing sensitivity.

6. Intraoral Photograph

Obtain a photograph of both the upper and lower teeth. This front view will show the teeth in the smile line. The photography must include a shade guide tab that is matched to the

---

Informed Consent for Professionally Applied Power Whitening (Light/Heat Activated) Chairside Treatment

The product our dentist/dental hygienist will be applying to your teeth is **Hydrogen Peroxide**＿＿＿＿＿＿(Percentage) with an activator. Your tissues will be isolated and the material will be applied to the tooth surfaces requiring whitening. A light/heat source will be activated to initiate the whitening. A series of three applications of the hydrogen peroxide material with light/heat activation will occur. Immediate whitening results should occur.

The most frequently reported side effects of peroxide tooth whitening are sensitivity and irritation to the gums. Sore throat and nausea may occur if product is accidentally swallowed. In rare cases pulpal necrosis (tooth death) could occur.

Patient Consent: I＿＿＿＿＿＿＿＿＿＿＿＿＿＿＿＿
(Full name), hereby give consent to treatment allowing the dentist/dental hygienist to apply a whitening agent to my teeth. I have been informed of the potential benefits and side effects of the treatment, and affirm that I have read and understand the instructions below.

Signed:＿＿＿＿＿＿＿＿＿＿＿＿＿＿＿＿＿＿＿

Witness:＿＿＿＿＿＿＿＿＿＿＿＿＿＿＿＿＿＿

Date:＿＿＿＿＿＿＿＿＿＿＿＿＿＿＿＿＿＿＿

One Copy for Patient
One Copy for Patient's Record

FIGURE 31.11. Sample of the consent form for power whitening.

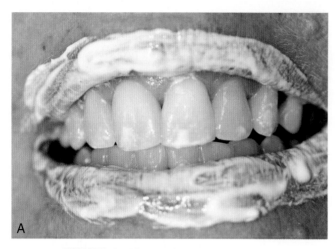 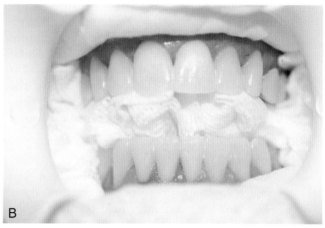

FIGURE 31.12.   **A.** Patient's lips with applied sunscreen. **B.** Isolation of teeth with check retractions, cotton rolls, gauze, and napkin.

tooth shade of the anterior teeth. Tabs may be positioned to the incisal edge of a central incisor (see *Fig. 31.2A*). A spectrophotometer or other color-measuring device could also be used (see *Fig. 31.2B*). The photo will document the initial tooth color for the patient record.

7. Isolate and Condition Patient's Soft Tissue
If lights are used, apply sunscreen to patient's lips and nose if they are possibly in the area to be exposed (see *Fig. 31.12A*). Retract lips and cheeks and isolate tissues with gauze and cotton rolls as in *Figure 31.12B*. No anesthesia should be used as the patient must be able to sense when chemicals or heat is irritating soft tissues or the pulp.

8. Paint-on Resin Dam
Carefully apply **paint-on resin dam** to all exposed gingival tissues in a 1 to 1 ½ mm width at gingival margin. Efforts should be paid to cover all exposed gingiva in the whitening area. Light-cure the material. Reapply to any gingival areas still exposed (see *Fig. 31.13A, B & C*).

9. Protective Eyewear
To avoid exposure to damaging light, both operator and patient must be wearing eyewear. Although splatter does not usually occur, the eyewear can protect from potential splash hazards. Protective eyewear can incorporate a filter specifically for the activation light.

10. Application of Whitening Agent
If necessary, mix whitening agent as per manufacturer's directions. Whitening agent is applied to all facial surfaces that are exposed when the patient smiles. The agent is syringed to the surface and then spread evenly over the tooth as shown in *Figure 31.14*. Brushes or swabs may be used to apply the agent evenly across the tooth surfaces.

11. Light Activation of Whitener
If the whitener requires light activation, activate for 15 to 20 minutes as per manufacturers' recommendation. Frequently, check for patient comfort to avoid chemical or thermal burns. Rinse, evacuate whitener, and reapply whitener. Repeat sequence two more times, totaling three applications and three light activations for the entire procedure. If a curing light is used, the light must be placed individually for 30 seconds for each tooth whitened. Between each application give the patient the chance to rest or opt to discontinue if uncomfortable. The procedure can be repeated at a second power whitening appointment at least 3 days after the first. Follow manufacturer's directions for frequency and time intervals.

12. At the end of the procedure, rinse, evacuate the whitening, and remove the paint-on dam and isolation materials.

13. Second Intraoral Photograph
A second intraoral photograph should be taken at the completion of procedure to document final results. Again, the shade guide should be used to determine whitening effects (*Fig. 31.2A*).

14. Patient Instructions
At this time, patient must be informed of side effects. An instruction sheet should be given to the patient. An example is included in *Figure 31.15*. Patient must realize that tooth sensitivity and gingival irritation could occur. Examine tissue for any gingival irritation. Instruct patient on the use of vitamin E oil for gingival irritation. A nonsteroidal antiinflammatory drug (NSAID) may be recommended for tooth sensitivity. NSAIDs are often recommended prior

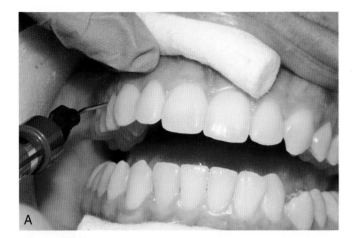

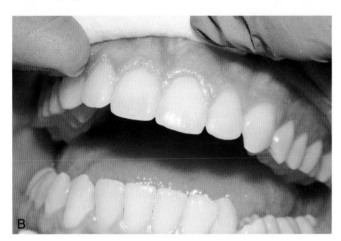

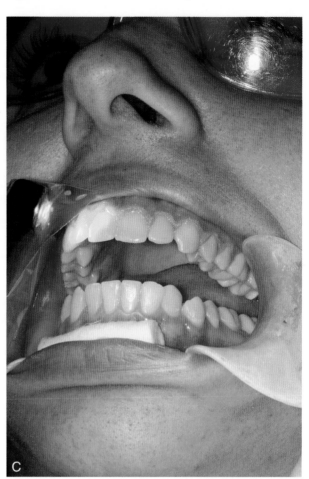

FIGURE 31.13. **A.** Cotton roll isolation and painting resin dam on gingiva. **B.** Resin dam in place. **C.** Light-curing resin dam.

to the procedure. Advise patient to avoid eating colored foods/drinks that may stain the dentition (e.g., tea, coffee, mustard, and red sauces). Smoking should also be avoided. Neutral sodium fluoride gel or potassium nitrate can be used in bleaching trays for 30 minutes twice per day. A sample of these trays is shown in *Figure 31.16*. Additional bleaching enhancement may

take place with the use of nightguard bleaching trays often created prior to the power whitening procedure. Allowing for no sensitivity, the patient may choose to further enhance the whitening by using the trays for a few nights after the power procedure. Any pain lasting more than 24 to 48 hours should be reported immediately to the dental office.

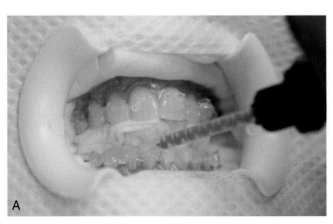

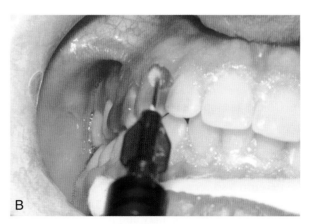

FIGURE 31.14. **A and B.** Applying hydrogen peroxide gel products Tonto facial surfaces.

Instructions for Post Power Whitening

You should see immediate whitening results. If you wish to further enhance the whitening you may use night guard bleaching trays for 2 to 3 days. Follow the manufacture's directions for tray use.

- Brush and floss your teeth in the usual manner.
- Avoid foods that stain such as tea, coffee, mustard, red sauces.
- If tooth sensitivity occurs, use neutral sodium fluoride gel or potassium nitrate in trays twice/day for 30 minutes.
- Prophylactic use of NSAIDS (Ibuprofen, aspirin) may be used for sensitivity.
- Gingival irritations can be treated with Vitamin E oil.
- Night guard whitening may be undertaken to enhance results.
- Whitening maintenance can be achieved with whitening mouthrinses and dentifrices.
- Touch up maintenance can be achieved in the future with night guard whitening trays.

FIGURE 31.15. Patient instructions to be given after power whitening.

15. Documentation

Document the procedure in the patient records. Include medical history, intraoral evaluation, informed consent, photograph, material used, the amount of time light-activated, and the beginning and ending shade guide results.

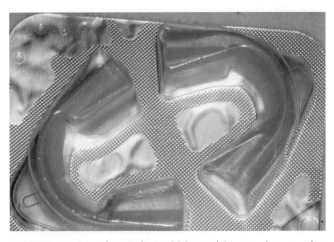

FIGURE 31.16. UltraEZ desensitizing gel in trays for use after power whitening procedure.

B. Evaluation Appointment

Before the evaluation, a telephone call could be made to the patient to confirm patient's comfort with the procedure. The patient may then return within 1 week for a follow-up appointment. At this time, the gingival tissues and the whitening results could be evaluated. Anterior restorations in need of replacement can be scheduled 1 week later allowing for the 2 weeks postwhitening. Any lingering sensitivities should be addressed at this time.

VI. Clinical Procedure for Professionally Applied Whitening Varnish

Philips Zoom QuickPro whitening varnish is a dual-layer whitening varnish product applied in the dental office similar to other power whitening procedures described earlier. Two layers are painted on the teeth to be whitened much like other "power" whitening procedures. The first layer contains peroxide whitener. The second layer protects the first from oral fluids. After 30 minutes, the patient removes the varnish by brushing or wiping off the varnish.

Summary

Clinical Procedures for Patient-Applied Professionally Supervised Whitening

First Appointment
- Obtain a complete medical history for the patient.
- Obtain the patient's signed informed consent after a full explanation.
- Perform a complete oral exam of all hard and soft tissues.
- Perform a scale and polish procedure.
- Obtain intraoral photographs, including a shade guide tab, of the maxillary and mandibular teeth.

- Take impression for model and tray construction.

Second Appointment
- Try the custom tray in the patient's mouth; make any adjustments.
- Provide the patient with instructions for using the tray.
- Provide the patient with written instructions, and schedule a follow-up appointment.

Third Appointment
- Examine the teeth for results; record the hours of treatment and any side effects.

- Provide more whitening if desired. Schedule another appointment.
- Take a posttreatment intraoral photograph, again including a shade guide tab.

Laboratory Procedures

1. Construct a stone model, and then trim it, making the base small and thin.
2. Place blockout resin (and cure) on the desired teeth in the proper location and thickness.
3. Heat the resin material until it sags 1 inch below the frame.
4. Turn on the vacuum, and immediately pull down the frame. Vacuum for 1 minute.
5. Trim any excess vinyl from the model with scissors.
6. Trim the tray again, up to gingival margins.
7. Heat the cut edges of the tray with a microtorch or warm instrument.
8. Replace the tray on the model, and readapt the edges to the model.

Clinical Procedures for Professionally Applied Power Whitening

1. Obtain a complete medical history.
2. Obtain the patient's signed informed consent.
3. Perform a complete intraoral evaluation.
4. Perform an oral prophylaxis.
5. Obtain intraoral photographs with shade guide included.
6. Retraction and isolation of soft tissues.
7. Apply paint-on resin dam.
8. Apply whitening agent.
9. Activate with light for 15 to 20 minutes as per manufacturers' directions.
10. Rinse and evacuate whitening agent.
11. Apply whitening agent for the second time.
12. Activate with light a second time for 15 to 20 minutes.
13. Rinse and evacuate whitening agent.
14. Apply whitening agent for the third time.
15. Activate with light for the third time for 15 to 20 minutes.
16. Rinse and evacuate whitening agent.
17. Remove retractors, isolation gauze, cotton rolls, and paint-on dam.
18. Obtain second intraoral photograph with shade guide.
19. Document procedure in the patient's record.
20. Explain and give written instructions to patient.
21. Reevaluate results at second appointment.

Review Questions

Question 1. **Which of the following is the professionally applied whitening material?**

a. Whitening dentifrice
b. Nightguard whitening agents
c. Power (light-/heat-activated) whitening agent
d. Whitening mouth rinse

Question 2. **Which of the following would be used as a carrier for nightguard tooth whitening agents?**

a. Boil and bite mouth guard
b. Fluoride tray
c. Custom vinyl tray
d. Athletic custom mouth guard

Question 3. **Which of the following helps prevent gingival irritation while nightguard whitening?**

a. Using a scalloped tray
b. Using a small dot of whitening in facial surfaces of tray
c. Using a mouth rinse prior to whitening
d. Both a and b

Question 4. **Why is the intraoral photograph with the shade guide necessary?**

a. To document the initial tooth color
b. To document the final tooth color
c. To document for patient records
d. All of the above

Question 5. **Application of a paint-on resin dam prior to power whitening helps:**

a. Isolate teeth and protect gingival tissue
b. Activate the whitening agent
c. Hydrate the teeth and tissue
d. Nourish the teeth and tissue

Question 6. **Which of the following would be considered a contraindication to tooth whitening?**

a. Severe intrinsic stain
b. Root or dentin sensitivity
c. Body dysmorphic dysfunction
d. All of the above

Debonding Orthodontic Resins

Objectives

After performing the laboratory/clinical exercises, the student will be able to do the following:

1. Explain the rationale for removing composite adhesive resin from the teeth following orthodontic treatment.
2. Discuss the clinical objectives for debonding.
3. Describe the effects of using improper debonding techniques or materials on enamel.
4. Demonstrate each step in the debonding procedure.
5. Self-evaluate the effectiveness of the debonding procedure.
6. Explain three follow-up considerations to be discussed with the newly debonded orthodontic patient.

Key Words/Phrases

debonding

orthodontic brackets

Introduction

Adhesive composite materials are commonly used to attach **orthodontic brackets** to enamel surfaces. These brackets hold the arch wire in place by means of elastics or ligature wires, as illustrated in Figure 13.1. Common orthodontic materials are discussed in Chapter 13, Specialty Materials. The orthodontist generally removes the fixed appliances and the adhesive resin at the end of orthodontic treatment. **Debonding** is the complete removal of composite and cement material from enamel surfaces after these appliances are removed. Generally, the orthodontist performs this procedure. However, if the orthodontic practice employs a dental hygienist, then he or she usually debonds the patient. Patients are normally referred to their general dentist for a complete dental examination, radiographs, and prophylaxis after the debonding appointment. The dental hygienist in the general practice is often the first person to see the patient after the active phase of orthodontic treatment is completed. Occasionally, fine remnants of adhesive resin remain on the facial surfaces of the patient's anterior and premolar teeth where the orthodontic brackets had been attached. The task of eliminating the residual composite material is then the responsibility of the general practice dental hygienist. It is important to completely remove all composite resin material to avoid the following:

- Plaque accumulation
- Stain
- Poor esthetics
- Demineralization and/or caries formation
- Gingival inflammation
- Mucosal response from rough resin

All debonding methods remove some enamel. The dental hygienist must select the least traumatic instruments and methods to accomplish the resin removal.

I. Objective of Debonding

The primary objective of debonding is to return the enamel surface to its natural, pretreatment appearance. A secondary objective is to return the enamel surface to its pretreatment texture or feel.

II. Problems with Improper Debonding Techniques and Materials

A number of hand and rotary instruments as well as a variety of abrasives have been investigated for use in debonding. Most studies indicate that some enamel alteration results from the debonding process. In addition, decalcified enamel surfaces (white spots) are much more likely to exhibit enamel loss than intact enamel. Faster techniques and coarser abrasives cause more damage to the enamel surfaces. Researchers generally agree that diamond burs, green stones, white stones, sandpaper discs, manual or ultrasonic scalers, pliers, and band removers should not be used to remove the composite adhesive resin that remains after bracket removal.

III. Debonding Procedure

Enamel surfaces that are gouged or scratched as a result of improper debonding methods or materials may cause the same problems that would result from leaving remnants of adhesive resin on the tooth. It is critical for the dental hygienist to follow the steps in the debonding procedure in sequential order to provide a smooth enamel surface. The materials needed for debonding are listed in Table 32.1.

A. Identification of the Resin

Identification of the remaining composite adhesive resin is necessary to avoid causing inadvertent damage to the enamel surface during resin removal. The resin that remains immediately after bracket and band removal (*Fig. 32.1*) is easily

TABLE 32.1. Armamentarium for Debonding Orthodontic Adhesive Resin

Mirror

Explorer

Low-speed handpiece

Tapered, plain-cut, tungsten carbide finishing bur

Aluminum oxide composite polishing cups and points

Rubber cup

Wet slurry of fine flour of pumice

Gauze

Disclosing solution

Dappen dish

Cotton-tipped applicator

Prophy angle

Contra angle

Safety glasses (for patient and clinician)

Personal protective equipment

Floss

Air/water syringe tip

Saliva ejector

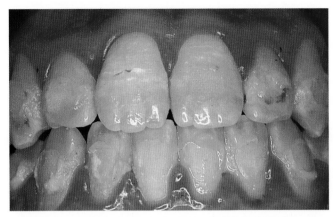

FIGURE 32.1. Facial view of anterior teeth with adhesive resin still remaining after removal of orthodontic brackets. (Reprinted from Gutmann ME. Composite adhesive resin removal following active orthodontic treatment. *J Pract Hyg.* 1996;5(3):16–19, with permission; ©1996, Montage Media Corporation.)

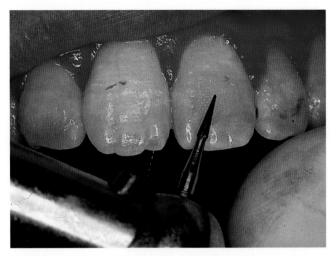

FIGURE 32.2. Use of finishing bur on a low-speed handpiece to remove the bulk of adhesive resin. (Reprinted from Gutmann ME. Composite adhesive resin removal following active orthodontic treatment. *J Pract Hyg.* 1996;5(3):16–19, with permission; ©1996, Montage Media Corporation.)

visible compared to the residual remnants that are frequently seen in general practice settings. The clinician may use one of the following methods to identify the location and amount of remaining resin:

1. Dry the tooth with air to see the resin. The resin appears as a square, opaque substance on the tooth surface.
2. Apply disclosing solution to the tooth with a cotton-tipped applicator. The composite material may stain the same as plaque.
3. Examine the tooth surface with an explorer. Resin will feel rough compared to smooth enamel. Some composite materials may also abrade the metal explorer, leaving a gray line on the surface.
4. Ask the patient to rub his or her tongue over the tooth surface to identify the exact location of the resin.

B. Removal of the Resin Bulk

Removal of the resin bulk requires use of a slow-speed handpiece and a tapered, plain-cut, tungsten carbide finishing bur. A slow-speed handpiece is preferred for better access and control.

Avoid decalcified areas that frequently surround the adhesive resin due to inadequate plaque/biofilm removal by the patient during active orthodontic treatment. Use the bur on the adhesive resin only and avoid the decalcified enamel as much as possible. In cases of significant decalcification, complete removal of bonding material may exacerbate the problem. An alternative procedure is (1) gross removal of bonding material, (2) followed by remineralization via fluoride treatments or other remineralization treatments, and (3) complete resin removal and enamel polishing

after 3 months. This alternative should reduce loss of tooth structure.

1. Use a brush-like stroke in one direction only.
2. Begin at the cervical aspect of the resin, and move to the incisal (*Fig. 32.2*).
3. As the resin is removed with the bur, it will resemble fine white shavings.
4. Rinse the tooth with water frequently, and then dry the surface to evaluate progress and to avoid using the bur on intact enamel. The resin remnant appears opaque and dull next to the glossy enamel surface.
5. The dental hygienist should strive to reach a balance between smoothness of the enamel surface and enamel removal. More enamel is removed as the surfaces become smoother. It is critical to frequently evaluate the tooth surface for remaining resin deposits. When none are visible, you are ready to proceed to the final finishing of the enamel surface.
6. During the procedure, ask the patient for feedback regarding smoothness.
7. A final check with the explorer and disclosing solution will confirm if all the resin has been removed.

C. Final Finishing

When no visible resin remains, the enamel surface is then finished and polished to restore its pretreatment appearance:

1. Use aluminum oxide composite finishing cups and points (Enhance Caulk/Dentsply, Milford, DE) at low speed over the resin-free enamel surface ▪ (*Figs. 32.3 and 32.4*).

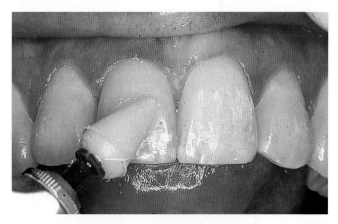

FIGURE 32.3. Aluminum oxide finishing point used to remove any enamel scarring resulting from burs. (Reprinted from Gutmann ME. Composite adhesive resin removal following active orthodontic treatment. *J Pract Hyg.* 1996;5(3):16–19, with permission; ©1996, Montage Media Corporation.)

2. Polish each tooth with a fine pumice slurry and a rubber prophylaxis cup (*Fig. 32.5*).

Tips for the Clinician

- During use of the bur, apply air frequently to dry the tooth and examine the surface; do not keep using the bur unnecessarily.
- Make sure that the patient moves his or her tongue over each tooth surface slowly to detect any residual resin.
- Emphasize the importance of office and home fluoride to remineralize enamel after debonding.

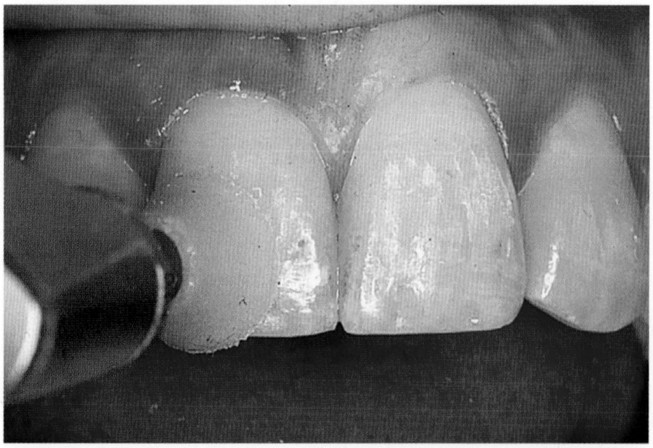

Precautions

- Begin the stroke with the bur at the cervical portion of the resin, and move toward the incisal or occlusal surface to avoid accidental trauma to the gingiva.
- To avoid enamel damage, do not try to remove composite adhesive resin with curets, scalers, diamond burs, high-speed handpieces, sandpaper discs, green stones, white stones, orthodontic pliers and band removers, or ultrasonic instruments.
- Because aerosols are produced during debonding, it is important to wear a face mask.
- During use of the bur, flying particles of resin may cause injury to the eyes, hence safety glasses for the patient and the clinician are essential.
- Composite polishing points, cups, and disks may generate significant heat. Employ these abrasives with caution if using them dry.

D. Evaluation

Use the Skill Performance Evaluation sheet in Appendix 2 to assess the effectiveness of the debonding procedure. Provide the patient with a hand mirror to view the results.

IV. Post-debonding Considerations

As with other dental hygiene care, educating the patient is important and should be included as part of the procedure. Include the following in your instructions:

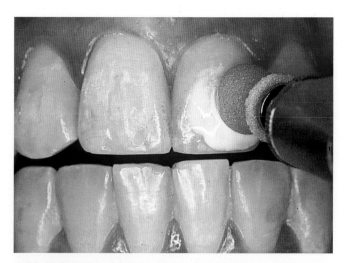

FIGURE 32.4. Aluminum oxide finishing cup used to remove any enamel scarring resulting from burs. (Reprinted from Gutmann ME. Composite adhesive resin removal following active orthodontic treatment. *J Pract Hyg.* 1996;5(3):16–19, with permission; ©1996, Montage Media Corporation.)

FIGURE 32.5. Polishing with fine pumice slurry and rubber cup. (Reprinted from Gutmann ME. Composite adhesive resin removal following active orthodontic treatment. *J Pract Hyg.* 1996;5(3):16–19, with permission; ©1996, Montage Media Corporation.)

A. Recommend a topical fluoride treatment or application of fluoride varnish to replenish the outer most fluoride rich layer of enamel.

B. Reinforce use of a fluoride dentifrice. Recommend use of a fluoride rinse on a daily basis.

C. Consider the use of 5,000 ppm toothpaste or recalcification products such as MI paste.

D. Schedule a maintenance appointment for a complete examination, radiographs, prophylaxis, and other preventive services as indicated by the patient's oral conditions (if the debonding procedure is performed in the orthodontic office). If residual composite material is found during the maintenance appointment in the general practice, it can be removed during that visit.

V. Acknowledgment

The authors thank Dr. Glen Boyles, Clinical Associate Professor of Orthodontics at West Virginia University School of Dentistry, for his review of this chapter.

Summary

1. Use air, an explorer, disclosing solution, and patient feedback to identify the resin.
2. Use a tapered, tungsten carbide finishing bur in a low-speed handpiece.
3. Move the bur from the cervical to the incisal surface of the resin in a light, brush-like stroke.
4. Evaluate resin reduction frequently by rinsing and drying, exploring, disclosing, and asking the patient to evaluate smoothness with his or her tongue.
5. After the resin is removed, polish the enamel with aluminum oxide polishing points.
6. Follow step 5 with aluminum oxide polishing cups.
7. Polish each surface with a fine pumice slurry, using a rubber cup and a slow-speed handpiece.
8. Use intermittent strokes to avoid heat generation.
9. Provide the patient with appropriate self-care instructions.

 ## Review Questions

Question 1. **Which of the following should be used to correctly debond?**

a. Tapered plain-cut finishing bur and a high-speed handpiece
b. Tapered plain-cut finishing bur and a low-speed handpiece
c. Tapered cross-cut finishing bur and a low-speed handpiece
d. Straight fissure, plain-cut bur, and a high-speed handpiece
e. Straight fissure, cross-cut bur, and a low-speed handpiece

Question 2. **All debonding methods remove some enamel. It is the responsibility of the hygienist to select the least traumatic method for resin removal.**

a. The first statement is true; the second statement is false.
b. The first statement is false; the second statement is true.
c. Both statements are true.
d. Both statements are false.

Question 3. **The direction of the stroke of the bur during debonding should be toward the:**

a. Gingival margin
b. Proximal surface
c. Embrasure spaces
d. Incisal or occlusal

Question 4. **It is important to remove all composite resin material during debonding to avoid all of the following *except* one. Which one is the EXCEPTION?**

a. Changes in occlusion
b. Gingival inflammation
c. Stain
d. Plaque accumulation

Question 5. **During the debonding procedure, which of the following should be done to avoid unnecessary use of the bur?**

a. Change to a new bur after the resin is removed on two teeth
b. Apply air frequently and examine the surface
c. Polish with the pumice slurry after 5 seconds of bur use
d. Use a constant circular motion with the bur

Placement of the Periodontal Dressing

Ashlee Sowards, M.S.D.H., T.T.S. and
Cathryn Frere, B.S.D.H., M.S.Ed.

33

Objectives

After performing the laboratory/clinical exercises in this chapter, the student will be able to do the following:

1. Correctly dispense and mix a periodontal dressing.
2. Properly apply the dressing.
3. Differentiate between four types of periodontal dressings.

Key Words/Phrases

hemostasis
periodontal dressing

Introduction

Periodontal dressings are physical barrier that is placed on surgical sites to protect the healing tissues from the forces produced during mastication, thereby providing patient comfort. These dressings also provide some splinting of mobile teeth during healing. After periodontal surgery, they help shape newly forming tissues by maintaining close adaptation of mucosal flaps and gingival grafts to the underlying tissues. Periodontal dressings help prevent postsurgical bleeding by keeping the initial blood clot in place. At present, no periodontal dressings are manufactured that contain therapeutic agents to aid in healing.

I. Purpose

The dental hygienist may be given the responsibility of placing a periodontal dressing when assisting the dentist during surgery, when performing postoperative care, or when a patient returns to the practice with a postsurgical emergency. Necessary items for placing a periodontal dressing are listed in Table 33.1.

II. Dressing Types

A. Zinc Oxide–Eugenol (ZOE) Dressing

Early periodontal dressings were made by mixing zinc oxide with eugenol. These are described in Chapter 7, Dental Cements. Because some patients experience adverse reactions to the eugenol, these dressings are seldom used today.

TABLE 33.1. Armamentarium for Placement of a Periodontal Dressing

Plastic-coated paper mixing pad

Wooden tongue depressor or broad, flexible, stainless steel spatula

Tube of Coe-Pak accelerator

Tube of Coe-Pak base

Petroleum jelly

Plastic instrument

Curet

Gauze squares

Dentoform (for laboratory exercises)

TABLE 33.2. Postoperative Instructions for Patients with a Noneugenol–Zinc Oxide Dressing

1. To prevent disturbance of the dressing while it is setting, avoid the following for 2 hours after the surgery:
   - Smoking, excessive talking, eating warm foodstuffs, or drinking warm beverages
   - Rubbing or applying pressure to the face in the area of surgery
   - Pushing on the dressing with the tongue
2. If a small piece of the dressing crumbles off, simply discard it.
3. If a piece of dressing breaks off, creating a sharp edge or exposing a sensitive area of the surgical site, call the treating dentist.

B. Noneugenol–Zinc Oxide Packs

Coe-Pak (G.C. America, Inc.) is one of the most commonly placed periodontal dressings. Its clinical preparation and application are discussed in this chapter. Compared to the ZOE dressings, this is a more pliable and smoother dressing. However, it must be prepared at the time it is used. Postoperative instructions for patients with a noneugenol–zinc oxide dressing are listed in Table 33.2.

C. Visible Light–Activated Surgical Packs

A urethane dimethacrylate resin-based material (e.g., Barricaid, Dentsply International, Inc.) is available in a syringe carrier for direct placement. There is no mixing of pastes or powder required. The material is activated by a visible light, giving the operator control over manipulation and setting time. On activation, a nonbrittle, protective, tasteless, translucent, elastic covering is formed. This dressing is especially useful in the anterior region, where esthetics are a concern.

D. Cyanoacrylate Dressing

N-Butyl cyanoacrylate is a liquid that polymerizes shortly after contact with the moisture of the oral tissues. An example of this dressing is PeriAcryl (GluStitch, Inc.), which is available in single-dose applicators (*Fig. 33.1*) or multiuse kits with a dispensing tray and applicator pipettes. This clear dressing adheres to the tissues and is hemostatic, bacteriostatic, and biodegradable. It does not need to be removed at a postsurgical follow-up. It is useful for securing the gingival margin after placement of intrasulcular local delivery antimicrobials and as a dressing for postbiopsy sites. Although it has many applications in periodontal surgery, it is not widely used at present.

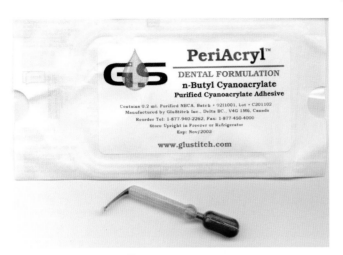

FIGURE 33.1. Single-dose applicator of PeriAcryl (GluStitch, Inc.), a cyanoacrylate dressing.

III. Preparation and Placement of the Noneugenol–Zinc Oxide Pack

A. Dispensing

1. Coe-Pak is supplied as two pastes, which are mixed immediately before placement.
2. The larger tube, containing the base paste, is composed primarily of petrolatum, rosin, and fatty acids.
3. The smaller tube, containing the accelerator, is a mixture of zinc and magnesium oxides and vegetable oils.
4. Equal lengths of base and accelerator are expressed onto the mixing pad, as shown in *Figure 33.2A*. The diameters of the expressed pastes (but not the lengths) will differ, corresponding to the size of the tube orifice. Usually, strips equal in length to the span of the surgical site are adequate to provide coverage.
5. Coe-Pak is also packaged as an automix material similar to impression materials. Simply express the mixed material onto a pad and allow mixed material to develop the proper consistency for use as described below.

B. Mixing

1. Using the center of the mixing pad, mix the base and accelerator with a tongue depressor (*Fig. 33.2B and C*) or metal spatula until the mixture is uniform in color, such as that illustrated in *Figure 33.2D*. Spatulation should take from 30 to 45 seconds. A capsule of tetracycline may be added during mixing to give antimicrobial properties to the dressing.
2. Gather the mixture into a compact mass (*Fig. 33.2E*), and let it rest for 2 to 3 minutes.

3. Lightly lubricate your fingers with petroleum jelly or sterile saline, and test the dressing. When the dressing is no longer tacky but is still soft and pliable, it is ready to be applied.

C. Placement

1. **Hemostasis**, the control of bleeding, should be achieved before a dressing is placed. Blot-dry the surgical site and the teeth in the area with sterile gauze. There should not be excessive bleeding. A dry application site will help with dressing retention.
2. If the surgical site is in the posterior region of the mouth, roll the dressing with lightly lubricated fingers into a rope about the diameter of a pencil. The rolled dressing is shown in *Figure 33.2F*.
3. Starting in the anterior facial area, place the roll on the cervical area of the teeth. Flatten the pack against the involved soft tissues and the cervical third of the teeth. Loop it around the distal of the terminal tooth, and continue covering the involved lingual tissues, pressing the lingual and facial interproximal segments firmly together.
4. If the surgical site is in the anterior portion of the mouth, divide the pack material into two equal portions, and place the strips on the facial and lingual sites.
5. Adapt the interproximal areas with a plastic instrument or the back of a curet, as shown in *Figure 33.3A*. These interproximal projections create mechanical retention for the dressing. The dressing should be only thick enough to give strength to the material and should cover only the surgical wound.
6. To help with retention in areas with open embrasures, small pieces of the dressing material can be shaped to wedge into the interproximal spaces before the dressing is applied.
7. When the surgical site includes a small edentulous area, the dressing is continued over that space, with the facial and lingual portions joining at the alveolar crest.
8. To aid in retention, include at least four or five teeth in the dressed area.
9. The final placement is shown in *Figure 33.3B*. The dressing should be only 2 to 3 mm in thickness at the area of greatest depth and only 8 to 10 mm in total width.
10. Working time for Coe-Pak dressing is 10 to 15 minutes for the regular set and 5 to 8 minutes for the fast set.
11. Assess placement of periodontal dressings by using the Skill Performance Evaluation sheet in Appendix 2.

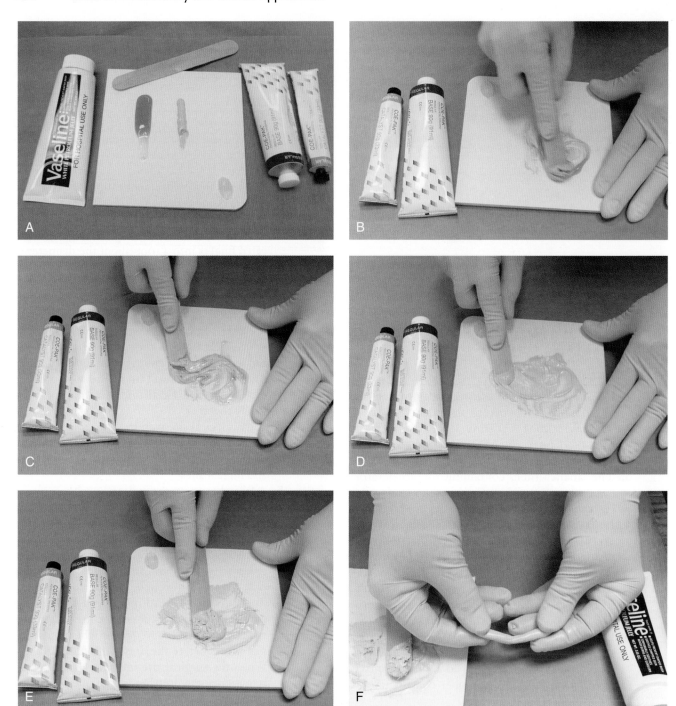

FIGURE 33.2. Mixing and placement of the periodontal dressing. **A.** Equal lengths of base and accelerator are dispensed on the mixing pad. **B–D.** The base and accelerator are mixed on the mixing pad until uniform in color. **E.** The mixture is gathered into a compact mass. **F.** When the dressing is no longer tacky, it is rolled into a "rope."

IV. Characteristics of a Well-Placed Dressing

A. The dressing should be nonmobile and rigid. A pack that moves is irritating to the tissues and may cause prolonged bleeding.

B. The pack should not extend coronally beyond the cervical third of the teeth. There should be no occlusal contact with the pack during mastication.

C. The wound should be covered without unnecessary overextension. The dressing should not extend more than 2 mm apical to the surgical site.

D. Dressing material should not extend into the vestibule or impinge on frenum attachments. Trim excess material that interferes with muscle movement.

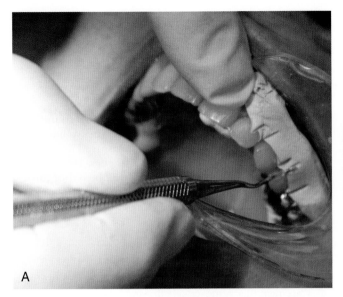
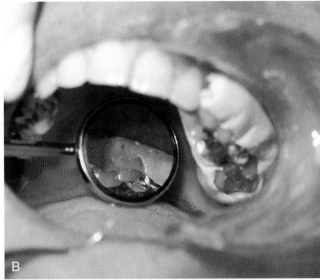

FIGURE 33.3. **A.** The dressing is pressed onto the surgical site and necks of the teeth. The dressing is pressed into the interproximal areas with the back of a curet or plastic instrument to create mechanical retention. **B.** Final placement. The dressing is removed from occlusal surfaces.

E. There should be as little bulk as necessary to give rigidity.

F. The surface should be smooth and edges tapered to provide patient comfort and to discourage plaque retention.

Tips for the Clinician

- Keep gloves moistened to prevent the dressing from adhering to your fingers.
- Retract the tissues in the area of the dressing to check for interference with muscle attachments.
- Have the patient try retraction, protraction, and lateral movements to check for occlusal interference.

Precautions

- Avoid using cyanoacrylate dressings for patients reporting sensitivity to cyanoacrylate and formaldehyde.
- Both the clinician and the patient should wear eye protection when the cyanoacrylate dressing is used, to prevent adhesion of the ocular tissues.
- Avoid placement of the Coe-Pak in patients with known allergies to pine tar products and peanuts.

Summary

1. Dispense equal lengths of base and accelerator onto a mixing pad.
2. Mix for 30 to 45 seconds to achieve a uniform color.
3. Gather the mixture into a compact mass, and let it rest until the dressing is no longer tacky.
4. Dry the surgical site and teeth in the area with sterile gauze.
5. Roll the dressing into a "rope" about the diameter of a pencil and equal in length to the span of the surgical site.
6. Starting at the anterior facial area of the surgical site, flatten the pack against the involved soft tissues and the cervical third of the teeth. Include at least four or five teeth in the dressing.
7. Apply the dressing to the lingual surface of the surgical site, pressing the lingual and facial interproximal segments together.
8. Adapt the interproximal areas with a smooth instrument surface to create retention.
9. Trim any excess dressing away from muscle attachments and occlusal surfaces, and smooth the edges.

Review Questions

Question 1. Which of the following would be a purpose for using the noneugenol–mineral oxide surgical dressing?

a. To decrease healing time
b. To stop postsurgical bleeding
c. To help hold the healing tissues in place
d. To keep bacteria away from the healing tissues

Question 2. The noneugenol–zinc oxide dressing is held in place by:

a. Physical retention
b. Adhesion to the tissues
c. Sutures

Question 3. The finished noneugenol–zinc oxide dressing placed after flap surgery should be:

a. Extended to the occlusal surface
b. Extended to the depth of the vestibule
c. Extended to fill interdental space
d. Rigid with tapered edges

Question 4. A patient is in the office to have a round 5-mm growth excised from the attached gingiva between the maxillary left lateral and central incisors. The patient is concerned about the subsequent esthetics. He is a consultant with many companies and will be out of town with work for the next 2 months. Which of the following would be the best choice of surgical site care for this patient?

a. Recommending warm saltwater rinses three times a day
b. Placement of a noneugenol–zinc oxide surgical dressing
c. Placement of a visible light–activated surgical dressing
d. Placement of a cyanoacrylate dressing

Question 5. All of the following statements regarding the noneugenol–zinc oxide dressing would be included in postsurgical instructions following periodontal flap surgery except one. Which one is the EXCEPTION?

a. Do not consume warm foodstuffs for 2 hours following surgery
b. If a piece of the dressing breaks off increasing postoperative discomfort, return to the office immediately for emergency care
c. If a small piece of dressing crumbles off, simply discard it
d. Do not smoke for 2 hours following the surgery

Removal of the Periodontal Dressing and Sutures

34

Objectives

After performing the laboratory/clinical exercises in this chapter, the student will be able to do the following:

1. Remove a surgical dressing without damage to the oral tissues.
2. Debride both hard and soft tissues after dressing removal.
3. Remove all placed sutures without contamination of or damage to the tissues.
4. List the information recorded in the patient's chart when removing a dressing or sutures.
5. Identify and name common suture patterns used in dentistry, and give an example of their application.
6. Describe the classification of suture materials.

Key Words/Phrases

absorbable sutures

chromic gut

continuous suture

interrupted sutures

nonabsorbable sutures

surgical gut

suture abscess

sutures

swaged

Introduction

Following periodontal surgery, the patient is frequently scheduled with the dental hygienist for a "post-op" appointment. Collagen deposition and primitive epithelium have usually repaired a surgical site by the end of the first postsurgical week. This provides enough strength to the wound to allow for dressing and suture removal. Therefore, the patient returns for a follow-up evaluation 7 to 10 days after the surgery. If the dressing has not been lost, the hygienist will remove the periodontal pack followed by suture removal and documentation of the healing state.

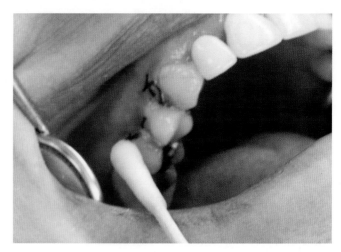

FIGURE 34.1. Teeth and tissues are swabbed with a disinfectant.

I. Removal of the Periodontal Dressing

A. A sturdy, blunt instrument, such as a surgical hoe, plastic instrument, or curet, is inserted under the edge of the dressing with a smooth surface against the tissue. Gentle lateral pressure is applied, and the pack is carefully loosened. Sutures that may have become incorporated into the dressing material must be detected and cut before each piece of pack can be removed. Remove the dressing pieces with forceps, being careful not to scratch the sensitive tissues. Suture removal is discussed later in this chapter, and the necessary items for removal of the periodontal dressing are listed in Table 34.1.

B. After the dressing has been removed, the teeth and tissues are swabbed gently with diluted disinfectant mouthwash or hydrogen peroxide on a cotton-tipped applicator to loosen food and bacterial debris, as shown in *Figure 34.1*. The area is

then rinsed with warm water. This may need to be repeated to debride the area.

C. Inspect the surgical site for approximation of incision edges and absence of drainage, inflammation, and edema. The healing state is evaluated and noted in the patient's chart. The tissues that had been surgically manipulated should be epithelialized (covered with epithelium); however, the epithelium will be friable at this early stage of healing. These tissues may appear redder than the surrounding tissues due to the greater vascularity and lesser degree of keratinization. Red, head-like projections of granulation tissue are an indication of residual calculus. If healing is delayed and the tissues are sensitive, another periodontal dressing may be placed for a 2nd week.

D. Residual dressing material and any visible calculus are removed, taking care not to disturb the fragile epithelium.

E. Assess periodontal pack removal by using the Skill Performance Evaluation sheet in Appendix 2.

TABLE 34.1. Armamentarium for Removal of the Periodontal Dressing and Sutures

Gauze squares

Cotton-tipped applicators

1:1 dilution of chlorhexidine gluconate mouthwash or hydrogen peroxide

Cotton pliers

Scaling instruments

Suture scissors or Dean scissors

Orange solvent (for laboratory exercises)

Skinless chicken breast with interrupted sutures (for laboratory exercises)

II. Suture Removal

Sutures are stitches that are used to control bleeding and to hold body tissues in a desired position until healing has progressed to the point at which sutures are no longer needed. This healing normally takes place in 5 to 7 days for oral tissues. Removal of the sutures is usually performed at the 7- to 10-day postsurgical follow-up visit. All sutures that are not removed at this time act as a foreign body and promote inflammation to varying degrees. An infection at the sight of a suture is called a **suture abscess** or a **stitch abscess**.

A. Classifications of Suture Materials

Suture materials are discussed in Chapter 13. A typical suture package is shown in *Figure 34.2A*.

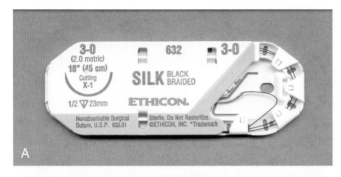

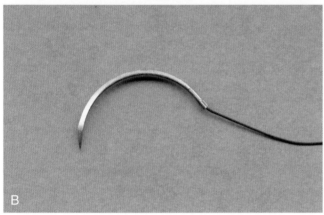

FIGURE 34.2. **A.** Silk suture material. **B.** Swaged suture needle.

Tips for Periodontal Dressing Removal (Laboratory Exercise)

- If the dressing is placed on a Dentoform for a laboratory exercise, prompt removal of the pack will facilitate cleaning of the Dentoform.
- Large pieces of retained material can be removed with a scaling instrument.
- The last traces of pack on the Dentoform can then be dissolved with orange solvent on a gauze square.

Precautions—Periodontal Dressing Removal

- Remove the surgical dressing with controlled force, checking for and cutting imbedded sutures.
- Loosened pieces of dressing are best removed with forceps to prevent scratching of the primitive epithelium.

1. Suture materials can be monofilaments (one strand of material) or multifilaments (multiple threads twisted or braided together in a strand). Greater capillary action, or "wicking effect," is created by the multifilaments, which draw more bacteria into the tissues and create a greater inflammatory reaction than the monofilaments. Multifilament sutures are often coated and can elicit less tissue response. Sutures may also be dyed to make them easier to see.

2. Suture materials can be natural or synthetic. Natural suture materials elicit a strong inflammatory response because of the presence of foreign proteins.

3. Suture materials can be divided into two broad categories: absorbable and nonabsorbable. Absorbable sutures are broken down and absorbed by the body. They may not need to be removed at a following appointment. Those that have not been completely absorbed before the postsurgical evaluation visit are usually removed for patient comfort. A follow-up appointment is necessary to remove nonabsorbable sutures.

4. Absorbable Sutures
   a. Natural **absorbable sutures** are absorbed by the process of phagocytosis and enzymatic resorption. Some synthetic materials are resorbed by hydrolysis, causing less inflammatory response.
      i. **Surgical gut** or "gut" is a monofilament made from the connective tissue of sheep or cattle intestinal mucosa.
      ii. **Chromic gut** is surgical gut that has been treated with chromic salts to inhibit enzymatic resorption. These sutures stay in place for 14 days or longer.
   b. Synthetic, biodegradable sutures are commonly being used in dentistry today. These may be braided polymer fibers of polylactic acid or polyglycolic acid. Monofilaments of other polymers having more flexibility are also available.

5. Nonabsorbable Sutures
   Nonabsorbable sutures can also be of natural or man-made materials. These materials will not be absorbed by the body; they must be removed at the postsurgical visit.
   a. Silk sutures are braided fibers of protein excreted by the silkworm. Although made of a natural, biodegradable protein, the absorption of silk progresses much more slowly than does the healing process. Therefore, silk sutures are classified as nonabsorbable because they must be removed.
   b. Synthetic, nonabsorbable sutures may be made of polypropylene, polyester, nylon, or Gore-Tex. Gore-Tex is made of polytetrafluoroethylene; the same polymer used for Teflon.

6. In the United States, sutures are sized according to diameter and are labeled numerically. As the number of zeros increases, the diameter decreases. For example, a "000" suture is larger in diameter than a "0000" suture. The "000" suture can also be expressed as "3-0" suture and is pronounced as "three ought" or "three zero." The suture sizes used most commonly in dentistry are 3-0 to 5-0.

7. The European system of sizing simply states the metric diameter of the suture.

8. The suture material can be supplied separate from the suture needles, or it can be manufactured attached to the needle, creating a continuous unit of suture and needle. The latter option is termed **swaged**. A swaged needle with silk suture material is shown in *Figure 34.2B.*

B. Suturing Techniques

1. Sutures that are placed in such a way that each stitch is tied and knotted separately are termed **interrupted sutures**. Examples are the single interrupted suture (*Fig. 34.3A*) and the mattress interrupted suture (*Fig. 34.3B*).

2. The uninterrupted or **continuous suture** is a series of stitches made with one thread, and it is tied at the beginning and at the end of the run. Examples of continuous sutures are the continuous blanket (*Fig. 34.3C*) and the simple continuous suture (*Fig. 34.3D*).

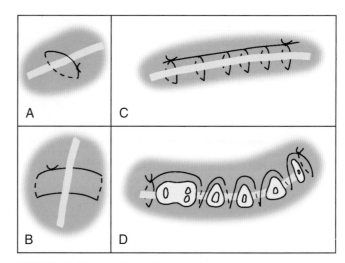

FIGURE 34.3. **A.** Single interrupted suture. **B.** Mattress interrupted suture. **C.** Continuous blanket suture. **D.** Simple continuous suture. The *wide gray lines* represent the incision. The *solid line* represents the suture above the tissues. The *dashed lines* represent the suture below the tissues.

Precautions–Suture Removal

- Use an intraoral or an extraoral rest when cutting sutures.
- Identify the placement pattern that was used when removing sutures, taking care not to leave residual material submerged in the tissues.

Tips for the Clinician–Suture Removal

- Identify the number of sutures to be removed by checking the patient's chart for the number of sutures that were placed.
- A topical anesthetic can be used to provide patient comfort during suture removal.
- If scissors cannot get under the loop, a # 11 scalpel blade may be used.
- When using a chicken breast for the laboratory simulation exercise, keep the sutures moist so that they will better imitate the oral cavity and facilitate removal.

C. Procedure for Removing the Single Interrupted Suture

The single interrupted suture is the most versatile suture. It can be used in most flap and graft surgeries.

1. The periodontal dressing is removed, and the surgical area is cleaned as discussed earlier in the chapter (*Fig. 34.1*).

2. Holding the forceps in the nondominant hand, the suture knot is grasped with the forceps, taking care not to pinch the tissues.

3. The knot is lifted away from the tissues, to create an opening to insert a scissors blade. This also exposes a portion of previously submerged suture material. Suture material that has been beneath the surface is considered to be free of bacteria.

4. With the dominant hand, insert one cutting tip of the suture scissors into the opening of the suture loop (*Fig. 34.4A*). Dean scissors are also commonly used for suture removal. Maintaining an intraoral or extraoral rest will provide stability and control of the hand holding the scissors.

5. In the section of suture material that was previously submerged, snip only one thread close to the tissue. Cutting both "ends" of the suture may result in suture material being left in the tissues

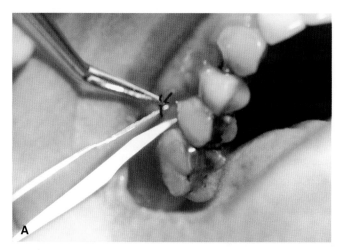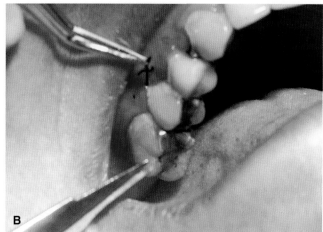

FIGURE 34.4. Suture removal. **A.** The suture knot is gently pulled away from the tissues, and the scissors tip is inserted into the suture loop. **B.** One thread is cut, and the suture is pulled out in one piece.

and, possibly, causing a suture abscess. Take care not to cut the soft tissues. If scissors are used with blades that are curved, the blade is inserted in the loop with the tip curved away from the tissues.

6. In a continuous, smooth action, pull the suture out in one piece (*Fig. 34.4B*), and place the suture on a gauze square.

7. Do not pass the knot (ouch) or suture material, previously exposed in the oral cavity, through the tissue. The knot or suture material will contaminate subepithelial tissues with bacteria.

8. Continue removing all visible sutures and placing them on the gauze square. Bleeding of the suture sites can be controlled by gauze applied with moderate pressure.

9. When finished, count the removed sutures. This count should equal the number of sutures that were placed and recorded in the patient's chart during the surgical appointment. Record the number of sutures removed in the chart.

10. Assess suture removal by using the Skill Performance Evaluation sheet in Appendix 2.

Summary

Periodontal Dressing Removal

1. A sturdy, blunt instrument is inserted under the edge of the dressing.
2. Gentle, lateral pressure is carefully applied to loosen the pack.
3. Check for and cut the sutures that have become incorporated into the dressing.
4. Remove dressing pieces with forceps.
5. Swab teeth and tissues with a disinfectant mouthwash and rinse.
6. Evaluate and record the healing state of the tissues.
7. Scale residual dressing material and residual calculus.

Suture Removal

1. The suture knot is grasped with forceps (held in the nondominant hand) and lifted.
2. Insert one blade of the scissors (held in the dominant hand) into the opening of the suture loop, and cut the suture in the section that was previously submerged.
3. Pull the suture out in a continuous, smooth action.
4. Count the number of removed sutures, and record this in the patient's chart.

Review Questions

Question 1. Which of the following methods is the best way to loosen and remove a periodontal dressing?

a. A rigid curet with slow, controlled movement

b. A sickle scaler with slow, controlled movement

c. A periodontal probe with quick lateral movement

d. A surgical hoe with quick lateral movement

Question 2. Seventy-eight-year-old Mrs. Wilson has come to the dental office as an emergency appointment with discomfort in a recent surgical site. Two weeks previously, she was in for a postsurgical appointment at which the dressing and sutures were removed. Reviewing the chart, you notice that Mrs. Wilson is a controlled diabetic and has hypertension controlled with medication. She had reported that a portion of the pack had been lost a few days after placement. Eight sutures were placed; however, only seven sutures were able to be found and were removed. Clinically, you find a localized red and edematous area distal to the maxillary second molar. Pus exudes from the area when pressure is applied. What is most likely the cause of the inflamed area?

a. She is healing poorly due to her age

b. She is healing poorly due to her diabetes

c. There is a retained suture

d. There is retained calculus in the area

Question 3. All of the following are procedures that correctly follow removal of the periodontal dressing except one. Which one is the EXCEPTION?

a. The area is swabbed with a disinfectant and rinsed to remove food and bacterial debris

b. The tissues are checked for the healing response and noted in the chart

c. Residual pieces of dressing in and around the tissues are removed

d. Areas of residual calculus are charted for removal at the next scale and polish appointment

Question 4. To remove a single interrupted suture, the suture knot is grasped with forceps and gently lifted away from the tissues before being cut for all of the following reasons except one. Which one is the EXCEPTION?

a. To create an opening in which to insert the scissors blade

b. To keep the introduction of bacteria into the tissues to a minimum

c. To allow the clinician to cut the knot away from the rest of the suture material

d. To prevent passing the knot through the tissues

Question 5. You are preparing a surgical tray for the dentist who has asked for "four-ought" or smaller size nonabsorbable suture material. You find the following suture materials in the supply cabinet. Which one do you choose?

a. 00000 chromic gut

b. 000 polylactic acid

c. 5-0 silk

d. 3-0 polytetrafluoroethylene

Temporary Crowns

35

Objectives

After performing the laboratory/clinical exercises in this chapter, the student will be able to do the following:

1. List at least three reasons for placing a temporary crown.
2. Describe the materials used to construct temporary crowns.
3. Describe a method to make a temporary crown with acrylic resin.

Key Words/Phrases

preformed shell crown

provisional

supererupt

temporary crowns

Introduction

A crown is a restoration that provides complete coverage of the coronal portion of a tooth. It may be composed of a variety of materials. Steps in the construction of a crown are shown in Figure 1.10. After diagnosis and treatment planning, the tooth is prepared. A temporary crown is made and then "worn" between the preparation appointment and the cementation appointment. **Temporary crowns** are made for patient comfort and esthetics. The temporary crown will protect the pulp from temperature extremes and other irritants. Temporary crowns are cemented with temporary cement and are removed when the permanent crown is ready to be placed. Temporary restorations are also used while making other indirect restorations, such as an inlay or bridge. The terms "interim" and "**provisional**" are replacing the term "temporary" in some dental circles; however, they basically mean the same thing. Necessary items for constructing a temporary crown are listed in Table 35.1.

I. Methods

A. Aspects to Consider

Three aspects must be considered when making a temporary crown (*Fig. 35.1*).

1. The outer surface of the crown should reproduce the anatomy of the tooth that is being restored. The shape of the crown includes occlusal contacts, proximal contacts, and side contours. The occlusal contacts must not be heavy (high), or the tooth will become sore from excessive biting forces. However, if the temporary crown has no occlusal contact, the tooth may drift occlusally or "**supererupt.**" Supereruption of the tooth will require excess occlusal adjustment of the permanent crown. Proximal contacts (*dark arrows* in *Fig. 35.1*) are also important. If the proximal contacts are too tight, the excessive force may push (orthodontically move) the adjacent teeth in a mesial or distal direction. The permanent crown will not have good contact, and food will impact between the teeth, causing periodontal problems. If the interproximal contacts of the temporary crown are open, food will again impact and cause periodontal problems. Proper interproximal contacts and side contours will facilitate periodontal health.

2. The inner surface of the temporary crown must closely follow the shape of the prepared tooth for retention. As with a permanent crown, the preparation should be covered by the temporary crown to prevent postoperative sensitivity. The margins

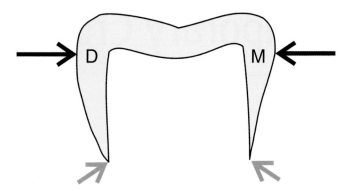

FIGURE 35.1. Cross section of a crown. *Dark arrows* point toward the mesial (*M*) and distal (*D*) contacts. *Light arrows* point toward the margins.

of the temporary crown (*light arrows* in *Fig. 35.1*) should be smooth and properly contoured to promote periodontal health and esthetics.

3. The temporary crown material must be thick enough and strong enough to withstand occlusal forces for several weeks.

B. Temporary Crown Surfaces

The outer surface of a temporary crown can be made in several ways. It is either part of a **preformed shell crown**, as shown in *Figure 35.2*, or it is constructed with use of a "mold" (negative shape). The mold can be made in the mouth before the tooth is prepared, or it can be made on a cast. The inner surface of the temporary crown conforms to the preparation because the temporary crown is typically made in the mouth, directly on the prepared tooth. Chemically activated acrylic resins were the most popular material for the construction of temporary crowns but have been replaced by resin systems called "bis-acryl" materials (see *Fig. 35.3A*). Bis-acryl materials can be described as having a chemical structure that is intermediate between that of acrylic resin and those of dental composite

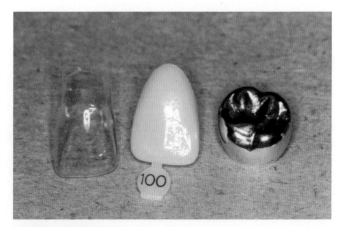

FIGURE 35.2. Types of preformed crowns, a celluloid crown form (*left*), a polycarbonate shell crown (*middle*), and an aluminum shell crown (*right*).

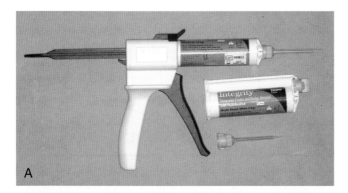

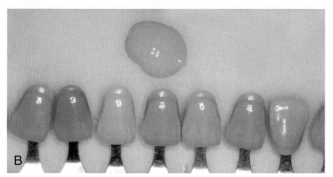

FIGURE 35.3. A. A bis-acryl resin automix product. **B.** A sample of shade A3 material next to a shade guide.

materials. They often contain some filler. Both acrylic resin and bis-acryl resins are available in a variety of shades (see *Fig. 35.3B*).

C. Techniques

The various techniques for construction of a temporary crown use a variety of materials and products. Each patient is unique, and he or she presents specific challenges to the dentist. Each clinician also has favorite materials and techniques, several of which are presented in this chapter.

One popular technique uses a disposable triple tray impression (Fig. 8.5B). The impression is taken before preparing the tooth. After preparing the tooth, the impression of the unprepared tooth of interest is filled with the temporary material in a doughy state. The impression is replaced in the patient's mouth. The patient closes into the normal bite, seating the impression (the form for the temporary crown) into place. The material sets. The patient opens, and the impression is removed. The temporary crown is removed from the impression or tooth and trimmed. Because the form is precisely seated by the opposing arch, the occlusion of the temporary crown is nearly perfect.

II. Preformed Temporary Crowns

Preformed crowns are shown in *Figure 35.2*. The preformed crown becomes the outer surface of the temporary crown.

Tips for the Clinician

- Mix the acrylic material, and wait for the doughy stage before seating the material on the prepared tooth. If the material is too runny, it will flow excessively.
- Remove and replace the temporary crown several times during the setting process to prevent the material from becoming locked in the interproximal undercuts.

Precautions

- Methyl methacrylate is irritating to the skin. Coat your hands with petroleum jelly.
- Methyl methacrylate is highly flammable. Do not use this material around a flame.

A. Use

1. Some preformed crowns can be directly luted with a "stronger" temporary cement, such as reinforced zinc oxide–eugenol (ZOE). The cement forms the inner surface.

2. Alternatively, the preformed crown can be first lined with a chemically activated polymer system. First, the resin system is mixed and placed inside the preformed crown. Next, the filled crown form is seated on the prepared tooth. The resin lining sets and forms the inner surface of the temporary crown. The lined crown is trimmed and then luted with temporary cement.

B. Preformed Crown Materials

1. Polycarbonate Crowns
   Polycarbonate crowns are supplied as maxillary and mandibular incisors, canines, and premolars. Each crown comes in a variety of widths, but only one shade is usually available. They are usually lined with acrylic resin, which will bond to the polycarbonate material. If polycarboxylate crowns are not lined with a resin, the color of the cement may show through.

2. Metal Shell Crowns
   At one time, aluminum shell crowns were popular, but other soft metals, such as tin, have now replaced aluminum. Soft metal shell crowns are similar in shape, but are much easier to adapt than stainless steel crowns. Stainless steel crowns are discussed in Specialty Materials. Metal shell crowns are typically used for molars

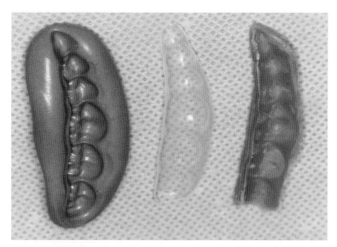

FIGURE 35.4. Molds (negative shapes) made of impression putty (*left*), a thermoplastic resin (*middle*), and wax (*right*).

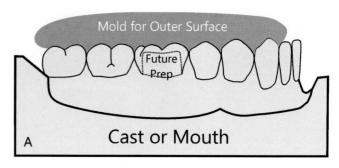

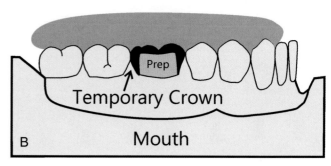

FIGURE 35.5. Section views of **A.** A mold made before the tooth is prepared. **B.** Tooth after preparation using the mold to construct the temporary crown. (*Black area* represents the original shape of the tooth's crown before preparation.)

and premolars because these crowns are not considered to be esthetic. Typically, they are lined with a polymer material before cementing. At times, however, they are not lined and are cemented with a thick mix of reinforced ZOE.

III. Constructed Temporary Crowns

    A. The "constructed" temporary crown is made in the mouth on the prepared tooth by using a mold to form the outer surface. The mold can be made on a cast or in the mouth before the tooth is prepared. The mold should have an "ideal" shape.

    B. The mold may be made from wax, elastic impression material, or a thermoplastic polymer, as shown in *Figure 35.4*. The material must first be soft so that it can be adapted to the "ideal" form. The material then sets or cools and becomes semisolid, forming a negative of the ideally shaped tooth, as shown in *Figure 35.5A*. When the temporary crown is made, the mold forms the outer surface.

    C. Next, a resin system is mixed and placed in the mold. The mold is seated in the mouth over the prepared tooth, matching the positive surfaces of adjacent unprepared teeth with the negative surfaces of the mold, as illustrated in *Figure 35.5B*. The material then sets. The mold is removed, and the set material is removed. Excess set material is trimmed to form the temporary crown.

IV. Celluloid Crown Forms

A clear, thin, preformed celluloid crown, as shown on the left in *Figure 35.2*, can be used as a mold. The mold is filled with acrylic or other resin material, as done with other types of molds. Celluloid is not affected by, and does not bond to, acrylic materials. Celluloid is thermoplastic;

it can be warmed and stretched to enlarge the opening. Celluloid crown forms can be made smaller by cutting a slit, overlapping the edges, and then joining the overlap with a drop of acetone. They are filled with an acrylic material, as previously discussed. The thin celluloid material is stripped off (removed) before trimming and cementing of the temporary crown.

V. Laboratory-Constructed Temporary Crowns

A dental laboratory may make a temporary crown or bridge for a complex case. Casts of the teeth to be restored are sent to the lab. The teeth on the cast are minimally prepared at the lab, and a temporary "shell" crown is made. In the mouth, after the teeth are prepared, the temporary shell crown is lined with acrylic resin. The crown is trimmed and cemented as done with other techniques.

VI. Constructing a Temporary Crown

A temporary crown can be constructed on a Dentoform by using a "vacuum-formed" mold and chemically activated acrylic resin. Necessary items are listed in Table 35.1. Both an unprepared and a prepared tooth for the Dentoform are used. Techniques for taking an alginate impression, pouring and trimming the model, and use of the vacuum former are presented in other chapters.

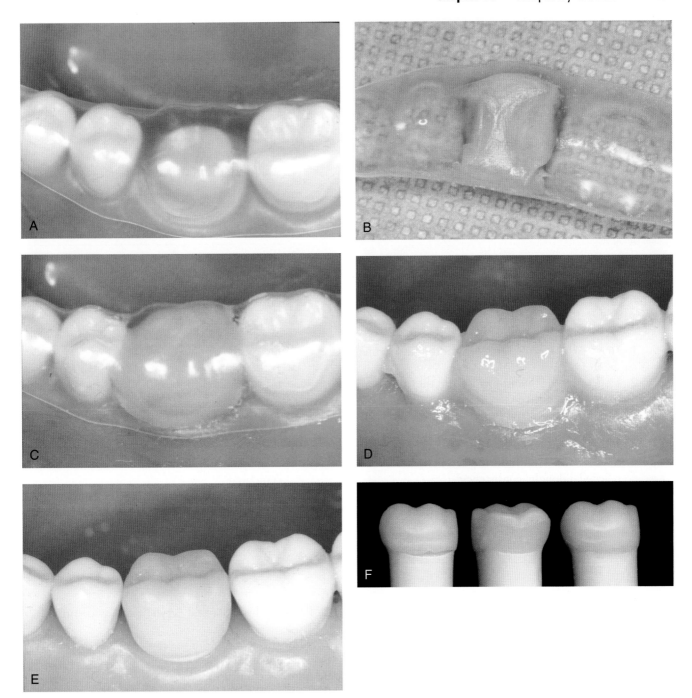

FIGURE 35.6. Steps in the construction of a temporary crown. **A.** Vacuum-formed mold on the Dentoform with crown prep in place. **B.** Vacuum-formed mold filled with freshly mixed acrylic resin in the area of the prepared tooth. **C.** Mold and acrylic resin seated on the prepared tooth. **D.** Vacuum-formed mold removed, leaving the acrylic resin on the prepared tooth. **E.** The trimmed and polished temporary crown. **F.** Margins of a temporary crown (from *left* to *right*): open buccal margin, acceptable lingual margin, and the same buccal margin now repaired.

A. Making the Thermoplastic Vacuum-Formed Mold

1. Make a cast of the Dentoform, using the original, unprepared tooth.
2. Heat the plastic sheet, and apply it to the cast as presented in Chapter 31, Vital Tooth Whitening: Patient–Applied, Professionally Supervised Clinical and Laboratory Procedures.

While the plastic is still hot, use an instrument such as a wax spatula to force the plastic into the four interproximal areas of the tooth of interest.

3. Trim the mold to include several teeth mesial and distal to the tooth of interest. Trim to the gingival margin of the crown of interest. A vacuum-formed mold on the Dentoform is shown in *Figure 35.6A*.

TABLE 35.1. Armamentarium for Constructing a Temporary Crown

Dentoform with a prepared tooth (a cast may be substituted)

Cast of the Dentoform with an unprepared tooth

Vacuum-formed material (0.02 inch in thickness)

Scissors

Wax spatula

Sharp knife or scalpel

Petroleum jelly

Acrylic powder and liquid

Lab handpiece

Pumice, miscellaneous discs, stones, and polishing devices

Articulating paper (optional)

B. Constructing the Temporary Crown

1. Insert the "crown prep" tooth into your Dentoform.
2. Lubricate the Dentoform with the prepared tooth (including the teeth) with petroleum jelly.
3. Mix the powder and liquid of the acrylic resin system to a thick consistency.
4. Fill the mold in the area of the prepared tooth (*Fig. 35.6B*). Wait until the acrylic material has reached a doughy consistency.
5. Seat the material on the prepared tooth on the Dentoform (*Fig. 35.6C*). The material may ooze over the gingiva, but do not try to remove it at this time.
6. Allow the material to set to a semirigid state. Remove the vacuum-formed mold and acrylic material from the Dentoform (*Fig. 35.6D*).
7. Trim any gross excess with scissors. Trim any excess in the interproximal areas with a sharp-bladed instrument or the curved scissors. Reseat the temporary crown on the Dentoform, and wait until the acrylic resin has become hard and rigid.

C. Trimming Excess Flash with a Handpiece, Burs, and Discs

1. Trim any excess flash, creating proper interproximal contacts (*Fig. 35.6E*).
2. Trim any excess flash at the margins. The temporary crown should end at the margin of the preparation. The contour of the crown at the margin should be in line with that of the remaining tooth structure.
3. If the temporary crown has a short margin, add more material to "repair" the temporary crown (*Fig. 35.6F*).
4. If desired, adjust the occlusion by using articulating paper and the opposing Dentoform arch.
5. Polish the temporary crown with pumice or other polishing materials. It is now ready to be cemented.
6. Assess the temporary crown by using the Skill Performance Evaluation sheet in Appendix 2.

Summary

1. Assemble the necessary materials.
2. Coat the Dentoform with petroleum jelly.
3. Mix the acrylic material.
4. Place the material in the previously made tooth-form mold.
5. Seat the filled mold on the Dentoform.
6. Remove the mold and acrylic resin, and trim any gross excess.
7. Allow the acrylic resin to set.
8. Trim any excess.
9. Adjust the occlusion.
10. Finish and polish.

Review Questions

Question 1. **Another name for a temporary crown is a:**

a. "One size fits all" crown

b. Provisional restoration

c. Suck-down crown

d. Resin crown

Question 2. **Important contacts of a temporary crown include:**

a. Occlusal

b. Interproximal

c. Both

d. Neither

Question 3. **Temporary crowns are placed for:**

a. Patient comfort

b. Esthetics

c. Function

d. All of the above

e. None of the above

Composite Finishing and Polishing

A. Todd Walls, D.D.S.

Objectives

After performing the laboratory/clinical exercises in this chapter, the student will be able to do the following:

1. Explain the rationale for composite finishing and polishing.
2. Recall the benefits of properly finished and polished composite restorations.
3. List two indications for finishing and polishing composite restorations.
4. Discuss the detrimental effects of poor composite placement and finishing.
5. Assess a composite restoration to determine whether it needs replacement or refinishing and polishing.
6. Differentiate between the procedures of composite finishing and polishing.
7. Evaluate a well-finished and polished composite restoration according to the criteria provided in this chapter.

Key Words/Phrases

finishing

flash

polishing

Introduction

The use of composite resin as an esthetic restorative material continues to expand. Once relegated to primarily anterior regions of the dentition where esthetics is a chief concern, composites are now being used to restore the entire dentition in a variety of situations. With this in mind, it is imperative that the dental hygienist be aware of the proper maintenance of composite materials to ensure periodontal health and prevent dental disease.

I. Purpose of Finishing and Polishing

The primary purpose of finishing and polishing composite restorations is to create a restoration that is smooth, uniform, and easily cleaned by the patient. This, in turn, can increase the longevity of the restoration, decrease the incidence of recurrent caries, and promote the health of surrounding tissues. Occasionally, patients will need to have their composite restorations polished and less often refinished.

A. Advantages of Finishing and Polishing

The following conditions result from proper finishing and polishing:
- Smooth, undetectable margins
- Plaque-resistant surface
- Healthier gingival tissues
- Increased longevity
- Enhanced esthetics
- Proper contours

B. Methods by Which These Benefits Are Achieved

These benefits are achieved by properly smoothing the cavosurface margins, reconstructing functional anatomy, and creating a surface that is smooth and free of voids. A smooth surface is necessary to simulate the high gloss of enamel.

II. Evaluation of Composite Restorations

Unlike amalgam restorations, composites can be completely finished and polished immediately after they are placed. Improper placement, incomplete finishing and polishing, or normal wear and tear increases the risk of recurrent caries, plaque retention, periodontal disease, and restoration failure. Composite restorations are evaluated as part of the dental examination. Some restorations may need to be finished and polished. In other instances, the restoration will need to be repaired or replaced.

A. Indications for Finishing and Polishing

1. Overextension or **flash**
2. Premature occlusal contact
3. Overhang
4. Limited stain
5. Limited recontouring of anatomy
6. Small chips or defects

B. Indications for Repair or Replacement

1. Gross overextension or overhang
2. Open margin
3. Fracture
4. Extensive stain
5. Recurrent caries
6. Open proximal contact
7. Larger defects

III. Finishing and Polishing Considerations

Similar to amalgam finishing and polishing discussed in Chapter 26, the process of finishing and polishing composite restorations can be considered two different procedures or two steps of a single procedure. During the **finishing** procedure, contours are corrected while margins and irregularities are smoothed. The **polishing** procedure should produce a smooth lustrous finish.

A variety of products are available ranging from burs, finishing strips, finishing disks, points, cups, pastes, and brushes, as pictured in *Figure 36.1*. Many manufacturers even market their own polishing systems. Some of the most common products are discussed in this chapter. The theory and process of finishing and polishing composites is consistent with that of other materials; a progression from coarse to finer abrasives is described in Chapter 16, Polishing Materials and Abrasion.

Heat generation during finishing and polishing must be controlled. The thermal conductivity of composite is not as high as that of amalgam, but the risk of pulpal irritation or injury from increased temperatures must be considered.

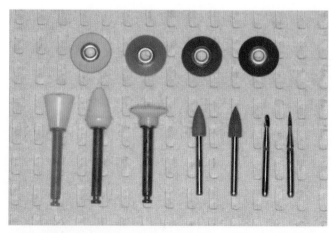

FIGURE 36.1. Abrasive disks, points, a cup, and burs used to finish and polish composite restorations.

The use of a slow-speed handpiece, water as a coolant, and intermittent strokes is recommended to avoid heat buildup and transmission.

Finally, care must be taken not to damage adjacent teeth or soft tissues. Isolate the tooth or teeth with cotton rolls, dry angles, or a rubber dam to prevent iatrogenic injury to surrounding tissues.

IV. Procedure for Composite Finishing and Polishing

A. Evaluate Restoration

Because dental composites are tooth colored and often difficult to see, it is useful to thoroughly dry the restored tooth with a light stream of air from the air–water syringe. With the restoration dry, visually inspect the contours to detect proper anatomical form, chips, voids, stains, or defects. Occlusal contacts can be evaluated using articulating paper. Use an explorer to gently examine all of the margins of the restoration. Proximal surfaces can also be evaluated with an explorer. Proper contacts and gingival margins can be confirmed with dental floss.

B. Discuss Procedure with Patient

Explain the rationale of composite finishing and polishing and review the steps of the procedure with the patient. Inform the patient of sensations he or she may experience during the process, especially those of finishing burs with a low-speed handpiece.

C. Gather Necessary Equipment

Select instruments based on the restoration and the clinician's preference. A list of equipment is included as Table 36.1.

TABLE 36.1. Armamentarium for Finishing and Polishing Composite Restorations

Mouth mirror

Articulating paper

Explorer

Slow-speed handpiece

Air–water syringe

Cotton rolls, dry angles, or rubber dam

Finishing burs

Finishing strips

Curved scalpel blade and handle

Finishing and polishing disks, cups, and points

Dental floss

Tips for the Clinician

- Effective lighting and dried surfaces allow for improved evaluation of surface irregularities.
- The sequence of steps is crucial. Do not proceed to the next step until the previous step has been completed.

Precautions

- Iatrogenic injury may occur to adjacent teeth or gingiva if the operator is not cautious.
- Heat can be generated rapidly on the tooth during composite finishing and polishing.
- Aerosols are created frequently when polishing with disks.
- An exposed metal shank or center of a disk will scratch and discolor the composite surface. Use care in positioning the disk.

D. Finish, Evaluate, Polish, and Reevaluate Restoration

Isolate the area with cotton rolls or a rubber dam. Finish and polish as described in the following sections. Reevaluate the restoration.

V. Finish the Composite Restoration

A. Proximal Surfaces

Overhangs are most frequently encountered in proximal areas. Access to proximal surfaces can be challenging and often dictates which finishing and polishing procedures can be incorporated.

1. Scalpel Blade

A curved scalpel blade is the most effective instrument to remove interproximal overhangs and flash. Use of a scalpel blade is shown in *Figure 36.2*. It is important that the operator uses a curved blade with a single cutting edge on the inside curve. The outer edge of the blade that contacts the gingiva lacks a cutting edge; therefore, the outer edge is not likely to traumatize the soft tissues. The blade is carefully held at a slight acute angle with the cutting edge in contact with the tooth surface. The blade is guided by tooth contours, and shaves rather than carves the excess composite material. If the hygienist is not comfortable using the scalpel or this is not in the scope of the state's practice act, the hygienist should use an alternative technique or ask for assistance from the dentist.

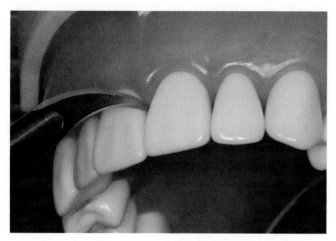

FIGURE 36.2. Removal of an interproximal overhang with a curved scalpel blade.

Use of a scalpel blade to remove a composite overhang is quite similar to debridement of a root surface with a curette.

2. Flame-Shaped Finishing Burs
Flame-shaped finishing burs can be used to smooth contours and margins, and remove overhangs, as shown in *Figure 36.3*. As with disks, move from tooth structure to restoration using smooth, deliberate, intermittent brush strokes. Stay in constant motion while engaging the surface to prevent gouging the restoration or tooth surfaces.

3. Finishing Disks
Finishing disks are useful when the restoration extends onto the facial or lingual surface, thereby allowing access to the area. Some manufacturers produce a series of abrasive disks that are color coded and gradually progress from coarse to fine. An example of a common disk system is Sof-Lex

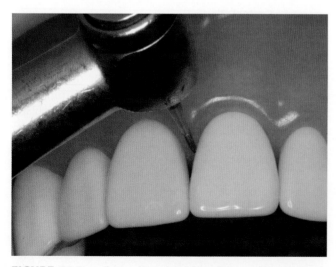

FIGURE 36.3. A flame-shaped finishing bur used in the proximal area.

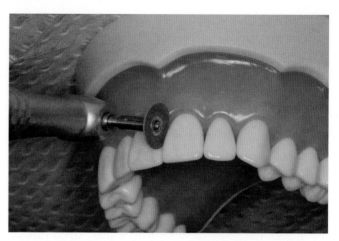

FIGURE 36.4. An abrasive disk used to finish the proximal area.

Discs (3M-ESPE, St. Paul, MN), shown in Figure 16.6. Use a smooth, deliberate, intermittent brush stroke. Starting from tooth structure, move over the surface of the restoration to smooth the surface and remove flash (see *Fig. 36.4*).

4. Finishing Strips
The center of the finishing strip contains no abrasives. Carefully pull or "floss" this portion of the strip through the proximal contact. Position the strip both on tooth structure and the restoration, and gently pull the strip over the surface or margin of the restoration, as pictured in *Figure 36.5*. Repeat this procedure as needed. Always confirm that the finishing strip is situated gingival to the proximal contact to avoid opening the contact.

B. Occlusal Surfaces

Occlusal finishing includes smoothing of margins, refining anatomy, and removing flash.

1. Egg- or Football-Shaped Finishing Burs
Egg- or football-shaped finishing burs can be used to complete practically all occlusal

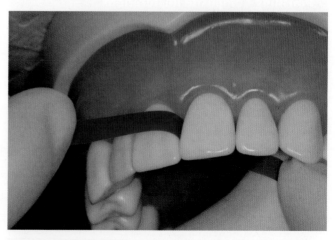

FIGURE 36.5. A finishing strip used to refine the proximal area.

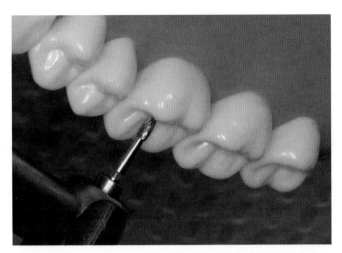

FIGURE 36.6. A finishing bur used to refine the occlusal surface.

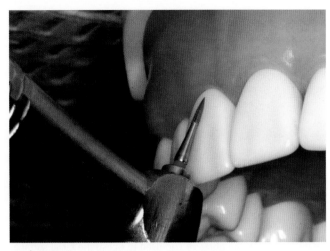

FIGURE 36.8. A finishing bur used to refine the contours of the facial surface.

finishing. Use of a bur is shown in *Figure 36.6*. Existing tooth structure is used to guide the bur over triangular ridges or the tip into grooves and fossae. Maintain smooth, intermittent brush strokes over the restored surface.

2. **Finishing Points and Cups**
   Finishing points or cups are used to smooth the surface and grooves, such as those shown in *Figure 36.7*. Maintain smooth, intermittent brushstrokes over the restored surface.

C. Facial and Lingual Surfaces

Finishing of facial and lingual surfaces, smoothes margins, refines axial contours, removes flash, and eliminates surface stains.

1. **Flame-Shaped Finishing Burs**
   Flame-shaped finishing burs can be used to contour surfaces, smooth margins, and remove flash (see *Fig. 36.8*). As with other abrasives,

move from tooth structure to restoration using smooth, deliberate, intermittent brush strokes. Stay in constant motion while engaging the surface to prevent gouging the restoration or tooth surfaces.

2. **Egg- or Football-Shaped Finishing Burs**
   Egg- or football-shaped finishing burs are often used on the lingual surfaces of anterior teeth. Their shape matches the lingual concavity of anterior teeth. Use existing tooth structure to guide the bur. Maintain smooth, intermittent brush strokes over the restored surface.

3. **Finishing Disks, Points, and Cups**
   Finishing disks and cups (*Figs. 36.9 and 36.10*) are useful on the facial surfaces of anterior teeth, while finishing points and cups are used on lingual surfaces of anterior teeth. A combination of disks, points, and cups is appropriate for posterior teeth. Use a smooth, deliberate, intermittent brush stroke. Starting from tooth

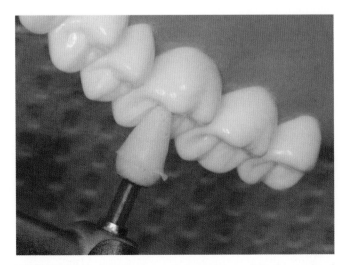

FIGURE 36.7. An abrasive point used to polish the occlusal surface.

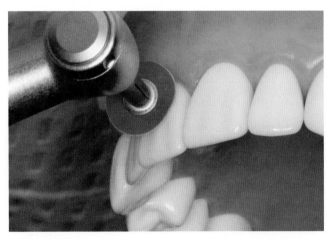

FIGURE 36.9. An abrasive disk used to finish the facial surface.

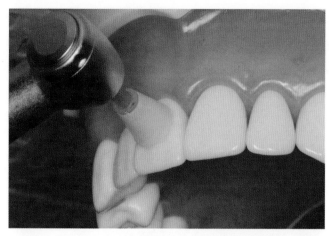

FIGURE 36.10. An abrasive cup used to polish the facial surface.

structure, move to the surface of the restoration. Use great care on the facial surfaces of anterior teeth, as esthetics is very important there.

D. Evaluate the Finishing Procedure

Assess the finishing procedure by using the criteria listed in the Skill Performance Evaluation Sheet in Appendix 2. *Do not proceed to the polishing procedure until these criteria have been met. Polishing will not accomplish a smooth surface unless each step during the finishing process has been successfully accomplished.*

VI. Polish the Composite Restoration

The process of polishing composite restorations is very similar to the finishing process. The major differences include the following: fine abrasives are used, less material is removed, and a lustrous surface results. Some abrasive devices are used to both finish and polish composites.

A. Polishing the Proximal Surfaces

Fine abrasive disks and strips or rubber polishing disks, points, and cups are used in the polishing procedure. Use a smooth, deliberate, intermittent

brush stroke. Starting from tooth structure, move over the surface of the restoration to produce a surface with a smooth, high luster.

B. Polishing Occlusal Surfaces

Polishing points or cups are used for the final polishing procedure. Move across the surface using smooth and deliberate strokes.

C. Polishing Facial and Lingual Surfaces

Polishing points, disks, or cups are used for the final polishing procedure. Again, keep moving across the surface using smooth and deliberate strokes.

D. Composite Polishing Pastes

For some clinicians, the final polishing step uses a rubber cup with a polishing paste shown in as Figure 16.17. These pastes create a lustrous surface to maximize esthetics.

E. Evaluate the Polishing Procedure

Assess the polished composite restoration using a mouth mirror, explorer, and the Skill Performance Evaluation Sheet in Appendix 2. The composite restoration should appear smooth and highly polished and should have a lustrous shine. There should be no damage to the adjacent tooth structure.

VII. Conclusion

At each patient recall appointment, composite restorations should be evaluated for recurrent caries, voids, and any need for refinishing and polishing. If indicated, this procedure may be performed during the recall visit, or scheduled as a separate appointment. When composite restorations are properly maintained, there will be less plaque retention, and subsequently, a lower incidence of periodontal disease and caries. In addition, finishing and polishing will increase the esthetics of the restoration and therefore patient satisfaction.

Summary

Composite Finishing and Polishing

Finishing

1. Evaluate restoration (margins, occlusion, proximal areas).
2. Discuss the procedure with the patient.
3. Isolate the area with cotton rolls or rubber dam
4. Smooth proximal surfaces if necessary (with burs, disks, strips).

5. Remove occlusal excess and eliminate flash with burs.
6. Define occlusal anatomy with burs.
7. Smooth cavosurface margins and occlusal surface.
8. Smooth facial and lingual surfaces.

Polishing

1. Use fine abrasive disks, strips, cups, and points to polish occlusal, proximal, facial, and lingual surfaces.
2. Rinse, dry, and evacuate composite restoration.

Learning Activities

1. In the dental materials laboratory, observe existing composites in extracted teeth. Evaluate margins and contours.

2. During patient assessment, evaluate composite restorations with an explorer, mouth mirror, and floss.

3. In the dental materials laboratory, using a typodont tooth with an existing cavity prep, place a composite restoration. Finish and polish the restoration.

4. Make a 5- × 10-mm sample of composite material. Polish as described in the Chapter 16, Learning Activities in Polishing Materials and Abrasion, using medium, fine, and superfine Sof-Lex Discs.

Review Questions

Question 1. The most effective method to prevent overheating of the pulp when polishing a composite is to:

a. Use light strokes

b. Maintain a moist tooth and composite

c. Lubricate with petroleum jelly

d. Use fine grit abrasives first

Question 2. Ideally, composite restorations should be finished:

a. After 1 week

b. After 24 hours

c. After 2 hours

d. At the placement appointment

Question 3. During composite finishing and polishing, coarser abrasive disks should be followed by finer abrasive disks. This allows for initially more rapid removal of larger scratches in the composite surface followed by less aggressive removal of material containing the smaller scratches.

a. The first statement is true; the second statement is false.

b. The first statement is false; the second statement is true.

c. Both statements are true.

d. Both statements are false.

Question 4. Finishing and polishing composite restorations improves all of the following *except* one. Which one is the EXCEPTION?

a. Surface luster

b. Gingival health

c. Marginal flash

d. Excessive corrosion

Question 5. When finishing the lingual of a composite restoration in an anterior tooth, the most effective abrasive would be a:

a. Finishing disk

b. Finishing cup

c. Flame-shaped finishing bur

d. Egg-/football-shaped finishing bur

Tips for the New Hygienist

John H. Tucker, D.M.D.

Objectives

After studying this chapter, the student will be able to do the following:

1. Discuss the role of the hygienist in the promotion of oral health in private practice dentistry.
2. Summarize the hygienist's role in the communication of treatment options to the patient.
3. Explain the importance of being a contributing, involved dental team member.

Introduction

A note from the authors: Currently, not many textbooks give tips to the graduate when entering dental hygiene practice. A contributing author who has practiced several years and has employed many dental hygienists has valuable information to share. And we, as authors of this text, wholeheartedly agree and have included his thoughts. Chances are that you would have been presented the same messages in your practice management coursework.

I. The Philosophy of the Practice

The hygienist will need to know the philosophy of the dental practice in which he or she works. Many dental offices are owned and run by one practitioner. This philosophy would include the technology, techniques, and protocols currently favored and any changes planned to be incorporated in the future. What does the dentist believe and why does he or she believe it? What are his strengths and weaknesses? What procedures does he or she routinely refer to specialists? What are his beliefs and attitudes about procedures such as orthodontics by a general dentist, implants, take-home and in-office whitening, laser treatment, all ceramic crowns, gold crowns, just to name a few?

If you know his dental practice philosophy (and hopefully agree), the hygienist can be a valuable asset in promoting the recommended treatment for the patient. If two people know what the other believes and are in agreement with these beliefs, isn't it easier to convey them to a third person? This is a very elementary principle, but in many cases, the dentist does not make the philosophy of the practice clear to the hygienist, nor does the hygienist make a point of asking.

II. The Patient's Awareness of His or Her Oral Condition

It is well accepted that patient education is one of the primary responsibilities of the dental hygienist. In most cases, this education is centered on the theme of oral hygiene home care procedures and disease prevention. When is the patient educated on his or her present oral condition? When is he or she given an update of the mouth? Does he or she know what kind of restorations he or she has and what material was used? Does he or she know the present condition of these restorations? Are they worn, fractured, or ragged?

The use of the intraoral camera is ideal to show the patient the areas of missing teeth, broken down restorations, cracked teeth, caries, and periodontal concerns. Since one's dentition must serve him or her for a lifetime, take the time to educate the patient on the present condition of teeth. I think you would be surprised at how many patients think that their teeth are fine and they are only worried about new cavities, when, in reality, the entire dentition may be in the process of breaking down. Deterioration can lead to arch collapse and possibly other more serious issues. There are a variety of multimedia patient education programs one must have in the office to inform patients about the various treatments available. This now leads to the next bit of advice.

III. The Promotion of Dental Services

You must understand that patients often will trust the opinion of the assistant or the hygienist before that of the dentist. This comes from what the social psychologists call the Approach/Inhibition Theory of Power, which suggests that the patient may be more wary of the person "in power" (in this case the dentist) than the hygienist. The patient would act differently (his or her behavior would be more trusting) with the dental assistant or hygienist as compared to the dentist. Because you are a professional, but with less "power" than the dentist, they will place a great deal of trust in you. They know that you do not have a vested financial interest in the decision and they will readily ask, "What would you do if it were you?" This now sets the stage for the opportunity to promote dentistry in the sense of encouraging the best treatment plan for that particular patient. One of our ethical principles we abide by as professionals is beneficence, which is to promote good. We need to promote good restorative care as well as good oral hygiene care. At the same time, it must be made clear that we are *not* "selling" dental treatment, especially treatment that is not truly needed. Unfortunately there are a few dental practitioners out there who seem to engage in the unethical practice of convincing the patient to spend money on dental treatment that is unwarranted, solely for the dentist's financial gain.

The promotion of quality dentistry is actually more complicated. There are dental needs that should be addressed immediately, such as infections. Others are less urgent. The hygienist who understands the philosophy of the practice can counsel the patient when financial and other limitations place the entire treatment plan beyond the patient's resources. Often, the crown that a mom needs takes a back seat to the son's or daughter's braces. The hygienist can address the benefits of accepting the treatment plan (the crown for the mom) and the risks involved when treatment is delayed.

Our promotion of what is needed now opens the door to another debated issue and that is the dental diagnosis by the hygienist. By no means do we advocate that the hygienist be the professional in the office who informs the patient of a prescribed treatment plan on what they *think* the patient should have done. The majority of the state dental practice laws forbid dental diagnosis by the hygienist because it is obviously out of the scope of practice of the hygienist's education. However, the hygienist could reinforce and promote the prescribed treatment. An acceptable scenario could be: the dentist informs the patient of his or her diagnosis and treatment plan, and if the dentist leaves the room, the patient may turn to the hygienist for his or her opinion. This, then, is the golden opportunity in which the hygienist, because he or she agrees with the dentist's practice philosophy, can validate and encourage the patient to partake in the prescribed treatment.

IV. The Patient's Best Interest

As mentioned previously, the entire office personnel want the best treatment and care for the patient. The hygienist has now become the patient's advocate. This also extends to insurance companies. Most insurance companies have limits on the amount of money that will be paid for a procedure. It may not be enough to pay for that particular restoration. Whether or not insurance pays for the needed restorative care, it should never deter the dental hygienist to encourage the patient to accept and complete the prescribed restorative treatment. Ethically, the patient's insurance status should not be a concern for the dental hygienist. The financial aspect of care is usually the responsibility of the patient and the dental receptionist or the office manager.

V. Office Technology

The practice will be best served if all employees are familiar with all of the office technology. Be familiar with the computer system and software. This would include the software that not only you and the dentist may use but the receptionist's too. It will make for a smooth, competent operation. Understand the use of all new, technologically advanced instruments and equipment that are utilized in the office. This knowledge and comfort with technology by all the employees will reflect in a very positive way in the eyes of the patients.

VI. A Member of the Dental Team

This has probably been presented to you before, in a variety of aspects. The entire practice should be revolving around the patient. "The patient is our first priority" may be a familiar motto that your program advocates. It takes ALL employees of the practice to fulfill this belief. Everyone in the office has their job responsibilities that contribute to making the patients the first priority. Once the patient's needs are met, the hygienist should be willing to help others when there is a cancellation in the schedule. He or she should not sit idle. Do not hesitate to ask others, such as the dental assistant or office manager, what you can do to contribute to office efficiency, organization, and cleanliness. Being a dental hygiene professional extends far beyond cleaning teeth. It is important to promote goodwill not only to patients but to other team members. A hygienist's poor attitude and laziness reflect negatively on the employer and other staff members. Certainly, patients will become aware of disharmony in the office. Doesn't the work day go by faster when you have been busy compared to one where there is idle time? And think of all the good you have done!

VII. Conclusion

Hopefully this short chapter has provided some insight for your future practice. Often it has been said that "experience is the best teacher," but having a few tips ahead of time can make adapting to a new practice more pleasurable.

Case
Studies

Introduction

The cases presented in this section are designed to stimulate discussion of the various dental materials that are used to restore or replace teeth. The questions involve not only dental materials but clinical dental hygiene as well. Maintenance of restorations, prostheses, and oral tissues should also be considered.

Case 1

The patient is a 63-year-old woman with a maxillary denture, and the appliance is presented in Figure CS1.1. She lives on a very limited income but visits the dental office yearly for a thorough dental examination and oral prophylaxis. At this visit, she presents with little plaque and stain but with a small amount of calculus on the supragingival, lingual surface of the remaining natural teeth.

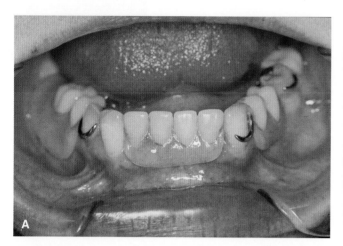

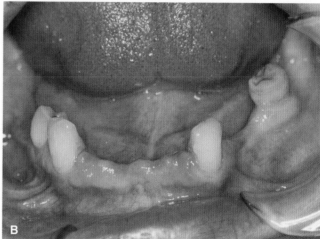

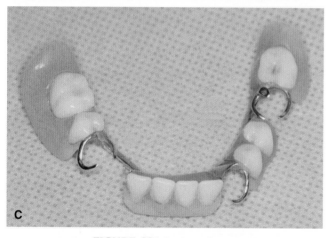

FIGURE CS1.1. **A.** Patient wearing dental appliance. **B.** Patient without appliance. **C.** Appliance.

QUESTIONS

Question 1. **The remaining natural teeth on the mandible include:**

a. Teeth #18, #22, #27, and #28

b. Teeth #19, #21, #25, and #26

c. Teeth #19, #22, #27, and #28

d. Teeth #18, #21, #26, and #27

Question 2. **The replacement prosthesis is correctly termed:**

a. A removable bridge

b. A removable partial denture

c. A partial

d. A fixed partial denture

Question 3. **The clasps of the prosthesis encircle which of the following teeth?**

a. Teeth #19, #22, and #27

b. Teeth #18, #21, and #26

c. Teeth #18, #22, and #28

d. Teeth #19, #22, and #28

Question 4. **The composition of the prosthesis may include as many as _____ dental materials.**

a. 2

b. 3

c. 4

d. 5

Question 5. **The polishing agent of choice for the patient's natural teeth should be:**

a. A pumice slurry

b. A coarse prophylaxis paste

c. A fine prophylaxis paste for all teeth

d. Selectively polish the stained teeth

Question 6. **After scaling and polishing the natural teeth, cleaning the dental prosthesis, and providing thorough patient education about calculus formation and removal, an appropriate recall recommendation would be:**

a. To continue the yearly recall date

b. To change to a 6-month recall because of the calculus formation

c. To keep the yearly recall but note in her record to closely assess the calculus formation and, if necessary, change the recall date accordingly

d. To encourage the patient to accept a 4-month recall so that calculus formation can be closely monitored

Case 2

The photographs (Fig. CS2.1) show a 25-year-old man having three restorations placed during his appointment. His gums bleed easily, and the probing depths for this quadrant are noted on the charting in Figure CS2.2. His oral hygiene home care consists of brushing two or three times a week and swishing with Scope mouthwash on the days he does not brush. Flossing is not a part of his oral hygiene regimen.

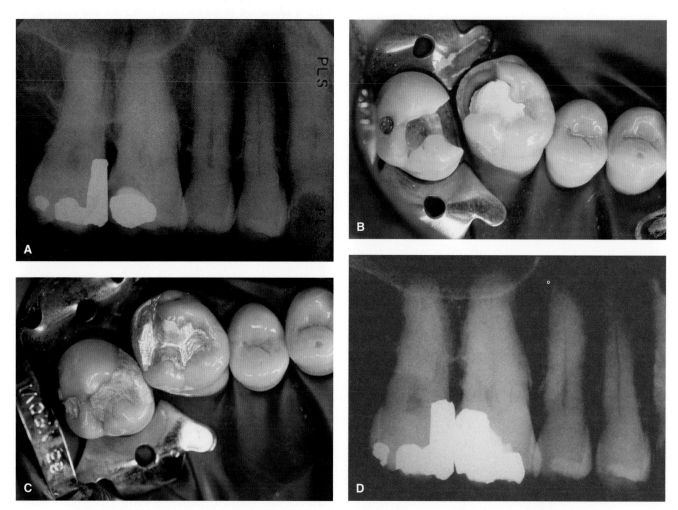

FIGURE CS2.1. A. Preoperative radiograph. **B.** Rubber dam isolation, ready to restore with amalgam. **C.** Amalgam restorations. **D.** Postoperative radiograph (Courtesy of Dr. Henry Miller, Martinsburg, WV).

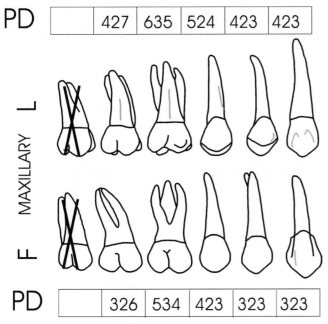

FIGURE CS2.2. Periodontal measurements of the teeth shown above.

QUESTIONS

Question 1. The teeth being restored in the photographs below are:

a. #2 and #3

b. #14 and #15

c. #13 and #14

d. #1 and #2

Question 2. In Figure CS2.1A, the "white" material on the floor of the preparation of the second tooth from the left is considered to be a _____, and its purpose is _____.

a. Liner; to provide strength and thermal insulation

b. Base; to provide strength and thermal insulation

c. Liner; to protect the pulp from chemical irritation

d. Base; to protect the pulp from chemical irritation

Question 3. From the most distal surface of the last tooth and moving mesially, the amalgam restorations would be named:

a. Disto-occlusal (DO), mesio-occlusal (MO), and disto-occluso-lingual (DOL)

b. Occlusal (O), MO, and DO

c. O, MO, and DOL

d. MO, DO, and DOL

Question 4. What two conditions also exist in this patient?

a. Pulpal involvement and periodontal disease

b. Premolar occlusal stain and gingivitis

c. Root calculus and gingivitis

d. Root calculus and periodontal disease

Question 5. In between the patient's restorative appointments, he has an appointment with you for the necessary dental hygiene care. Assuming that the dental and dental hygiene assessments and diagnoses have been made, implementation of the dental hygiene care would include:

a. Scaling and polishing

b. Scaling, root debridement, and polishing

c. Radiographs, root debridement, and polishing

d. Scaling, root debridement, polishing, and evaluation

Question 6. The new amalgams could best be finished and polished with:

a. Slurries of pumice and tin oxide

b. A slurry of tin oxide

c. Finishing burs and then slurries of pumice and whiting

d. Coarse and then fine prophylaxis pastes

Question 7. Which of the following teeth should be closely "periodontally monitored"?

a. #2

b. #2 and #3

c. #2, #3 and #4

d. All teeth in the case presentation should be monitored in the same way.

Case 3

The patient is a 31-year-old woman who is very self-conscious of a malformed tooth that everyone can see. She has yearly dental exams and also sees the hygienist during the same appointment. Her oral home care is excellent. She is most interested in having this tooth "look a lot better than it does." The procedure to restore this tooth is illustrated in Figure CS3.1.

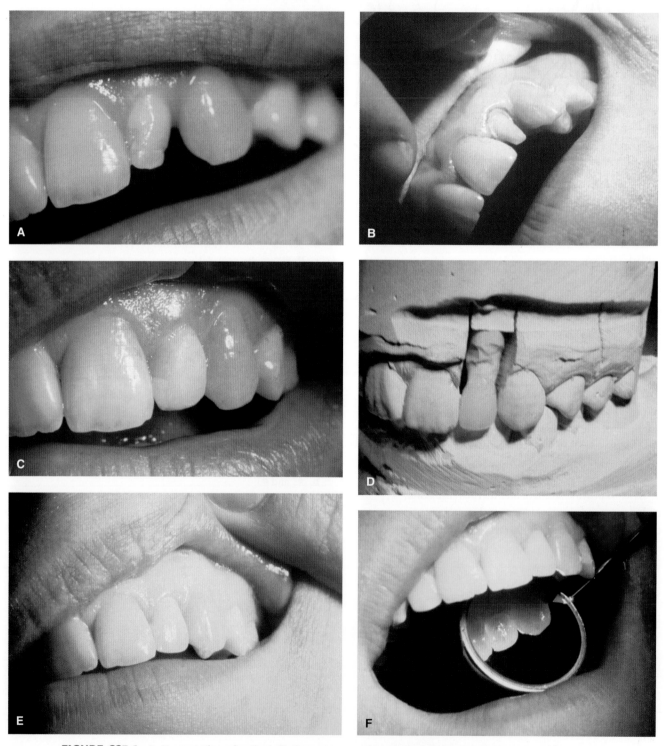

FIGURE CS3.1. **A.** Presentation of patient. **B.** Crown preparation. **C.** Temporary crown. **D.** Casts with ceramic crown. **E.** Permanent crown placed (facial). **F.** Permanent crown placed (lingual).

QUESTIONS

Question 1. Tooth #10 in Figure CS3.1A is commonly called:

a. Fusion
b. Traumatic injury
c. Peg lateral
d. Erosion

Question 2. The final restoration is said to be a _____ restoration, and the restorative procedure used to fabricate this particular restoration is called a(n) _____ technique.

a. Removable; direct
b. Fixed; indirect
c. Removable; indirect
d. Fixed; direct

Question 3. After the crown preparation is made, the patient leaves with a restoration as the one shown in Figure CS3.1C. This is known as a _____ restoration.

a. Interim
b. Provisional
c. Permanent
d. Substitute

Question 4. We can assume that the crown shown in Figure CS3.1E and F contains no metallic materials. Therefore, the dental material usually used in this technique is a:

a. Cold-curing resin
b. Special restorative cement
c. Composite material
d. Ceramic material

Question 5. The "polishing agent of choice" for the dental material selected in question 4 is:

a. Toothpaste only
b. A "mild" Prophy Paste
c. A slurry of whiting
d. Any typical Prophy Paste

Question 6. The most desirable characteristic of the dental material selected in question 4 is:

a. Translucency
b. Abrasion resistance (hardness)
c. Fracture toughness
d. Availability of many shades

Question 7. If the patient in this case had discolored teeth and wanted to have them whitened besides having the new restoration fabricated, when should the whitening take place?

a. Before the restoration is fabricated
b. After the restoration is fabricated
c. Between the fabrication appointments
d. Whitening is contraindicated in this case

Case 4

Wesley Mullins, D.D.S.

This patient is a 43-year-old woman with an unremarkable medical history. The patient reports that she brushes and flosses two times each day. She says that her gums bleed sometimes and that she really wants to "get my teeth in good shape and keep them that way."

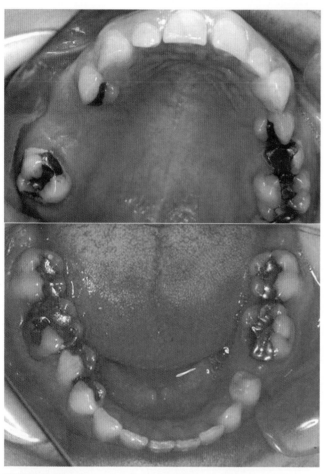

FIGURE CS4.1. Occlusal photographs of maxillary and mandibular arches. (Courtesy of Dr. Wes Mullins, Knoxville, TN.)

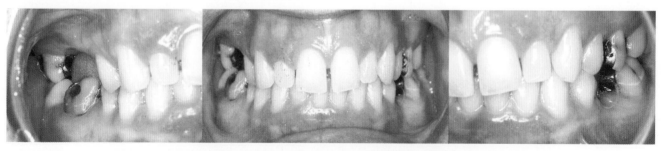

FIGURE CS4.2. Lateral and frontal photographs. (Courtesy of Dr. Wes Mullins, Knoxville, TN.)

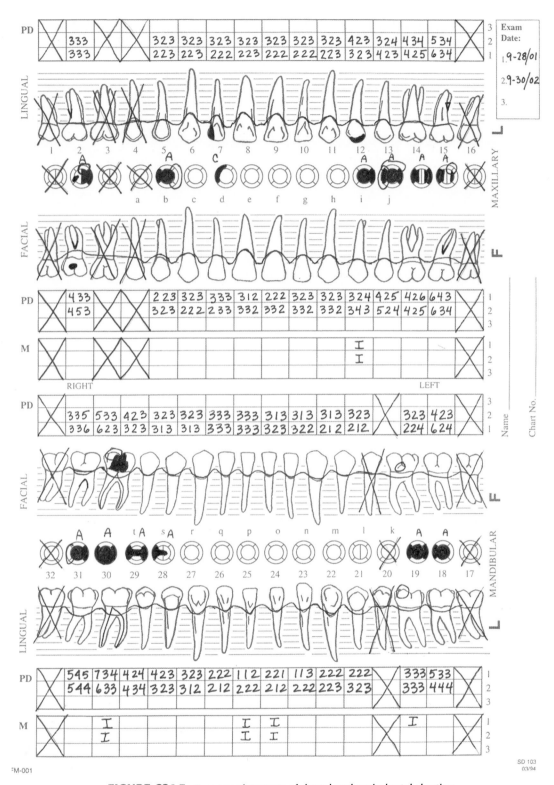

FIGURE CS4.3. Two appointments of dental and periodontal charting.

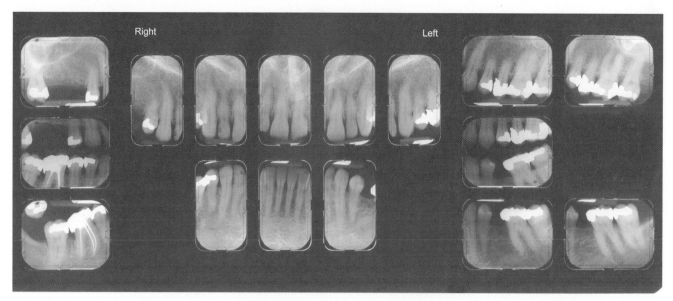

FIGURE CS4.4. Full mouth radiographs.

QUESTIONS

Question 1. **Periodontally, the patient's gingival health has _____ compared to the original baseline probing.**

a. Greatly improved
b. Slightly improved
c. Not changed
d. Slightly deteriorated
e. Greatly deteriorated

Question 2. **Fractures are evident on which of the following teeth?**

a. Tooth #19
b. Teeth #19 and #31
c. Teeth #13 and #19
d. Teeth #19 and #30
e. Teeth #13, #19, and #31

Question 3. **Radiographically, tooth #30 has _____ roots and _____ canals.**

a. 2; 2
b. 3; 2
c. 3; 3
d. 2; 3

Question 4. **Multiple restorations can be placed on one tooth. From this patient's records, examples are present on teeth #2, #14, and #15.**

a. The first statement is true; the second statement is false.
b. The first statement is false; the second statement is true.
c. Both statements are true.
d. Both statements are false.

Question 5. **What can be said about tooth #30 distal and tooth #31 mesial amalgam margins?**

a. Tooth #30 is open; tooth #31 is overextended.
b. Tooth #30 is overextended; tooth #31 is open.
c. Both margins are overextended.
d. Both margins are open.

Question 6. **The canals in tooth #30 are filled with _____ material(s).**

a. The same
b. Two
c. Three
d. Temporary

Question 7. **Supereruption is apparent on what tooth?**

a. Tooth #19
b. Tooth #21
c. Tooth #30
d. Tooth #31

Question 8. **According to the periodontal chart, the recession on tooth #31 has at least _____ mm of gingival recession.**

a. 2
b. 3
c. 4
d. 5

Case 5

This patient is a 73-year-old woman with controlled hypertension without dry mouth who takes medication for osteoporosis. She mentions that she smokes four or five cigarettes a week because of anxiety. Her oral home care consists of brushing and flossing two times each day. She says her gums rarely bleed, she has no sensitivity, and she really wants to "keep my teeth in the best shape as possible." She is happy with her smile.

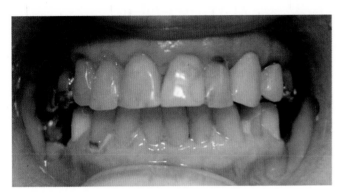

FIGURE CS5.1. Photograph of anterior teeth in occlusion.

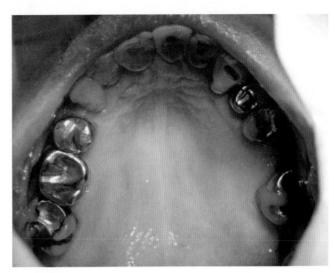

FIGURE CS5.3. Occlusal photograph of maxillary arch.

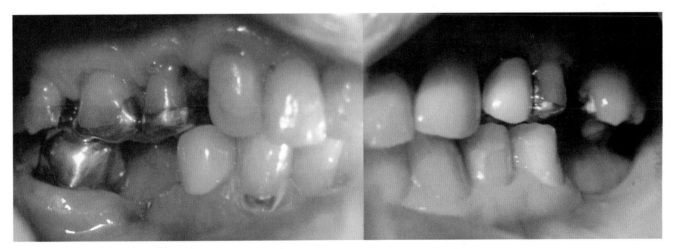

FIGURE CS5.2. Photograph of posterior teeth in occlusion.

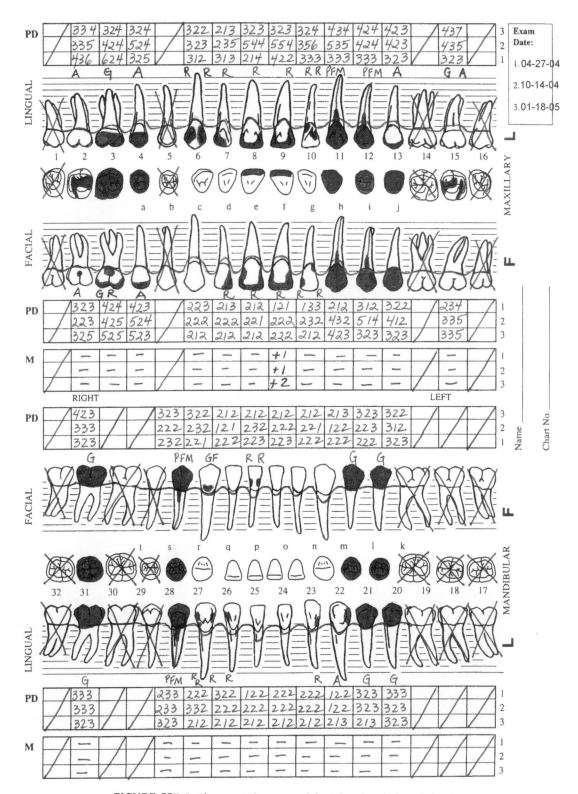

FIGURE CS5.4. Three appointments of dental and periodontal charting.

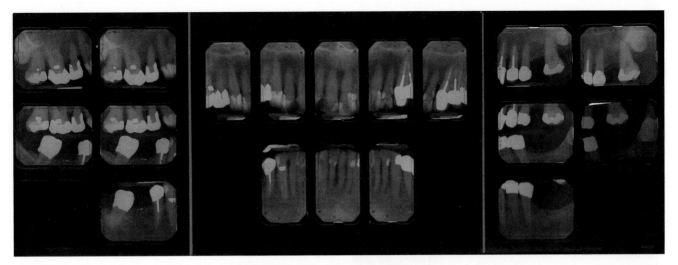

FIGURE CS5.5. Full mouth radiographs.

QUESTIONS

Question 1. From the information presented, which arch of this patient is in better periodontal health?

a. Maxillary
b. Mandibular
c. Both arches are in "periodontically identical health"
d. Both arches are "periodontically unhealthy"

Question 2. How many kinds of dental restorations have been placed in this patient's mouth?

a. 2
b. 3
c. 4
d. 5

Question 3. When the patient reports she is on medication for osteoporosis, what possible oral ramifications come to mind?

a. Necrotizing stomatitis
b. Xerostomia
c. Bisphosphonate-induced osteonecrosis
d. Increased caries susceptibility

Question 4. After learning the patient's medications, medical conditions, and habits, your chairside patient education should include information on:

a. Nutritional counseling
b. Pit and fissure sealants
c. Tobacco cessation
d. Tooth whitening

Question 5. After performing an oral exam, reviewing the radiographs and dental history, an appropriate recommendation for this patient would be:

a. Fluoride varnish on teeth #s 9, 22, 25, and 26
b. The use of patient applied fluoride
c. Pit and fissure sealants
d. The use of saliva substitutes

Question 6. The largest restoration on tooth #15 is a (an):

a. MO amalgam
b. MO gold inlay
c. DO amalgam
d. Occlusal gold inlay
e. DO gold inlay

Question 7. Teeth #s 11, 12, and 28 have:

a. Root canals and post and cores
b. Root canals and PFM crowns
c. Post and cores and PFM crowns
d. Root canals, post and cores, and PFM crowns

Case 6

John H. Tucker, D.M.D.

This patient is a 62-year-old woman with controlled type II diabetes. The patient reports that she brushes in the morning and evening but only flosses in the evening. She has excellent plaque control and has had regular dental care throughout the years. She is unhappy with her smile. The patient presents with a crown that fractured off of tooth #28 and shares with the dentist that she thought her "upper front teeth look fake" and her "lower front teeth look worn out." The photographs include pretreatment, preparation, and posttreatment. The dental and periodontal charts were recorded before the upcoming restorative treatment.

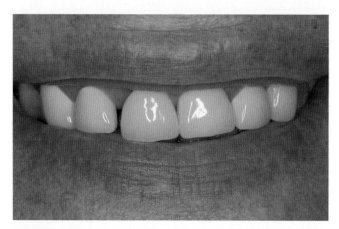

FIGURE CS6.1. Preoperative photograph of maxillary anterior teeth.

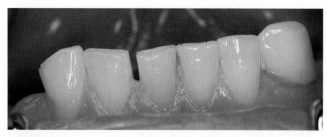

FIGURE CS6.2. Preoperative photograph of mandibular anterior teeth.

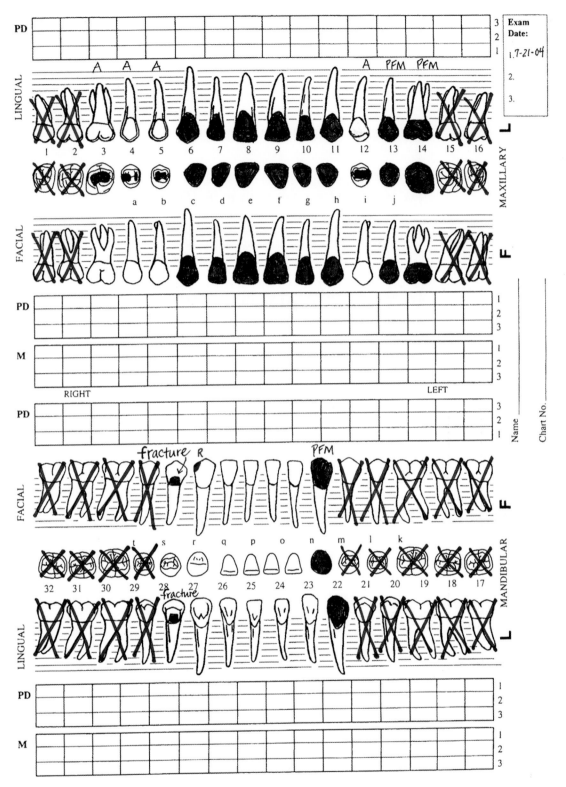

FIGURE CS6.3. Preoperative dental charting.

Periodontal Chart

FLORIDA
PROBE

Chart #:

Name:

Examiner:

Date: July 21, 2004

PSR

| 0 | 0 | 0 |
| 0 | 0 | 0 |

Right   Left

Recession: 1 2 1   211   111   111   111   1 1 1   1 1 1   111   111   111   212   2 2 2
Depth   3 2 3   323   323   323   323   3 2 3   3 2 3   323   333   333   233   3 3 3

GM

Facial

Tooth #   1   2   3   4   5   6   7   8   9   10   11   12   13   14   15   16

GM

Lingual

Depth   3 2 3   323   323   323   323   3 2 3   3 2 3   323   333   333   233   3 3 3
Recession: 2 2 2   221   111   111   111   1 1 1   1 1 1   111   111   111   212   2 2 2
Mobility

Mobility
Recession: 2 1 2   211   111   111   112   3 3 3
Depth   3 2 2   322   333   333   222   3 3 3

GM

Lingual

Tooth #   32   31   30   29   28   27   26   25   24   23   22   21   20   19   18   17

GM

Facial

Depth   3 2 2   322   333   333   222   3 3 3
Recession: 2 2 2   111   111   111   111   3 3 3

Diagnosis

Gingivitis
(04500-Type I)
☐ Mild
☐ Moderate
☐ Severe

Periodontitis
☐ Early
(04600 Type II)
☐ Moderate
(04700 Type III)
☐ Advanced
(04800 Type IV)
☐ Refractory
(04900 Type V)

Legend

Pocket Depth Change
Deeper
↓ >1mm and <2mm
↓ >2mm
Improvement
↑ >1mm and <2mm
↑ >2mm

Depth Bar Indicators
▯ Depth > 10mm
▮ Depth >= 4.0mm
▮ Depth < 4.0mm
▯ Recession
▯ Recession > 10mm

⅋ Minimal Attached
Gingiva
∅ No Attached Gingiva

◆ Bleeding
◇ Suppurating
◈ Bleeding And
Suppurating
● Plaque

Furcation
⩔ Furcation = 1
⩔ Furcation = 2
⩔ Furcation = 3

Summary

Patient has 18 teeth, 0 of 108 sites or 0% of the pocket depths are greater than 4.0 mm

Bleeding: 0 sites (0%) bleeding, 0 buccal and 0 lingual.
Recession: 18 teeth had some recession with 8 having recession equal to or greater than 2.0 mm
Furcations: 0 furcations were found.
Mobility: 0 teeth had some degree of mobility.
Plaque: 0 total sites have plaque/calculus, 0 interproximal, 0 lingual and 0 buccal.

Plaque Sites

Left   Right

FIGURE CS6.4. Preoperative periodontal charting.

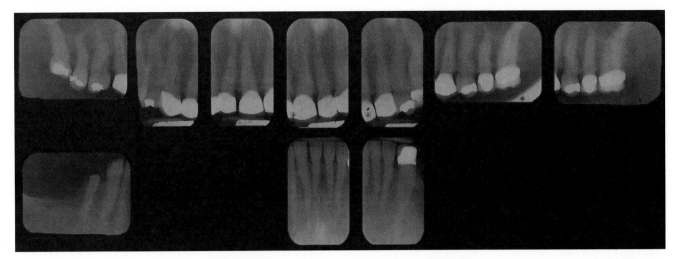

FIGURE CS6.5. Preoperative full mouth radiographs.

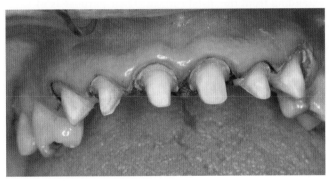

FIGURE CS6.6. Photograph of preparations of maxillary anterior teeth.

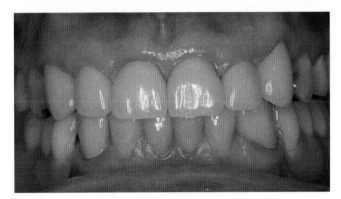

FIGURE CS6.7. Postoperative photograph of anterior teeth.

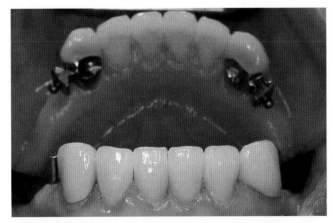

FIGURE CS6.8. Postoperative photograph of mandibular anterior teeth showing rest seats and precision attachments.

QUESTIONS

Question 1. **The patient said, "My upper front teeth look fake." This would professionally translate that her original maxillary ceramometal crowns are:**

a. Overcontoured and very opaque

b. Overcontoured and too translucent

c. Undercontoured and very opaque

d. Undercontoured and too translucent

Question 2. **The treatment plan called for porcelain veneers on teeth 23, 24, 25, and 26. These would be recorded on the dental chart:**

a. The same way a porcelain crown is charted

b. By outlining the lingual surface on these teeth

c. By outlining the facial surface on these teeth

d. By outlining the facial and lingual surfaces on these teeth

Question 3. **From the information provided in this case, the gingival health of this patient is considered to be:**

a. Poor

b. Acceptable

c. Very good

d. Cannot be determined with the information provided

Question 4. **Which tooth exhibits the developmental condition of dilaceration?**

a. 3

b. 4

c. 5

d. 6

Question 5. **The radiolucency on the distal of #27 is a (an):**

a. Amalgam restoration

b. Gold inlay

c. Carious lesion

d. Composite restoration

Question 6. **The veneers that were placed on #23 to #26 (Figs. CS6.7 and CS6.8) were most likely luted with a _____ cement.**

a. Zinc oxide and eugenol

b. Polycarboxylate

c. Glass ionomer

d. Composite

e. Zinc phosphate

Question 7. **In the mandibular posttreatment photograph (Fig. CS6.8), teeth 22 and 27 have metallic projections extending from the distal surface. Their purpose is to attach to the:**

a. Future implant restoration

b. Provisional (temporary) posterior teeth

c. New partial denture

d. Orthodontic retainer

Case 7

Patricia Inks, B.S.D.H., M.S.

A 35-year-old African American male presents to the dental office. He says he has not been to a dentist in several years. A comprehensive medical history is taken, and he is classified as an ASA Class I. The photos were taken following periodontal debridement by quadrant.

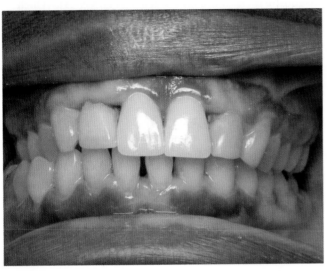

FIGURE CS7.1. Photograph of anterior teeth in occlusion.

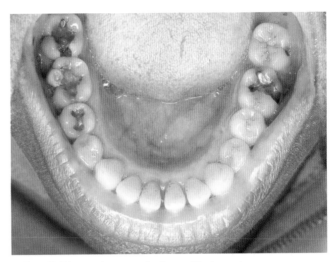

FIGURE CS7.3. Photograph of mandibular arch.

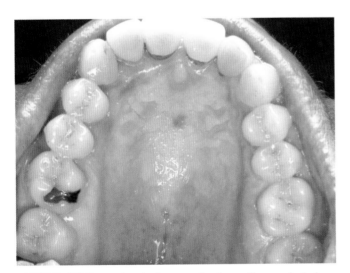

FIGURE CS7.2. Occlusal photograph of maxillary arch (mirror view).

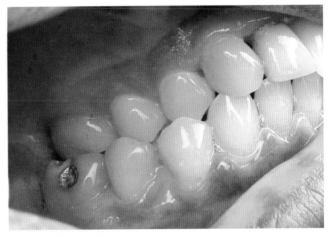

FIGURE CS7.4. Photograph of right posterior teeth in occlusion.

QUESTIONS

Question 1. What types of restorations are seen on tooth #s 8 and 9?

a. Porcelain veneers

b. Porcelain jacket crowns

c. Porcelain fused to metal crown

d. Acrylic crowns

e. There are no restorations on #8 and #9

Question 2. Using Figures CS7.1 and CS7.4, identify Angle's classification of occlusion.

a. Class I

b. Class II, Division I

c. Class II, Division II

d. Class III

Question 3. The manner in which the posterior teeth on the right side (Fig. CS7.4) are occluding is termed:

a. Cross bite

b. Over jet

c. Overbite

d. Deep bite

Question 4. Tooth # 3 (Fig. CS7.2) has been restored with a Class _____ amalgam restoration.

a. I

b. II

c. V

d. VI

Question 5. The patient is complaining of pain and sensitivity to hot and cold when eating. Which quadrant of the mouth would most likely be the area causing the pain?

a. Maxillary right (Q #1)

b. Maxillary left (Q #2)

c. Mandibular left (Q # 3)

d. Mandibular right (Q # 4)

Question 6. All but one of the following is appropriate diagnostic tools to use on tooth # 31(Fig. CS7.3). Which one is NOT an appropriate diagnostic tool for this tooth?

a. Visual inspection

b. Pulp testing

c. Laser/light fluorescence

d. Periapical radiograph

Question 7. A(an) _____ would be an appropriate supplemental oral hygiene aid for the anterior cervical embrasures.

a. End-tuft brush

b. Interproximal brush (proxy brush)

c. Unwaxed fine floss

d. Rubber tip

Case 8

Maryfrances Cummins, R.D.H., M.P.H.

This patient is a 47-year-old male who is 6 ft tall and weighs 220 lb. Floss catches in the upper right side. His blood pressure is 135/85 mm Hg, pulse 70 bpm, and respiration 18. He is under the care of a physician for diabetes mellitus type 2 and has a penicillin allergy. He is currently taking metformin and insulin. He had spinal surgery in 2007.

Dental history: This patient has had dental restorative work including endodontic therapy. He has received only sporadic and emergency dental care in the past 7 years. His last dental visit was 2 years ago for a periodontal abscessed tooth, #3. Pus was drained through a gingival incision, and the patient was placed on an antibiotic. He did not return for the recommended follow-up care.

Social history: This patient is married and works as a bus driver. Although his physician has recommended smoking cessation, the patient still smokes a pack of cigarettes a day. Also, he has unhealthy dietary habits and limited physical activity due to his past back surgery.

Chief complaint: "My gums are receding and the spaces between my teeth seem to grow. Also, my teeth become sensitive to cold and my bad breath does not go away."

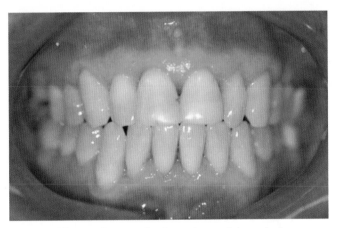

FIGURE CS8.1. Photograph of anterior teeth in occlusion.

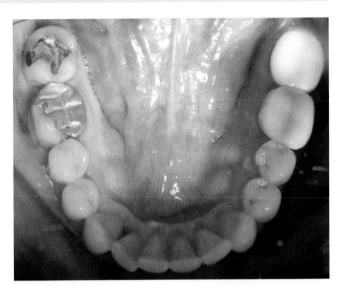

FIGURE CS8.3. Photograph of mandibular arch.

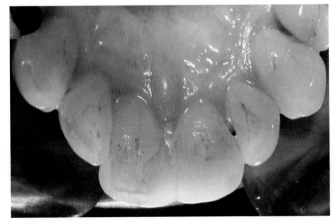

FIGURE CS8.2. Occlusal photograph of maxillary anterior teeth (mirror view).

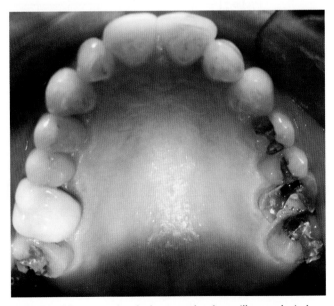

FIGURE CS8.4. Occlusal photograph of maxillary arch (mirror view).

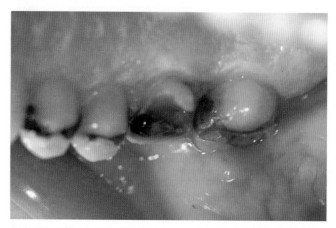

FIGURE CS8.5. Photograph of right maxillary posterior teeth, palatal view.

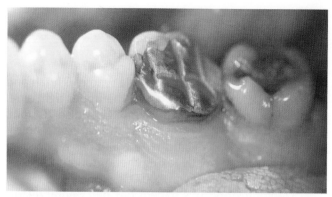

FIGURE CS8.6. Photograph of right mandibular posterior teeth, lingual view.

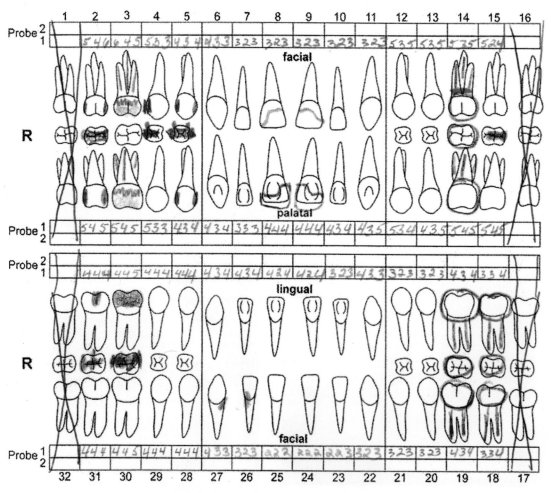

FIGURE CS8.7. Preoperative dental charting.

QUESTIONS

Question 1. Which of the following findings is most likely a contributing factor to the periodontal involvement of tooth #5?

a. Caries

b. Amalgam overhang

c. Subgingival calculus

d. Occlusion

Question 2. The fractured crown on tooth #3 is most likely due to all of the following except one. Which one is the EXCEPTION?

a. Caries

b. No restoration placed after endodontic therapy

c. Occlusal trauma

d. Bone loss

Question 3. What is the G.V. Black caries classification for the maxillary central incisors?

a. Class III

b. Class IV

c. Class V

d. Class VI

Question 4. The mandibular right first premolar (#28) has 3 mm of gingival recession on the lingual aspect. What would be the clinical attachment loss for this tooth?

a. 3 mm

b. 5 mm

c. 7 mm

d. 9 mm

Question 5. The patient chooses not to restore tooth #3 and wants it extracted. Which of the following is NOT an option for replacement after this tooth is extracted?

a. Removable partial denture

b. Implant and crown

c. Full upper denture

d. Three unit fixed partial denture (fixed bridge)

Question 6. Considering the patient's complaint of sensitivity to cold stated in the chief complaint section, what professional topical fluoride should the dental hygienist recommend for this patient?

a. 1.23% acidulated phosphate fluoride gel

b. 8% stannous fluoride gel

c. 5% sodium fluoride varnish

d. Any one of these may be recommended

e. None of the above products should be recommended

Case 9

Maryfrances Cummins, R.D.H., M.P.H.

This patient is a 48-year-old female. She is 5 ft 7 inches tall and weighs 135 lb. Her blood pressure is 124/84 mm Hg, pulse 72 bpm, and respiration 20. She reports taking "diet drugs" 15 years ago and claims she has an allergy to sulfa drugs, morphine, and codeine. She is currently taking amoxicillin, 1,000 mg twice daily, for a sore throat prescribed by her physician. She is under the care of a physician for drug and alcohol addiction.

Dental history: The patient has undergone dental restorative work in the past including endodontic therapy, post and core build up, and crowns. She has only received emergency care in the past 3 years due to lack of access to her family dentist.

Social history: Patient recently moved in with her parents who are 70 and 75 years old and in good health. She admits to having a drug habit for which she is currently being treated. She has unhealthy dietary habits and craves sweets. She smokes two packs of cigarettes a day.

Chief complaint: "I want to get my mouth back in shape."

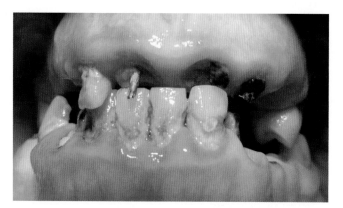

FIGURE CS9.1. Photograph of anterior teeth in occlusion.

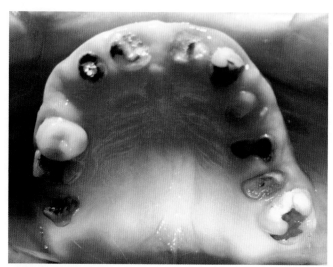

FIGURE CS9.3. Photograph of maxillary arch (mirror view).

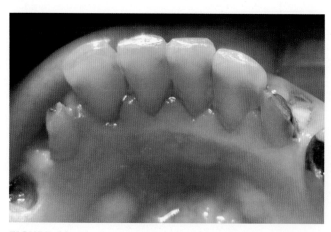

FIGURE CS9.2. Photograph of mandibular anterior teeth.

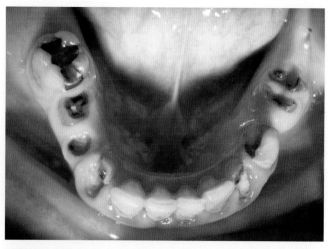

FIGURE CS9.4. Photograph of mandibular arch (mirror view).

ADULT CLINICAL EXAMINATION

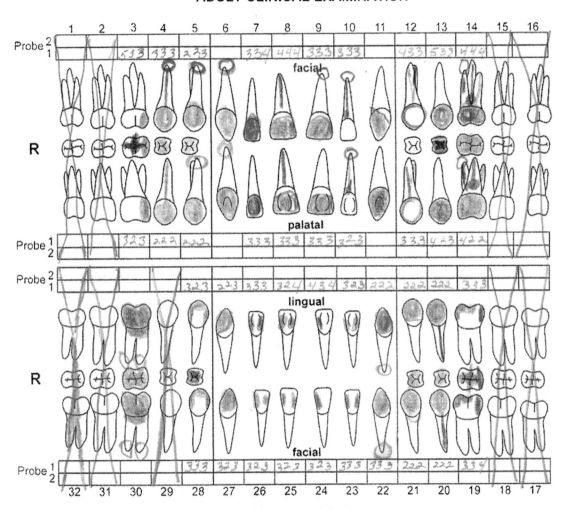

FIGURE CS9.5. Dental charting.

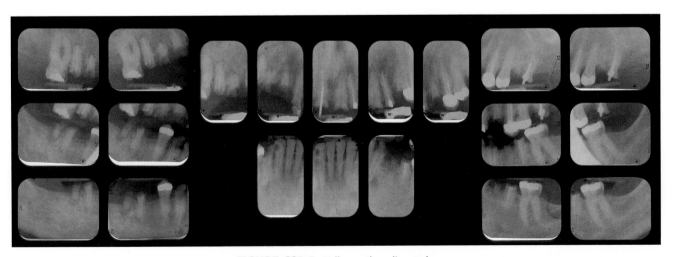

FIGURE CS9.6. Full mouth radiographs.

QUESTIONS

Question 1. Which teeth have a history of endodontic therapy?

a. 6, 7, 8

b. 8, 10, 20

c. 22, 23, 24

Question 2. All of the following are associated with "meth mouth" EXCEPT one. Which one is the exception?

a. Poor oral hygiene

b. Cracked teeth

c. Broken bones

d. Craving sweets

Question 3. Which set of teeth listed below have periapical radiolucencies?

a. 4, 5, 10

b. 3, 6, 12

c. 23, 24, 30

d. 22, 24, 27

Question 4. One treatment plan for this patient would be to do a full mouth extraction. All of the following would be included in the treatment plan EXCEPT one. Which one is the exception?

a. Oral hygiene instructions

b. Periodontal debridement

c. Amalgam polishing

d. All of the above should be in the treatment plan

Question 5. Were the radiographs and the photographs taken during the same appointment?

a. Yes

b. No

c. Unable to determine

Case 10

Andrea Warzynski, R.D.H., M.Ed.

The patient is a 61-year-old female who keeps regular 6-month prophylaxis and exam appointments. Her medical history reveals that she is a two-time cancer survivor. She was diagnosed with breast cancer several years ago and had a mastectomy of her left breast along with chemotherapy. In the recent past she had a reoccurrence of the cancer in the lymph nodes of her left arm. She had surgery to remove the lymph nodes along with radiation and chemotherapy. She is now in remission. Currently, she wears a compression sleeve on her left arm to reduce swelling. She is a former smoker, but has not had a cigarette in over 20 years.

Her current medications include Klonopin; Losartan; Zofran ODT; Protonix; Pyridium; Senokot; tamoxifen; vitamins B_{12}, B_6, and D_3; and calcium. She uses EMLA cream and nystatin topical powder as needed at surgical sights.

The initial dental exam reveals localized gingival inflammation, bleeding on probing, and localized subgingival interproximal calculus present in the posterior areas. According to her dental history, she recently had a root canal on tooth #19 and still has some pain associated with that tooth. She grinds her teeth and uses a custom-made fluoride tray with a 3% fluoride gel. Her previous dentist told her to complete the fluoride treatment at night before bed. She admits that she does not do it as often as she should.

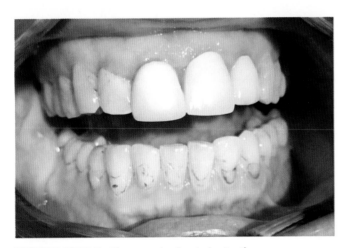

FIGURE CS10.1. Photograph of anterior teeth.

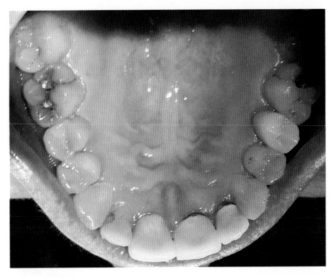

FIGURE CS10.2. Photograph of maxillary arch.

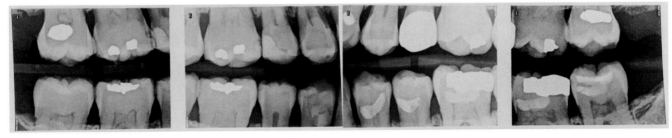

FIGURE CS10.3. Bitewing radiographs which predate root canal therapy for tooth #19.

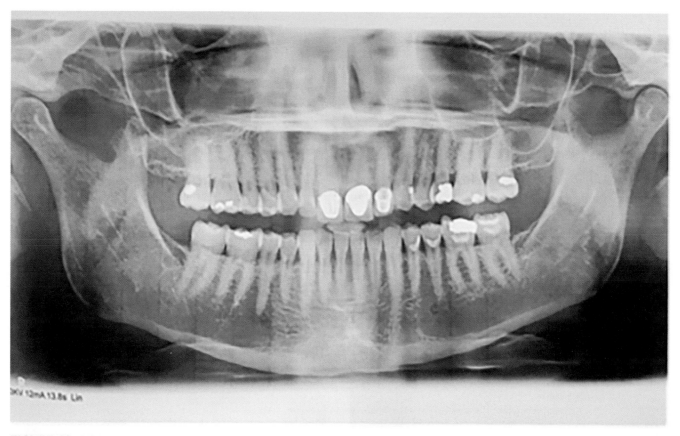

FIGURE CS10.4. Panorex radiograph, predates bitewing radiographs, photographs, and root canal therapy for tooth #19.

QUESTIONS

Question 1. Based on the photographs, how many crowns are present on the maxillary arch?

a. 2

b. 3

c. 4

d. 5

Question 2. It is most likely that the crown on tooth #9 is made of:

a. Composite

b. Composite and metal

c. Porcelain

d. Porcelain and metal

Question 3. What is the GV Black caries classification of the restoration on tooth #22?

a. I

b. II

c. III

d. IV

e. V

Question 4. What would be the best explanation for the missing cusp tips on the patient's right side?

a. Grinding habits

b. Decay

c. Esthetic restoration

d. Brushing habits

Question 5. According to the bitewing radiographs, tooth #3 has decay present. What tooth surface(s) will be included as part of the restoration?

a. Mesial

b. Buccal

c. Occlusal

d. Mesial and occlusal

e. Buccal and occlusal

Question 6. On the bitewing radiographs, tooth #19 is restored. Which one correctly describes the restoration(s) present?

a. One amalgam restoration

b. One amalgam restoration with a base material

c. Two composite restorations

d. Two restorations, one composite and one amalgam

e. Three restorations, two composite and one amalgam

Question 7. Does tooth #4 have a restoration? If so, describe it.

a. Yes; occlusal composite

b. Yes; DO-composite

c. Yes; DOL-composite

d. No restoration present

Question 8. The patient uses custom-made fluoride trays at home. What kind of impression material was most likely used to construct the trays?

a. Alginate

b. Agar

c. ZOE impression paste

d. Polysulfide

Question 9. Based on this patient's medical history, what is the best rationale for why this patient is using an at-home fluoride treatment?

a. Rampant decay

b. Periodontal disease

c. Cancer treatments

d. Gingival recession

Question 10. Which of the following medications is used to help reduce the production of stomach acid?

a. Klonopin

b. Losartan

c. Protonix

d. Zofran

Case 11

Michael Hanna, D.M.D.

Initial Exam: The patient is a 4-year-old Caucasian female. She is healthy with the exception of a history of low iron levels and a heart murmur. She is not taking any medications and is allergic to Suprax (cefixime), a cephalosporin antibiotic. The patient was referred by a local dental clinic due to disruptive behavior and extensive decay. Patient was held by mother during the exam and would not communicate. The exam reveals extensive decay and disruptive behavior. The child is routinely put to bed with a baby bottle containing milk. Home water is fluoridated. Complete oral rehabilitation under general anesthetia was discussed with mother including risks versus benifits. The mother approves the treatment plan as reviewed. Subsequently the patient was treated in the operating room.

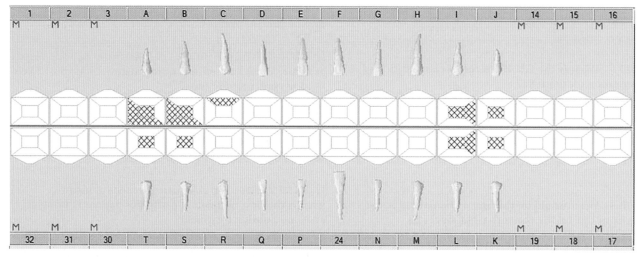

FIGURE CS11.1. Dental chart of teeth and caries present at initial exam.

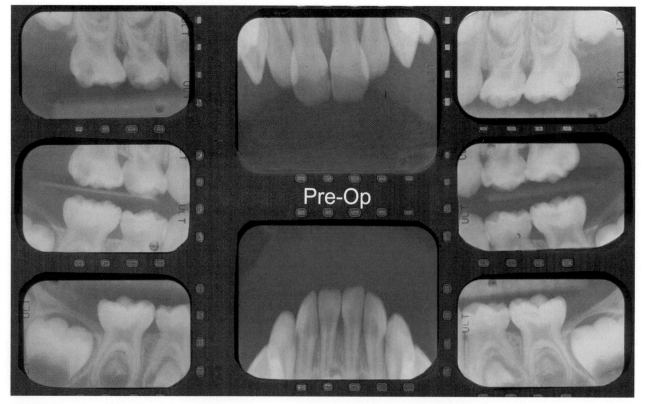

FIGURE CS11.2. Preoperative radiographs.

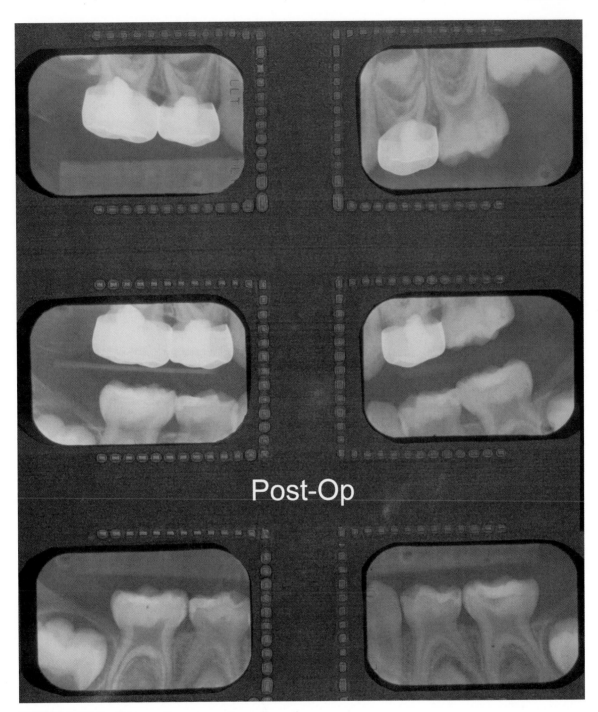

FIGURE CS11.3. Eight-month-postoperative radiographs.

QUESTIONS

Question 1. The extensive caries present at the initial exam is a result of:

a. Amount of sugar in the patient's diet
b. Frequency of sugar exposure
c. Low fluoride in the patient's home water supply
d. Lack of regular flossing

Question 2. Teeth #A and #B were restored with:

a. Porcelain bonded to metal crowns
b. Composite crowns
c. Stainless steel crowns
d. Ceramic crowns

Question 3. The removal of the coronal pulp of #A, #B, and #I is called a:

a. Pulpotomy
b. Root canal therapy
c. Direct pulp cap
d. Indirect pulp cap

Question 4. Restoring tooth #A is necessary to:

a. Maintain space in the arch for the eruption of tooth #4
b. Prevent tooth #3 from mesial drift during eruption
c. Both
d. Neither

Question 5. The child had caries in all eight primary molars. Regarding the eruption dates of primary molars, what can be said about the following?

The primary first molars, both maxillary and mandibular erupt basically at the same time. For the primary second molars, the mandibular molar usually erupts before the maxillary molar.

a. The first sentence is true; the second sentence is false.
b. The first sentence is false; the second sentence is true.
c. Both sentences are true.
d. Both sentences are false.

Question 6. It was stated in the case background that the patient had a history of low iron levels. An iron deficiency is usually associated with which of the following?

a. Neutropenia
b. Leukocytosis
c. Hemophilia
d. Anemia

APPENDIX

Answers and Justifications to Review Questions and Case Studies

1

CHAPTER 1

1. **b.** The FDA is the regulatory agency, whereas the ADA develops standards and administers those standards and guidelines. The AADR is a professional organization for dental researchers. The OSHA mandates the practice of standard (universal) precautions for blood-borne pathogens.

2. **c.** It is not within the scope of dental hygiene practice to choose the restorative material for the patient. This is the responsibility of the dentist. Understanding how dental materials behave, educating the patient, and assessing the patient are all patient care responsibilities of the hygienist.

3. **e.** Gingival third caries, anterior and posterior and both lingual and facial, are defined as Class V.

4. **c.** The degradation of teeth and dental materials, biocompatibility, biting forces, esthetic demands of the patient, and temperature changes are all restrictions that limit the use of dental materials.

5. **d.** When the temperature changes in the oral cavity, no dental material expands and contracts by exactly the same amount as the natural tooth structure. Over time, this expansion and contraction may cause leakage around the restoration and tooth sensitivity.

6. **c.** The periodontium supports the tooth in a stable condition and gives feedback on the forces being placed on the teeth. The gingival tissues seal out undesirable agents and attach to the teeth, forming a barrier. The pulp serves to respond to thermal stimuli, as it contains the nerve cells.

7. **a.** When a significant amount of tooth structure is missing from a particular tooth, a crown will encircle and support the remaining tooth structure. A pontic is the "false tooth" on a bridge, whereas an implant replaces the entire tooth, including the root. A fixed partial denture replaces teeth that may be missing in an arch and is cemented in place.

8. **a.** It is true that the cavity preparation design helps to secure the restoration in place. But because gold castings such as an inlay are cemented in place and must be first seated without cement as a "try-in," the walls must diverge so that it can be removed and then cemented. The converging walls of an amalgam preparation, as well as the added undercut areas, help to retain it in the cavity prep.

9. **b.** Technically, the only terms that would be interchangeable are study model and diagnostic cast. This replica is used to study the size and position of the oral tissues. If a restoration is constructed on the replica, it is called a cast.

10. **d.** Amalgam, composites, and glass ionomers are all direct restorative materials. They are placed directly into the cavity preparation once all the decay is removed. Porcelain materials must be fabricated in a dental laboratory because they are fired in an oven at high temperatures. Temporary restorations are usually made for the patient to be used between appointments while indirect restorations are being fabricated.

11. **c.** Class III devices are the most regulated and require premarket approval. Class I is the least regulated. There is no Class IV.

12. **a.** Calculus is visible on the distal surface of #2 but not others. Do not confuse the crestal bone with calculus. The teeth appear radiographically correct and no distortion has occurred during exposure.

CHAPTER 2

1. **d.** Window glass has strong atomic bonds but short-range order similar to that of liquids. The consistent spatial relationship between molecules is 5 to 10 neighbors apart. The short-range order is the reason why glass sometimes flows; an example is a window in a very old house where the bottom half of the window may be slightly thicker than the top half.

2. **b.** Metallic bonds are formed when the electrons are shared by all the atoms. Covalent bonds result when two atoms share a pair of electrons. Ionic bonds occur when an electron is "given up" by one atom and then accepted by another. Secondary bonds involve the uneven distribution of electrons. Partial charges result.

3. **a.** The valence electrons in a metallic bond are shared between atoms. Metals have distinct properties, which are the result of their atomic bond. The "negative cloud" and the "positive core" result in many weak, multidirectional primary bonds. In turn, this results in a strong material. Secondary bonds are formed when a partial charge results from an uneven distribution of electrons around an atom or molecule. Covalent bonds result when two atoms share a pair of electrons. Ionic bonds occur when an electron is "given up" by one atom and then accepted by another.

4. **b.** Translucent materials are those that allow some light to pass through, such as the incisal third area of anterior teeth. Dental ceramics can be matched in translucency and color to replace the natural tooth structure. A ceramic dental

455

restorative material is neither transparent (all light passes through) nor opaque (no light passes through). Brittleness is a disadvantage of ceramics as a dental restorative material.

5. **c.** The cross-linking not only adds to the strength, but the more cross-links that are present, the more rigid and stiff the material becomes. Polymers will stretch and recoil, similar to the movements of a "Slinky," if they have no or minimal cross-links.

6. **d.** Tin foil is a pure metal that has been compressed into a very thin film. The other materials listed are composed of two or more different materials. The resulting material has improved properties compared with those of either individual material.

7. **a.** A permanent dipole is a bond that has a permanent partial charge. Permanent dipoles form weak secondary bonds. The bonds in a fluctuating dipole are the result of an intermittent, uneven distribution of electrons around the atoms or molecules. Hydrogen bonds are "special" permanent dipoles because of the single electron. Primary bonds are strong bonds between atoms that involve the transfer or sharing of electrons.

8. **a.** In a metal, each positive core is surrounded by an electron cloud, and the core "feels" little difference when an atom slides by another atom. Since the surroundings (atomic bonding) do not change, neither do the properties. Ceramics would fracture when bent because of the ionic bonding and the resulting electron repulsion if a negative ion slides "one over" to another negative ion. Polymers may bend easily or may fracture depending on the bonding between the chains.

9. **b.** A composite is a material that is made from two or more different solid materials. A colloid is a mixture of gases, liquids, or solids at a microscopic level and is a suspension of one material in another. A solution is one material completely dissolved in another, whereas an emulsion is a type of colloid composed of two liquids that do not blend together to form one liquid. Their stability when mixed together is usually temporary.

10. **c.** A covalent bond results when two atoms share a pair of electrons and is one of three types of primary bonds. An ionic bond results when an atom gives up an electron and another accepts it. A metallic bond is a primary bond in which valence electrons are shared, but by all the atoms in the object, not just two. Secondary bonds are the result of partial charges from an uneven distribution of electrons around an atom or molecule.

CHAPTER 3

1. **c.** Good wetting indicates that the adhesive is in very close contact with the adherend, forming a low-contact angle. Poor wetting "stays as a drop," and a high-contact angle is formed.

2. **d.** Tension is a pulling or stretching stress, which many times is referred to as tensile stress. Compression is a crushing or pushing force. Torsion is a twisting stress, and shear is a sliding stress.

3. **c.** The higher the modulus of elasticity, the stiffer is the material. The modulus is a measure of flexibility. A rubber band has a low modulus; a mouth mirror has a high modulus. Resilience is the ability of a material to absorb energy without

deforming, whereas toughness is the ability of a material to absorb energy up to and including failure or fracture.

4. **c.** Nearly all materials will contract (sometimes ever so slightly) when cooled and expand when heated. Measuring this change in size (volume) in relation to the change in temperature is called the coefficient of thermal expansion. In dentistry, this property holds importance because, ideally, the tooth structure and the restorative material should expand and contract the same amount.

5. **b.** Remember that you cannot have stress (load) without strain (change in length). They occur together. When they are proportional, as illustrated on a graph, it is a straight line. As we increase the load (by adding more monkey charms), eventually, the spring will not go back to the original length. This stress is no longer proportional to the strain. We have reached the yield strength on the graph, and the line begins to curve.

6. **a.** The modulus of elasticity is defined as the stress divided by the strain in the linear portion of the stress–strain graph.

7. **a.** Other examples of physical properties are color and thermal conductivity. Strength and stiffness are mechanical properties, and setting reactions are chemical properties.

8. **d.** Torsion is a twisting stress, such as turning a doorknob. Shear stress occurs when parts of an object slide past each other. Tension is a pulling stress, and bending is a combination of compression, tension, and shear stresses.

9. **c.** Solubility is calculated as the amount of material that dissolves in a given time. Viscosity is the ability of a material to flow. Water sorption is the ability of a material to absorb water. Wetting is the interaction of a liquid with a surface.

10. **b.** Mechanical properties include stress, strain, resilience, toughness, fatigue, and elasticity, to name a few. Physical properties include thermal conductivity, heat capacity, vapor pressure, viscosity, hardness, and many more. Chemical properties describe setting reactions and decay and degradation. Biologic properties are the effects materials have on living tissue.

11. **d.** Thermal conductivity is the rate of heat flow through a material. It is measured as heat flow over time. Heat capacity is a measure of the amount of thermal energy a material can hoard (like a microwave trivet), whereas heat of fusion is the amount of energy required to melt a material. The coefficient of thermal expansion is a measure of change in volume in relation to the temperature change.

12. **b.** The definitions of these four properties are described in #11 above. The composite resin restorative material expands and contracts at a different rate than enamel and dentin. Over time, a gap is created between the tooth and restoration when it contracts (from cold beverage) and then closes when the soup is eaten. This process is called percolation and may result in microleakage, tooth sensitivity, and recurrent decay.

13. **a.** Those liquids that act as solvents and evaporate readily have a high vapor pressure. Materials with low vapor pressure do not evaporate quickly. All liquids have some degree of vapor pressure. A liquid's vapor pressure is a constant and does not vary. Therefore, it cannot be "intermittent."

14. **b.** Compression is defined as "a pushing or crushing stress." The pressing of the plastic mass of amalgam by the amalgam condenser instrument is an example of compression.

15. **a.** Solubility is a measure of a materials' ability to dissolve in water. The dental cement has a low solubility and serves

the patient well by not dissolving for a long period of time in the patient's mouth. Cements have the most demanding requirements of any material.

16. **c.** Stress concentration occurs near voids, pits, and cracks. Stress concentration may cause breaks and fractures at a much lower stress than if they were not present.

CHAPTER 4

1. **a.** The sticky material, or the bonding material that sticks the stamp to the envelope, is called the adhesive. The stamp and the envelope are referred to as adherends.

2. **c.** If the bracket breaks off cleanly between the bonding material and the enamel surface, it is called an adhesive failure. When the fracture or failure occurs within the bonding material, it is termed a cohesive failure. Residual bonding material would be present on both the bracket and the tooth surface.

3. The numbers for the correct sequence are 2, 5, 7, 1, 3, 6, 8, and 4. The tooth surface must first be cleaned and then rinsed and dried before the etchant can be placed. Next, the etchant is placed for 15 to 30 seconds. This, too, must be thoroughly rinsed and gently dried. The bonding resin is then applied, and it flows into the enamel micropores. The restorative material is applied last and bonds to the previously placed bonding resin.

4. **c.** A 37% concentration of orthophosphoric acid is commonly used. Lower concentrations have been tested but tend to be too weak. Higher concentrations are too aggressive.

5. **d.** The enamel rods are arranged less regularly than on permanent teeth. The surface must be etched longer to assure that the bonding (resin) material will be retained.

6. **a.** The micropores formed by the etchant are too small to be seen by the naked eye, so this bonding process is known as micromechanical bonding. Secondary, rather than primary, bonds are formed because the unset bonding resin flows around the decalcified collagen fibers and sets, thus entangling the two molecular chains together without primary bonds. Secondary bonds promote this entanglement.

7. **b.** This layer of "dentin debris" not only remains on the surface but also extends into the dentinal tubules. It is similar to sticky, sappy pinewood saw dust, and it adheres to the newly cut surface. After the smear layer is removed with etchant, a primer layer is applied and flows into the open tubules of etched dentin. The adhesive (layer) is a low-viscosity resin and sets similarly to enamel-bonding resin.

8. **b.** The adhesion/bonding mechanism reduces microleakage, which decreases the likelihood of recurrent decay. Bonding agents seal off the space between the tooth and the restoration. This protects the interface area not only from microleakage but also from postoperative sensitivity.

9. **d.** The hybrid layer is a combination of the resin adhesive and decalcified dentin. The dentin becomes decalcified during the etching process. A bond is formed when the collagen fibers (the organic component of the dentin) are surrounded by and become embedded in the resin adhesive material. Enamel tissue is not a part of the hybrid layer, and the smear layer is actually the "dentin debris" left by the dental bur.

10. **c.** It is a current belief that the smear layer is created when dentin tissue is cut during tooth preparation (see #7 above).

Composites do not irritate the pulp; the microleakage of composites causes the irritation. Etching of dentin does not irritate the pulp tissue, and the smear layer does not need to be preserved.

CHAPTER 5

1. **d.** The coefficient of thermal expansion for restorative resins can be 2 to 10 times greater than tooth structure. Repeated expansion and contraction can open and close the gaps at the margin of the restoration. Other problems with resins include polymerization shrinkage and lack of abrasion resistance.

2. **c.** The silane coupling agent coats the filler particles of the composite and is chemically compatible with both the filler and the resin phases. It also transfers the stress from the weaker resin phase to the stronger filler phase. The matrix is composed of a soft resin, which has little strength and wears easily. The filler particles are made of "engineered" glass and add strength to the restoration. Polymers are another name for plastics, and adhesives are materials that will stick to a flat surface or bond two flat surfaces together. (These are discussed in Chapter 4, Adhesive Materials.)

3. **b.** Because of the very small particle size, microfills finish and polish better than any other type of composite. They have, however, a high coefficient of thermal expansion, low strength, and a low percentage of filler (40–50%).

4. **c.** With chemical-cure materials, two pastes are mixed and set by a chemical reaction. This limits the operator's working time. There is also a possibility of incorporating air bubbles while mixing. Many contain more matrix material and less filler than light-cure products.

5. **a.** Depth of cure is the amount or increment of composite that can be successfully cured by a light source. Incremental addition refers to adding and curing small amounts of composite material in the cavity preparation.

6. **d.** The smaller the particle size of the filler, the better will be the finish and polish of the surface of the restoration. Smaller particles are less likely to break down and fall out of the resin matrix, thus leaving a roughened surface to accumulate stain and debris. The size of the filler particle does not affect the polymerization reaction, the technique for adding increments, or the etching time.

7. **c.** A decreased filler content decreases the viscosity of the material and, therefore, increases the "flowability." This makes placement easier for the dentist. Flowable composites are usually placed under a hybrid composite material. Condensable composites aid in placement by inhibiting filler particles from sliding by one another. This makes them feel stiffer and thicker than the typical composites. Hybrid composites contain several particle sizes to create a material that has superior strength and that polishes well.

8. **b.** Hybrid composites are used in restorations undergoing moderate stress in which strength and wear resistance are more important than surface luster. For low-stress areas, high surface luster, and Class V restorations, microfill composites are used.

9. **d.** Preventive resin restorations combine a pit-and-fissure sealant and a composite restoration. The composite is placed first, with any remaining pits and fissures being covered by the sealant material. Compomers are a mix of glass ionomer

and composite materials. Flowable composites will "flow" into the preparation because of lower viscosity. Condensable composites contain filler particles that inhibit them from sliding past each other for a "stiffer, thicker" feel. This consistency allows for easier placement.

10. **d.** Abrasion resistance for hybrid composites is very good compared to the other composite types. Abrasion resistance is poor for the older, macrofilled composites.

11. **a.** Thermal expansion is poor for microfill composites. For hybrid composites, thermal expansion is considered to be good.

12. **b.** Hybrid composites have 75–80% filler by weight. Microfills have 40–50%, and macrofills have 70–75%. Flowable composites are 50% filler by weight.

13. **c.** Light-activated composites are supplied as a single paste, with no mixing required. Polymerization does not begin until the material is exposed to a very bright light. They are popular among dentists because they will "set on demand" (dentist has control of setting time). The chemically activated materials are usually a two-paste system that has to be mixed together to have the polymerization reaction begin. Once mixing begins, the reaction takes place until a set (hard) product forms.

14. **c.** Compomers bond and set like composite resins, but initially release fluoride-like glass ionomers. Flowable composites are those that have a lower viscosity due to decreased filler content. Condensable composites are those that have a "thicker, stiffer feel," which possibly makes condensation easier. Preventive resin restorations are a combination of pit and fissure sealants and composite restorations; the composite is placed first, then the rest of the area is sealed.

15. **d.** Microfill composites have filler particles sized from 0.03 to 0.5 μm, low strength, good abrasion resistance, and have very good polishability. Macrofill composites have 10- to 25-μm particle sizes, fair strength, poor abrasion resistance, and poor polishability. Hybrid composites range in particle size from 0.5 to 1 μm, good strength, very good abrasion resistance, and good polishability.

CHAPTER 6

1. **d.** Remember that the dental amalgam is composed of mercury and amalgam alloy, approximately 50% each. It was mentioned that silver (Ag) comprises 65% of the alloy, but this is 65% of the 50% of the alloy component of the dental amalgam. This reasoning is also true for copper (Cu) and tin (Sn). Aluminum (Al) is not found in dental amalgam.

2. **c.** Amalgam has a high compressive strength, but tensile and shear strengths are comparatively low. Bending strength is a combination of tensile and compression strengths and is low as well.

3. **c.** Tin–mercury comprises the gamma-two (γ_2) phase of the setting reaction of low-copper (traditional) dental amalgams. "Gamma" is used to designate the silver–tin (Ag–Sn) phase. "Gamma-one" is used to designate the silver–mercury phase (Ag–Hg). There is no tin–tin compound in the setting reaction of amalgam.

4. **b.** Silver causes setting expansion and increases the strength and corrosion resistance. Zinc will minimize oxidation. Tin will reduce strength and corrosion resistance and will maximize oxidation.

5. **b.** Lowering the mercury content increases the strength and results in less marginal breakdown. Increasing the mercury content decreases the strength and results in more marginal breakdown.

6. **b.** The marginal seal of corrosion products that forms over time, between the inner surface of the tooth and the restoration (interface), is the feature that makes amalgam a successful restorative material. The price and the ease of use are advantages, but they do not account for its success as a restorative material. Finishing and polishing can extend the service of the restoration, but the seal at the interface is the most important feature contributing to its success.

7. **c.** The proper trituration technique is controlled by the dentist, whereas the composition of the alloy, rate of the setting reaction, particle shape, and particle size of the alloy are controlled by the manufacturer.

8. **f.** An amalgam restoration that has been finished and polished reduces the ability for plaque to adhere, resists tarnish and corrosion, and is more likely to have continuous margins with tooth structure. Voids in the restoration are the result of the condensation technique of the clinician. They are not related to finishing and polishing.

9. **b.** In the high-copper amalgam reaction, tin reacts with copper rather than with mercury. This eliminates the undesirable gamma-two phase. Tin reacts with silver to form the gamma phase, an Ag–Sn compound. Tin reacts with mercury in the low-copper (traditional) setting reaction to form gamma-two. Zinc, if present, reduces oxidation of the other metals in the alloy.

10. **a.** The life expectancy of an amalgam restoration is indirectly related to the size of the restoration. As the restoration increases in size, so do the internal stresses, thus decreasing the life expectancy.

11. **a.** Amalgams using lathe-cut alloy particles require more force during condensation because these particles are rough and do not slide past each other easily. In contrast, spherical particles have a soft, "mushy" feel, and a condenser may push through the mass easily. The blended or admixed alloy particles would have an in-between consistency or "feel," that of spherical or lathe-cut.

12. **b.** Overtriturated amalgam is difficult to condense, exhibits a shortened working time, and tends to crumble. Undertriturated amalgam has a mushy-grainy feel and is difficult to properly condense. It may also appear soupy. Properly triturated amalgam is cohesive, smooth, and plastic. The mercury–alloy ratio is set and proportioned by the manufacturer and is usually not the cause of a poor consistency and decreased setting time.

13. **d.** Amalgam is a cost-effective restorative material that provides good service over a reasonably long time. It is used for amalgam cores, tooth fractures, and cingulum pits on anterior teeth. It is commonly used for Class I, II, V, and VI caries. It is seldom used for Class III and IV caries because the "silver" color can be seen in the interproximal and facial areas.

14. **c.** One-tenth of 1% (0.1) of the population has a true allergy to mercury. Therefore, for the vast majority of patients, mercury toxicity is not a problem.

15. **b.** When properly placed, direct gold, or gold foil, is a long-lasting restoration. It is placed by condensing it into the cavity preparation. Its cost is reasonable, but the cost of labor

to place it can be expensive. A disadvantage is the lack of strength when compared to other metallic restorations.

CHAPTER 7

1. **d.** Glass ionomer is the most common cement at this time that is supplied in capsule form and mixed in the amalgamator.

2. **e.** Glass ionomer and ZOE cements are used for caries control. Glass ionomer cements leach fluoride that inhibits caries. ZOE has an obtundent effect on the pulp; this is an advantage when caries are deep. Other cements do not have these advantages.

3. **a.** Only glass ionomer cements release fluoride. ZOE does, however, protect and soothe the pulp, but it is weak and lacks long-term strength compared to other cements.

4. **c.** In addition to its lack of strength, ZOE is the most soluble compared to glass ionomer, zinc phosphate, and polycarboxylate. Glass ionomer is the least soluble, with zinc phosphate and polycarboxylate ranking second and third, respectively, in their ability to resist solubility.

5. **b.** Glass ionomer must be mixed within 1 minute to achieve the correct consistency. It must also possess a shiny appearance on luting to maintain maximum adhesion.

6. **a.** In oral fluids, cements are much more soluble than gold alloy, porcelain, or porcelain-fused-to-metal restorations.

7. **d.** Because zinc phosphate produces an exothermic reaction during manipulation, it is important to release this heat during mixing. This is done by spreading the mix over the entire surface of the slab so that the heat can dissipate. This technique is not necessary for ZOE, polycarboxylate, or glass ionomer.

8. **c.** Calcium hydroxide promotes the formation of secondary dentin. Silicates, temporary cements, and composite cements do not promote the formation of secondary dentin.

9. **b.** Fluoride is added to the raw materials of certain cements to make manufacturing of the glass powder easier. An added clinical benefit is the leaching and incorporation of fluoride into dentin and enamel, which serves as a deterrent to secondary decay.

10. **d.** Composite cement would be the luting agent of choice because it directly bonds the ceramic restoration to tooth structure. It is assumed that a dentinal bonding system is used before the cement is applied. Composite cements are also called resin cements. Zinc phosphate and polycarboxylate are more opaque and tend to "defeat the purpose" of the esthetic, translucent properties of the ceramic. ZOE is also opaque but can only serve as a temporary luting agent due to its low strength and high solubility.

11. **a.** The advantages of polycarboxylate cement are its ability to bond to tooth structure (one of the first) and its biocompatibility. It is usually used as a luting cement and an intermediate base. Its disadvantages are lack of strength and moderate solubility.

12. **g.** Zinc oxide and eugenol cement serves many purposes for the dental patient. Formulations of ZOE are used for luting temporary crowns, temporary restorations, and intermediate bases under permanent restorations. It is soluble and lacks strength, so it is not recommended as a permanent restorative material or a luting agent for permanent crowns.

CHAPTER 8

1. **b.** A major advantage of alginate impression material is the ease of use. It is also fairly inexpensive. It is very much affected by the gain or loss of water. It should be poured as soon as possible because of its lack of stability.

2. **b.** Elastomeric impression materials, or elastomers, are flexible and may be deformed and then return to their original shape. Thermoplastic impression materials may be elastic or inelastic. They set by a physical change when cooled. Inelastic materials cannot be stretched; they also are rigid. Resins, by definition, are rigid polymers.

3. **d.** An increase in the water temperature will increase the rate of setting or shorten the gelation time. The mix is still usable regardless of water temperature as long as there is adequate working time.

4. **d.** "Aqueous" refers to water. Therefore, the impression material must be water based. In dentistry, there are two such materials: reversible and irreversible hydrocolloid. Irreversible is the only water-based choice. Polysulfides and addition silicones are elastomers. Impression compound is much like wax. ZOE impression material is an inelastic material and contains no water in its composition.

5. **b.** The brown paste in polysulfide impression material is the accelerator; the white paste is the base. Retarders are chemicals added to materials to decrease the setting rate. Fillers are added to the pastes to control the viscosity.

6. **d.** Dental impression compound is a thermoplastic material. It can be heated and softened repeatedly. Alginate is an example of an irreversible material. Once it has set, it cannot be resoftened. The other terms, chemoplastic and hydroelastic, are not used to describe impression materials.

7. **b.** ZOE impression paste sets into a hard, brittle mass. This makes it inelastic (or not elastic). Polysulfide and addition silicone are elastomers (they are elastic and will flex). Alginate also sets into an elastic material.

8. **d.** The hydrocolloids, alginate and agar, set by changing from a sol to a gel. This setting process is called gelation. Gypsum products (Chapter 9) set by a crystallization process, and elastomeric impression materials set by polymerization. In dentistry, curing is another term for polymerization.

9. **b.** The use of agar impression material does require special equipment, but the impression material is very reasonably priced. The detail reproduction is excellent, and the impression is easy to pour compared to elastomeric impression material.

10. **c.** The shrinkage and exudation of water is syneresis. Imbibition occurs when the impression absorbs water, such as during long exposure to disinfecting solutions. Gelation is the term given to the setting process of hydrocolloid material. Hysteresis refers to a material's characteristic of having a melting temperature different from its gelling temperature.

11. **a.** Addition silicones are the most popular of the elastomeric impression materials, but cost is not the reason. They are expensive. The ease of use and the excellent characteristics and properties account for their popularity.

12. **c.** The accurate fit of the custom tray to the patient's oral tissues requires an existing model. Therefore, an alginate impression is usually taken and poured with a gypsum product (stone or plaster), and the custom tray is then made on the study model.

13. **b.** Alginate would be the impression material of choice for these impressions. They are poured in dental stone and used for diagnosis and treatment planning. The accuracy of alginate is adequate for this purpose but not for final impressions. Agar and elastomeric impression materials are final impression materials, which means that casts and dies are made from these impressions on which restorations are fabricated. Dental impression compound is used for the fabrication of dentures.

14. **c.** With a triple tray, three "records" can be obtained: the prepared tooth, the bite registration, and the impression of the opposing tooth. It is considered a special use tray. A custom tray is made on a model of the patient's arch with an acrylic resin. It is custom-made by a dental professional. A stock tray is an "off the shelf" tray and can be purchased in a variety of shapes, sizes, and materials. Bite registration trays, another special use tray, record the occlusal surfaces of both arches.

15. **a.** ZOE, alginate, and addition silicone impression materials all set by a chemical reaction. Wax used as an impression material, agar, and impression compound set by a physical change and will solidify or gel when cooled. These are said to be thermoplastic materials.

CHAPTER 9

1. **a.** The amount of water added to a gypsum product is directly related to its strength. The higher the W/P ratio, as in plaster, the softer and weaker is the resulting gypsum product.

2. **d.** Potassium sulfate is a common accelerator for gypsum products, as is borax, a retarder. Oleic acid, glycerin, and ethyl alcohol are not used to change the setting time of gypsum products.

3. **d.** High-strength stone may also be called die stone, improved stone, Type IV gypsum, Densite, or modified alpha-hemihydrate. Plaster is referred to as beta-hemihydrate or Type II gypsum. Dental stone may also be called Hydrocal, Type III gypsum, or alpha-hemihydrate.

4. **b.** As a standard setting time for gypsum products, 30 to 45 minutes for a final set is given. The Gillmore needle (or fingernail) should not leave indentations and can be used to determine a final setting time.

5. **b.** For 50 g of stone, 14 to 15 mL of water is required. For 100 g of stone, 28 to 30 mL of water is used. For 50 g of improved stone, 10 to 12 mL of water is used. For 100 g of plaster, 45 to 50 mL of water is needed.

6. **c.** Study models are used for observation, diagnosis, and treatment planning. Restorations or appliances are not made on them, as they are usually constructed from weaker gypsum products. Casts are replicas that are usually constructed with improved stone, and appliances and restorations are fabricated on them. A die is a working replica of a single tooth and is usually part of a cast.

7. **a.** Increasing the setting time would mean that it takes more time for a product to set. Thus, decreasing the setting time results in a product that sets faster, requiring less time to set. Manipulating the setting time does not enhance the properties of a gypsum product; in fact, it can be deleterious to them.

8. **c.** Because plaster requires the most water for a correct mix (proper W/P ratio), it would be the weakest, softest, and most porous of the three common gypsum products. Improved stone would be the most dense and the strongest, and dental stone would fall between plaster and improved stone.

9. **b.** Dry strength refers to the strength when excess water is not present. This may be two or three times the wet strength. The wet strength is measured at the final set (30–45 minutes). The initial strength occurs when loss of gloss is present and is an indication of the working time.

10. **c.** It is recommended to first add the water and then the powder to the mixing bowl. As a result, less air is incorporated into the mix. "Eyeballing" is not recommended because the W/P ratio will not be correct and an inferior product will result. Adding water to the powder or adding powder and water to the bowl simultaneously tend to increase the porosity of the resulting mix.

11. **d.** Final setting time can be determined by attempting to penetrate the material with a dull instrument or a fingernail. Initial setting time is said to occur when the material loses its shine, or "loss of gloss." Final setting time takes approximately 30 to 45 minutes. The change from wet to dry strength usually occurs after 8 hours.

12. **a.** When setting time is increased, it takes the material longer to set. A decreased setting time yields a faster setting material or takes less time to set. If the setting reaction is decreased, the material will take longer to set, and if it is increased, it will take less time to set.

CHAPTER 10

1. **c.** The gypsum investment material that comprises the mold must be expanded to compensate exactly for the shrinkage of the metal casting. Otherwise, the cast restoration will not fit the preparation of the patient's tooth.

2. **c.** The mold (investment) must expand and provide compensation for the metal contraction during casting. The main, obvious purpose of the investment, however, is to create a mold from the wax pattern in the casting process.

3. **c.** Porcelain has outstanding esthetic properties, such as translucency and life-like appearance. It is very brittle, however, and may fracture when subjected to high occlusal forces. It is recommended for veneers and low-stress crowns for anterior teeth, such as maxillary lateral incisors.

4. **b.** The "crown" portion of a dental bridge is called a retainer. Joined to the retainers are the artificial, replacement teeth called pontics. The prepared teeth onto which the bridge is cemented are called abutments.

5. **e.** Inlay wax is used for casting procedures. It leaves no residue in the burnout process and has a higher melting temperature. It is also harder than other dental waxes. Sticky wax is also a hard wax that melts at a higher temperature, but this wax is used as an "attachment medium," such as attaching a sprue to a pattern. Boxing wax is used to pour impressions, and baseplate wax is used in the fabrication of dentures.

6. **c.** Burnout during casting is done to eliminate the wax pattern and create a mold space for the molten metal. Investment covers the wax pattern that has been mounted within the casting ring with a sprue. The crucible becomes heated when the solid casting metal is melted and turned into liquid, but it is an adjunct to the melting of the metal. Shrinkage compensation is necessary for the mold; it must expand the exact amount that the metal will shrink during casting.

7. **a.** Once the pattern is waxed, the sprue is gently attached with inlay or sticky wax. It is then placed into the crucible former (also called the sprue base). Next, a gypsum investment is usually vacuum mixed and poured into the casting ring that contains the wax pattern (investing process). After the casting ring is "burned out," the metal is melted and forced into the casting ring (casting).

8. **c.** Thirty-three percent of 1,000 parts is 333. Fineness is described in parts per 1,000; hence, 33% gold alloy would be expressed as 333 fine or 8 carat. A 50% gold alloy would be 500 fine or 12 carat.

9. **b.** Changing porcelain powder to a solid is called sintering. The powder is not melted, so the shape of the restoration is maintained. Burnishing involves pushing the metal toward the tooth to close gaps between the casting and the tooth. Investing is covering a wax pattern mounted in a casting ring with a mixed gypsum product (investment).

10. **a.** It is true that castable glass is one type of an all-ceramic restoration. All-ceramic restorations are not superior to ceramometal restorations in the aspect of strength and that makes the second statement false.

11. **c.** Amalgam, gold foil, and composite restorations are direct restorations, which mean that they are constructed directly in the oral cavity. It usually involves placing the restorative material "directly" into the cavity preparation. Other restorations, such as inlays, onlays, crowns, and bridges, are constructed outside of the oral cavity, in a dental laboratory. Hence, they are referred to as "indirect" restorations. The term "fixed" is used to designate that it is not removable because it is cemented, or luted, in place. A fixed restoration is not removable by the patient.

12. **b.** A veneer is a thin layer of material that covers another material. In dentistry, it is a restoration that is placed on the facial surface of anterior teeth to cover, or "veneer," esthetic problems. A buildup (core) is when the crown of a tooth is broken down to the point of needing to be "rebuilt" to hold the final restoration. A coping is the metal substructure that supports the porcelain layers in a ceramometal restoration. A pontic is a replacement tooth.

13. **d.** A provisional crown is the appropriate, professional name (especially used by prosthodontists) for a temporary crown.

14. **c.** Precious metals include the noble metals and silver. The noble metals are gold, platinum, and palladium. Nonprecious metals are those that do not contain any noble elements. High-noble metals contain 60% or more gold and other noble elements.

15. **a.** Bonding porcelain to metal in a ceramometal restoration provides a precise fit to the prepared tooth structure. The disadvantage is the opacity, because of the metal. There is no difference in the patient's ability to remove plaque whether it be an all ceramic or ceramometal crown.

CHAPTER 11

1. **b.** Once the denture teeth are set in the wax rims, it is called a denture setup. The other terms are not used to describe this step of denture fabrication and are listed as distracters.

2. **a.** A thin layer of material is ground away. The monomer is applied to dissolve some of the set material. One end of the dissolved polymer remains embedded in the acrylic denture resin. New material is then mixed and applied, and the new polymer chains entangle with the old dissolved chains.

Applying monomer to the surface does not affect the setting reaction, finishing and polishing, or color of the denture.

3. **d.** The major difference between heat-activated and chemically activated resin systems is that no chemical activator is present in the liquid of the heat-activated resins. Heat-activated resins have more strength than chemically activated resins, and there is less, not more, inhibitor in the heat-activated liquid.

4. **a.** Today's denture teeth are usually acrylic rather than porcelain. Porcelain teeth are, however, harder than acrylic teeth and cause excessive wear to the natural opposing teeth.

5. **c.** Partial denture frameworks usually include clasps, connectors, and mesh. The denture base and teeth are not considered to be part of the framework, although they are a part of the removable partial denture.

6. **b.** Toughness is the ability of a material to absorb energy beyond the yield point, up to the failure point. Resilience is the ability to absorb energy and not become deformed until it reaches the yield point. Fatigue is the failure of an object after being stressed repeatedly for a long time. Creep is the small change in shape that results when an object is under continuous compression.

7. **b.** A maxillary denture is much easier to wear than a mandibular denture because of the extension of the borders of the denture (which helps to create the seal) and the larger surface-bearing area. Saliva helps to achieve the seal and improve the suction.

8. **d.** The wax rims serve many purposes. They are used to determine the patient's midline, plane of occlusion, and the size of the denture teeth needed.

9. **c.** Partial dentures are processed the same way as a complete denture except that the acrylic resin must flow through and around the mesh of the framework. The finishing, polishing, and processing techniques take approximately the same amount of time.

10. **Answer: 3, 6, 8, 5, 7, 1, 10, 2, 9, and 4.** After a master cast is made from patient impressions, a chemically activated resin baseplate and wax rims are constructed on it. These are tried in the patient's mouth and used to mount the master casts on an articulator. Next, the denture teeth are set in wax. This "wax denture" is called the denture setup and is inserted into the patient's mouth as the "wax try-in." Once the dentist and patient are satisfied with the fit, occlusion, function, esthetics, and phonetics, the master cast and denture setup are embedded in stone within the denture flask. The flask is heated in hot water and the wax is flushed out, creating a mold space. The denture teeth remain embedded in stone. The acrylic resin is mixed and placed in the mold, and the mold is then compressed. The closed mold is heated in a water bath to activate the resin. After processing, the denture is removed from the mold, finished, polished, and disinfected.

CHAPTER 12

1. **d.** Endosseous or tooth form implants are screwed or pressed into a cut hole in the bone. Transosseous or staple implants include a plate and bolts that go through the mandible in the anterior region. Subperiosteal implants involve two surgeries, an impression, cast, and a metal framework.

2. **c.** A healing cap is placed on the implant during the second surgery. It extends out of the mucosa into the oral cavity. Once this heals and epithelial tissues are formed, the healing cap is removed, and an abutment is placed. Impressions may be necessary before treatment is completed, but they are not taken during the second surgery. Osseointegration is not measured during either surgery.

3. **b.** The patient must maintain excellent plaque control and practice frequent and effective oral hygiene to ensure longevity of the implant. The dentist would adjust and monitor the occlusion of the implant with the opposing teeth. Fluoride applications at home are not typical for maintenance of implants.

4. **d.** The temperature of the bone must not be greater than 117°F or 47°C when the surgical handpiece is being used. The bone can be heated a little past body temperature (98.6°F). The temperature of 117°C is equivalent to 243°F and would definitely damage the bone tissue.

5. **a.** Patients with systemic diseases, such as diabetes, are contraindicated for dental implants. Smokers and patients practicing poor oral hygiene are also poor candidates for implants. Recurrent caries are not associated with contraindications for dental implants.

6. **c.** It is true that titanium is very difficult to cast and does not have high strength compared to other metals. The strength of titanium is adequate for implants and will osseointegrate with bone.

7. **b.** An alveolar ridge having no teeth is said to be edentulous. In most cases, when the mandibular arch atrophies, it becomes smaller in size due to aging. An atrophic edentulous mandible is one that has no teeth, is very "low" and small, and would not be adequate to support a denture. The word "iatrogenic" means "caused by a professional by accident" and the word "dentulous" means "with, or having, teeth."

8. **c.** The patient's home care regimen may consist of only a toothbrush and floss, or a variety of many auxiliary aids. The hygienist will work with the patient to select the proper aids and instruct in their use to accomplish the necessary removal of plaque. Many appointments may be needed to achieve this. Plaque removal by the patient is critical for the health and longevity of the implant. Without excellent homecare maintenance, the implant may fail over time.

9. **d.** In the first surgery, an implant is placed. In the next surgery, a healing cap is placed, which is exposed to the oral cavity. Later, the healing cap is removed and an abutment is placed on the implant. It acts as an abutment of a bridge and supports the prosthesis. A cylinder is then placed on the abutment, and then, a crown is placed on the cylinder. All of these attachments are depicted in *Figure 12.4*.

10. **c.** The scope of practice of a dental hygienist does not include selecting restorative materials for tooth restoration. However, a very important role of the hygienist is patient education, determining the time between dental hygiene visits, and selecting the best auxiliary aids for the patient to achieve optimal plaque removal.

CHAPTER 13

1. **b.** Obturate refers to the filling and sealing of the root canal once the pulp tissue is removed. Accessing the canal means to create an opening through the tooth to the pulp chamber. This is done with a handpiece and bur.

2. **b.** Macrofilled composite resins have large filler particles compared to microfills and hybrids. A metal instrument drawn across residual composite will result in a gray line. The filler particles in the resin are harder than the metal explorer and will abrade the metal tip, thus leaving a metal residue (gray line) on the remaining composite. The filler particles in microfill and hybrid composites are much smaller than the macrofill particles, and they may not leave a gray line.

3. **d.** An apicoectomy surgically removes 1 to 3 mm of the root apex. A retrofill is preparing, filling, and sealing of the apical end of the root. A root resection, another surgical procedure, is the removal of an entire root of a multirooted tooth. Retreatment is root canal therapy performed a second time.

4. **c.** Irrigants are aqueous solutions used to disinfect the canal system. Common irrigants are sodium hypochlorite, saline, and chlorhexidine gluconate. Paper points are used to dry the root canal. Sealers are a type of cement used to coat the canal and to fill in voids between the canal wall and gutta–percha. Gutta–percha is a polymeric material with zinc oxide and barium sulfate added.

5. **d.** A retainer is a fixed (bonded) or removable appliance to prevent relapse after active orthodontic treatment is completed. A bracket is a small metal, ceramic, or polymer material that has a centered, horizontal slot. The archwire fits into the slot of each bracket, usually across the entire arch. A ligature, either wire or elastic, secures the archwire into the bracket slot.

6. **a.** Brackets are secured to the tooth surface by acid etching and composite resin. Dental cements may be used to secure bands to the tooth (molars). Chemically activated resins are used to make custom trays and denture fabrication and repairs. Ligatures secure the archwire into the bracket slot.

7. **d.** Lateral condensation is used to fill the root canal with gutta–percha. Condensation is a term used in dentistry to describe the method of compressing and filling a small area in a tooth, such as a preparation or root canal. Of all the answers, this one is most appropriate.

8. **a.** For permanent molars, a pulpotomy is a temporary procedure and is followed by root canal therapy. For primary molars, it is a permanent procedure and is restored with a stainless-steel crown. This will maintain space and function until the permanent molar takes its place.

9. **b.** Orthodontic brackets are bonded onto the facial surfaces and hold an arch wire in place on each tooth in the arch. The brackets transfer the forces of the wire, springs, and elastics to the teeth. Bands encircle the crown and are used on molars because they require more force to move compared to other teeth. Retainers are used to prevent relapse after treatment. Composite resin is used to attach the bracket to the tooth surface.

10. **c.** Surgical silk suture is nonabsorbable and must be removed at a later appointment. Absorbable sutures are usually placed on the inside of the body, and since the body resorbs them, a later appointment for removal is not necessary. Surgical gut suture is one type of absorbable suture.

CHAPTER 14

1. **c.** Glass ionomers, ceramic materials, and composite are the restorative materials that could be adversely affected by acidulated phosphate fluoride (APF). Because glass is a component of each of these materials, the APF could etch these surfaces and result in a dull appearance and diminished luster.

2. **c.** When scalers and curettes are used around cast gold margins, use of a horizontal or oblique stroke, rather than a vertical one, is recommended. Vertical strokes have a tendency to "lift" the tightly adapted gold margins next to tooth structure. Posterior instruments are recommended for posterior teeth. Sonic and ultrasonic scalers are not recommended for use on cemented castings because they could fracture the cement underneath.

3. **d.** A dull sound would be heard from an explorer on composites and glass ionomers. Sharp sounds would be heard from gold foil, base metal alloys, enamel, dentin, amalgam, and cast gold.

4. **d.** Tactile sensitivity is derived from the sense of touch. When the clinician *lightly* holds an instrument, such as an explorer, the character of a surface is transmitted from the tip through the shank and then through the handle and into the clinician's fingertips. Therefore, the clinician would be distinguishing rough from smooth surfaces. Distinguishing dull sounds from sharp addresses auditory capabilities, or the sense of hearing; glossy from dull is a visual determination; and opaque from translucent are characteristics pertaining to radiographs.

5. **b.** When high heat is created during amalgam polishing, surface characteristics will be altered when temperatures reach or exceed 140°F. At high temperatures, mercury is released from the amalgam, which causes accelerated (not arrested) corrosion and marginal breakdown. Surfaces should be smoother, not rougher, after finishing and polishing. Tactile, rather than auditory, sensitivity is the criterion that best describes polishing (from rough surface to smooth), rather than a "dull" compared to a "sharp" sound.

6. **a.** The agents of choice for a final polish of a gold crown intraorally are silex and tin oxide. Brown and green polishing points are used for the initial steps. Aluminum oxide discs are used on composites, and prophylaxis pastes are used for porcelain.

7. **a.** There is much less heat production when a wet or moist abrasive or polishing agent is used compared to when it is dry. Swallowing and rinsing does not play a major role when using a moist polishing agent. In actuality, a dry polishing agent would remove stain faster than a moist one.

8. **b.** When the margins of a cast gold restoration have been marginated, it means the dentist has used hand instruments to adapt the edges of the restoration tightly to the preparation. The term "try-in" is used to describe if a casting fits precisely into the preparation before cementation. Margination and marginal ridges have very little in common. Marginal ridges are the mesial and distal boundaries of the occlusal surface. The gingival margin is the edge of the gingiva nearest to the incisal or occlusal surface.

9. **b.** Because gold and/or gold foil are metallic restorations, like amalgam, they may be polished in a similar manner. The surface hardness of glass ionomer and composite are softer, and the abrasives used on gold would be too abrasive for these materials. The porcelain on a PFM restoration could essentially be polished with porcelain polishing points; the metal portion would be polished similar to amalgam or gold.

10. **d.** Because glass ionomer, porcelain, and composite are made of glass particles or particles very similar to glass, the acidulated fluoride will etch the outer surface and cause a loss of reflection or possibly dull the appearance of the restoration.

CHAPTER 15

1. **b.** Dental hygienists must collect and assess data to formulate a dental hygiene diagnosis. They must recognize anatomy, landmarks, and restorations to identify normal from abnormal, both clinically and radiographically. Dental hygienists do not legally provide a definitive diagnosis to the patient or prescribe radiographs.

2. **c.** The radiographic appearance for contrast of different objects in the mouth depends on the thickness and composition of the object/material. Very dense (compact) objects/materials absorb or attenuate more of the x-rays, thus allowing less of the primary beam to hit the film emulsion and fewer silver halide crystals to be exposed.

3. **d.** Less dense (compact) objects/materials absorb fewer x-rays and appear radiolucent on the radiograph. More dense objects appear radiopaque.

4. **a.** Gutta-percha, although not a dense material, has fillers added to make it more dense and radiopaque.

5. **a.** Porcelain is radiolucent, and metal is radiopaque. When the two materials are combined in the fabrication of a crown (PFM), both the opacity and the lucency can be viewed. This is because of the density of the metal and the less-compact porcelain materials.

6. **b.** Orthodontic bands are metal and are radiographically opaque. Because the band encircles the entire tooth, it prohibits the practitioner from viewing the proximal or occlusal surfaces of the tooth on a radiographic film. Whether the band is bonded or cemented on the tooth does not make a difference. Fogging would appear radiolucent, not radiopaque.

7. **c.** A resorbable periodontal material used to heal and/or repair is not dense or compact enough to be viewed on a radiograph. What can be viewed as a radiolucency is the loss of periodontal bone. In the healing or repairing process, the alveolar bone "fills in" with new bone, which will be viewed as radiopaque.

8. **c.** A base is somewhat dense because it is radiographically visible. Yet, the base is not as dense as the metal restoration. As a result, some x-rays pass through the base material to expose the silver halide crystals in the gelatin. This is not true of the metal restoration because the x-rays are absorbed (attenuated) by the metal, not allowing them to pass through, thus resulting in an opaque image. If an object is translucent, it means you can see through it, as light will pass through. If an object is opaque, you will not be able to see through it.

9. **c.** It is important to be able to distinguish dental materials from tooth tissues. Therefore, the shape of materials placed on and in the tooth should be somewhat different from the expected anatomy of the tooth. The composition, size, or

amount of the restorative material is not a radiographically distinguishing critical feature when differentiating a radiopaque dental material from tooth tissues.

10. **c.** The composition and the amount of filler particles add density to the material when viewed radiographically. This density makes them more radiopaque, which distinguishes them from carious lesions. Compressive strength, elasticity, and coefficients of thermal expansion have nothing to do with the radiographic appearance of the restoration.

CHAPTER 16

1. **d.** Emery is the abrasive that is sometimes referred to as corundum. It is a natural form of aluminum oxide and appears as grayish-black sand. Tin oxide and pumice are abrasive powders, and garnet is a dark-red abrasive that is usually found on coated disks.

2. **b.** Pumice is a silica-like volcanic glass that is used to polish enamel, gold foil, amalgam, and acrylic denture bases. Aluminum oxide is another name for emery. Sand is a form of quartz, may be of various colors, and is bonded to paper disks for grinding metals and plastics. Zirconium silicate is a common abrasive in dentifrices.

3. **b.** Calcium carbonate is also called chalk or whiting. It is a mild abrasive, usually supplied in powder form, and mixed with a "vehicle" (liquid) to produce a slurry. Silex and pumice are used in the same manner. Aluminum oxide is an abrasive that is found in many grits, bonded onto disks and strips, and impregnated into rubber wheels and points.

4. **a.** The abrasive particle must be harder than the surface being abraded to achieve the desired result. If it is softer, the surface meant to be abraded will not be, and instead, the abrasive will be worn away.

5. **d.** Hardness of the abrasive particle, particle size, particle shape, pressure, speed, and lubrication used, all affect the rate of abrasion. Bonded and coated abrasives encompass a wide variety of agents. They are usually bonded, impregnated, or coated onto disks, strips, points, rubber wheels, burs, or stones.

6. **d.** Finishing is the term used when producing the final shape and contour of a restoration. Polishing is the abrasion of a surface to reduce the size of the scratches until the surface appears shiny. Abrasion is the wearing away of a surface. Cutting is removing material by a shearing-off process. Examples of cutting are milling, machining, or drilling.

7. **c.** "Vehicles," usually liquids, are used with powders to create a slurry. Examples of vehicles used with powders include water, glycerin, alcohol, and mouthwash. Rubber cups and brushes as well as felt cones are devices used in polishing teeth and dental appliances.

8. **c.** Both statements are true. Abrasives are used in a series (most abrasive to least abrasive) during polishing. The same agent (from larger grit to smaller grit) or different agents (from most abrasive to least abrasive) may be used. The size of the scratches becomes smaller as the chosen abrasive becomes finer, until the scratches finally are smaller than the wavelength of visible light. When the scratches are this size, the surface appears shiny.

9. **b.** It has been documented in the literature that up to 3 to 4 μm of enamel may be removed when polishing with pumice. This coronal portion of the tooth is the fluoride-rich layer of enamel that has been absorbing fluoride from various sources, including food, water, dentifrices, and topical fluoride applications.

10. **d.** Ideal prophylaxis pastes should possess the characteristics of high polish and low abrasion. A high polish produces the shiny, smooth surface as a result of polishing, and low abrasion refers to the grit of the abrasive within the paste and the resulting "scratches" that it leaves on the surface after "polishing."

11. **a.** Table 16.1 lists restorative materials, abrasives, and tooth tissues in the order of their hardness. Pumice is harder than enamel, but amalgam, composite, and gold alloy are all softer than enamel.

12. **b.** Air powder polishing is designed to remove plaque, biofilm (soft deposits), and stain. This equipment is unlike a sonic or ultrasonic scaler that would remove calculus. It is designed as a "polisher" combining air, water, and an abrasive agent under pressure.

13. **c.** Silica is the most frequently used abrasive in dentifrices. The other two dentifrices used in recent years are phosphates and carbonates.

14. **c.** A finely ground diamond powder would be used to polish esthetic restorations. Calcium carbonate and pumice would be found in specific traditional prophylaxis pastes. Emery is an abrasive that is mostly used in dental laboratory procedures.

15. **a.** The traditional prophy paste would be used on the stain on the natural teeth. The tin oxide is recommended for the gold, and the polishing agent for the esthetic restorations would be used on the composite restorations. Pumice and silex have been used to remove heavy stains on natural teeth in the past and are also used for polishing amalgams. In the selection of polishing agents for restorations and natural teeth, it is important to remove the deposit with the least abrasive agent.

CHAPTER 17

1. **d.** A nonvital tooth is one that does not have a live (vital) pulp. The pulp may be present but necrotic, missing, or replaced with a root canal filling material.

2. **b.** Tooth structure must be removed to obtain an opening into the pulp chamber of a nonvital tooth. A facial veneer requires removal of facial tooth structure, and a porcelain-bonded-to-metal crown requires removal of tooth structure from all surfaces.

3. **c.** Carbamide peroxide is more stable than hydrogen peroxide. It is used only in the vital tooth whitening technique. It decomposes into hydrogen peroxide and is used in concentrations from 10% to 20%. Hydrogen peroxide decomposes into water and oxygen radicals.

4. **a.** Any number of teeth can be treated at the same time. A full arch of teeth can be treated in the same time as one tooth in the same arch. The strength of the product, the type of stain, and the time of exposure all affect the success of the bleaching process.

5. **d.** Extrinsic stains are more effectively treated than intrinsic stains and discolorations. Tetracycline-stained teeth and teeth with fluorosis are difficult to treat.

6. **b.** Tooth sensitivity, the most common side effect associated with tooth whitening, is usually reversible. After the treatment is discontinued, it should be absent in a few days. Potassium nitrate and neutral sodium fluoride are common topical agents used in the active treatment of tooth sensitivity. A tray made of rigid material frequently produces pressure on one or more teeth to cause sensitivity.

7. **d.** Esthetic dental procedures are increasing in popularity, but the procedure most commonly used today is tooth whitening.

8. **a.** Brushing with a potassium nitrate–containing dentifrice will aid in reducing tooth sensitivity that may occur during/after whitening. Anesthesia should not be used during power bleaching so that a patient could respond to any painful stimuli possibly produced by excessive heat created during the procedure.

9. **d.** The restoration should not be placed sooner than 1 to 2 weeks, preferably 2 weeks. The bonding capabilities of composite are initially weaker post bleaching and usually return after 1 week. The tooth initially lightens but tends to darken and remains a stable color around 2 weeks posttreatment. Any sooner placement will result in a composite that may not match or may not adhere to tooth structure.

10. **d.** All of the conditions except previous use of the nightguard bleaching system is contraindicated. Patients using photosensitive drugs, undergoing chemotherapy or radiation therapy, or having a history of melanoma are all at additional risks of medical complications with light-activated bleaching systems. Many patients move from the use of nightguard tray systems to the light-activated systems in search of better and quicker whitening results.

11. **d.** Currently, the aqueous cleaning technology is only available in swabs. Tray whiteners may come in gel. The aqueous cleaning technology is a liquid and is dispensed in a swab. This product does not come in a strip form.

12. **c.** Although manufacturers' pamphlets and SDS information may address safety issues, dental professionals should be aware that a nonbiased statement on safety and effectiveness of whitening products is available on the ADA Web site. The ADHA has no such statement.

CHAPTER 18

1. **d.** The goal of oral appliance therapy is to enlarge the airway and to reduce its collapsibility to maintain an adequate airway during sleep. Reducing the airway would make it more difficult to maintain adequate breathing.

2. **d.** According to published research, patients wearing an oral appliance during sleep have demonstrated no changes in their periodontal health. There have been no increases in periodontal conditions or diseases reported with use of the oral appliance.

3. **c.** Athletic mouthguards, when worn correctly and consistently, may prevent a concussion by aiding absorption of the dynamic pressures of head trauma.

4. **b.** Nightguards are worn to alleviate tooth surface wear by absorbing occlusal pressure that occurs from grinding of teeth during sleep. Nightguards have not been reported to decrease dental caries. Orthodontic appliances may be worn to provide minor tooth movement or teeth stabilization. Space maintainers temporarily hold teeth in position.

5. **d.** Stock mouthguards are premade, in various sizes, and may be purchased at athletic and department stores. Custom mouthguards are fabricated by dental professionals to fit the patient's arch; they require an impression and cast.

6. **a.** Thermoplastic material will soften on heating and reharden on cooling. This makes them ideal for adapting to an individual's dentition.

7. **a.** Wet, soft-bristled toothbrushes are recommended to clean oral appliances. Commercial liquid cleaners are also available for soaking. Hot water is not recommended because of possible distortion of the appliance.

8. **d.** Mouth protectors can be custom-made by the dental professional, bought at a store in a pre-sized selection (stock mouthguard), and prepared through the "boil and bite" method by the individual.

9. **c.** Space maintainers are used to temporarily hold teeth in position. For example, if a deciduous molar is prematurely lost, a space maintainer may be used to keep the adjacent teeth from moving into that area where the tooth is missing. Nightguards are worn to alleviate bruxism. Custom whitening trays are designed to hold whitening solutions. Sleep apnea is alleviated by an appliance that enlarges the airway.

10. **a.** It is vital that the athletic mouthguard be compatible with the athlete's dentition, so that the force can be absorbed by the appliance and the athlete will be more likely to wear the appliance when needed. In most cases, athletic mouthguards are fabricated for maxillary teeth.

11. **c.** The gingival contours of teeth should be detailed or replicated in an oral appliance because they are needed to help the appliance fit properly and aid with retention. The sulcus and periodontal ligament are essentially subgingival and do not aid in retention of the appliance. The soft palate is located posterior to the hard palate and is not adjacent to the teeth, so it would not help to retain the appliance.

12. **c.** An adult patient undergoing radiation for head or neck cancer is at increased risk for dental caries. The radiation damages the salivary glands, resulting in xerostomia, which in turn contributes to caries. Fluoride will not aid in the treatment of halitosis or periodontal disease. A 3-year-old may not be compliant in the use of custom trays, and there is an increased risk of ingesting fluoride.

CHAPTER 19

1. **b.** Tarnish is a corrosive attack that produces a film or layer on a metal surface. Corrosion is a process in which a metal is changed to a metal oxide. Electrochemical corrosion is a combination of a chemical reaction and the flow of an electric current. Galvanic corrosion is an electrochemical process in a wet environment. Two dissimilar metals and an electrolyte solution cause a current to flow, which results in corrosion.

2. **c.** Passivation is done in the manufacture of instruments and creates a layer of chromium oxide on the instrument surface to protect it from corrosion. Electroplating is the process of coating with metal by means of an electric current. Electropolishing produces a smooth, highly polished finish that is less likely to corrode. Alloys are made by combining two or more metals in a molten state.

3. **d.** The standard protocol for chemical vapor sterilization is 270°F, 20 to 40 psi, for at least 20 minutes (not 10 minutes, as in choice "c"). Steam autoclaving occurs at 270°F, 27 psi, for at least 6 minutes. Dry heat sterilization involves 2 hours and a temperature of 320°F.

4. **a.** Risks are involved when re-tipping instruments, but frequent breakage between the shank and tip is not listed as one of the many risks. These risks include detachment, contamination, imbalance, and wear rates.

5. **b.** Three questions need to be asked to determine when instruments should be sharpened: First, "How many times a day did I, or will I, use that instrument?" Second, "What degree of difficulty did I, or will I, encounter while using this instrument?" Third, "For what procedures did I use, or will I be using, the instrument?"

6. **d.** The major components of stainless steel alloy are iron, chromium, and nickel.

7. **a.** The disadvantage of using noble metals in the fabrication of instruments is cost. They are very expensive compared to stainless steel or carbon steel. Pitting and corrosion will not occur with noble metals and would be ideal for instrument composition. A faster wear rate may occur with "noble metal instruments" compared to carbon steel and stainless steel instruments, but it is not the major disadvantage.

8. **c.** Dry heat sterilization is used when items to be sterilized cannot withstand compressed steam conditions. Unsaturated chemical vapor sterilization is recommended for carbon steel instruments, but disadvantages include odor and a need for ventilation. The temperature for steam autoclaving is 270°F, and for dry heat, it is 320°F; therefore, materials that cannot withstand these heat sterilization processes should be sterilized with chemical solutions.

9. **c.** The correct sequence in the instrument maintenance cycle is to use sterile instruments, inspect them after use, clean them appropriately, sterilize them, and then sharpen sterile instruments. The safest time to sharpen instruments is after sterilization, immediately before use.

10. **b.** Electropolishing is the procedure that produces a highly polished finish. Passivation is the creation of a corrosion-resistant chromium oxide layer. Cryogenics is the science of very low temperatures, far below the freezing point of water. Heat treatment is a combination of heating and cooling operations timed and applied to a metal or alloy, that result in desired mechanical properties.

CHAPTER 20

1. **c.** PPE must not be worn out of the treatment area because it is contaminated from splatter and aerosol and, thus, is a source of infection.

2. **b.** Nonsterile exam gloves are sufficient for most dental procedures. Sterile surgeon's gloves are necessary only during invasive (surgical) procedures. Neither copolymer gloves nor utility gloves are acceptable for any intraoral procedure.

3. **c.** Because of the potential for leakage of gloves, hands should be washed before donning and after removing the gloves. In October 2002, the CDC endorsed the use of alcohol-based products for hand cleaning as long as the hands are not visibly contaminated.

4. **c.** Utility gloves are the thickest gloves and provide more protection against potential injury from a sharp instrument.

5. **c.** If a patient with a highly infectious disease spread by aerosol is treated, a HEPA mask must be worn to filter out microbes. Standard masks do not have a high-enough filtration capability. The use of surgeon's gloves does not protect against aerosol, and a face shield allows for suction of aerosol up under the shield.

6. **a.** Sharp objects must be disposed of in hard, puncture-resistant containers and not in cardboard boxes or plastic bags.

7. **e.** Glutaraldehydes are high-level disinfectants in which items must be immersed. They are too toxic to be sprayed.

8. **c.** Both statements are true. An acceptable disinfectant must kill both hydrophilic and lipophilic viruses. The protein coating on hydrophilic viruses makes them much more difficult to kill compared to lipophilic viruses.

9. **a.** According to Spaulding's classification, any item with the potential to penetrate soft tissue or bone is considered to be a "critical" item and must be heat sterilized only.

10. **c.** Neither disinfection nor sterilization will occur if bioburden is not first removed from the object being disinfected or sterilized.

11. **c.** This amount of time is necessary for antibody detection and is recommended by the CDC. If seroconversion is going to occur, it will happen within 2 months. Waiting several months to a year without knowledge of seroconversion, the individual may become susceptible to hepatitis.

12. **a.** The CDC recommends that biological monitoring be conducted at least weekly, any time an implant is sterilized, or sooner if sterilizer malfunction is ed. Monitoring is the only way sterilization can be assured.

13. **c.** Steel-toed shoes will protect the feet from falling objects but are not common in dental offices. Fire extinguishers, GFCI outlets, neoprene (rubber) gloves, and eye protection are common.

14. **e.** Mercury, disinfectants, latex gloves, and nitrous oxide have all caused problems to health care workers. Fluorescent lighting has not.

15. **c.** A variety of chemicals in the dental office can penetrate latex gloves. Information regarding the proper protective gloves is found in the safety data sheet.

16. **c.** Poor lighting, poor posture, and repetitive motions contribute to musculoskeletal problems. Use of indirect vision contributes to proper posture and lower strain on the back and neck.

17. **a.** Mercury (Hg) vapor is the most hazardous form of Hg encountered in a dental office. It is readily absorbed by the lungs. Liquid Hg is also hazardous because it has a high vapor pressure. Dental amalgam is safe, however, because the Hg is bound in a metallic compound. The same is true for amalgam scrap.

CHAPTER 21

1. **c.** All blood and saliva must be cleaned from any item before application of a disinfectant because they inhibit disinfection.

2. **c.** Disinfecting appliances is not indicated when adjustments at chairside are performed as long as sterile handpieces, burs, and rag wheels are used.

3. **b.** Do not clean ultrasonically by placing appliances directly into solution in the ultrasonic holding tank. All other statements must be followed. When cleaning the appliance in an ultrasonic unit, however, the appliance must be placed in a leak-proof, zippered bag or sterile glass beaker that contains fresh ultrasonic solution. Then, the bag or beaker is placed in the solution in the holding tank. This will prevent cross-contamination during cleaning.

4. **b.** Neither statement nor reason is correct. Even though a dental prosthesis is disinfected before making adjustments with a rag wheel in the laboratory and before returning the prosthesis to the patient, there is the potential for cross-contamination between patients if a sterile rag wheel is not used for each patient's prosthesis.

5. **c.** A zippered plastic bag containing mouthwash and water is the recommended storage method. Water is needed for hydration and to prevent distortion. The mouthwash provides a pleasant taste for the patient. The patient's stone cast would not be clean. An individualized, closed container (denture cup) must have a liquid in it to prevent distortion of the prostheses.

6. **c.** The primary goal is to prevent cross-contamination. This includes protecting the patient and laboratory personnel from each other, as well as the dental office staff and laboratory equipment.

7. **c.** When using a spray, constant contact with all the surfaces cannot be assured. Spraying twice is not a recommended method, and only the aerosol of glutaraldehydes is considered toxic.

CHAPTER 22

1. **c.** The tubes of paste/paste materials have openings sized to dispense the proper ratio of pastes when equal lengths are utilized.

2. **c.** It is important to read, understand, and follow directions. Understanding the procedures involved when using a material will reduce the likelihood of an error.

3. **c.** Dental materials well set faster in the mouth than on the countertop of bracket tray. The increased temperature of the mouth will accelerate the set. The other three statements are true.

4. **d.** Dental materials should be mixed aggressively, as they cannot be harmed or damaged. Mixing slowly or in increments (for most materials) may affect the setting rate and characteristics of the material.

CHAPTER 23

1. **c.** Both calcium hydroxide and ZOE are significantly accelerated by humidity as water increases ionization of the components and thus setting.

2. **b.** ZOE has a sedative or obtundent effect on the dental pulp. Calcium hydroxide and glass ionomer are fairly neutral, whereas zinc phosphate is initially irritating.

3. **c.** Zinc phosphate cement is mixed slowly to dissipate the heat of the setting reaction. ZOE takes time to mix because of the effort required to incorporate sufficient powder. Calcium hydroxide and glass ionomer cements are mixed quickly.

4. **d.** Glass ionomer cements should be used before they lose their glossy appearance. If the cement is dull, the setting reaction may have progressed to the point where adhesion is decreased.

5. **a.** To be useful as a dental material, set dental cements must be insoluble in water and therefore cannot be cleaned with soap and water. Cleaning is much easier before these materials set as they can be wiped off instruments and washed with soap and water.

6. **a.** Resin composite cements can be bonded to tooth structures with the same bonding systems, which are used to bond a resin composite restoration to dentin and enamel. ZOE and zinc phosphate do not bond to tooth structure. Glass ionomer is self-adhesive.

CHAPTER 24

1. **b.** 6 × 6 inch square is the most common pre-cut size of rubber dam material. The 5 × 5 inch square is used for primary dentition or anterior teeth.

2. **e.** All of the above are used on the removal of the rubber dam, see Table 24.2.

3. **c.** If possible, the treatment tooth is mesial to the anchor to allow access without interference by the clamp. If the treatment tooth was distal to the anchor tooth, the clamp would interfere with access during treatment.

4. **c.** The rubber dam is contraindicated for patients with severe asthma. Visibility, patient protection, and moisture control are all indications for rubber dam placement.

5. **c.** The butterfly-shaped clamp is used to isolate the facial surfaces of anterior and some posterior teeth and retract the adjacent gingiva.

CHAPTER 25

1. **c.** Dental sealants are effective in preventing dental caries by eliminating sites difficult to clean with normal patient oral hygiene. They do not contribute to remineralization of tooth structure, so they do not reverse decay or restore enamel integrity.

2. **b.** Enamel appears chalky white when properly etched because the surface is microscopically rough. The etched surface scatters light-like ground glass rather than reflecting it like a smooth mirror.

3. **c.** After placing, the sealant should be checked for both high occlusal contacts with articulating paper and open interproximal contacts with floss.

4. **b.** It is recommended that the liquid etchants should be rinsed between 10 and 15 seconds and gel etchants at least 30 seconds. Not removing etchant thoroughly will result in inadequate retention.

5. **a.** Many times an occlusal adjustment is needed with filled sealants. However, using articulating paper and a #6 or #8 round bur is not the only acceptable method. The clinician may also use a green or white stone with articulating paper.

CHAPTER 26

1. **b.** A Class II preparation lacks the necessary box-like shape and therefore requires a matrix band to complete the needed shape. Class I and V preparations have a box-like shape. Class III and IV preparations are usually restored with composite materials. A metal matrix band would prevent light-activated polymerization.

2. **b.** The soft putty-like amalgam material is pushed into the cavity preparation to compress the various increments onto each other to minimize voids. The unset material is too thick to flow. Shear, pull, or rotation movements of the condenser will not produce the desired density.

3. **b.** Tin oxide is used as a polishing agent to produce a high luster on amalgam restorations. Due to the larger size of abrasive particles, alumina, zirconium silicate, and flour of pumice do not produce a high luster.

4. **d.** Excessive heat generation may produce an increased susceptibility to breakdown and corrosion. Pulpal injury, a release of mercury to the surface, and a dull appearance all may result from overheating the amalgam.

5. **b.** The surface is discolored. Tarnish is a removable surface film or discoloration on the amalgam. It does not affect the internal integrity of the restoration.

6. **c.** Both statements are true. It is important to begin with coarser abrasives and progress to less abrasive materials. Coarse abrasives produce larger scratches and as the operator progresses to smaller abrasives, the larger scratches become less defined.

7. **b.** Ideally, all amalgam restorations should be finished and polished 24 hours after placement. This allows for correction of problems or conditions incurred during placement, thereby reducing plaque accumulation.

8. **a.** The primary purpose of finishing and polishing amalgams is to produce a smooth surface, free of voids, that is less likely to tarnish or corrode.

9. **a.** A submarginal area is a term used when an internal wall of the preparation is exposed, most likely due to an overcarved amalgam. An open margin is a space between the amalgam and tooth surfaces. Overextension or flash are terms used when a thin ledge of amalgam extends beyond the cavosurface margin.

10. **c.** During the finishing of amalgam restorations, it is important to maintain the original anatomy of the restoration to assure functional anatomy.

11. **d.** Corrosion is a surface or subsurface chemical deterioration that occurs on or within the amalgam restoration. Finishing and polishing are unable to improve the excessive corrosion defects within the amalgam alloy.

12. **c.** Green and brown points and cups are used to produce a smooth satin and shiny surface to the amalgam restoration. They are used only for polishing and not for finishing. Finishing burs and stones are used to remove surface irregularities or to remove a bulky contact area. Preparation of the amalgam surface is not needed prior to the use of finishing burs.

CHAPTER 27

1. **f.** All of these procedures should be accomplished before the impression is taken. Clothing should be protected with a napkin, and the patient should be upright to minimize gagging. Appliances should be removed so they are not captured in the impression. The mouthwash will reduce organism count for the operator and dental lab technicians.

2. **c.** The 11:00 position for the maxillary impression gives the operator the best access and control over the patient and helps to ensure the best results. The operator would be at 7:00 position for the mandibular arch. For the left-handed operator, the maxillary impression would be taken at the 1:00 position and the mandibular at the 5:00 position.

3. **b.** Add the powder to the water to ensure the proper mix and best result. It is believed that adding water to powder would increase the chance of incorporating air bubbles into the mix.

4. **d.** It is true that the cooler water will increase, or lengthen, the time the operator has to work with the material. Conversely, warmer water will decrease, or shorten, the working time. Working time begins when the powder and water come in contact with each other.

5. **b.** The mixing time is usually 1 minute to mix the material, fill the tray, and seat the impression. For regular set, the setting time is usually 3 to 4 minutes.

CHAPTER 28

1. **b.** The first pour will have initially set before the second pour is done, which helps to prevent distortion. It may take longer than a single-pour or boxing wax technique. There is no difference in reproduction quality among the different types of pours.

2. **a.** Loss of gloss (the cast or model is no longer shiny) is an indication that the initial setting time is near, usually 10 minutes after the initial pour. Resilience and elasticity are characteristics that do not apply to gypsum products. As a gypsum product sets, the compressive strength would increase, rather than decrease.

3. **b.** This combined height is most esthetically pleasing while maintaining the integrity of the oral structures. Choices a and b would mean that the models have no or very little base; the last choice, an overall height of 3.0 to 3.5 inches, would indicate models with extremely thick bases.

4. Answer: 3, 5, 1, 6, 7, 2, and 4 is the correct sequence for the steps in model trimming.

CHAPTER 29

1. **b.** Custom trays CAN be constructed to record anatomical features such as tori. Since the operator has control of all aspects of tray fabrication, most anatomical anomalies can be easily accommodated. A custom tray better ensures an even impression material thickness, can be used again for the same patient, and has more stability than stock trays.

2. **c.** The accuracy of the final impression is influenced by the thickness of impression material. To ensure the proper thickness, there should be 2 to 3 mm of space between the impression tray and the cast during fabrication. 0.5 to 1 mm is not enough space, and 4 to 6 mm is too much.

3. **b.** The extension of the custom tray resin 3 to 4 mm beyond the gingival margin onto the tissues is to capture all of the anatomy of the necessary teeth and supporting gingiva. Excessively extending the resin over the land area will make the set tray difficult to seat and will need a lot of trimming in the lab. The tray thickness should not be thin because it could fracture in use. Ideally, the final thickness should be uniform and approximately 2 to 3 mm and not 6 to 7 mm. A tray that is too short will not control the flow of the impression materials. The resulting impression could lack

all of the anatomic features necessary to fabricate the final prosthesis.

4. **a.** When taking the final impression, occlusal stops allow the dentist to confirm that the tray has been fully seated and stable in the mouth. This allows a consistent and proper thickness of impression material around the prepared tooth or teeth. Stops are indicated for both maxillary and mandibular arch trays. They would not be placed on the centric cusps because the accuracy of the impression in this critical area could be reduced.

5. **a.** Custom tray borders should always be checked with your fingers to verify that the borders are smooth, continuous, and rounded. Remember, these borders will be engaging the soft tissues of the patient's mouth. Square, rough, or sharp edges can traumatize the soft tissues.

CHAPTER 30

1. **c.** The impression tray must be held in place for 5 to 7 minutes so that the tray material and the syringe material can join and set properly. It is very important to follow the manufacturer's directions.

2. **d.** Using this material ensures stability, accuracy, ease of clean up, and allows the impression to be poured at a later date. Even though it is more expensive than other impression materials, many dentists feel that the advantages outweigh the cost.

3. **b.** Two people should be involved in preparing addition silicone impression material. One person fills the tray, while the other is working with the syringe material. Once the syringe material is injected around the area of interest, the tray material is immediately seated on top of it.

4. **c.** The warmer temperature of the palm will accelerate or decrease the setting time of the impression material. Using the fingertips allows for proper working and setting time. The material does not stain the operator's hands nor is it difficult to remove from the surface of the skin.

5. **d.** In most instances, the tray adhesive will dry in the impression tray in 10 minutes.

CHAPTER 31

1. **c.** The power (light/heat-activated) whitening agent is the professionally applied whitening material. The nightguard whitening agents may be professionally supervised but are patient applied. Dentifrices and mouthrinses are over-the-counter and patient-applied materials.

2. **c.** The custom vinyl tray would be used to apply nightguard whitening. Boil and bite and athletic mouthguards would be too bulky. Fluoride trays would not fit snugly for the whitening material.

3. **d.** Using a scalloped tray and using a small dot of whitening in the facial surfaces of tray will help keep the material from leaching onto gingival tissues. There is no evidence that rinsing prior to whitening would eliminate gingival irritation. Mouth rinses containing alcohol may cause gingival irritation.

4. **d.** All of the above. To observe results and record them accurately, a photograph is necessary with a shade guide, both initially and after bleaching has been completed.

5. **a.** Teeth must be isolated to limit the whitening agent to tooth surfaces only. The gingival tissue must also be protected from irritation by the whitening agents. The whitening agent is activated by light or heat. Teeth and tissue are not hydrated but actually dehydrated during the procedure. There are no known nutrients in the resin dam material.

6. **d.** All of the listed choices are contraindicated for tooth whitening.

CHAPTER 32

1. **b.** The recommended bur is the tapered plain-cut finishing bur. It should be used with a low-speed handpiece for better access and control. In addition, in most state practice acts, use of high-speed handpieces is not permitted by hygienists. There are no tapered cross-cut finishing burs. Straight fissure plain-cut and cross-cut burs are designed to take away much more surface than finishing burs and therefore are not indicated for debonding.

2. **c.** It is true that all debonding methods remove some enamel. Some methods remove much more than others. It is the responsibility of the hygienist to select the least damaging method for resin removal.

3. **d.** The stroke of the debonding bur should be toward the incisal or occlusal surface to avoid accidental trauma to the gingiva. One would not intentionally use the bur in the gingival direction because of the possibility of tissue injury. It is not recommended to use the bur toward the interproximal/embrasure surface. It may be efficient in one direction (i.e., toward the mesial), but it may not be in the other direction (toward the distal).

4. **a.** All-composite resin material should be removed to avoid gingival inflammation, stain, plaque, poor esthetics, decalcification/caries formation, and mucosal response from rough resin. Resin left from the bonding of orthodontic brackets should not affect the patient's occlusion.

5. **b.** Compressed air should be applied frequently and the surface examined visually to determine if the surface is free of resin. Having the patient rub his or her tongue over the surface will also aid in residual resin detection. The bur should be used in brush-like strokes, and there is no determined time limit in its use. In most cases, burs do not need to be changed before one patient is completed. In heavy cases, a new bur may be needed for each patient.

CHAPTER 33

1. **c.** The dressing will help control postsurgical bleeding by holding the initial clot and healing tissues in place. This is particularly important in graft and flap surgeries. Postsurgical healing proceeds at a normal rate with or without a dressing. Bleeding of the surgical site is stopped before the dressing is placed. A surgical dressing cannot "sterilize" the surgical site. Bacteria and food particles will find their way under the dressing, although a smooth surface will make the dressing less plaque retentive. Also, the presence of the dressing does provide a physical barrier to friction during eating and speaking, thus providing comfort for the patient.

2. **a.** As the dressing is being placed, pressure is applied in the interdental spaces to help force dressing between the teeth, providing physical or mechanical retention. The dressing is not adhesive. Sutures are used to position soft tissues, not retain the dressing. Sutures should not be embedded in the dressing as this would make removal of the dressing more difficult and painful.

3. **d.** The properly placed dressing should be smooth with tapered edges and have just enough bulk to provide rigidity. The surgical site should be covered, but extending a surgical pack to the occlusal surface is not necessary. This over extension will likely interfere with occlusion, which would be disconcerting to the patient and may jeopardize the integrity of the dressing. Extension to the depth of the vestibule would also cause discomfort. The noneugenol metallic oxide dressing is maintained in place by mechanical retention, thus interlocking in the interdental embrasures is needed for retention. Filling the interdental space will likely impinge on the healing tissues and make removal difficult.

4. **d.** The cyanoacrylate dressing gives esthetically acceptable coverage without bulk and is biodegradable. Saltwater rinses alone may not provide adequate comfort for the patient. The noneugenol zinc oxide dressing would be too bulky, and aesthetics would be of concern. Although the visible light-activated surgical dressing may be aesthetically acceptable, the dressing would need to be removed at a follow-up appointment in less than 2 weeks.

5. **b.** If a piece of the dressing is broken away, one needs to return to the office for care only when this causes discomfort but not immediately. If a small piece of dressing crumbles off, it is usually of no consequence and can simply be discarded. Exposing the dressing to warm liquids or warm foods may soften the dressing. Smoking also exposes the dressing to heat. (It also delays healing.)

CHAPTER 34

1. **a.** Surgical pack removal is done by inserting a sturdy, blunt instrument under the edge of the dressing and applying steady controlled movement. The surface of the instrument that is against the friable soft tissue should be smooth. The pressure applied to the dressing should be steady and controlled in case suture material has incorporated into the dressing material. These sutures will need to be cut to allow dressing removal.

2. **c.** Healing is not compromised by age alone nor is it compromised when diabetes is well controlled. Retained calculus would most likely cause overgrowth of beady granulation tissue. The cause is most likely due to a suture that was overlooked in the posterior of the maxillary vestibule.

3. **d.** Areas of residual calculus are removed at the postsurgical appointment to allow for healing of the tissues.

4. **c.** Care should be taken not to cut the knot away from the submerged suture material. This could result in suture material that is completely submerged and not retrievable. One blade of the scissors is inserted into the opening created under the knot, and only one end of the suture is cut.

5. **c.** Chromic gut and polylactic suture materials are absorbable. A "smaller" sized suture material would be 5-0 (00000) or more 0s. A 3-0 sized suture material would be larger than the requested 4-0 suture material.

CHAPTER 35

1. **b.** An alternative term used to describe a temporary crown is provisional restoration. Temporary crowns are made of acrylic or other resin materials and are custom fitted to the tooth. They are made with suck-down molds and acrylic resins materials.

2. **c.** Proper occlusal and interproximal contacts of a temporary crown are important. If the occlusal contacts are high, the patient will likely return with a sore tooth from hyperocclusion. If they are low, the tooth may drift up (down) into occlusion and the permanent crown will need a great deal of adjustment. The interproximal contacts need to be properly adjusted so the tooth does not move mesial or distal, which will result in excessively tight or open contacts for the permanent crown.

3. **d.** A well-constructed temporary crown will improve patient comfort, esthetics, and function. A tooth prepared for a crown will likely feel very odd to the tongue, be sensitive to hot and cold, appear very small or malformed, and will not function well when eating.

CHAPTER 36

1. **b.** The most effective method to prevent overheating of the pulp when polishing a composite is to keep the tooth and composite moist with water spray or irrigation. Light strokes will help, but overheating can occur rapidly with abrasive rubber points. Petroleum jelly is not as effective as water. Fine grit abrasives are used last, not first.

2. **d.** Ideally, composite restorations should be finished and polished at the placement appointment. Composites obtain the great majority of their strength when polymerized. Therefore, there is no need to wait before finishing and polishing. Delaying finishing and polishing could negatively affect plaque retention and esthetics.

3. **c.** Coarser abrasive disks should be followed by finer abrasive disks to initially remove material containing the larger scratches and defects in the composite surface. Less aggressive finishing of the composite surface is needed to remove the remaining smaller scratches.

4. **d.** Composite materials are made of a polymer filled with a ceramic material. Neither component corrodes as metals do. Finishing and polishing composites does improve the surface luster, marginal contours, and thus gingival health.

5. **d.** The egg/football-shaped finishing bur most closely matches the desired shape of the anatomy of the lingual surface of an anterior tooth and therefore is the most effective abrasive to use.

CASE 1

1. **c.** The remaining natural teeth are the mandibular right first premolar (tooth #28) and canine (tooth #27), the left canine (tooth #22), and the left first molar (tooth #19). It is easiest to see this tooth arrangement if you look at the removable appliance in Photo C.

2. **b.** The correct terminology for this appliance is "removable partial denture." Bridges are usually a fixed appliance. "Partial"

is a commonly used name, shortened from the correct term. It is not a fixed partial denture, however, because the patient can remove it.

3. **d.** The clasps on this appliance encircle the mandibular right second premolar (tooth #28), the left canine (tooth #22), and the left first molar (tooth #19).

4. **b.** If the appliance contains porcelain teeth, it would have three materials: porcelain, the metal framework, and the resin base. If the teeth are resin (somewhat different than the denture base resin), the appliance could still be said to be composed of three materials.

5. **d.** The information presented in the case states that the patient has very little plaque and stain. The patient will be best served by closely examining the teeth after scaling to determine which teeth warrant polishing because they are extrinsically stained. The other agents contain an abrasive (even the fine paste) that is more than what the patient would need to clean the surfaces of the teeth.

6. **c.** Keeping the patient's limited income in mind and making thorough notes in the chart, you could see if the patient education resulted in a lower deposit accumulation at the next recall. If it did, keep the recall date at 1 year; if it did not, change the recall date to 6 months.

CASE 2

1. **a.** The prepared teeth in the photographs are the maxillary right second (tooth #2) and first (tooth #3) molars. The dental anatomy, as well as the radiographs, help the observer to identify these teeth. The roots and the sinus cavity help to determine the arch, and the narrowed occlusal outline helps to distinguish left from right.

2. **b.** Base materials are usually thick in dimension so that they can provide strength and thermal insulation from hot and cold foods and liquids. Liners are usually thin and protect the pulp from chemical irritation, such as that from acid etching.

3. **c.** From the most distal surface going mesially, the names of the cavity preparations are occlusal (O), mesio-occlusal (MO), and disto-occluso-lingual (DOL). The most distal prep (the distal pit of the occlusal surface) is not a DO, even though it may appear that way. The marginal ridge has not been prepared—hence, an occlusal preparation.

4. **d.** Besides the restorative needs, the patient also exhibits root calculus on the distal of tooth #2 and significant bone loss. The bone loss and deposits are evidence of periodontal disease. The patient may have gingivitis as well. The photographs B and C show the patient wearing a rubber dam; therefore, evidence of gingivitis cannot be seen. Gingivitis is never evident on a radiograph.

5. **d.** The root calculus indicates the need for root planing. This may need to be done with local anesthesia in several appointments. Ideally, a reevaluation appointment is scheduled after all the debridement is complete to check the tissue, presence of deposits, and the patient's home care regimen. Polishing may or may not be performed in this appointment.

6. **c.** The use of a finishing bur, polishing first with a slurry of pumice, and then one of tin oxide is a typical technique used in polishing amalgams. Using finishing burs will provide a smooth finished surface before polishing. Using tin oxide

alone is not an adequate abrasive, and prophylaxis pastes are designed to remove stain on natural teeth rather than provide a smooth surface and a high shine that we hope to achieve for amalgam restorations.

7. **c.** Monitoring all the teeth would not necessarily be an incorrect approach to take, but knowing that the probing depths on teeth #2, #3, and #4 range from 5 to 7 mm, it would seem logical to monitor these very closely with frequent baseline recordings and prescribed radiographs. As we know, teeth with measurements of 4 mm or less can be successfully managed by the patient's oral home care regimen.

CASE 3

1. **c.** The lateral incisors are usually the teeth that develop in a "peg" shape. Fusion is the joining of two teeth into one during development. Erosion is a result of acidic substances wearing away the enamel, such as that occurs in a person who frequently sucks on lemons.

2. **b.** When a permanent crown is cemented in place, it is said to be "fixed" (or not removable). The indirect technique is the method of fabrication involving an impression, stone casts, or dies and a casting or firing process. The fabrication is done "indirectly," meaning the patient is not in the chair. The patient must have a temporary restoration when this technique is used. Examples of the direct technique are those restorations such as amalgam and composites, in which the restoration is "made" (or placed) directly in the patient's mouth, usually in one appointment.

3. **b.** A provisional (or temporary) restoration is one that is planned to be replaced in a short time. An interim restoration is a "long-term" temporary restoration. After an existing condition is resolved, a permanent restoration is placed. Permanent restorations are those that are not planned to be replaced in a particular time period.

4. **d.** In this case, the lingual aspect of the crown is visible (with use of the mouth mirror). Looking closely, translucency is evident. When metal is not included as part of an anterior crown, one can assume that the material used is a ceramic material.

5. **d.** Because porcelain is "fired" at very high temperatures, it results in a very hard surface. It can tolerate most grits of Prophy pastes. This is not the case for other tooth-colored restorative materials, such as composite resins and glass ionomer. For those materials, mild abrasive and polishing agents should be used.

6. **a.** The most desirable characteristic of porcelain is its esthetic properties, specifically the translucency, like that of tooth enamel. True, many shades are available, but other tooth-colored restorative materials have a wide shade selection as well. The hardness and low fracture toughness of porcelain are undesirable characteristics. In fact, porcelain is so hard that it will wear away the opposing natural enamel, and it is so brittle that it will fracture quite easily.

7. **a.** Whitening procedures should be done before the restoration is fabricated so that the color of the porcelain will match the natural teeth. Whitening is contraindicated for situations such as root sensitivity, unrealistic expectations, pregnancy, patients younger than the age of 18 years, and heavy smokers. From time to time, the patient will have to use the whitening agent again so that the color will be maintained.

CASE 4

1. **b.** As seen on the periodontal charting, the areas of 5, 6, and 7 mm on the first visit have slightly improved or stayed the same. These are the areas a clinician would look at first to determine the progression of the periodontal condition.

2. **c.** As seen on the intraoral photographs, the maxillary left second premolar and the mandibular left first molar both have cuspal fractures on the lingual surface.

3. **d.** Tooth #30, the mandibular right first molar, has two roots. The mesial root has two canals. The mesial canals are filled with a different material (silver points) than the distal canal (gutta-percha). The two materials appear radiopaque; the silver points appear more radiopaque than the gutta-percha. Maxillary molars usually have three roots.

4. **c.** It is not uncommon for a single tooth to have multiple restorations. As indicated on the patient's record, especially the dental charting, teeth #2, #14, and #15 have two restorations. Remember that on maxillary molars, attempts will be made to preserve the oblique ridge. This ridge provides strength to the tooth. Therefore, you would most likely see an MO and a DO rather than an MOD restoration.

5. **c.** Both amalgam margins are overextended in the interproximal area. These are commonly termed "amalgam overhangs." An open margin may be described as a gap between the tooth and the restoration in which the explorer catches in both directions, from tooth to restoration and restoration to tooth. A submarginal area exists when the preparation is underfilled and the explorer catches from restoration to tooth.

6. **b.** Two different filling materials were used to fill the three root canals. This is evident by the different radiopacity of the materials in the canals for tooth #30 on the radiographs. Both materials are permanent root canal filling materials.

7. **c.** Supereruption occurs when a tooth does not have an opposing tooth in the opposite arch. The tooth will erupt above the occlusal plane. This patient does not have teeth #3 and #4. Therefore, tooth #30 has no opposing contact. The radiographs illustrate the obvious extent of the supereruption of tooth #30.

8. **b.** Each line in the apical section of this periodontal chart is marked off in increments of 2 mm. The line drawn over tooth #31 goes just past the first line, meaning that it is at least 3 mm. You may have "read up" to the next increment and answered 4, but drawings on a chart should be made as exact as possible.

CASE 5

1. **b.** From the periodontal chart, one can see the 7-mm pocket on #15 and the increased mobility on #9. Both arches have gingival recession. The probing depths on the mandibular arch are all within normal limits. Therefore, the mandibular arch is "periodontally healthier" than the maxillary.

2. **d.** Five types of dental restorations are present in this patient. They are amalgam, gold, composite resin, gold foil (or cohesive gold), and porcelain (fused to metal).

3. **c.** The patient may be prone to bisphosphonate-induced osteonecrosis especially if she has undergone procedures such as periodontal surgery, extractions, or implant placement.

The hygienist should perform thorough dental exams, have the patient in the best periodontal health as possible, evaluate oral hard and soft tissues every 3 to 6 months, and evaluate the fit of all oral prostheses.

4. **c.** The patient shared her habit of cigarette smoking. Your oral hygiene home care instruction should include information on tobacco cessation. Tooth whitening, pit and fissure sealants, and nutritional counseling are not indicated for this patient.

5. **b.** Looking at the patient's dental charting, one can see a multitude of restorations. Of the choices listed, the patient would benefit most from patient-applied fluoride. Even though the gingiva on #9, #22, #25, and #26 is recessed, the patient reports no sensitivity, so fluoride varnish is not indicated. No dry mouth is reported, so salivary substitutes are not needed. The patient would not need sealants because all posterior occlusal surfaces are either restored or missing.

6. **b.** The large restoration on #15 is a mesio-occlusal gold inlay. It is labeled "G" on the chart, and the restoration drawn on the occlusal view of the chart is drawn to the outside line on the left side, indicating a mesio-occlusal restoration. This "MO" can also be viewed in the photograph. The amalgam restoration extends from the occlusal to the lingual.

7. **d.** Teeth #s11, 12, and 28 all have had root canal therapy, post and cores placed, and have been restored with porcelain-fused-to-metal crowns. "PFM" is labeled on the dental chart. The apical portions of these root canals have had gutta-percha (less radiolucent), and the post (more radiopaque) fills the remainder of the canal.

CASE 6

1. **a.** Ceramometal crowns tend to look "fake" or unnatural when they are overcontoured and very opaque in color. This happens because the lab may have had to add many layers of porcelain to sufficiently cover the metal coping underneath. The result is a "bulky looking" tooth and with all the porcelain layers, the translucent properties are lost, and thus the tooth becomes opaque.

2. **c.** In most dental and dental hygiene educational curriculums, esthetic veneers are charted by only outlining the facial surface on the tooth on the chart.

3. **c.** From the case information, we learn that the patient is 62 years old. We can see from the periodontal chart that there is a limited amount of recession. However, the probing depths are very much within normal limits. It is well accepted that gingival recession is a common oral finding in older individuals. Therefore, taking all the aforementioned into consideration, the patient's gingival health may be considered as being "very good."

4. **b.** The root of tooth #4 is dilacerated. This can be seen radiographically and is quite obvious. As you may recall, dilaceration is a developmental disturbance in the shape of teeth. It refers to an angulation, or a sharp bend or curve, in the root of a formed tooth.

5. **d.** The radiolucency on the distal of #27 is a composite resin. As you can see from these cases, the radiographic appearance of composite resins can vary greatly depending on the composition of the resin material. Some are quite radiopaque, whereas others are very radiolucent. Metals, such as amalgam or gold, will always appear opaque. The radiographic

appearance of composites when compared to caries is that composite restorations will have a more defined outline.

6. **d.** Composite cements are usually used to attach ceramic veneers to the tooth surface. They employ the acid-etch technique and have the property of translucency when set as compared to polycarboxylate and zinc phosphate. Glass ionomers can be used but do not have the benefits of acid etching.

7. **c.** The projections on the distal surface of teeth 22 and 27 are precision attachments designed to retain the new removable partial denture to the natural teeth. These attachments do not have a retention arm that can be visible on the facial surfaces of the canines. Neither an orthodontic retainer nor dental implants use these types of retention.

CASE 7

1. **c.** Looking at *Figure CS 7.2*, you can see the metal at the gingival margins of the linguals of #8 and #9. The porcelain has been fused to the metal substructure in the laboratory, hence, porcelain fused to metal crown restorations. Porcelain veneers cover only the facial and sometimes incisal surfaces. Porcelain jacket crowns are more translucent and do not have any metal in them. It is obvious that #8 and #9 are restored because of the visible metal at the gingival margin.

2. **b.** In Class II Division I occlusion, the MB cusp of the maxillary first molar occludes mesial to the buccal groove of the mandibular first molar and the maxillary anterior incisors are proclined and a large overjet is present. In Class II Division II occlusion (not as common), the molars are the same, but the anterior incisors are retroclined and a deep overbite exists. In Class I occlusion, the MB cusp of the maxillary first molar occludes with the central groove of the mandibular first molar. In Class III occlusion, the MB cusp of the maxillary first molar is distal to the central groove of the mandibular first molar.

3. **a.** In *Figure CS 7.4*, the maxillary teeth are positioned lingual to the mandibular teeth. This relationship is termed "cross bite." Overjet, overbite, and deep bite all refer to the relationship of anterior teeth. Overjet refers to the horizontal measurement of the distance between the facial surface of the mandibular incisors and the lingual surface of the maxillary incisors. Overbite and deep bite both refer to the vertical overlap of the maxillary and mandibular incisors. The maxillary incisors overlap the incisal third of the mandibular incisors in a normal overbite.

4. **a.** According to GV Black's classification, a restoration in the pits and fissures of the occlusal, lingual, or buccal surfaces is a Class I restoration. Class II restorations involve the proximal surfaces of the posterior teeth. Restorations on the gingival third on the facial and lingual in the posteriors and anteriors define Class V restorations. Class VI restorations involve the cusp tips and incisal edges.

5. **d.** There is an obvious defective restoration on tooth #31. It also appears as if there is new decay around the restoration. This is the most likely cause of pain, but without more information, pain could be from another area.

6. **c.** Visual inspection, pulp testing, and a periapical radiograph would each give us information about tooth #31. Laser or light fluorescence technology does not need to be used on a tooth that has obvious defects.

7. **b.** An interproximal brush will clean the embrasure area very well. The dental professional could choose the appropriate size and shape to fit the embrasure. An end-tuft brush may fit in the embrasure but will not clean the interproximal surface as effectively. The rubber tip is most effective at stimulating and massaging the gingiva, and fine floss will not clean the root surface as effectively as the interproximal brush.

CASE 8

1. **b.** With the floss catching in that area as stated in the chief complaint section of the background information, and by reviewing the dental chart, one can assume that the patient's inability to clean that area thoroughly because of the amalgam overhang can lead to periodontal involvement.

2. **d.** Bone loss alone does not cause the crown portion of the tooth to fracture. However, caries, occlusal trauma, or not placing a permanent restoration after endodontic therapy (or any of these in combination) may result in the fracture of the tooth.

3. **b.** Dr. G.V. Black classified the most common sites for dental caries. Class III includes proximals of the anterior teeth that does NOT include the incisal angle. Class IV includes the proximals of anterior teeth and the incisal angle. This patient has restorations on the incisal angle including the facial and lingual third of these teeth. A Class V involves the gingival third, while a Class VI involves a cusp tip or incisal edge.

4. **c.** The attachment loss is measured by adding together the recession of 3 mm and the probing depth of 4 mm (from baseline probing on dental chart) to get the sum of 7 mm.

5. **c.** Hopefully, neither the dentist nor the patient would encourage the removal of ALL teeth (to accommodate a full upper denture) when only one tooth is affected. Only one tooth needs to be replaced. Choices a, b, and d are all possible modalities to replace this tooth.

6. **c.** Sodium fluoride varnishes are approved as Class II medical devices for use as a tooth desensitizer. Fluoride varnishes are the agent of choice for reduction of sensitivity for such patients as described in this case. The APF and NaF gels would not have the extended contact time with the tooth to reduce the sensitivity as the varnish would.

CASE 9

1. **b.** Look closely at the radiographic full mouth series. You can see the radiopaque filling material in the canal portion of these specific teeth.

2. **c.** Broken bones are not associated with "meth mouth." It is typical that drug addicts are victims of self-neglect, including their oral hygiene. Their teeth will often crack from repeated clenching and bruxing, and some methamphetamine users crave sweets. Another oral manifestation of meth mouth is xerostomia, from a lack of normal secretions.

3. **a.** On the chart, and in the films, teeth #s 4, 5, and 10 should be obvious to the dental care provider. However, #s 22 and 27 on the films may be the mental foramens.

4. **c.** There is no need to polish existing amalgams if teeth are to be extracted. Periodontal debridement, and oral hygiene instructions before the teeth are extracted, will aid in the healing process by reducing the bacterial count.

5. **b.** Tooth #12 has a restoration on the radiograph, but the photograph shows the crown of the tooth fractured at the gingival line. It is important to compare clinical photographs with radiographs and the dates on each to determine the most recent and accurate record.

CASE 10

1. **c.** There are four crowns on the patient's maxillary arch. These are tooth #s 8, 9, 10, and 13. Looking at the photograph, these teeth tend to appear more opaque than the translucent natural teeth. And often, the metal "underlayer," called the coping, will show near the lingual gingival margin. These are two typical characteristics of full coverage crowns.

2. **d.** Tooth #9, a central incisor, has been fabricated from metal and porcelain. This can be determined by looking at the radiographs. The metal under layer (the coping) appears radiopaque, while the porcelain appears radiolucent. A full porcelain or some composite crowns will appear totally radiolucent, and at this time, composite and metal crowns are not routinely made.

3. **e.** The restoration on #22 is a Class V. The gingival third of facial and lingual surfaces of both anterior and posterior teeth comprise Class V caries and restorations. They can be restored with composite, amalgam, or gold foil. Class I are the pits and fissures of teeth, while Class II are defined as the proximal surfaces on posterior teeth. Class III involves the proximal surfaces of anterior teeth, and Class IV also appears on anterior teeth, but involves the proximal and incisal surfaces.

4. **a.** Missing cusp tips are an indication of bruxism, or habitual grinding of the teeth. Decay and esthetic restorations would not result in cusp tip wear in any respect, and toothbrush abrasion (brushing horizontally near the gumline) occurs at the cervical third of the tooth rather than the cusp tip.

5. **d.** Parts of the mesial and occlusal surfaces will be restored when the decay is removed. The dentist will use a dental bur and a handpiece to remove the decay from the occlusal. To remove the decay on the mesial, he will have to cut through the mesial marginal ridge from the occlusal and create a "proximal box." This is the typical design for a Class II restoration; the occlusal section connects to the proximal box. Examples of Class II cavity preparations and restorations are shown in Chapter 1, *Figure 1.9*. The buccal surface would remain intact, since it is not affected by decay.

6. **d.** There are two restorations present, one amalgam and one composite. The amalgam is two surfaces, the distal and occlusal. The composite is only one surface, the buccal. Many larger restorations may have a based placed under it to protect the pulp, but this one does not. Due to the angulation of the premolar bitewing, the composite looks like it sits directly underneath the amalgam, therefore resembling a base. The molar bitewing shows a more accurate positioning of both restorations, and it shows that they are two separate entities.

7. **b.** As seen in the bitewing radiographs, the panorex, and the intraoral photographs, tooth #4 has a two surface, DO, composite restoration. The margins do not extend onto the buccal or lingual surfaces.

8. **a.** Alginate would be the best option for impressions due to its ease of use, availability, short setting time, and the amount of detail necessary for fluoride trays. Agar requires special equipment and a detailed preparation technique, which would make it not suitable for this procedure. ZOE impression material sets to a hard and brittle mass, which limits their use to edentulous ridges. Polysulfide impression material has a very long working time, 4 to 6 minutes (which can be an advantage), but a long setting time in the mouth, 15 minutes. They also have a disagreeable odor and taste and will stain clothing.

9. **c.** Many cancer treatments consist of oral medication, chemotherapy, and radiation. All of these can cause excessive dry mouth, and regular fluoride treatments may help prevent caries development. Fluoride treatments can be used in cases of gingival recession, but this patient has minimal recession, and these treatments would typically not be recommended. Rampant decay is not present in this case. Fluoride trays are not used in the treatment of periodontal disease.

10. **c.** Protonix is a proton pump inhibitor, which decreases the amount of stomach acid being produced. Klonopin is a seizure medication that can also be used to treat anxiety. Losartan is an antihypertensive medication used to lower blood pressure. Zofran is a 5-HT3 antagonist used to prevent nausea and vomiting, which can be caused by chemotherapy and radiation. 5-HT3 antagonists inhibit serotonin receptors in the vomiting center of the brain and small intestines.

CASE 11

1. **b.** The use of the baby bottle with sugar-containing liquid, such as milk, during the night encourages caries producing bacteria. "Baby Bottle Caries" results from this repeated exposure to sugar not the amount. Flossing cannot clean the occlusal surfaces, which are carious. While fluoride can reduce caries, when the pH drops below the critical pH of fluorapatite, decalcification results.

2. **c.** Compare the postoperative radiographs to *Figure 13.11C*. The partially radiolucent appearance suggests a stainless steel crown. Also review the crown in *Figure 1.5C* and the large composite in *Figure 15.13*.

3. **a.** A pulpotomy removes the coronal portion of the dental pulp, while root canal therapy removes the entire pulp. A pulp cap, direct or indirect, does not remove pulp tissue. A pulp cap places a liner material directly on the pulp tissue or indirectly on dentin.

4. **c.** Restoring tooth #A both maintains space for #4 and prevents #3 from mesial drift. Without #A in the arch, space would be lost, and it is likely crowding will occur. The likelihood of needed orthodontic treatment will increase if tooth #A is extracted rather than restored.

5. **c.** Both sentences are true. The maxillary and mandibular first molars erupt approximately at the same time, usually at 16 months. However, for the second molars, the mandibular second molars usually erupts first, at 27 months, and then the maxillary second molar erupts a little later, at 29 months. These time frames are averages.

6. **d.** Anemia is defined as a reduction in the normal level of red blood cells. There are different classes of anemia, iron deficiency anemia being one. Leukocytosis is an increase in the number of circulating white blood cells, and hemophilia is caused by low levels or an absence of a blood protein essential for clotting. Neutropenia is an abnormally low level of neutrophils in the blood. Neutrophils are a common type of white blood cell important for fighting infections.

Skill Performance Evaluations

Chapter 23

MIXING ZINC PHOSPHATE CEMENT FOR LUTING AND BASE CONSISTENCY

Satisfactory performance of this lab/clinical skill is expected. The student self-evaluates his/her performance under the column marked "STUDENT" by using an "√" for each criterion in either the satisfactory (S) column or unsatisfactory (U) column. Next, the student folds back the "STUDENT" section *before* the faculty evaluates under the "INSTRUCTOR" columns. After the instructor evaluates, the skill performance is discussed based on both evaluations.

If satisfactory, the skill evaluation is complete. If unsatisfactory, remediation will occur until criteria are performed satisfactorily.

	INSTRUCTOR		STUDENT	
CRITERIA	S	U	S	U
1. Luting Consistency:				
a. Powder is properly incorporated into the liquid.				
b. Mix is completed within the specified mixing time.				
c. Mix will form a "1-inch string" between the spatula and slab.				
2. Base Consistency:				
a. Powder is properly incorporated into the liquid.				
b. Mix is completed within specified mixing time.				
c. Mix is thick, putty-like, and shaped into a ball.				

(Fold Back)

Faculty, please identify minimum lab and clinical competency levels:

Laboratory: #_____ criteria must be performed satisfactorily.

Clinical: #_____ criteria must be performed satisfactorily.

Time Started: _____ Time Completed: _____

Instructor: _____

Suggestions/Comments:

_____

_____

_____

Chapter 23

MIXING GLASS IONOMER CEMENT–LUTING CONSISTENCY

Satisfactory performance of this lab/clinical skill is expected. The student self-evaluates his/her performance under the column marked "STUDENT" by using an "√" for each criterion in either the satisfactory (S) column or unsatisfactory (U) column. Next, the student folds back the "STUDENT" section *before* the faculty evaluates under the "INSTRUCTOR" columns. After the instructor evaluates, the skill performance is discussed based on both evaluations.

If satisfactory, the skill evaluation is complete. If unsatisfactory, remediation will occur until criteria are performed satisfactorily.

CRITERIA	INSTRUCTOR		STUDENT	
	S	U	S	U
1. The powder is incorporated into the liquid in one portion.				
2. The mix is completed within the specified time.				

(Fold Back)

Faculty, please identify minimum lab and clinical competency levels:

Laboratory: #_____ criteria must be performed satisfactorily.

Clinical: #_____ criteria must be performed satisfactorily.

Time Started: _____ Time Completed: _____

Instructor: _____

Suggestions/Comments:

_____

_____

_____

Chapter 23

MIXING ZINC OXIDE–EUGENOL AS A BASE OR TEMPORARY RESTORATIVE MATERIAL

Satisfactory performance of this lab/clinical skill is expected. The student self-evaluates his/her performance under the column marked "STUDENT" by using an "√" for each criterion in either the satisfactory (S) column or unsatisfactory (U) column. Next, the student folds back the "STUDENT" section *before* the faculty evaluates under the "INSTRUCTOR" columns. After the instructor evaluates, the skill performance is discussed based on both evaluations.

If satisfactory, the skill evaluation is complete. If unsatisfactory, remediation will occur until criteria are performed satisfactorily.

	INSTRUCTOR		STUDENT	
CRITERIA	S	U	S	U
1. Powder and liquid are properly incorporated into the mix.				
2. Mix is consistent and has a putty-like appearance.				
3. Mix is completed within 1.5 minutes.				

(Fold Back)

Faculty, please identify minimum lab and clinical competency levels:

Laboratory: #_____ criteria must be performed satisfactorily.

Clinical: #_____ criteria must be performed satisfactorily.

Time Started: _____ Time Completed: _____

Instructor: _____

Suggestions/Comments:

_____

_____

_____

Chapter 24

RUBBER DAM APPLICATION AND REMOVAL

Satisfactory performance of this lab/clinical skill is expected. The student self-evaluates his/her performance under the column marked "STUDENT" by using an "√" for each criterion in either the satisfactory (S) column or unsatisfactory (U) column. Next, the student folds back the "STUDENT" section *before* the faculty evaluates under the "INSTRUCTOR" columns. After the instructor evaluates, the skill performance is discussed based on both evaluations.

If satisfactory, the skill evaluation is complete. If unsatisfactory, remediation will occur until criteria are performed satisfactorily.

	INSTRUCTOR		STUDENT	
CRITERIA	S	U	S	U
Application				
1. Rubber dam is punched correctly.				
2. Clamp is ligated and seated properly.				
3. Rubber dam is inverted around isolated teeth.				
4. Rubber dam is smooth and tear free.				
5. Frame is properly placed and centered.				
Removal				
1. Dam material and frame are removed as one unit.				
2. Interproximals are free of rubber dam remnants.				

(Fold Back)

Faculty, please identify minimum lab and clinical competency levels:

Laboratory: #_____ criteria must be performed satisfactorily.

Clinical: #_____ criteria must be performed satisfactorily.

Time Started: _____ Time Completed: _____

Instructor: _____

Suggestions/Comments:

_____

_____

_____

Chapter 25

PIT AND FISSURE SEALANTS

Satisfactory performance of this lab/clinical skill is expected. The student self-evaluates his/her performance under the column marked "STUDENT" by using an "√" for each criterion in either the satisfactory (S) column or unsatisfactory (U) column. Next, the student folds back the "STUDENT" section *before* the faculty evaluates under the "INSTRUCTOR" columns. After the instructor evaluates, the skill performance is discussed based on both evaluations.

If satisfactory, the skill evaluation is complete. If unsatisfactory, remediation will occur until criteria are performed satisfactorily.

	INSTRUCTOR		STUDENT	
CRITERIA	S	U	S	U
1. Tooth surface is plaque free.				
2. Tooth is adequately isolated.				
3. Etched surfaces appear chalky white.				
4. Sealant covers all areas indicated for placement.				
5. Bubbles, voids, and defects are not present.				
6. Interproximal areas remain open and "unsealed."				
7. Sealant does not interfere with occlusion.				

(Fold Back)

Faculty, please identify minimum lab and clinical competency levels:

Laboratory: #_____ criteria must be performed satisfactorily.

Clinical: #_____ criteria must be performed satisfactorily.

Time Started: _____ Time Completed: _____

Instructor: _____

Suggestions/Comments:

_____

_____

_____

Chapter 26

AMALGAM PLACEMENT AND CARVING

Satisfactory performance of this lab/clinical skill is expected. The student self-evaluates his/her performance under the column marked "STUDENT" by using an "√" for each criterion in either the satisfactory (S) column or unsatisfactory (U) column. Next, the student folds back the "STUDENT" section *before* the faculty evaluates under the "INSTRUCTOR" columns. After the instructor evaluates, the skill performance is discussed based on both evaluations.

If satisfactory, the skill evaluation is complete. If unsatisfactory, remediation will occur until criteria are performed satisfactorily.

CRITERIA	INSTRUCTOR		STUDENT	
	S	U	S	U
1. Amalgam Placement:				
a. Matrix, if needed, is properly placed and wedged.				
b. Amalgam is correctly mixed and condensed without voids.				
2. Amalgam Carving:				
a. All margins are carved flush to the adjacent tooth structure.				
b. Contact areas are restored, if preparation included a proximal surface.				
c. Occlusal anatomy is carved to reproduce proper tooth form (anatomy).				
d. Occlusal anatomy is carved to reproduce proper tooth function, no interferences.				

(Fold Back)

Faculty, please identify minimum lab and clinical competency levels:

Laboratory: #_____ criteria must be performed satisfactorily.

Clinical: #_____ criteria must be performed satisfactorily.

Time Started: _____ Time Completed: _____

Instructor: _____

Suggestions/Comments:

_____

_____

_____

Student Name: _____   Date: _____

Chapter 26

AMALGAM FINISHING AND POLISHING

Satisfactory performance of this lab/clinical skill is expected. The student self-evaluates his/her performance under the column marked "STUDENT" by using an "√" for each criterion in either the satisfactory (S) column or unsatisfactory (U) column. Next, the student folds back the "STUDENT" section *before* the faculty evaluates under the "INSTRUCTOR" columns. After the instructor evaluates, the skill performance is discussed based on both evaluations.

If satisfactory, the skill evaluation is complete. If unsatisfactory, remediation will occur until criteria are performed satisfactorily.

CRITERIA	INSTRUCTOR		STUDENT	
	S	U	S	U
Finishing				
1. Excessive amalgam has been removed from cavosurface margins.				
2. Amalgam appears smooth.				
3. Occlusion registers properly with articulating paper.				
4. Occlusal and marginal anatomies are well defined.				
5. Porosity and pits have been removed.				
6. Contour of the restoration approximates the original contour of the tooth.				
7. Adjacent tooth structure is left undamaged.				
Polishing				
1. Amalgam is without scratches and appears smooth.				
2. Amalgam has a high polish and lustrous shine.				
3. Adjacent tooth structure is left undamaged.				
4. Time utilization is satisfactory.				

(Fold Back)

Faculty, please identify minimum lab and clinical competency levels:

Laboratory: #_____ criteria must be performed satisfactorily.

Clinical: #_____ criteria must be performed satisfactorily.

Time Started: _____ Time Completed: _____

Instructor: _____

Suggestions/Comments:

_____

_____

_____

Student Name: _____ Date:_____

Chapter 27

ALGINATE IMPRESSIONS

Satisfactory performance of this lab/clinical skill is expected. The student self-evaluates his/her performance under the column marked "STUDENT" by using an "√" for each criterion in either the satisfactory (S) column or unsatisfactory (U) column. Next, the student folds back the "STUDENT" section *before* the faculty evaluates under the "INSTRUCTOR" columns. After the instructor evaluates, the skill performance is discussed based on both evaluations.

If satisfactory, the skill evaluation is complete. If unsatisfactory, remediation will occur until criteria are performed satisfactorily.

	INSTRUCTOR		STUDENT	
CRITERIA	S	U	S	U
1. All teeth are present without voids or air bubbles in critical areas.				
2. All edentulous ridges/spaces are present.				
3. All vestibular areas are present and intact.				
4. All frena and muscle attachments are present and intact.				
5. All interpapillary spaces are present with minimal tearing.				
6. No voids in critical areas: palate, floor of mouth, vestibular areas, and tray showing through impression.				
7. Impression is stable; alginate is attached to the tray.				
8. Adequately extended; retromolar area included.				
9. Appropriate infection control procedures: bowls, spatula, impression.				

(Fold Back)

Faculty, please identify minimum lab and clinical competency levels:

     Laboratory: #_____ criteria must be performed satisfactorily.

     Clinical: #_____ criteria must be performed satisfactorily.

Time Started: _____ Time Completed: _____

Instructor: _____

Suggestions/Comments:

_____

_____

_____

Chapter 28

TRIMMING AND FINISHING STUDY MODELS

STUDENT		Study Models	FACULTY	
MAX	MAND		MAX	MAND
		OVERALL		
		1. All teeth and anatomy are preserved (none removed through trimming; no broken or chipped teeth).		
		2. Stone is smooth; no voids or blebs >1 mm; cleared of dust and trimming debris.		
		BASES		
		3. Occluded models and occlusal plane are parallel to the benchtop, height does not differ by >1/8 inch (3 mm).		
		4. Bases are smooth and flat; no bevels; does not rock (a nail file will not slide under).		
		5. Height of occluded models is 2.0–2.5 inches (50–60 mm).		
		6. Bases are 1/3 of height; anatomy is 2/3 of height in the anterior region.		
		BORDERS		
		7. Posterior borders are flat and bite will not open when occluded models are placed on their backs (<1 mm).		
		8. Arch length extends at least 0.25 inch (6 mm) beyond most posterior teeth, not removing maxillary tuberosity, hamular notch, or mandibular retromolar areas.		
		9. Back of maxillary model is perpendicular to median line (<3 degree).		
		10. The vestibule is not removed by trimming.		
		11. Sides are flush, flat, and smooth.		
		OTHER		
		12. Tongue area is flat and smooth without removing any anatomy.		
		13. Models are labeled with student's (or patient's) name and date.		

(Fold Back)

Laboratory: #_____ criteria must be performed satisfactorily.

Instructor: _____

Chapter 29

CUSTOM IMPRESSION TRAY

Satisfactory performance of this lab/clinical skill is expected. The student self-evaluates his/her performance under the column marked "STUDENT" by using an "√" for each criterion in either the satisfactory (S) column or unsatisfactory (U) column. Next, the student folds back the "STUDENT" section *before* the faculty evaluates under the "INSTRUCTOR" columns. After the instructor evaluates, the skill performance is discussed based on both evaluations.

If satisfactory, the skill evaluation is complete. If unsatisfactory, remediation will occur until criteria are performed satisfactorily.

	INSTRUCTOR		STUDENT	
CRITERIA	S	U	S	U
1. Tray has uniform thickness.				
2. Tray is smooth.				
3. Placements of stops are appropriate.				
4. Sizes of stops are adequate.				
5. Handle size is acceptable.				
6. Handle location is acceptable.				

(Fold Back)

Faculty, please identify minimum lab and clinical competency levels:

Laboratory: #_____ criteria must be performed satisfactorily.

Clinical: #_____ criteria must be performed satisfactorily.

Time Started: _____ Time Completed: _____

Instructor: _____

Suggestions/Comments:

_____

_____

Chapter 30

ELASTOMERIC IMPRESSIONS

Satisfactory performance of this lab/clinical skill is expected. The student self-evaluates his/her performance under the column marked "STUDENT" by using an "√" for each criterion in either the satisfactory (S) column or unsatisfactory (U) column. Next, the student folds back the "STUDENT" section *before* the faculty evaluates under the "INSTRUCTOR" columns. After the instructor evaluates, the skill performance is discussed based on both evaluations.

If satisfactory, the skill evaluation is complete. If unsatisfactory, remediation will occur until criteria are performed satisfactorily.

	INSTRUCTOR		STUDENT	
CRITERIA	S	U	S	U
1. No bubbles or voids are present in critical areas.				
2. Impression is not distorted.				
3. All critical areas are reproduced.				
4. No critical areas are torn.				

(Fold Back)

Faculty, please identify minimum lab and clinical competency levels:

　　　Laboratory:　　#_____ criteria must be performed satisfactorily.

　　　Clinical:　　#_____ criteria must be performed satisfactorily.

Time Started: _____ Time Completed: _____

Instructor: _____

Suggestions/Comments:

_____

_____

_____

Chapter 31

BLEACHING TRAY CONSTRUCTION—CLINICAL PROCEDURE

Satisfactory performance of this lab/clinical skill is expected. The student self-evaluates his/her performance under the column marked "STUDENT" by using an "√" for each criterion in either the satisfactory (S) column or unsatisfactory (U) column. Next, the student folds back the "STUDENT" section *before* the faculty evaluates under the "INSTRUCTOR" columns. After the instructor evaluates, the skill performance is discussed based on both evaluations.

If satisfactory, the skill evaluation is complete. If unsatisfactory, remediation will occur until criteria are performed satisfactorily.

	INSTRUCTOR		STUDENT	
CRITERIA	S	U	S	U
1. Medical history is completed.				
2. Informed consent is explained to and signed by the patient.				
3. Pretreatment intraoral examination is completed.				
4. Prophylaxis is completed.				
5. Intraoral photography is completed with matching shade guide tab in place.				
6. Full-arch alginate impression is taken.				
7. Gypsum casts are produced and trimmed.				
8. Block-out resin is applied and cured to facial surfaces of teeth to be whitened.				
9. Resin tray is constructed and trimmed to specification.				
10. Patient is instructed regarding the use of tray for the application of whitening agent.				
11. Follow-up examination is completed and retreatment assigned as necessary.				
12. Posttreatment intraoral photography is completed with matching shade guide tab in place.				

(Fold Back)

Faculty, please identify minimum lab and clinical competency levels:

Laboratory: #_____ criteria must be performed satisfactorily.

Clinical: #_____ criteria must be performed satisfactorily.

Time Started: _____ Time Completed: _____

Instructor: _____

Suggestions/Comments:

_____

_____

_____

Chapter 32

DEBONDING ORTHODONTIC RESINS

Satisfactory performance of this lab/clinical skill is expected. The student self-evaluates his/her performance under the column marked "STUDENT" by using an "√" for each criterion in either the satisfactory (S) column or unsatisfactory (U) column. Next, the student folds back the "STUDENT" section *before* the faculty evaluates under the "INSTRUCTOR" columns. After the instructor evaluates, the skill performance is discussed based on both evaluations.

If satisfactory, the skill evaluation is complete. If unsatisfactory, remediation will occur until criteria are performed satisfactorily.

	INSTRUCTOR		STUDENT	
CRITERIA	S	U	S	U
1. The enamel contains no gouges or scarring.				
2. No resin remains on the tooth.				
3. The enamel appears glossy when dried with air.				
4. The enamel feels smooth and glass-like with the explorer.				
5. Disclosing solution does not adhere to the remaining resin.				
6. Patient reports a smooth enamel feel with the tongue.				

(Fold Back)

Faculty, please identify minimum lab and clinical competency levels:

Laboratory: #_____ criteria must be performed satisfactorily.

Clinical: #_____ criteria must be performed satisfactorily.

Time Started: _____ Time Completed: _____

Instructor: _____

Suggestions/Comments:

_____

_____

_____

Chapter 33

PLACEMENT OF THE PERIODONTAL DRESSING

Satisfactory performance of this lab/clinical skill is expected. The student self-evaluates his/her performance under the column marked "STUDENT" by using an "√" for each criterion in either the satisfactory (S) column or unsatisfactory (U) column. Next, the student folds back the "STUDENT" section *before* the faculty evaluates under the "INSTRUCTOR" columns. After the instructor evaluates, the skill performance is discussed based on both evaluations.

If satisfactory, the skill evaluation is complete. If unsatisfactory, remediation will occur until criteria are performed satisfactorily.

CRITERIA	INSTRUCTOR		STUDENT	
	S	U	S	U
1. Dressing material is dispensed and mixed until uniform in color.				
2. Dressing has set sufficiently to allow for easy manipulation.				
3. Dressing is 3–4 mm at its thickest area.				
4. Dressing is 8–10 mm wide.				
5. Surface of the dressing is smooth with tapered edges (i.e., no slices or cracks).				
6. Dressing is placed with interproximal retention.				
7. Dressing does not interfere with muscle attachments.				
8. Dressing does not extend beyond the cervical 1/3 of the crown (height of contour).				
9. At least four teeth are incorporated in the dressed area.				

(Fold Back)

Faculty, please identify minimum lab and clinical competency levels:

Laboratory: #_____ criteria must be performed satisfactorily.

Clinical: #_____ criteria must be performed satisfactorily.

Time Started: _____ Time Completed: _____

Instructor: _____

Suggestions/Comments:

_____

_____

_____

Chapter 34

REMOVAL OF PERIODONTAL DRESSING

Satisfactory performance of this lab/clinical skill is expected. The student self-evaluates his/her performance under the column marked "STUDENT" by using an "√" for each criterion in either the satisfactory (S) column or unsatisfactory (U) column. Next, the student folds back the "STUDENT" section *before* the faculty evaluates under the "INSTRUCTOR" columns. After the instructor evaluates, the skill performance is discussed based on both evaluations.

If satisfactory, the skill evaluation is complete. If unsatisfactory, remediation will occur until criteria are performed satisfactorily.

CRITERIA	INSTRUCTOR		STUDENT	
	S	U	S	U
1. A constant, controlled lateral pressure is applied to remove the dressing.				
2. Dressing material is thoroughly removed.				
3. Teeth and tissues are swabbed with disinfectant mouthwash, then rinsed.				

(Fold Back)

Faculty, please identify minimum lab and clinical competency levels:

Laboratory: #_____ criteria must be performed satisfactorily.

Clinical: #_____ criteria must be performed satisfactorily.

Time Started: _____ Time Completed: _____

Instructor: _____

Suggestions/Comments:

_____

_____

_____

Chapter 34

SUTURE REMOVAL

Satisfactory performance of this lab/clinical skill is expected. The student self-evaluates his/her performance under the column marked "STUDENT" by using an "√" for each criterion in either the satisfactory (S) column or unsatisfactory (U) column. Next, the student folds back the "STUDENT" section *before* the faculty evaluates under the "INSTRUCTOR" columns. After the instructor evaluates, the skill performance is discussed based on both evaluations.

If satisfactory, the skill evaluation is complete. If unsatisfactory, remediation will occur until criteria are performed satisfactorily.

	INSTRUCTOR		STUDENT	
CRITERIA	S	U	S	U
1. The suture is properly retracted from the tissue.				
2. A fulcrum or rest is used when cutting the suture.				
3. Only one "end" of the suture is cut.				
4. The suture is cut close to the tissue, in the area previously submerged, without tissue damage.				
5. The suture is removed with a smooth, continuous motion.				
6. Removed sutures are inspected and the number is recorded in the chart.				

(Fold Back)

Faculty, please identify minimum lab and clinical competency levels:

Laboratory: #_____ criteria must be performed satisfactorily.

Clinical: #_____ criteria must be performed satisfactorily.

Time Started: _____ Time Completed: _____

Instructor: _____

Suggestions/Comments:

_____

_____

_____

Chapter 35

CONSTRUCTING A TEMPORARY CROWN

Satisfactory performance of this lab/clinical skill is expected. The student self-evaluates his/her performance under the column marked "STUDENT" by using an "√" for each criterion in either the satisfactory (S) column or unsatisfactory (U) column. Next, the student folds back the "STUDENT" section *before* the faculty evaluates under the "INSTRUCTOR" columns. After the instructor evaluates, the skill performance is discussed based on both evaluations.

If satisfactory, the skill evaluation is complete. If unsatisfactory, remediation will occur until criteria are performed satisfactorily.

CRITERIA	INSTRUCTOR		STUDENT	
	S	U	S	U
1. Mesial and distal contacts are not open. Cannot see light through the contacts.				
2. Shape approximates that of the original tooth.				
3. All margins are closed.				
4. No voids >1 mm are present.				
5. Optional–Occlusal contacts are similar to adjacent teeth.				

(Fold Back)

Faculty, please identify minimum lab and clinical competency levels:

Laboratory: #_____ criteria must be performed satisfactorily.

Clinical: #_____ criteria must be performed satisfactorily.

Time Started: _____ Time Completed: _____

Instructor: _____

Suggestions/Comments:

_____

_____

_____

Chapter 36

COMPOSITE FINISHING AND POLISHING

Satisfactory performance of this lab/clinical skill is expected. The student self-evaluates his/her performance under the column marked "STUDENT" by using an "√" for each criterion in either the satisfactory (S) column or unsatisfactory (U) column. Next, the student folds back the "STUDENT" section *before* the faculty evaluates under the "INSTRUCTOR" columns. After the instructor evaluates, the skill performance is discussed based on both evaluations.

If satisfactory, the skill evaluation is complete. If unsatisfactory, remediation will occur until criteria are performed satisfactorily.

CRITERIA	INSTRUCTOR		STUDENT	
	S	U	S	U
Finishing:				
1. Excessive composite has been removed from cavosurface margins.				
2. Composite appears to be smooth.				
3. Occlusion registers properly with articulating paper.				
4. Occlusal and marginal anatomy is well defined.				
5. Porosity and pits have been removed.				
6. Contour of the restoration approximates the original contour of the tooth.				
7. Adjacent tooth structure is left undamaged.				
Polishing				
1. Composite is void of scratches and appears smooth.				
2. Composite has a lustrous shine.				
3. Adjacent tooth structure is left undamaged.				
4. Time utilization is satisfactory.				

(Fold Back)

Faculty, please identify minimum lab and clinical competency levels:

Laboratory: #_____ criteria must be performed satisfactorily

Clinical: #_____ criteria must be performed satisfactorily

Time Started: _____ Time Completed: _____

Instructor: _____

Suggestions/Comments:

_____

_____

_____

Index

Note: Page numbers followed by "t" indicates table; those followed by "f" indicates figures.